**General Practice**

# An Approach to Differential Diagnosis

# General Practice
# An Approach to Differential Diagnosis


***Editors***

**Jyotirmoy Pal**
MBBS MD(General Medicine) FRCP FICP FACP WHO Fellow
Professor (General Medicine)
Department of Medicine
College of Medicine and Sagore Dutta Hospital
Kamarhati, West Bengal, India
Dean, Indian College of Physicians (ICP)
President-Elect, Association of Physicians (API)

**Nandini Chatterjee**
MD FRCP(Glasgow, London) FICP
Professor
Department of Medicine
Institute of Postgraduate Medical
Education and Research (IPGMER) and SSKM Hospital
Kolkata, West Bengal, India
Ex-Editor Journal of Indian Medical Association (JIMA)
Editor-in-Chief Bengal Physician Journal (Association of Physicians of India)

***Foreword***

**Girish Mathur**


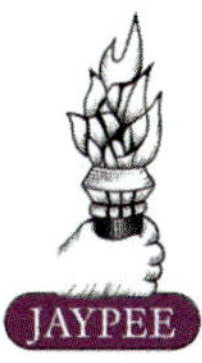



JAYPEE BROTHERS MEDICAL PUBLISHERS
*The Health Sciences Publisher*
**New Delhi | London**

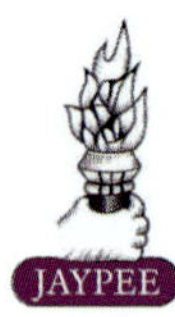

**Jaypee Brothers Medical Publishers (P) Ltd**

**Headquarters**
EMCA House
23/23-B, Ansari Road, Daryaganj
New Delhi 110 002, India
Landline: +91-11-23272143, +91-11-23272703
+91-11-23282021, +91-11-23245672
E-mail: jaypee@jaypeebrothers.com

**Corporate Office**
4838/24, Ansari Road, Daryaganj
New Delhi 110 002, India
Phone: +91-11-43574357
Fax: +91-11-43574314
E-mail: jaypee@jaypeebrothers.com

**Overseas Office**
J.P. Medical Ltd
83 Victoria Street, London
SW1H 0HW (UK)
Phone: +44 20 3170 8910
E-mail: info@jpmedpub.com

**EU GPSR** Authorised Representative
Logos Europe, 9 rue Nicolas Poussin
17000, La Rochelle, France
Phone: +33 (0) 6 67 93 73 78
E-mail: contact@logoseurope.eu

Website: www.jaypeebrothers.com
Website: www.jaypeedigital.com



**Inquiries for bulk sales may be solicited at:** jaypee@jaypeebrothers.com

***General Practice: An Approach to Differential Diagnosis* / Jyotirmoy Pal, Nandini Chatterjee**

*First Edition:* **2024**
*Reprint:* 2025
ISBN: 978-93-5696-313-9

*Printed in India*

# Contributors


**Abhinaba Datta** MBBS MD PGT MD(Medicine)
Department of Medicine
Medical College Kolkata
Kolkata, West Bengal, India

**Agnibha Maiti** MBBS MD(Medicine)
Assistant Professor
Department of Medicine
IPGMER and SSKM Hospital
Kolkata, West Bengal, India

**Amanjot Kaur** MD
Senior Resident
Department of Medicine
Dr BR Ambedkar State Institute of Medical Sciences (AIMS)
Ajitgarh
SAS Nagar, Punjab, India

**Amit Kalwar** MD(Medicine)
Assistant Professor
Department of Medicine
Silchar Medical College and Hospital
Silchar, Assam, India

**Amlan Kusum Datta**
MBBS MD(General Medicine) DM(Neurology) DrNB(Neurology)
Consultant
Department of Neurology
Bangur Institute of Neuroscience
IPGMER and SSKM Hospital
Kolkata, West Bengal, India

**Anirban Dalui** MBBS MD(Community Medicine)
Fellow of College of General Practitioners
Community Medicine and Family Medicine
Barasat Government Medical College and Hospital
Barasat, West Bengal, India

**Apu Adhikary** MBBS MD
Assistant Professor
Department of General Medicine
MJN Medical College
Kolkata, West Bengal, India

**Aritra Ray** MBBS MD(General Medicine)
Senior Resident
General Medicine
RG Kar Medical College and Hospital
Kolkata, West Bengal, India

**Arshdeep Maman** MD
Assistant Professor
Department of Medicine
Dr BR Ambedkar State Institute of Medical Sciences (AIMS)
Ajitgarh
SAS Nagar, Punjab, India

**Arunima Dhabal**
MD(Dermatology)
Senior Resident
College of Medicine and Sagore Dutta Hospital
Kolkata, West Bengal, India

**Ashish Goel** MD MPH
Professor and Head
Department of Medicine
Dr BR Ambedkar State Institute of Medical Sciences (AIMS)
Ajitgarh
SAS Nagar, Punjab, India

**Ashish Jindal** MD
Assistant Professor
Department of Medicine
Dr BR Ambedkar State Institute of Medical Sciences (AIMS)
Ajitgarh
SAS Nagar, Punjab, India

**Bickram Pradhan** MD FACP
Professor and Head
Department of Gastroenterology and Hepatology
BP Koirala Institute of Health Sciences
Dharan, Nepal

**Biswajit Banik** MBBS(Honours) MD(General Medicine) DM(Medical Gastroenterology, Gold Medalist)
Senior Resident
Department of Gastroenterology
IPGMER and SSKM Hospital
Kolkata, West Bengal, India

**Biva Bhakat** MD(General Medicine) MBBS
Senior Resident
General Medicine
Nil Ratan Sircar Medical College and Hospital
Kolkata, West Bengal, India

**Boudhayan Das Munshi** MBBS DNB(General Medicine) Fellowship in Diabetology(JIPMER) MNAMS
Assistant Professor
General Medicine
All India Institute of Medical Sciences (AIIMS)
Kalyani, West Bengal, India

**BR Bansode** MD(Medicine)
Ex-President API, Head
Department of Medicine
Babasaheb Ambedkar Railway Hospital
Mumbai, Maharashtra, India

**Chandan Chatterjee** MD
Professor and Head
Registrar Academic
Department of Pharmacology
ESI-PGIMSR, ESIC MC
Kolkata, West Bengal, India

**Debmalya Bhattacharyya**
DM(Clinical Hematology)
MD(General Medicine)
Consultant
Apollo Multispeciality Hospital
Kolkata, West Bengal, India

**Dipankar Datta** MBBS MS(ENT)
Consultant ENT and Sleep
Apnoea Surgeon
Belle Vue Clinic
Kolkata, West Bengal, India

**Dippyoman Ghosh** MBBS
Junior Resident
ESI-PGIMSR, ESIC Medical
College
Kolkata, West Bengal, India

**Disha Chakraborty**
MBBS(Honours) MD
Senior Resident
Dermatology
Calcutta National Medical
College and Hospital
Kolkata, West Bengal, India

**Dishari Haldar** MBBS MD
Senior Resident
Dermatology
Calcutta National Medical
College and Hospital
Kolkata, West Bengal, India

**Gautam Raghu** MS(ENT)
Senior Resident
Department of ENT
Medical College and Hospital
Kolkata, West Bengal, India

**Md Hamid Ali** MD(Medicine)
Associate Professor
Murshidabad Medical College
and Hospital
Murshidabad, West Bengal, India

**Indrashis Podder**
MD(Dermatology)
Assistant Professor
College of Medicine and Sagore
Dutta Hospital
Kolkata, West Bengal, India

**Jasprabh Karanjit Kaur** MD
Senior Resident
Department of Medicine
Dr BR Ambedkar State Institute of
Medical Sciences (AIMS), Ajitgarh
SAS Nagar, Punjab, India

**Joydeep Mukherjee** MBBS DNB
DM MNAMS FICP
RMO cum Clinical Tutor
Department of Neurology
NRS Medical College and
Hospital
Kolkata, West Bengal, India

**Jyoti Bajpai** MD(Pulmonary
Medicine)
Assistant Professor
Department of Respiratory
Medicine
King George's Medical University
Lucknow, Uttar Pradesh, India

**Jyotirmoy Pal** MBBS MD(General
Medicine) FRCP FICP FACP WHO Fellow
Professor (General Medicine)
Department of Medicine
College of Medicine and Sagore
Dutta Hospital
Kamarhati, West Bengal, India
Dean, Indian College of
Physicians (ICP)
President-Elect, Association of
Physicians (API)

**Kaushik Hazra** MBBS DTCD MD
Associate Professor
Department of General Medicine
JIMSH
Kolkata, West Bengal, India

**Komal Aggarwal** MD(DVL)
SCE(Dermatology)
Senior Resident
Department of Dermatology
Calcutta National Medical
College and Hospital
Kolkata, West Bengal, India

**Koushik Bhattacharya**
DM(Nephrology)
Assistant Professor
Department of Nephrology
IPGMER and SSKM Hospital
Kolkata, West Bengal, India

**Kripasindhu Gantait** MBBS MD
FICP FIACM FIAMS
Professor and Head
Department of Medicine
Jhargram Government
Medical College
Professor of Medicine and Head
in Rheumatology Division of
Midnapore Medical College
(MMC)
Ex-President
Indian Medical Association
Midnapore, West Bengal, India

**Mainak Mukhopadhyay**
MBBS MD(Medicine) MRCP(Ireland)
DM(Cardiology)
Interventional Cardiologist
AMRI Hospital, Saltlake
Kolkata, West Bengal, India

**Monidipa Ghosh** MBBS
Post Graduate Trainee (MD
Radiodiagnosis)
KPC Medical College and Hospital
Kolkata, West Bengal, India

**Nandini Chatterjee** MD
FRCP(Glasgow, London) FICP
Professor
Department of Medicine
Institute of Postgraduate
Medical Education and Research
(IPGMER) and SSKM Hospital
Kolkata, West Bengal, India
Ex-Editor Journal of Indian
Medical Association (JIMA)
Editor-in-Chief Bengal Physician
Journal (Association of
Physicians of India)

**Nilay Kanti Das**
MD(Dermatology) MAMS
FRCP(London)
Professor and Head
College of Medicine and
Sagore Dutta Hospital
Kolkata, West Bengal, India

**Oendri Bhattacharyya** MBBS
1st Year DNB PGT
Department of General Medicine
JIMSH
Kolkata, West Bengal, India

**Onkar Awadhiya** MBBS MD(General Medicine)
Assistant Professor
Department of General Medicine
AIIMS Nagpur
Nagpur, Maharashtra, India

**Parinita Ranjit** MBBS MD(General Medicine)
Assistant Professor
General Medicine
Calcutta National Medical College and Hospital
Kolkata, West Bengal, India

**Pasang Lahmu Sherpa** MBBS MD FICP
Associate Professor
North Bengal Medical College and Hospital
Siliguri, West Bengal, India

**Pranab Kumar Maity** MBSS MD
Associate Professor
Department of Medicine
RG Kar Medical College
Kolkata, West Bengal, India

**Purbasha Biswas** MBBS MD
Postdoctoral Trainee
Department of Neurology
NIMHANS
Bengaluru, Karnataka, India

**Raja Dhar** MBBS MD(Chest Medicine) FRCP(London, UK) FCCP(USA) CCT(Respiratory and General Medicine, UK) MSc(Evidence Based Medicine, UK)
Director and Head
Department of Pulmonology
Calcutta Medical Research Institute
Kolkata, West Bengal, India

**Rakesh Kumar** MBBS MD
Professor and Head
Department of Community Medicine
IQ City Medical College
Durgapur, West Bengal, India
Director, Dr. Kumar's Diabetes and Lifestyle Clinic

**Rana Bhattacharjee** MD (Medicine) MRCP DM(Endocrinology) FICP FRCP FACE
Department of Endocrinology and Metabolism
IPGMER and SSKM Hospital
Kolkata, West Bengal, India

**Ranjan Bhattacharyya** MD(Psychiatry, Gold Medal) DNB(Psychiatry) MNAMS
Associate Professor and Head
Department of Psychiatry
Murshidabad Medical College and Hospital
West Bengal Medical Education Services
Director
Charak Square Diagnostic and Research Center
Direct Council Member (2021–2024)
Indian Psychiatric Society
Honorary Assistant Secretary, Indian Medical Association, Bengal State Branch

**Ratul Seal** MBBS MD
Senior Resident
Department of General Medicine
JIMSH
Kolkata, West Bengal, India

**Ritu Attri** MD
Assistant Professor
Department of Medicine
Dr BR Ambedkar State Institute of Medical Sciences (AIMS)
Ajitgarh
SAS Nagar, Punjab, India

**Rojina Choudhury** MBBS MD(General Medicine) DNB(General Medicine)
RMO cum Clinical Tutor
Department of Medicine
NRS Medical College
Kolkata, West Bengal, India

**Ruchit Shah** DNB(Medicine) DNB(Cardiology) FESC
Interventional Cardiologist
Valves (TAVR, Mitraclip Tricuspid clip) – LA, USA
Imaging (IVUS, OCT, FFR) – Seoul, South Korea
Breach Candy, Saifee, Jaslok, Wockhardt, Prince Aly Khan, KJ Somaiya Hospital
Mumbai, Maharashtra, India

**Rupsa Mukhopadhyay** MBBS
Junior Resident (MBBS)
ESI-PGIMSR, ESIC Medical College
Kolkata, West Bengal, India

**Saikat Datta** MD(Medicine) FRCP(Glasgow) FICP FIACM
Professor and Head
Department of Medicine
MJN Medical College
Cooch Behar, West Bengal, India

**Saikat Mondal** MD(Medicine)
Associate Professor
Department of Medicine
AIIMS Kalyani
Kolkata, West Bengal, India

**Sanjay Bandyopadhyay (Banerjee)** MBBS MD DNB DM(Gastroenterology) MNAMS FRCP
Head
Department of Gastroenterology
ILS Hospital, Dumdum
Kolkata, West Bengal, India

**Saibal Das** MBBS MD(Pharmacology) DM(Clinical Pharmacology)
Scientist D (Medical)
ICMR – Centre for Ageing and Mental Health
Kolkata, West Bengal, India

**Santanu Banerjee** MBBS MS(Orthopedics)
Consultant Orthopedics
Department of Orthopedics
Panacea Nursing Home
Kolkata, West Bengal, India

**Satabdi Datta** MBBS DNB(Anesthesiology)
Senior Resident
Department of Anesthesiology and Critical Care
Chittaranjan National Cancer Institute (CNCI), Rajarhat
Kolkata, West Bengal, India

**Sattik Siddhanta** MBBS(Honours) MD(Medicine) DM(Endocrinology) PG Dip Diabetology(England) FICP
Associate Professor
Department of Medicine
IPGMER and SSKM Hospital
Kolkata, West Bengal, India

**Saumitra Ray** MBBS MD FRC FCSI FICP FACC FESC SCAI
Ex-Professor
Vivekananda Institute of Medical Sciences
Director of Intervention Cardiology, AMRI(S)
Kolkata, West Bengal, India

**Saumya Singh**
Junior Research Fellow
Department of Medicine
University College of Medical Sciences
New Delhi, India

**Shambo Samrat Samajdar**
MBBS MD DM(Clinical Pharmacology) Fellowship Respiratory and Critical Care(WBUHS) Fellow Allergy-Asthma Specialist Course (AAAAI) Diploma Allergy Asthma Immunology PG Diploma Endocrinology and Diabetes (RCP)
Independent Clinical Pharmacologist and Consultant Physician
Diabetes and Allergy-Asthma Therapeutics Specialty Clinic
Kolkata, West Bengal, India

**Shashank R Joshi** MD DM FICP FACP(USA) FACE(USA) FRCP (London, Edinburgh, Glasgow) (Padma Shri Awardee)
Consultant Endocrinologist
Joshi Clinic, Lilavati Hospital, Sir HN Reliance and Bhatia Hospitals, Mumbai, Maharashtra
Adjunct Faculty JSS Medical College, Mysore and Jaipur National University
Mysuru, Karnataka, India

**Shubham Sharma**
DNB(Respiratory Medicine)
Consultant Pulmonologist and Interventionalist
Gleneagles Hospital
Bengaluru, Karnataka, India

**Siladitya Dewasi** MBBS MD(Resident Emergency Medicine)
Final Year Resident
Department of Emergency Medicine
IPGMER and SSKM Hospital
Kolkata, West Bengal, India

**Sinjan Ghosh** MBBS MD(Internal Medicine) DM(Neurology)
Life Member – Indian Academy of Neurology and Cognitive Neurology Subsection
Clinical and Research Fellow, Behavioral Neurology
Division of Adult Neurology, Department of Medicine
Baycrest Health Sciences, University of Toronto
Toronto, Ontario, Canada

**SK Shahriar Ahmed**
MD(Dermatology)
Senior Resident
Calcutta National Medical College
Kolkata, West Bengal, India

**Smarajit Banik** MD FICP FIACM FRCP
Professor and Head of Internal Medicine
Japaiguri Medical College and Hospital
Jalpaiguri, West Bengal, India

**Smiti Rani Srivastava**
MS(Ophthalmology) FRCS(Glasgow)
Associate Professor
Ophthalmology
IPGMER and SSKM Hospital
Kolkata, West Bengal, India

**Sougata Sarkar** MBBS MD DM(Clinical Pharmacology)
Clinical Pharmacologist
Department of Clinical Pharmacology
Calcutta School of Tropical Medicine
Kolkata, West Bengal, India

**Srabani Ghosh** MD(Internal Medicine) DM(Neuromedicine)
Associate Professor
Institute of Post Graduate Medical Education and Research (IPGMER)
Kolkata, West Bengal, India

**Sramana Palit** MBBS
Junior Resident
ESI-PGIMSR, ESIC Medical College
Kolkata, West Bengal, India

**Subhankar Naskar** MBBS MD(General Medicine)
Assistant Professor
General Medicine
Calcutta National Medical College and Hospital
Kolkata, West Bengal, India

**Subhra Sankar Sen** MBBS MD(General Medicine)
Postdoctoral Trainee
Department of Neurology
Bangur Institute of Neurosciences
IPGMER and SSKM Hospital
Kolkata, West Bengal, India

**Sudip Das** MD(Dermatology and Venereology)
Head
Department of Dermatology
Calcutta National Medical College and Hospital
Kolkata, West Bengal, India

**Sudip Das** MS(ENT)
Professor
Department of ENT
Medical College and Hospital
Kolkata, West Bengal, India

**Sudip Ghosh** MBBS MD(Respiratory Medicine) DM(Pulmonary Medicine and Critical Care)
Assistant Professor
Pulmonary Medicine and Critical Care
AIIMS Kalyani
Kalyani, West Bengal, India

**Suman Ghosh** MD(General Medicine)
Resident Medical Officer (RMO)
Malda Medical College
Malda, West Bengal, India

**Sumit Chakraborty** MBBS MD(General Medicine) DM(Endocrinology)
Professor
General Medicine
North Bengal Medical College
Siliguri, West Bengal, India

**Supriya Sarkar** MD(Respiratory Medicine)
Fellow of Indian College of Physicians
Fellow of National College of Chest Physicians
Professor and Head
Department of Respiratory Medicine
College of Medicine and Sagore Dutta Hospital Kamarhati
Kolkata, West Bengal, India

**Surya Kant** MBBS MD(Gold Medalist) FCCP(USA) FACP(USA) FRCP(London) FRCP(Glasgow) FGAPIO FAPSR FISEB FAMS FIAMS FNCCP FCAI FIMSA FIAB FICS FUPDA FIACM FICP FCGP FISC FGSI
Professor and Head
Department of Respiratory Medicine
King George's Medical University
Lucknow, Uttar Pradesh, India

**Suryasnata Bhowmik** MSc(Biochemistry)
Pre-graduate Medical Intern (MBBS)
Nilratan Sircar Medical College
Kolkata, West Bengal, India

**Shuvra Neel Baul** MBBS MD(Medicine) DNB(Medicine) DM(Hematology)
Assistant Professor
Hematology
NRS Medical College and Hospital
Kolkata, West Bengal, India

**Swati Kumar** MD(Medicine) DM(Neurology) SCE Neurology RCP UK
Assistant Professor
Department of Neurology
Bangur Institute of Neurosciences
IPGMER and SSKM Hospital
Kolkata, West Bengal, India

**Tanuka Mandal** MD(General Medicine)
Consultant
Department of General Medicine
RG Kar Medical College and Hospital
Kolkata, West Bengal, India

**Tapas Bandyopadhyay** MD FICP PG Diploma Endocrinology and Diabetes
Consultant Physician
Department of Internal Medicine
Medica Superspecialty Hospital
Kolkata, West Bengal , India

**Udas Chandra Ghosh** MBBS MD(Medicine) DNB(Medicine) DNB(Respiratory Diseases) DTCD FICP FRCP(Glasgow)
Professor
Department of Medicine
Medical College Kolkata
Kolkata, West Bengal, India

**Uddalak Chakraborty** MD(Internal Medicine) DM(Neurology) Resident
Senior Resident
Department of Neurology
Bangur Institute of Neurosciences
IPGMER and SSKM Hospital
Kolkata, West Bengal, India

**Uttam Kumar Nath** MD(Internal Medicine) DFID(Fellowship in Diabetes Management) CCCS(Certificate Course in Cardiovascular Disease and Stroke)
Assistant Professor
Jorhat Medical College and Hospital
Jorhat, Assam, India

# Foreword

It gives me immense pleasure to present the book "*General Practice: An Approach to Differential Diagnosis*" with an aim to provide a practical approach to differential diagnosis and clinical analysis of disease presentation.

This book will be of immense help in day-to-day practice of our colleagues and a ready reckoner for the practitioners for decision-making and investigation.

I once again congratulate Professors Jyotirmoy Pal and Nandini Chatterjee for this wonderful effort and wish them all the best for the success of this publication.

**Girish Mathur**
**President**
**Association of Physicians of India, 2023**

# Preface

It is our pleasure to introduce this book on clinical approach to disease symptomatology. Clinical Medicine is the heart of medical practice and is fast becoming a lost art.

Mindless prescriptions of hoards of investigations lead not only to unnecessary financial burden but also oft-repeated interventions and radiation exposure.

An analytical approach to signs and symptoms with careful consideration of differential diagnosis is very important to find a potential diagnostic clue. Investigations should be individualized and focused depending on inferences derived from clinical evaluation.

We hope this book is helpful for physicians and students alike to enrich standard of care.

**Jyotirmoy Pal**
**Nandini Chatterjee**

# Contents

## SECTION 1: COMMON SIGNS AND SYMPTOMS

## SECTION 2: MEDICAL EMERGENCIES

# SECTION 1

# Common Signs and Symptoms

# PART 1

# Cardiology

# CHAPTER 1

# Chest Pain

*Raja Dhar, Shubham Sharma*

## INTRODUCTION

Chest pain is one of the most common chief complaints of patients presenting to emergency departments (EDs) annually.

Etiologies of chest pain range from life-threatening conditions to those that are relatively benign.

The most common causes of chest pain in outpatients are musculoskeletal and gastrointestinal conditions, while stable angina constitutes 10%, respiratory conditions 5%, and acute myocardial ischemia (including myocardial infarction) approximately 2–4%. Similarly, conditions presenting with chest pain that pose an immediate threat to life include acute coronary syndrome, aortic dissection, pulmonary embolism, tension pneumothorax, pericardial tamponade, and mediastinitis (e.g., esophageal rupture).

The initial goal in the emergency room should be to identify these life threats.

## ETIOLOGY

### Cardiac Causes of Chest Pain

#### *Myocardial Ischemia*

- Angina pectoris is described as chest pain attributable to ischemia of the myocardium.
- Stable angina presents as pressure, heaviness, tightness, or constriction in the center or left side of the chest that is precipitated on exertion and is relieved at rest.
- Associated symptoms include pain in the chest precipitating with emotional stress or cold, which radiates to the neck, jaw, and shoulder; dyspnea; nausea and vomiting; diaphoresis; presyncope; and palpitations **(Flowchart 1)**.

#### *Aortic Dissection (Table 1)*

- It is a rare condition but may be a surgical emergency as it could be life-threatening if left undiagnosed and untreated.
- Patients typically present with sudden onset of chest and back pain that is severe, sharp, and "tearing" in quality.
- Pain can radiate anywhere in the chest or into the abdomen.
- Aortic dissection can be complicated by cerebrovascular accident, syncope, myocardial infarction, which is typically and usually due to involvement of the right coronary artery (RCA) territory, and heart failure.
- Predisposing factors:
    - Aortic aneurysm
    - Hypertension (HTN)
    - Vasculitis

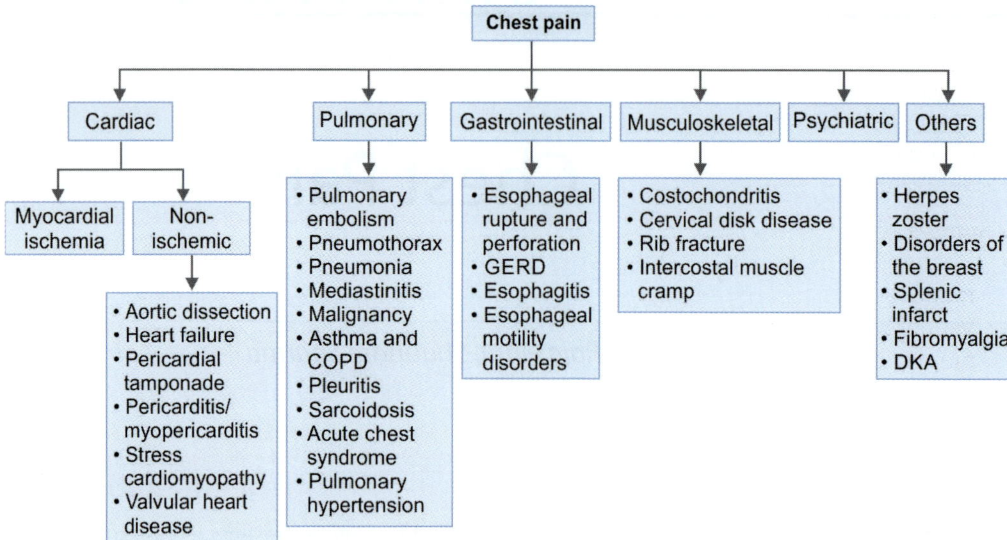


**FLOWCHART 1:** Etiology of chest pain.

(COPD: chronic obstructive pulmonary disease; DKA: diabetic ketoacidosis; GERD: gastroesophageal reflux disease)

**Table 1: Classifications of aortic dissection.**

| *Class* | *Description* |
|---|---|
| ***Stanford classification*** | |
| Type A | Dissection involving the ascending aorta, regardless of the site of the primary tear |
| Type B | Dissection of the descending aorta |
| ***DeBakey classification*** | |
| Type 1 | Dissection of the ascending and descending thoracic aorta |
| Type 2 | Dissection of the ascending aorta |
| Type 3 | Dissection of the descending aorta |
| ***Classification of different variants of aortic dissection*** | |
| Class 1 | Classic dissection with separation of intima/media; intimal flap between dual lumens (true and false dissection) |
| Class 2 | Medial disruption with intramural hematoma separation of intima/media; no intraluminal tear or flap imaged |
| Class 3 | Discrete/subtle dissection; intimal tear without hematoma (limited dissection) and eccentric bulge at tear site |
| Class 4 | Atherosclerotic penetrating ulcer; ulcer usually penetrating to adventitia with localized hematoma |
| Class 5 | Iatrogenic/traumatic dissection |

- Marfan's syndrome or other collagen diseases
- Coronary artery bypass grafting (CABG)/ cardiac catheterization
- Drugs (crack cocaine)
- Trauma

**Diagnosis of Aortic Dissection**

- History and physical examination may raise a suspicion.
- Variations in pulse or blood pressure (>20 mm Hg difference between right and left arms)
- *Electrocardiography (ECG)*: Usually inconclusive, unless other cardiac complications associated with the dissection
- Imaging **(Figs. 1A to C)**:
    - *Chest radiograph*: It may show mediastinal widening.
    - Computed tomography (CT) scan of the thorax
    - Transesophageal echocardiography (TEE)
    - Magnetic resonance imaging (MRI)
    - Transthoracic echocardiography (TTE)

Computed tomography scan of the thorax, TEE, and MRI are superior to TTE in terms of diagnostic accuracy.

**Management of Aortic Dissection**

- In an acute setting:
    - Intensive care unit (ICU) admission
    - *Pain control*: Morphine
    - Reduction of systolic blood pressure (SBP) with an aim of 100–120 mm Hg or lowest tolerated; heart rate (HR) aim should be <60bpm.
    - Intubate if unstable

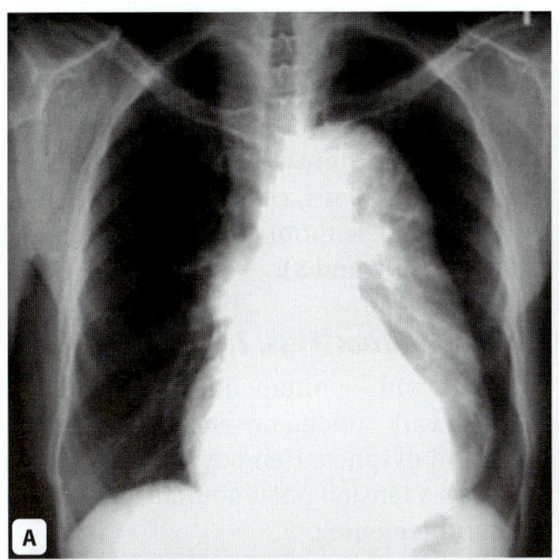


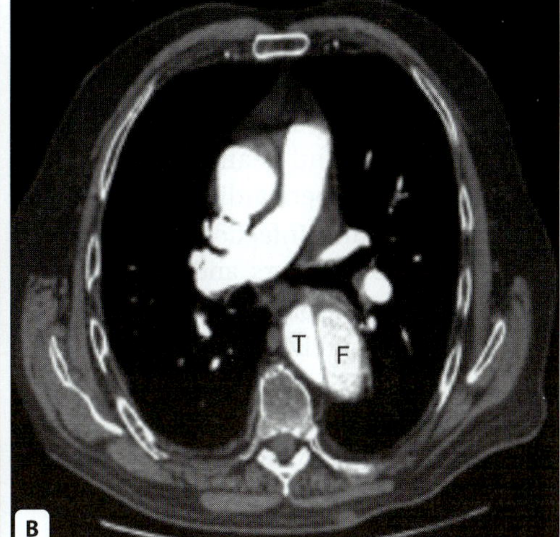


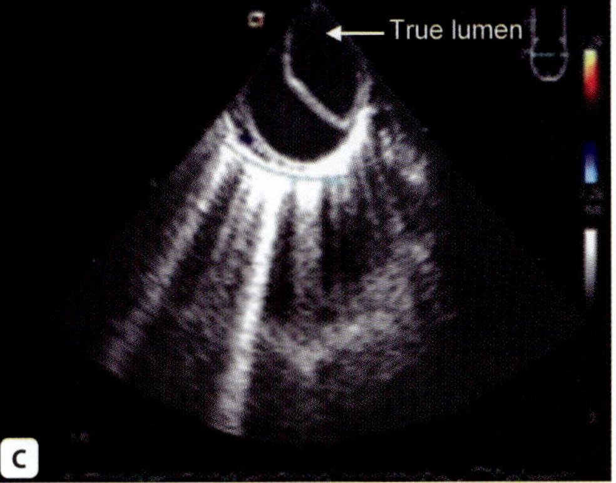


**FIGS. 1A TO C:** Aortic dissection.

- First-line treatment includes parenteral β-blockers (labetalol, propranolol, and esmolol).
- If HR <60bpm and SBP >100 mm Hg with good mentation and renal function, nitroprusside can be given.
- If the patient is hemodynamically unstable, look for blood loss, tamponade, or heart failure prior to volume replacement.

### *Heart Failure*

- Heart failure may also present with chest pain.
- Acute decompensated heart failure may present with chest discomfort along with progressive dyspnea, cough, fatigue, and peripheral edema.

### *Pericarditis/Myopericarditis*

- Pericarditis is the inflammation of the pericardial sac.
- Pleuritic chest pain that is improved by sitting up and leaning forward is characteristic of pericarditis.
- Etiologies include infection, medications, autoimmune disorders, and malignancy.
- Diagnosed on the basis of history, physical examination, and ECG findings.
- Myopericarditis indicates a primarily pericarditis syndrome with minor involvement of the underlying myocardium.

### *Stress Cardiomyopathy*

- Stress cardiomyopathy is also called takotsubo cardiomyopathy.
- It is a transient cardiac syndrome that involves left ventricular apical akinesis and mimics acute coronary syndrome.
- It often occurs in the setting of physical or emotional stress or critical illness.
- There is the presence of new ECG abnormalities such as ST segment elevation and/or T-inversion with mild elevation in cardiac enzymes. However, there is no significant coronary artery stenosis on coronary angiography.
- Left ventricular apical ballooning is present.

### *Mitral Valve Disease*

- Mitral stenosis can infrequently cause chest pain.
- It is often a result of pulmonary HTN and right ventricular hypertrophy.

## Pulmonary Causes of Chest Pain

Life-threatening pulmonary etiologies of chest pain include pulmonary embolism and tension pneumothorax. Patients with pulmonary etiologies for chest pain generally also have respiratory symptoms and may be hypoxemic **(Table 2)**.

### *Pulmonary Embolism*

Pulmonary embolism has variable presentation and should be suspected in any patient complaining of new onset or worsening dyspnea, chest pain, or prolonged hypotension without an obvious etiology **(Flowcharts 2 and 3)**.

### *Pneumothorax* (Figs. 2 and 3)

Patients with spontaneous pneumothorax present with sudden onset of pleuritic chest pain and dyspnea. Hemodynamic instability suggests a tension pneumothorax, which can be life-threatening.

Pneumothorax can be primary or secondary.

#### Primary Spontaneous Pneumothorax

- It is seen in patients without an underlying lung disease.
- It typically occurs in tall and thin males. Smoking, male gender, and Marfan's syndrome are risk factors.
- Patients are usually young (typically in their twenties) and present with sudden-onset dyspnea and pleuritic chest pain at rest.

**Table 2: Pulmonary causes of chest pain.**

| ***Pulmonary condition*** | | ***Other associated clinical features*** |
|---|---|---|
| Pneumonia | Pleuritic chest pain | Fever and productive cough |
| Malignancy | Chest pain is typically on the same side as primary tumor | Cough, dyspnea, and hemoptysis |
| Asthma and COPD | Feeling of chest tightness | Dyspnea |
| Pleuritis | Pain due to inflammation of the lung pleura. Causes include autoimmune disease (e.g., SLE) and drugs (e.g., procainamide, hydralazine, isoniazid) | Associated signs and symptoms of autoimmune disease such as fever, rash, arthralgias, and constitutional symptoms |
| Sarcoidosis | | Cough and dyspnea<br>Cardiac sarcoidosis can cause arrhythmias and sudden death, which may be heralded by chest pain, palpitations, syncope, or dizziness |
| Acute chest syndrome | In patients with sickle cell anemia | Fever, hypoxia, tachypnea, and cough |
| Pulmonary hypertension | Exertional chest pain | Exertional dyspnea and syncope |

(COPD: chronic obstructive pulmonary disease; SLE: systemic lupus erythematosus)

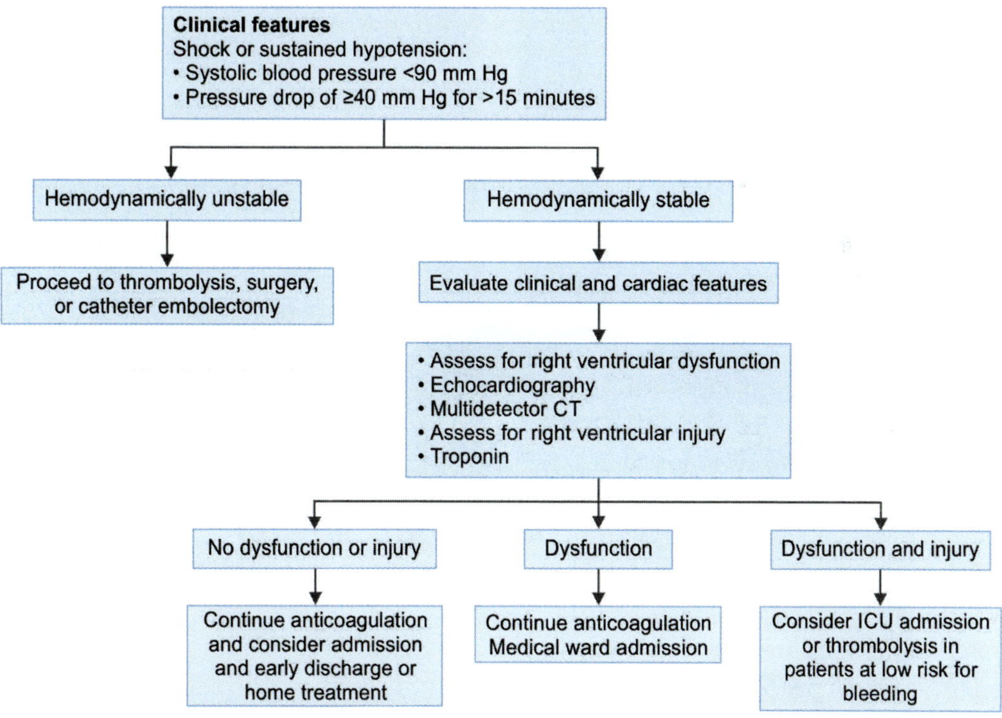


**FLOWCHART 2:** Diagnostic algorithm for pulmonary embolism.

(CT: computed tomography; ICU: intensive care unit)

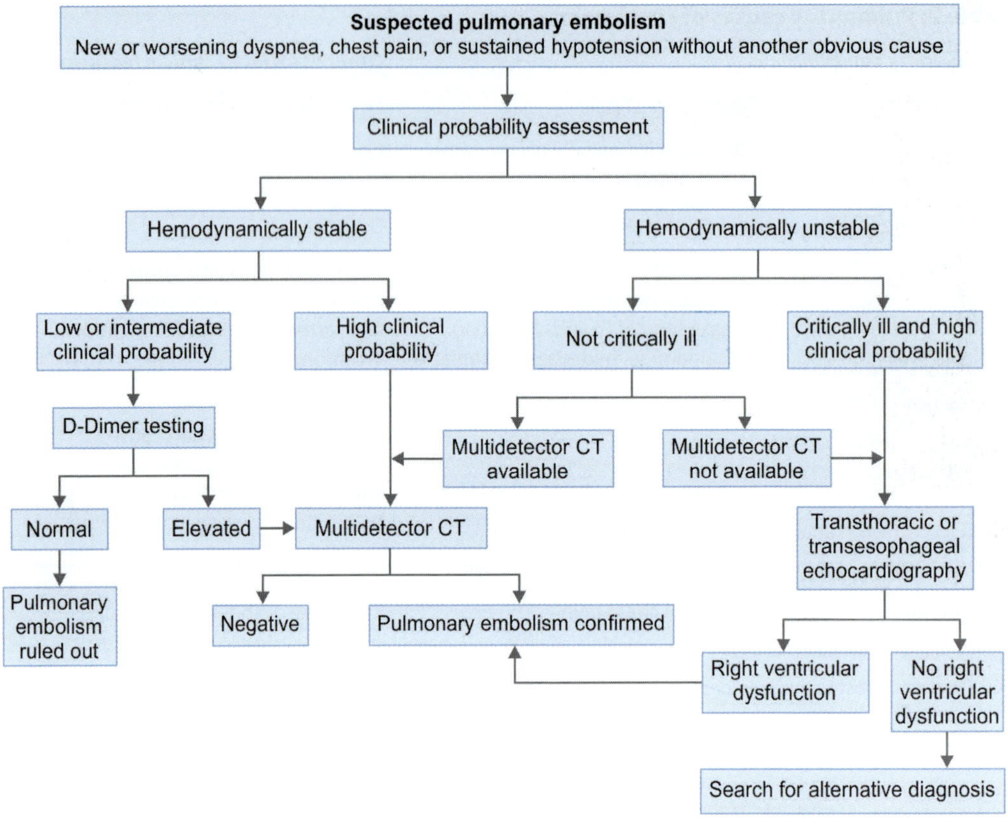

**Suspected pulmonary embolism**
New or worsening dyspnea, chest pain, or sustained hypotension without another obvious cause

↓

Clinical probability assessment

- Hemodynamically stable
  - Low or intermediate clinical probability → D-Dimer testing
    - Normal → Pulmonary embolism ruled out
    - Elevated → Multidetector CT
  - High clinical probability → Multidetector CT
- Hemodynamically unstable
  - Not critically ill
    - Multidetector CT available → Multidetector CT
    - Multidetector CT not available → Transthoracic or transesophageal echocardiography
  - Critically ill and high clinical probability → Transthoracic or transesophageal echocardiography

Multidetector CT
- Negative
- Pulmonary embolism confirmed

Transthoracic or transesophageal echocardiography
- Right ventricular dysfunction → Pulmonary embolism confirmed
- No right ventricular dysfunction → Search for alternative diagnosis

**FLOWCHART 3:** Management of pulmonary embolism.

(CT: computed tomography)

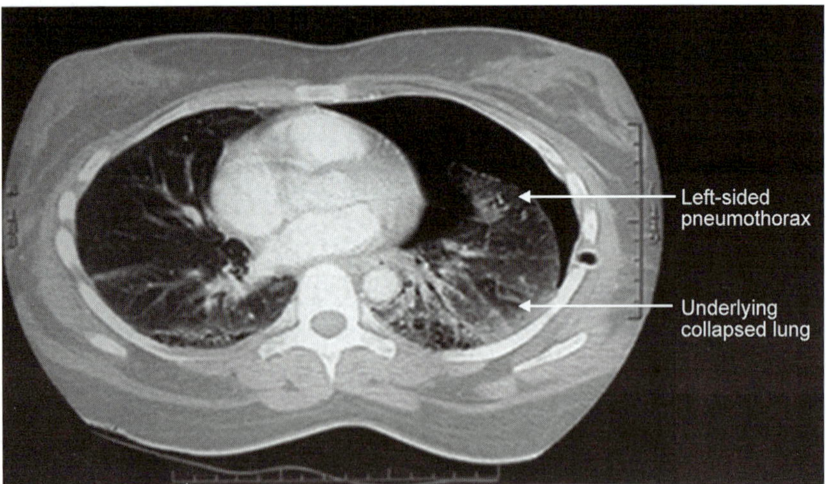


**FIG. 2:** Computed tomography scan of thorax showing left-sided pneumothorax with underlying collapsed lung. It can overestimate the size of the pneumothorax.

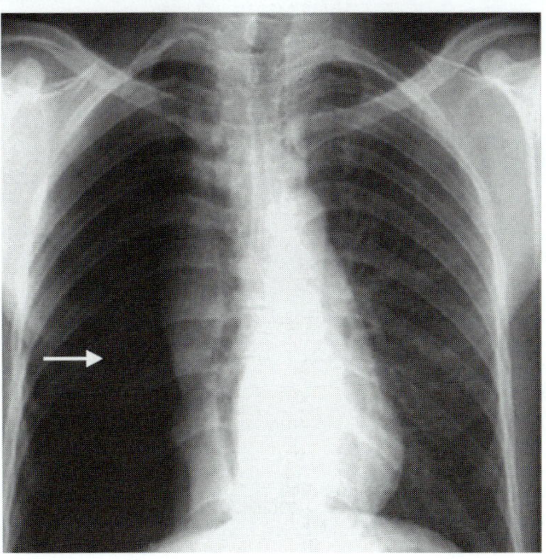

**FIG. 3:** Chest radiograph showing right-sided pneumothorax. Look for the pleural line. Such diagnosis can be difficult in patients with chronic obstructive pulmonary disease due to the underlying bulla that resemble a pneumothorax on a chest.

- Physical findings include decreased chest excursion, decreased breath sounds, and hyperresonance.
- Arterial blood gas (ABG) may be normal or may suggest type 1 respiratory failure. Hypercapnia is uncommon due to adequate ventilation of contralateral lung.

#### Secondary Spontaneous Pneumothorax

- It is seen in patients with an underlying lung disease.
- Any lung disease can predispose; however, chronic obstructive pulmonary disease (COPD) is most common and a major risk factor.
- *Pneumocystis carinii* pneumonia, cystic fibrosis, and tuberculosis are also common causes.
- Physical presentation is similar to primary spontaneous pneumothorax, but ABG is typically abnormal due to the underlying lung disease.

**Table 3: Gastrointestinal causes of chest pain.**

| ***Chest pain of gastrointestinal etiology*** | |
|---|---|
| Esophageal rupture and perforation | Spontaneous perforation of the esophagus results from a sudden increase in intraesophageal pressure, usually caused by straining or vomiting. Also called Boerhaave's syndrome<br>Can also be iatrogenic, as a result of instrumentation done in the gastrointestinal tract |
| Gastroesophageal reflux disease | Described as squeezing or burning type, located substernally, and radiates to back, neck, jaw, or arms and mimics the pain of myocardial ischemia. Usually resolves spontaneously or with antacids |
| Esophagitis | Can be medication induced |
| Other causes | Esophageal motility disorders and hiatus hernia |

## Gastrointestinal Causes of Chest Pain (Table 3)

Certain gastrointestinal conditions can also give rise to chest pain. Gastroesophageal reflux disease (GERD) is a common cause of noncardiac chest pain. Esophageal perforation, although rare, is a life-threatening etiology of chest pain.

### *Esophageal Rupture: Diagnosis and Management*

- Early chest radiographs show mediastinal or free peritoneal air.
- Hours to days later, widening of the mediastinum and pleural effusion can be seen.

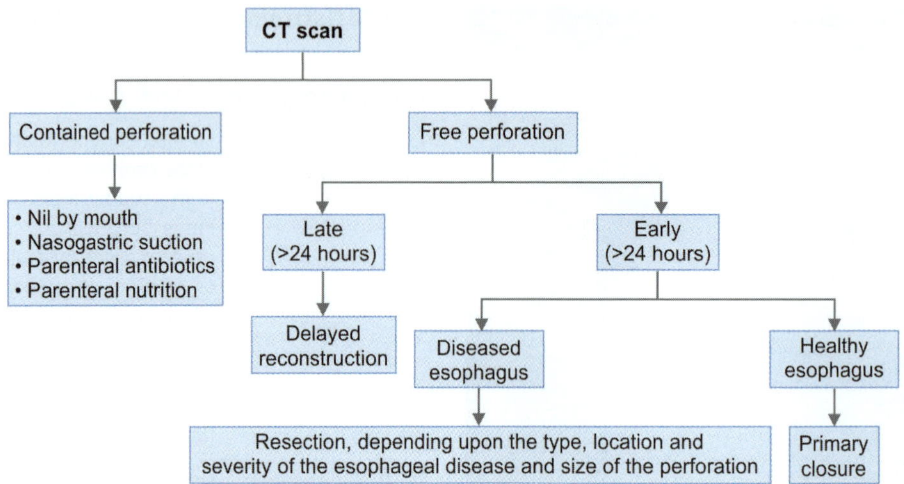


**FLOWCHART 4:** Computed tomography (CT) scan of esophageal rupture.

- CT scan shows esophageal edema, extra-esophageal air, and periesophageal fluid **(Flowchart 4)**.
- Esophagram will characteristically show the extravasation of contrast.
- There is no role for endoscopy, which introduces more air into the mediastinum.

## Musculoskeletal Causes of Chest Pain

- Chest pain due to musculoskeletal etiology is very common, besides gastrointestinal causes. Pain can be mild to severe but seldom life-threatening.
- It can occur due to various causes such as isolated musculoskeletal chest pain syndrome, most common cause of which being costochondritis and lower rib pain syndromes, or it can be due to rheumatoid arthritis and fibromyalgia.
- Rib fractures associated with pleuritic chest pain that is localized and reproducible with palpation. There is often a description of an associated injury.
- Chest wall trauma should be evaluated carefully because there could be an association of injury with the underlying lung parenchyma and major.

## Psychiatric Causes of Chest Pain

Chest pain is a common complaint among patients with psychiatric disorders, especially in panic attack and panic disorders. But such pain should also be evaluated carefully as such patients may develop or have coexisting coronary heart disease (CHD).

Depression and somatization syndrome are other psychiatric conditions wherein in patients may present with chest pain.

## Other Causes of Chest Pain

**Table 4** summarizes other causes of chest pain.

# CONCLUSION

Musculoskeletal and gastrointestinal conditions are the most common etiologies presenting with chest pain, but a clinician should always have an eye to identify the life-threatening etiologies, namely acute coronary syndrome, aortic dissection, pulmonary embolism, tension pneumothorax, pericardial tamponade, and mediastinitis.

Such patients tend to appear anxious and distressed and may be diaphoretic and dyspneic and often have unstable vital signs and should be referred to the ED immediately.

**Table 4: Other causes of chest pain.**

| | |
|---|---|
| Substance related | Cocaine use can result in myocardial ischemia (most common), besides aortic dissection, coronary artery aneurysm, myocarditis, cardiomyopathy, and arrhythmias. Chest pain due to cocaine use can also be due to pulmonary toxicity ("crack lung"), pneumothorax and pneumomediastinum, pulmonary vascular disease |
| Referred pain | Methamphetamine toxicity may cause similar features<br>For example, from abdominal organs (biliary colic) or from cervical disk disease<br>Occurs because the same spinal cord segment supplies the dermatomal areas of chest wall as well as parietal pleura or peritoneum |
| Herpes zoster | Pain is usually preceded by the characteristic rash and dysesthesia is usually present in the affected dermatome. Similarly, postherpetic neuralgia may also cause chest pain. |
| Trauma, domestic violence | |

While the clinical history and physical examination are the most important aspect of any disease evaluation, they are often not sufficient in distinguishing cardiac from noncardiac chest pain or life-threatening conditions from not so serious conditions.

Initial work-up should include an ECG and a chest radiograph, and further work-up and imaging can be decided by the clinician based on the suspicion of the most likely cause of the chest pain.

Atypical presentations also often occur, especially in the elderly, terminally ill, and patients with other comorbidities, and it is important to guard against premature diagnostic closure based upon the history.

## CLINICAL PEARLS

- Chest pain is a complaint with wide differential diagnosis
- Common causes include musculoskeletal and GI causes
- But the physician must keep in mind that life threatening causes like ACS aortic dissection tension pneumothorax.

## FURTHER READINGS

1. Chun AA, McGee SR. Bedside diagnosis of coronary artery disease: a systematic review. The American Journal of Medicine. 2004;117(5):334-43.
2. Schey R, Villarreal A, Fass R. Noncardiac chest pain: current treatment. Gastroenterology & Hepatology. 2007;3(4):255-62.
3. Bautz B, Schneider JI. High-Risk Chief Complaints I: Chest Pain-The Big Three (an Update). Emerg Med Clin North Am. 2020;38(2):453-98.

# CHAPTER 2

# Dyspnea

*Supriya Sarkar, Nandini Chatterjee*

## INTRODUCTION

Unlike cardiac activities, respiratory activities can be controlled voluntarily. Yet, we are not aware of our breathing as we take breathing for granted. But when we cannot breathe, nothing else matters. Dyspnea is classically described as unusually uncomfortable awareness of breathing. It may be described as chest tightness or constriction, increased work or effort of breathing, air hunger, need to breathe, urge to breathe, cannot get a deep breath, unsatisfying breath, heavy breathing, rapid breathing, or breathing more. We must be convinced about the symptom of dyspnea. For example, catch of breath may be due to pleuritic chest pain or heaviness of chest may be due to accumulation of pleural fluid, and these should be differentiated from dyspnea. It is always useful to understand what a patient means rather than what the patient describes.

## WHAT IS DYSPNEA?

The American Thoracic Society defines dyspnea as a "subjective experience of breathing discomfort that consists of qualitatively distinct sensations that vary in intensity. The experience derives from interactions among multiple physiological, psychological, social, and environmental factors and may induce secondary physiological and behavioral responses."

Dyspnea is a symptom and must be distinguished from the signs of increased work of breathing. Signs of increased work of breathing include increased rate and depth of respiration and use of accessory muscles of respiration—intercostal, suprasternal, and supraclavicular suction. As dyspnea is a subjective symptom, some patients may malinger, some may complain disproportionately of increased dyspnea as compared with his disease, and some patients may not complain even when they have signs of increased work of breathing (probably they ignore it or may be habituated with it or may accommodate dyspnea with lifestyle modification).

## MECHANISM OF DYSPNEA

### Receptors

As with other sensations, the sensation of dyspnea starts from receptors. These receptors are present in the airways, lung parenchyma, respiratory muscles, and other areas.

Chemoreceptors (both central and peripheral) can sense the changes in partial pressure of $CO_2$, $O_2$, and pH and ensure that alveolar ventilation can adapt to the metabolic changes. Hypoxia can cause dyspnea indirectly by increasing ventilatory drive. The mechanism of direct effect of hypoxia is poorly understood. It may be due to perceiving the sensation as it reaches directly to the level of consciousness. The direct effect may explain the beneficial role of oxygen on dyspnea. Hypoxic hyperventilation may cause air trapping and dynamic hyperinflation, which may produce dyspnea.

Pulmonary receptors are slowly adapting stretch receptors (SASRs), rapidly adapting receptors (RARs), and juxtapulmonary (J) receptors. SASRs present in large airways respond to increase in lung volume. RARs present in airway epithelium respond to particulate irritations, direct stimulations of the airways, and pulmonary congestion. Juxtapulmonary receptors present in the bronchial and laryngeal mucosa and pulmonary capillaries are nonmyelinated fibers. They are stimulated by different mechanical and chemical stimuli. Sensations from those pulmonary receptors are carried to the central respiratory centers via the vagus nerve. Pulmonary receptors, particularly juxtapulmonary receptors, are implicated as the generator of dyspnea.

Mechanoreceptors are mainly present in the respiratory muscles and have a negative effect on dyspnea. Stimulation of mechanoreceptors, contrary to our belief, generates a negative impact on the genesis of dyspnea and reduces its sensation. Mechanoreceptors for volume, flow, muscle shortening, muscle tension, and chest wall displacement provide peripheral sensory feedback. Ultimately, the intensity of central motor output at the central sensory level is modulated. Inspiratory chest wall vibration reduces the sense of dyspnea, whereas expiratory vibration has an opposite effect.

## Respiratory Effort and Central Corollary Discharge

Dyspnea is said to be arising from greater respiratory muscle activity or effort. Sense of effort is a central sensation related to increased central motor command, muscle load, or when muscles are weakened, fatigued, or paralyzed. When ventilation is increased, the increased motor command is sent to ventilatory muscles and the motor cortex. Simultaneously, a copy signal is sent to sensory cortex, which is termed central corollary discharge. A corollary discharge is also sent from brainstem centers, but they are weak, and they are usually sensed as air hunger. The sense of muscle effort and corollary discharge is dependent on the absolute magnitude and duration of load. Relative magnitude of load, compared with the maximum capacity of muscles, is also an important determinant of corollary discharge.

## Neuroventilatory Dissociation

We get distress when we achieve less than what we deserve. Similarly, dyspnea results from interaction between efferent and afferent signals, the neuroventilatory dissociation. Dyspnea occurs when more than expected respiratory effort is necessary to achieve a given amount of ventilation. The phenomenon is also described as length-tension inappropriateness, where length represents change in lung volume and in other way the ventilation whereas tension indicates respiratory muscle tension and in other way respiratory effort. Misbalance between them produces the sensation of dyspnea.

## Role of Central Nervous System

Dyspnea results from simultaneous and multiple sensory inputs. The role of the central nervous system is important in the integration of those complex sensations. Dyspnea arises from three distinct brain areas: Right anterior insula, cerebellar vermis, and medial pons. The sensation of dyspnea results from the sensorimotor integration and the modulation of the perceived intensity.

## WHAT ARE THE CAUSES OF DYSPNEA?

Dyspnea may occur due to increased work of breathing as a result of airway obstruction, stiff lung or hyperinflated lung, increased respiratory activity as a result of increased need of ventilation, and stimulation of receptors within lungs, pulmonary vessels, and extravascular structures. Cardiovascular diseases may cause dyspnea by accumulation of fluid in lungs. Some noncardiac/nonrespiratory conditions may also cause dyspnea. Finally, dyspnea may be psychological in origin.

### Dyspnea in Airway Diseases

Both asthma and chronic obstructive pulmonary disease (COPD) can cause dyspnea by expiratory airflow obstruction and dynamic hyperinflation of the lungs and chest wall, thereby increasing the work of breathing. Patients with acute bronchoconstriction may complain of a sense of tightness of chest. A ventilation-perfusion mismatch in obstructive airway diseases may cause hypoxemia, thereby increasing respiratory effort.

Classically, dyspnea in COPD is persistent (without a symptomless period) and progressive (increases its intensity relentlessly) with periods of exacerbations (periods of increased symptoms). On the other hand, dyspnea in asthma is usually episodic in nature with symptom-free intervals. Dyspnea of chronic asthma may have the same characteristics as those of COPD. Dyspnea of airway diseases is usually associated with wheeze (a musical wheezy sound heard by naked ears).

### Dyspnea of Lung Parenchymal Diseases

Diseases involving interstitium and lung parenchyma due to several mechanisms (infections, occupational dust exposures, autoimmune disorders, or by unknown mechanisms) cause stiffness of lung. As a result, lung compliance (distensibility of lungs) decreases and thereby work of breath increases. Hypoxemia due to ventilation-perfusion mismatch increases ventilatory drive. Stimulation of pulmonary receptors is also responsible for the pathogenesis of dyspnea in mild-to-moderate interstitial lung diseases.

### Diseases of the Chest Wall and Pleura

Diseases of the chest wall (kyphoscoliosis), weakness of respiratory muscles (myasthenia gravis or Guillain-Barré syndrome), and stiffness of chest wall (scleroderma) increase the effort of breathing. Similarly, pleural diseases (effusion or pneumothorax) cause dyspnea by increasing the work of breathing and by stimulating pulmonary receptors (due to underlying atelectasis).

### Dyspnea due to Diseases of Cardiovascular System

Left ventricular diseases resulting from coronary artery diseases, hypertensive heart diseases, and nonischemic cardiomyopathies cause pulmonary interstitial edema and thereby stimulate pulmonary receptors. Dyspnea may be augmented by hypoxemia (as a result of ventilation-perfusion mismatch) and increased ventilatory drive. Constrictive pericarditis and cardiac tamponade increase intracardiac pressure and pulmonary vascular pressures, and thereby cause dyspnea.

Pulmonary thromboembolic diseases and primary diseases of the pulmonary circulation (primary pulmonary hypertension and pulmonary vasculitis) can cause dyspnea. The underlying mechanism is thought to be due to stimulation of receptors in pulmonary vessels. Hypoxemia and hyperventilation may augment that process.

## Other Causes of Dyspnea

Anemia is associated with dyspnea, which may be due to stimulation of metaboreceptors. Dyspnea may be observed in hyperthyroidism as a result of increased metabolic activities and in hypothyroidism as a result of pleural or pericardial effusion.

# HOW TO APPROACH DYSPNEA?

## First Step

Firstly, we should identify different expressions of dyspnea as dyspnea may be expressed in different words according to a patient's understanding. It is also important to be sure whether the patient is actually complaining of dyspnea. Expressions of other symptoms may mimic those of dyspnea. For example, a catch of breath may be due to pleuritic chest pain. It is also important to recognize dyspnea even when a patient is not complaining about it. A patient with arthritis may have limited activities, and thereby he/she cannot recognize his/her symptoms. A patient with chronic dyspnea may adapt that problem by modifying his/her lifestyle.

## Second Step

Secondly, respiratory origin of dyspnea should be characterized by presence of seasonality and wheezing, be to differentiate from dyspnea arising from other diseases. Anemia, hyperthyroidism, or hypothyroidism can be easily identified clinically as well as with simple laboratory tests.

### *Psychological Dyspnea*

Psychological dyspnea is usually identified by detailed history, a patient's background, and meticulous observation of the patient's behavioral pattern. But in some cases, it is difficult to recognize, and then it is important to rule out organic diseases before diagnosing it as functional. It is also important to remember that psychological factors may precipitate attacks of dyspnea in organic diseases. For example, attacks of asthma may be precipitated by psychological stress.

### *Distinguishing Cardiovascular Dyspnea from Respiratory Dyspnea*

The differentiation is often difficult and sometimes may be impossible. Yet, an endeavor in this regard is always beneficial in clinical medicine. Differentiating dyspnea from respiratory diseases and cardiac diseases is an important step. The differentiation is often difficult as cardiac diseases cause dyspnea mainly by accumulation of fluid in lungs. Cardiac origin of dyspnea should be suspected if there is a history suggestive of cardiac disease, history of hypertension, ischemic heart disease, presence of palpitation, precordial chest pain, and history suggestive of paroxysmal nocturnal dyspnea. On the other hand, the presence of wheeze, cough with expectoration, hemoptysis, and nonprecordial chest pain is suggestive of respiratory origin of dyspnea. Wheeze may be found in left ventricular failure due to accumulation of fluid in the peribronchovascular spaces. Cough may be found in both conditions, but expectoration (mucoid and mucopurulent) is suggestive of respiratory disease and pink frothy expectoration is suggestive of left ventricular failure. Frank hemoptysis is always suggestive of respiratory diseases except mitral valvular diseases.

High blood pressure may suggest cardiac origin, but it is nonspecific. Physical findings such as gallop rhythm, murmur, abnormal heart sounds, and fine basal crackles are suggestive of cardiac origin of dyspnea. Right ventricular gallop and murmur arising from tricuspid and pulmonary valves may occur in cor pulmonale and are indicative of a respiratory cause of dyspnea. Basal crackles are also found in respiratory diseases, particularly in diffuse parenchymal lung diseases.

Cardiopulmonary exercise test may be an effective tool in differentiating respiratory from cardiac origin of dyspnea. Respiratory origin is evident when at peak exercise the patient demonstrates hypoxemia or the patient develops bronchospasm. Cardiac origin is suggested if the heart rate becomes >85% of predicted maximum, anaerobic threshold occurs early, blood pressure is extremely high or low, $O_2$ consumption per heart rate falls, or there is appearance of ischemic changes in electrocardiogram (ECG).

## Third Step

A detailed history taking has no substitute in the analysis of dyspnea. The onset of dyspnea is important as sudden onset usually indicates a vascular phenomenon (acute myocardial infarction and pulmonary thromboembolism) or pneumothorax. In children, sudden onset of dyspnea may occur in foreign body inhalation. Longer duration of dyspnea usually suggests obstructive airway diseases, interstitial lung diseases, chronic heart failure, or cardiomyopathy. Shorter duration of dyspnea may occur in infective diseases, pleural diseases, or acute cardiac diseases. Dyspnea may increase rapidly in tension pneumothorax, acute myocardial infarction, or gradually in pleural effusion or cardiomyopathy. Episodic dyspnea (with symptom-free intervals) usually suggests asthma, bronchospasm, intermittent myocardial ischemia, pulmonary embolism, etc. Acute increase in dyspnea in patients with relentlessly progressive dyspnea is suggestive of exacerbations of COPDs or interstitial lung diseases.

Dyspnea with wheeze usually suggests obstructive airway diseases. Nocturnal dyspnea can occur in left ventricular failure (due to increased venous return) and asthma (due to presence of allergens in bed). Exertional dyspnea is nonspecific and it only gives an early indication of respiratory or cardiac diseases. Orthopnea occurs in conditions such as congestive cardiac failure, gastroesophageal reflux diseases, and obesity. Platypnea (dyspnea in an upright position that relieve in supine position) occurs in left atrial myxoma or hepatopulmonary syndrome. Smoking history may be associated with both COPD and ischemic heart disease.

## Fourth Step

A meticulous physical examination may give important clues to the diagnosis. General survey should focus on pallor, cyanosis, jaundice, clubbing, neck vein, edema, etc. Signs of dyspnea such as tachypnea, use of accessory muscles of respiration, supraclavicular and intercostal retractions, and tripod position (sitting with one's hands braced on the knees) are important to note. Different breathing patterns (Cheyne–Stokes breathing, Biot's breathing, Kussmaul's breathing, etc.) should be appreciated. Pulsus paradoxus may be found in COPD or asthma. Examination of thorax (symmetry of hemithorax, movement of thorax, mediastinal position, percussion notes, breath sounds, added sounds, and vocal resonance) should be carefully done to diagnose the pathological changes of lungs, pleura, or thoracic cage. Engorgement of neck veins and their pulsatility are important and reflect right-sided cardiac events and diseases of superior vena cava. Cardiac examination should include examination of blood pressure, pulses, jugular veins, abnormalities of heart sounds, and murmurs. Abdomen should be carefully examined for paradoxical movement. Raynaud's phenomenon may suggest collagen vascular diseases.

## Fifth Step

Investigations should depend on clinical clues and clinical settings. They depend on the suspected origin of dyspnea. Routine blood examination, thyroid function tests, liver function tests, and lipid profile will eliminate anemia, thyroid disorders, hepatopulmonary syndrome, and risk of cardiovascular diseases.

When the cardiac cause of dyspnea is suspected, then the investigation should start with ECG and echocardiography. Special cardiac investigations such as 24-hour Holter monitoring or cardiac angiography should be done on a case-to-case basis. When respiratory causes are suspected, then investigations should start with chest X-ray posteroanterior (PA) view, spirometry, and sputum examination. High-resolution computed tomography (HRCT) of thorax should be done if preliminary investigations suggest interstitial lung disease, parenchymal lung disease, or airway disease. Contrast-enhanced computed tomography (CECT) of thorax should be done for pleural diseases, lung malignancies, and mediastinal diseases. Pleural fluid examination is an essential step for pleural effusion. It should be remembered that the most common cause of bilateral pleural effusion is congestive cardiac failure. Measurement of diffusion capacity of the lungs for carbon monoxide (DLCO) should be done for interstitial lung diseases and obstructive airway diseases. Bronchoprovocation test is rarely required for the diagnosis of asthma when symptoms are intermittent and spirometry is normal.

When no clue is available from history and clinical examination, then apart from routine blood biochemistry, chest X-ray PA view, ECG, echocardiography, and HRCT thorax should be done to start with. The next step will be determined by the results of preliminary investigation results.

## Sixth Step

It is important to assess the severity of dyspnea. Generally, dyspnea is classified as stage I (dyspnea occurring with more than habitual exercise), stage II (with habitual exercise), stage III (with less than habitual exercise), and stage IV (dyspnea occurring at rest). The Modified Medical Research Council (mMRC) dyspnea scale **(Table 1)** is widely used and standardized. A patient's descriptions of dyspnea are graded as "I only get breathlessness with strenuous exercise" (mMRC grade 0); "I get short of breath when hurrying on the level

**Table 1: Modified Medical Research Council (mMRC) scale for dyspnea.**

| *Please tick in the box that applied to you (one box only) (Grades 0–4)* | | |
|---|---|---|
| mMRC grade 0 | I only get breathless with strenuous exercise | ☐ |
| mMRC grade 1 | I get short of breath when hurrying on the level or walking up in a slight hill | ☐ |
| mMRC grade 2 | I walk slower than people of same age on the level because of breathlessness, or I have to stop for breath when walking on my own pace on the level | ☐ |
| mMRC grade 3 | I stop for breath after walking 100 m or after few minutes on the level | ☐ |
| mMRC grade 4 | I am too breathless to leave the house or I am breathless when dressing or undressing | ☐ |

*Continued*

*Continued*

| ***CAT assessment*** | | |
|---|---|---|
| For each item below, place a mark (x) in the box that best describes you currently. Be sure to only select one response for each question | | Score |
| I never cough | ⓪①②③④⑤ | I cough all the time |
| I have no phlegm (mucus) in the chest at all | ⓪①②③④⑤ | My chest is completely full of phlegm (mucus) |
| My chest does not feel tight at all | ⓪①②③④⑤ | My chest feels very tight |
| When I walk up a hill or one flight of stairs, I am not breathless | ⓪①②③④⑤ | When I walk up a hill or one flight of stairs, I am very breathless |
| I am not limited doing any activity at home | ⓪①②③④⑤ | I am very limited doing activity at home |
| I am confident leaving my home despite my lung condition | ⓪①②③④⑤ | I am not at all confident leaving my home because of my lung condition |
| I sleep sound | ⓪①②③④⑤ | I do not sleep sound because of my lung condition |
| I have lots of energy | ⓪①②③④⑤ | I have no energy at all |

(CAT: chronic obstructive pulmonary disease assessment test)

or walking up in a slight hill" (mMRC grade 1); "I walk slower than people of my age on the level because of breathlessness, or I have to stop for breath when walking on my own space on the level" (mMRC grade 2); "I stop for breath after walking 100 meters or after few minutes on the level" (mMRC grade 3); and "I am too breathless to leave the house or I am breathless when dressing or undressing" (mMRC Grade 4). COPD assessment score (CAT score) is an important tool for assessing dyspnea and other symptoms.

## MANAGEMENT OF DYSPNEA

Management of dyspnea depends on identification of cause and treatment of specific disease. Supplemental $O_2$ should be administered for resting or exercise-induced desaturation [oxygen saturation ($SpO_2$) <90%]. Pleural fluid aspiration may temporarily relieve dyspnea. When the disease is not curable or treatable, then symptomatic management may be an essential step. Pulmonary rehabilitation program may be helpful in patients with chronic dyspnea. Dyspnea due to malignancies may respond to opioids, particularly morphine. Assurance and sympathetic interventions are helpful in terminally ill patients.

## CONCLUSION

Dyspnea may arise from a wide variety of respiratory, cardiac, hematological, metabolic, and psychological diseases. Identification of the causes of dyspnea is an essential step. Detailed history, meticulous clinical examination, and routine investigations will identify the etiology in most of the cases. Sometimes, special investigations are required. Symptomatic management should go along with specific management of etiological disease. In terminally ill patients, assurance and opioids may alleviate symptoms.

## CLINICAL PEARLS

- Dyspnea can occur due to respiratory cardiac renal hematological metabolic and psychological causes.
- Each etiology may be recognized by following a systematic clinical approach of exclusion.
- The therapy is individualized according to etiology.

## FURTHER READINGS

1. Baron RM. Dyspnea. In: Loscalzo J, Fauci A, Kasper D, Hauser S, Longo D, Jameson JL, (Eds). Harrison's Principles of Internal Medicine 21e. McGraw Hill; 2022.
2. Viniol A, Beidatsch D, Frese T, Bergmann M, Grevenrath P, Schmidt L, et al. Studies of the symptom dyspnoea: a systematic review. BMC Fam Pract. 2015;16:152.

# CHAPTER 3

# Palpitation

*Mainak Mukhopadhyay*

## INTRODUCTION

Palpitation is one of the common complaints among patients consulting physicians.

## DEFINITION

Palpitation can be defined as an unusual awareness of own heartbeat, mimicking a "fluttering" sensation in the chest.

## CLASSIFICATION

- Intermittent
- Sustained
- Regular
- Irregular

## ETIOLOGY

- Cardiac—one-third
- Psychiatric—one-third
- Others—one-third

## CARDAIC CAUSES OF PALPITATION (TABLE 1)

*Rate and rhythm related*:
- *Sinus tachycardia* (appropriate or inappropriate)
- Arrhythmia

*Hyperdynamic circulation (any catecholaminergic state)*:
- Anemia
- Fever
- Thyrotoxicosis
- Arteriovenous (AV) fistula

*Increased preload*:
- Aortic regurgitation (AR)
- Mitral regurgitation (MR)

*Others*:
- Left atrial (LA) myxoma (postural palpitation and postural varying diastolic murmur)
- Mitral valve prolapse (MVP)
- Pulmonary embolism (PE)
- Postural orthostatic tachycardia syndrome (POTS)

## PSYCHIATRIC CAUSES OF PALPITATION

Psychiatric causes of palpitations include:
- Panic attacks (can mimic heart attack)
- Anxiety disorder
- Somatization

Patients with psychiatric causes for palpitations more commonly report a longer duration of the sensation (>15 minutes) and other accompanying symptoms than do patients with other causes.

**Table 1: Characteristics of palpitation in different cardiac arrhythmias.**

| | |
|---|---|
| Supraventricular or ventricular ectopics | Irregular palpitation, the feeling of a "skipped" heartbeat due to postextrasystolic potentiation |
| Paroxysmal supraventricular tachycardia | Intermittent regular palpitation |
| Ventricular tachycardia | Intermittent regular palpitation. Often with hemodynamic compromise. Associated with IHD, HCM, channelopathies, ARVC, and infiltrative cardiomyopathies |
| Atrial tachycardia and atrial flutter | Intermittent regular palpitation |
| Atrial fibrillation | Irregular palpitation. Associated with mitral valve disease, HCM, and atrial enlargement in HFpEF |
| Multifocal atrial tachycardia | Irregular palpitation. Associated with pulmonary diseases, e.g., COPD |

(ARVC: arrhythmogenic right ventricular cardiomyopathy; COPD: chronic obstructive pulmonary disease; HCM: hypertrophic cardiomyopathy; HFpEF: heart failure with preserved ejection fraction; IHD: ischemic heart disease)

## OTHER CAUSES OF PALPITATION

Other common causes of palpitations are:
- Thyrotoxicosis
- Drugs (thyroxine, aminophylline, cocaine, ethanol, tobacco, caffeine, atropine, and amphetamines)
- Spontaneous skeletal muscle contractions of the chest wall

## RELEVANT MEDICAL HISTORY

- Any history of coronary artery disease or its risk factors
- Any family history of sudden cardiac death suggesting channelopathies or arrhythmogenic cardiomyopathies
- Drug and addiction history
- Thyroid dysfunction
- Any recent history of tuberculosis or sarcoid [Both tubercular and sarcoid cardiomyopathy are strongly associated with ventricular tachycardia (VT)]
- Whether palpitation is associated with dyspnea or angina or syncope (strongly suggests an underlying serious cardiac cause)
- *Character of palpitation*: Regularity (patient can "tap out" the rhythm of the palpitations to reveal the regularity), related to work or at rest, onset and offset (abrupt onset and offset go in favor of reentrant tachyarrhythmia, whereas gradual onset and offset are more of sinus tachycardia)
- Any existing valvular pathology

## CLINICAL CLUES

- Pallor to rule out anemia
- Elevated temperature to rule out fever causing palpitation.
- *Pulse*: Increased rate with regular rhythm is found in sinus tachycardia, paroxysmal supraventricular tachycardia (PSVT), atrial tachycardia, and VT. Irregular rhythm can be due to supraventricular ectopics (SVEs) or ventricular ectopics (VEs), atrial fibrillation (AF), and multifocal atrial tachycardia (MAT).

  Pulsus alternans can hint toward LV dysfunction. High-volume pulse is found in AR.
- Blood pressure with its postural changes can give clues to hypertension or orthostatic hypotension (associated with pheochromocytoma) or POTS.

- Edema and neck veins evaluation to rule out heart failure
- Auscultation of precordium is mandatory, specifically for cardiac murmurs to rule out structural heart disease.
- Physical features of thyrotoxicosis

## EVALUATION

- Resting electrocardiogram (ECG) can document sustained arrhythmia or if recorded during the event of palpitation can also pick up the culprit arrhythmia. Otherwise, resting ECG can give clues to the possible cause of arrhythmia, for example, ischemic heart disease (IHD), left ventricular hypertrophy, atrial enlargement, long or short QT, Brugada, epsilon wave of arrhythmogenic right ventricular cardiomyopathy (ARVC), S1Q3T3 or right ventricular (RV) strain of PE, bifascicular heart block (VT in 5% cases), and pre-excitation.
- Exercise ECG can be helpful if palpitation is exertional only. It can help to diagnose catecholaminergic polymorphic ventricular tachycardia (CPVT) or accessory pathway-mediated tachycardia.
- Holter monitoring is not very effective unless there is a frequent symptom. Holter monitoring can be effective in psychogenic palpitation. In such cases, if the patient is advised to maintain a time-based palpitation symptom card during the Holter monitoring, the physician can document the near-normal heart rate and rhythm even during the complaint of palpitation.
- External loop recorder (ELR) or extended patch Holter monitoring is often helpful, at least when there is once-in-a-month symptom.
- Implantable loop recorder (ILR) with a battery life of around 3 years can be very helpful in less frequently symptomatic palpitations.
- Wearable devices such as smartwatches (e.g., Apple Watch) or AliveCor devices are very helpful in the diagnosis of arrhythmias, especially paroxysmal Af.
- Complete hemogram to rule out anemia
- Thyroid function test to rule out thyrotoxicosis
- Transthoracic echo Doppler study to rule out structural heart diseases, for example, heart failure, hypertrophic cardiomyopathy (HCM), IHD, and valve pathology.
- Electrophysiology study is helpful where all other methods fail to yield a definite cause.

## CONCLUSION

The primary aim of the clinical evaluation of palpitation is to exclude life-threatening arrhythmia. Hence, a systematic approach is necessary to reach a proper life-saving diagnosis.

## CLINICAL PEARLS

- Detailed history taking is extremely important in palpitation.
- Bedside clinical examination gives important clues to the diagnosis.
- Investigations must be rational and guided by the history and clinical findings.

## FURTHER READINGS

1. Libby P, Bonow RO, Mann DL, Tomaselli GF, Bhatt DL, Solomon SD, et al. Braunwald's heart disease a textbook of Cardiovascular Medicine. Philadelphia, PA: Elsevier; 2022.
2. Fuster V, Narula,Jagat, Vaishnava P, Leon MB, Callans DJ, Rumsfeld JS, et al. Fuster and Hurst's the heart: 15th edition. New York: Mc Graw Hill; 2022.
3. Loscalzo J, Kasper DL, Longo DL, Fauci AS, Hauser SL, Jameson JL, et al. Harrison's principles of Internal Medicine, twenty-First edition vol 1 & 2, New York: McGraw Hill; 2022.

# CHAPTER 4

# Syncope

*Mainak Mukhopadhyay*

## INTRODUCTION

Framingham studies revealed the etiology of syncope in the general population—21% due to reflex syncope, 9.4% due to orthostatic hypotension (OH), 9.5% due to cardiac syncope, and 9% are nonsyncopal transient loss of consciousness (TLOC). Despite detailed evaluation, 37% remained unexplained syncope.

## DEFINITION

Syncope is a TLOC, due to transient global cerebral hypoperfusion, characterized by rapid onset, short duration, and spontaneous complete recovery.

Transient loss of consciousness is a state of the real or apparent loss of consciousness with loss of awareness, characterized by amnesia for the period of unconsciousness, abnormal motor control, loss of responsiveness, and short duration.

## CLASSIFICATION

Transient loss of consciousness:
- TLOC due to head injury
- Nontraumatic TLOC
    - Syncope (reflex syncope, OH, cardiac syncope)
    - Epileptic seizure
    - Psychogenic pseudosyncope
    - Others

## SYNCOPE–SEIZURE DIFFERENTIATION

The differences between syncope and seizure are given in **Table 1**.

## BASIC APPROACH

- To identify true syncope, clinical history is the most important part. Statement of the witness and any event-video clip is of paramount importance. Unless physicians properly listen to the history of a suspected patient of syncope, it is impossible to reach the diagnosis with any other sophisticated test.
- To diagnose the exact type of syncope and treat it accordingly
- If definite diagnosis is not possible, then it is mandatory to risk stratify.
- High-risk patients must be admitted and thoroughly followed up.
- Investigations must be done to diagnose cardiac syncope properly as it has a mortality issue.

**Table 1: Syncope–seizure differentiation.**

| *Clinical feature* | *Syncope* | *Epileptic seizures* |
|---|---|---|
| ***Useful features*** | | |
| Presence of trigger | Very often | Rare |
| Nature of trigger | Emotions for VVS, specific trigger for traditional syncope, standing for OH | Flashing light is best known, also range of rare trigger |
| Prodromes | Autonomic activation in reflex syncope, light-headedness in OH, palpitation in cardiac syncope | • *Epileptic aura*: Repetitive (includes déjà vu)<br>• Epigastric aura and/or an unusual unpleasant smell |
| Myoclonus | • <10 irregular in amplitude, asynchronous, asymmetrical<br>• Starts after the onset of LOC | • 20–100, synchronous, symmetrical, hemilateral<br>• The onset mostly coincides with LOC<br>• Clear long-lasting automatisms as chewing or lip smacking at the mouth |
| Tongue bite | Rare, tip of tongue | Side of tongue (rarely bilateral) |
| Duration of LOC | 10–30 seconds | May be many minutes |
| Confusion after attack | No understanding of situation for <10 seconds in most syncope | Memory deficit, i.e., repeated questions imprinting for many minutes |
| ***Features of limited utility*** | | |
| Incontinence | Not uncommon | Common |
| Myoclonus | Very often | ~60% |
| Eyes open | Frequent | Nearly always |
| Fatigue and sleep afterwards | Common, particularly in children | Very common |

(LOC: loss of consciousness; OH: orthostatic hypotension; VVS: vasovagal syncope)

## REFLEX SYNCOPE

Reflex (neurally mediated) syncope is of the following types:

- Vasovagal (orthostatic and emotional)
- Situational (micturition, swallow, defecation, cough, sneeze)
- Postexercise
- Carotid sinus syndrome (CSS)

Clinical clues to reflex syncope are:

- Long history of recurrent syncope, occurring before the age of 40 years
- After unpleasant sight, sound, smell, or pain
- Prolonged standing
- During the meal
- Being in crowded and/or hot places
- Autonomic activation before syncope: Pallor, sweating, and/or nausea/vomiting
- With head rotation or pressure on the carotid sinus (as in tumors, shaving, tight collars)
- Absence of heart disease

## ORTHOSTATIC HYPOTENSION

Syncope due to OH is of the following types:

- Drug-induced OH (e.g., vasodilators, diuretics, phenothiazine, antidepressants)

- Volume depletion (hemorrhage, diarrhea, vomiting, etc.)
- Primary autonomic failure (pure autonomic failure, multiple system atrophy, Parkinson's disease, dementia with Lewy bodies)
- Secondary autonomic failure (diabetes, amyloidosis, spinal cord injuries, autoimmune autonomic neuropathy, paraneoplastic autonomic neuropathy, kidney failure)

Hypotension may be exacerbated by venous pooling during exercise (exercise-induced), after meals (postprandial hypotension), and after prolonged bed rest (deconditioning).

Clues to syncope due to OH are:

- While or after standing
- Prolonged standing
- Standing after exertion
- Postprandial hypotension
- Temporal relationship with start or changes of dosage of vasodepressive drugs or diuretics leading to hypotension
- Presence of autonomic neuropathy or Parkinsonism

## CARDIAC SYNCOPE

Cardiac syncope types are:

- Bradyarrhythmia (sinus node dysfunction, atrioventricular conduction system disease)
- Tachyarrhythmia
- Structural cardiac diseases [aortic stenosis, ischemic heart disease (IHD), hypertrophic cardiomyopathy, cardiac space-occupying lesions, pericardial disease/tamponade, congenital anomalies of coronary arteries, prosthetic valve dysfunction]
- Cardiopulmonary and great vessel diseases (pulmonary embolus, acute aortic dissection, pulmonary hypertension)

Clinical clues to cardiac syncope are:

- During exertion or when supine
- Presence of structural heart disease or coronary artery disease
- Family history of unexplained sudden death at a young age
- Sudden-onset palpitations immediately followed by syncope
- Electrocardiogram (ECG) findings are suggestive of arrhythmic syncope.

## RISK STRATIFICATION

Risk stratification is given in **Table 2**.

## CARDIOVASCULAR AUTONOMIC TESTING

- Active standing to rule out OH [fall in systolic blood pressures (BP) from baseline value > 20 mm Hg or diastolic BP (DBP) >10 mm Hg or a decrease in SBP to <90 mm Hg]
- Carotid sinus massage (CSM): CSM is indicated in patients > 40 years of age with syncope of unknown origin compatible with a reflex mechanism. Carotid sinus hypersensitivity (CSH) and CSS are close but different entities. With a proper approach (as depicted in **Flowchart 1**), cardioinhibitory (CI) and vasodepressor (VD) variants can be identified.
- Head up tilt table (HUTT) testing
- Ambulatory BP monitoring (ABPM) to rule out OH, nocturnal dipping pattern, and nocturnal hypertension
- Valsalva maneuver and deep breathing may also be considered to look for phasic BP and heart rate changes.

## INVESTIGATION IN SYNCOPE

- ECG
- Holter monitoring is yielding unless the frequency of the event is more than weekly.
- External loop recorder (ELR) is effective if the event frequency is less than monthly.
- Internal loop recorder (ILR) is indicated when the event is less frequent.

**Table 2: Risk stratification.**

| *Low-risk* | *High-risk (red flag)* |
|---|---|
| ***Syncopal event*** | |
| • Associated with prodrome typical of reflex syncope (e.g., light-headedness, feeling of warmth, sweating, nausea, vomiting)<br>• After sudden unexpected unpleasant sight, sound, smell, or pain<br>• After prolonged standing or crowded, hot places<br>• During a meal or postprandial<br>• Triggered by cough, defecation, or micturition<br>• With head rotation or pressure on carotid sinus (e.g., tumor, shaving, tight collars)<br>• Standing from supine/sitting position | *Major*<br>• New onset of chest discomfort, breathlessness, abdominal pain, or headache<br>• Syncope during exertion or when supine<br>• Sudden-onset palpitation immediately followed by syncope<br>*Minor* (high risk only if associated with structural heart disease or abnormal ECG)<br>• No warning symptoms or short (<10 seconds) prodrome<br>• Family history of SCD at a young age<br>• Syncope in the sitting position |
| ***Past medical history*** | |
| • Long history (years) of recurrent syncope with low-risk features with the same characteristics of the current episode<br>• Absence of structural heart disease | Major<br>• Severe structural or coronary artery disease (heart failure, low LVEF, or previous myocardial infarction) |
| ***Physical examination*** | |
| • Normal examination | *Major*<br>• Unexplained SBP in ED < 90 mm Hg<br>• Suggestion of gastrointestinal bleed on rectal examination<br>• Persistent bradycardia (<40 bpm) in awake state and in absence of physical training<br>• Undiagnosed systolic murmur |
| ***ECG*** | |
| • Normal ECG | • ECG changes consistent with acute ischemia<br>• Mobitz II second- and third-degree AV block<br>• Slow AF (<40 bpm)<br>• Persistent sinus bradycardia (<40 bpm)<br>• Bundle branch block or IVCD<br>• Q waves consistent with CAD or cardiomyopathy<br>• Sustained and nonsustained VT<br>• Dysfunction of a pacemaker or ICD<br>• Type 1 Brugada pattern<br>• Long QT |

*Continued*

*Continued*

| ***Low-risk*** | ***High-risk (red flag)*** |
|---|---|
| ***ECG*** | |
| | *Minor* (only if history suggests arrhythmic syncope)<br>• Mobitz I second-degree AV block and one-degree AV block with markedly prolonged PR interval<br>• Asymptomatic inappropriate mild sinus bradycardia (40–50 bpm) or slow AF (40–50 bpm)<br>• Paroxysmal SVT or atrial fibrillation<br>• Preexcited QRS complex<br>• Short QTc interval (≤340 ms)<br>• Atypical Brugada patterns<br>• Negative T waves suggestive of ARVC |

(AF: atrial fibrillation; ARVC: arrhythmogenic right ventricular cardiomyopathy; AV: atrioventricular; BP: systolic blood pressure; CAD: coronary artery disease; ECG: electrocardiogram; ED: emergency department; ICD: implantable cardioverter-defibrillator; IVCD: intraventricular conduction delay; LVEF: left ventricular ejection fraction; SCD: sudden cardiac death; SVT: supraventricular tachycardia; VT: ventricular tachycardia)

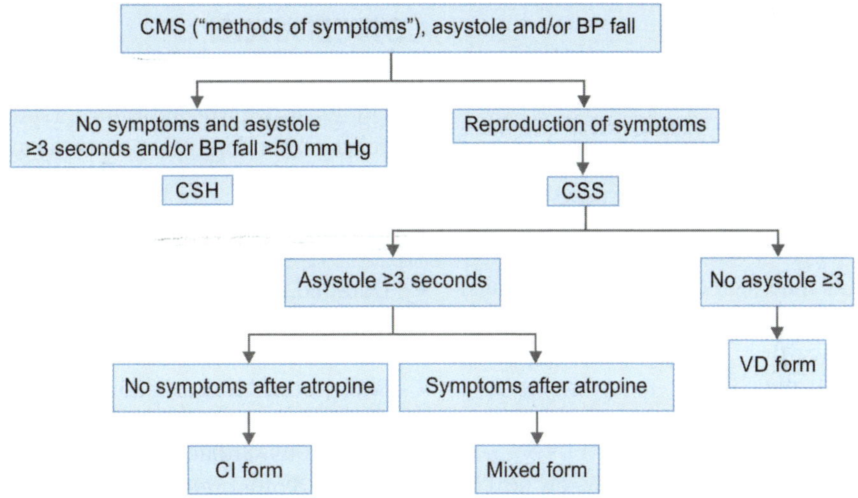


**FLOWCHART 1:** Carotid sinus massage (CSM).

(BP: blood pressure; CI: cardioinhibitory; CSH: carotid sinus hypersensitivity; CSS: carotid sinus syndrome; VD: vasodepressor)

- Exercise ECG is indicated only when the syncope is exertional to rule out exercise-induced arrhythmia.
- Echo Doppler study to rule out arrhythmogenic structural heart disease
- Coronary angiography is recommended for IHD.
- Electrophysiology study is recommended in unexplained syncope cases.

# BASIC MANAGEMENT PROTOCOL

Recommendations in reflex syncope and OH are:

- Reassurance and explanation of the risk of recurrence
- Avoidance of triggers and situations
- Adequate hydration and salt intake

- Modification or discontinuation of the hypotensive drug regimen should be considered.
- Abdominal binders and/or support stockings to reduce venous pooling should be considered.
- Midodrine and fludrocortisone may be considered if symptoms persist.
- Counter pressure maneuvers

In cardiac syncope, pacemaker or implantable cardioverter-defibrillator (ICD) is recommended depending on the cause.

## PSYCHOGENIC PSEUDOSYNCOPE

- Relatives or colleagues should know what a typical attack looks like (usually patients look as if they are asleep but cannot be woken).
- Relatives or colleagues should know beforehand what to do during a typical attack. The attacks are not a medical emergency, so it is not necessary to call an ambulance.
- The attacks will pass by themselves, but some patience is required.
- Patients may be moved during an attack, if necessary.
- While waiting for the attack to end, patients may be put in a comfortable position, such as lying on their side with a pillow under the head.
- People close to the patient may stay next to the patient and comfort them when they recover, as they are then often emotionally distressed.
- Humility and empathy are needed with these patients.

## DRIVING AND SYNCOPE

- Untreated arrhythmia patients are not allowed to drive.
- After successful treatment, reflex syncope and OH patients are allowed to drive.
- After pacemaker implantation, patients can drive.
- Professional drivers with implanted ICDs should not drive any longer.
- Patients who are at high risk for sudden cardiac death are not allowed to drive.

## CONCLUSION

The importance of the evaluation of syncope is to identify cardiac syncope. Hence, a systematic approach is mandatory for proper diagnosis.

## CLINICAL PEARLS

- Detailed history and observer's description are essential for the evaluation of transient loss of consciousness.
- Background clinical history and abnormal physical examination findings are clues to the serious cardiac cause of syncope.
- ECG and other relevant investigations are necessary to establish the proper diagnosis.

## FURTHER READINGS

1. Libby P, Bonow RO, Mann DL, Tomaselli GF, Braunwald E, Bhatt DL, et al. Braunwald's heart disease: A textbook of cardiovascular medicine. 12th ed. Philadelphia, PA: Elsevier; 2022.
2. Fuster V, Narula J, Vaishnava P, Leon MB, Callans DJ, Rumsfeld JS, et al. Fuster and Hurst's the heart: 15th edition. New York: Mc Graw Hill; 2022.
3. Loscalzo J, Fauci AS, Kasper DL, Hauser SL, Longo DL, Jameson JL. Harrison's principles of internal medicine. 21st ed. New York: McGraw Hill; 2022.
4. 2018 ESC guidelines for diagnosis and mana gement of syncope [Internet]. [cited 2024 Jan 4]. Available from: https://www.acc.org/latest-in-cardiology/ten-points-to-remember/2018/04/04/14/28/2018-esc-guidelines-for-syncope.

CHAPTER 5

# Intermittent Claudication

*Mainak Mukhopadhyay*

## INTRODUCTION

Presentations of peripheral arterial diseases (PADs) depend upon the involved territories, namely:

- Cerebrovascular diseases
- Upper extremity artery disease (UEAD)
- Mesenteric artery disease
- Renal artery disease (RAD)
- Lower extremity artery disease (LEAD)
- Manifestations of LEAD are:
    - Typical intermittent claudication
    - Chronic limb-threatening ischemia (CLTI)
    - Acute limb ischemia (ALI)

## PATHOPHYSIOLOGY OF LOWER EXTREMITY ARTERY DISEASE

The Latin verb *claudicare* means *to limp*. In 1858, Jean-Martin Charcot described pain in the lower extremities resulting from arterial insufficiency. Claudication means cramping pain in the leg induced by exercise, typically caused by progressive atherosclerosis obstructing the arteries (LEAD). Risk factors of LEAD are:

- Family history of cardiovascular disease (CVD)
- Hypertension
- Diabetes
- Dyslipidemia
- Chronic kidney disease (CKD)
- Obesity
- Elderly age group
- History of cancer radiation therapy
- Smoking (present and/or past), including passive smoking exposure
- Prior CVD

## MEDICAL HISTORY IN LOWER EXTREMITY ARTERY DISEASE

- Assess the risk factors of LEAD.
- *Symptoms related to LEAD*:
    - *Walking impairment/claudication*:
        - Type: Fatigue, aching, cramping, discomfort, burning
        - Location: Buttock and thigh (aortoiliac disease), calf and/or foot (femoral artery and distal branches). An elderly patient attending the clinic with a complaint of exertional pain in the leg and foot can be casually stamped as degenerative arthritis unless thoroughly approached to rule out LEAD.

        - Timing: Triggered by exercise, uphill rather than downhill, quickly relieved with rest; chronicity
        - Claudication onset distance
    - Extreme pain (including foot) at rest and evolution at upright or recumbent position (important point to differentiate from neurogenic claudication)
    - Poorly healing wounds of the extremities
- *Symptoms to rule out other vascular territory involvement*:
    - Arm exertion pain, particularly if associated with dizziness or vertigo
    - Angina, dyspnea
    - Postprandial abdominal pain and weight loss
    - Erectile dysfunction

## CLINICAL EVALUATION IN LOWER EXTREMITY ARTERY DISEASE

Abdominal palpation; palpation of femoral, popliteal, dorsalis pedis, and posterior tibial artery pulses; and temperature gradient assessment are to be done. Careful inspection of lower limbs, including feet (i.e., color difference, presence of any cutaneous lesion, calf hair loss, and muscle atrophy), is important. Peripheral neuropathy assessment in case of diabetes or LEAD must be ruled out. Auscultation at different levels including the flanks, periumbilical region, and groin is mandatory. Blood pressure measurement of all four limbs is essential.

## FUNCTIONAL CLASS ASSESSMENT IN LOWER EXTREMITY ARTERY DISEASE

Fontaine or Rutherford classification is used for the functional classification of LEAD **(Table 1)**.

## WORKUP IN LOWER EXTREMITY ARTERY DISEASE: RISK FACTOR ASSESSMENT

- *Body mass index (BMI)*: For obesity
- Fasting blood sugar (FBS), glycated hemoglobin (HbA1c): To rule out diabetes mellitus
- *Lipid profile*: To look for dyslipidemia
- *Urea, creatinine, and urine evaluation*: To exclude CKD

**Table 1: Functional classification of lower extremity artery disease.**

| ***Fontaine classification*** | | | | ***Rutherford classification*** | | |
|---|---|---|---|---|---|---|
| ***Stage*** | | ***Symptoms*** | | ***Grade*** | ***Category*** | ***Symptoms*** |
| I | | Asymptomatic | ⇔ | 0 | 0 | Asymptomatic |
| II | IIa | Nondisabling intermittent claudication | ⇔ | I | 1 | Mild claudication |
| | | | | I | 2 | Moderate claudication |
| | IIb | Disabling intermittent claudication | | I | 3 | Severe claudication |
| III | | Ischemic rest pain | ⇔ | II | 4 | Ischemic rest pain |
| IV | | Ulceration or gangrene | ⇔ | III | 5 | Minor tissue loss |
| | | | | III | 6 | Major tissue loss |

## ESTABLISHING THE DIAGNOSIS OF LOWER EXTREMITY ARTERY DISEASE

Lower extremity artery disease is diagnosed using the following modalities:

- Doppler ultrasound is the first investigation of choice (should also be used to rule out abdominal aortic aneurysms in patients of LEAD).
- Computed tomography (CT) angiography **(Fig. 1)**
- Magnetic resonance (MR) angiography

## ANKLE-BRACHIAL INDEX

Measurement of the ankle-brachial index (ABI) is indicated as a first-line noninvasive test for screening and diagnosis of LEAD.

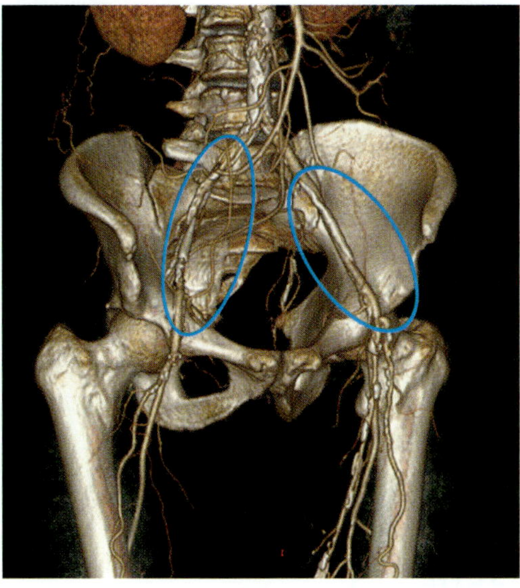

**FIG. 1:** Three-dimensional (3D) reconstructed computed tomography (CT) angiography of bilateral lower limbs showing lower extremity artery disease (LEAD) with vascular calcification starting from the aortoiliac segment downward in an elderly male smoker presenting with intermittent claudication with a prior history of coronary angioplasty.

In the case of incompressible ankle arteries or ABI > 1.40, alternative methods such as the toe-brachial index, Doppler waveform analysis, or pulse volume recording are indicated.

- Who should have an ABI measurement in clinical practice?
  - Patients with clinical suspicion for LEAD:
    - Lower extremities pulse abolition and/or arterial bruit
    - Typical intermittent claudication or symptoms suggestive for LEAD
    - Nonhealing lower extremity wound
  - Patients at risk for LEAD because of the following clinical conditions:
    - Atherosclerotic diseases: Coronary artery disease (CAD), any PADs
    - Other conditions: DM, CKD, heart failure
  - Asymptomatic individuals clinically free but at risk for LEAD:
    - Men and women aged >65 years
    - Men and women aged <65 years classified at high cardiovascular (CV) risk according to the European Society of Cardiology (ESC) guidelines
    - Men and women aged >50 years with family history for LEAD
- How to measure the ABI?

  The patient is placed in a supine position and cuff placed just above the ankle; wounded zones should be avoided. After a 5–10-minute rest, the systolic blood pressure (SBP) is measured by a Doppler probe (5–10 MHz) on the posterior and the anterior tibial (or dorsal pedis) arteries of each foot and on the brachial artery of each arm. Automated blood pressure (BP) cuffs are mostly not valid for ankle pressure and may overestimate results in case of low ankle pressure. The ABI of each leg is calculated by dividing the highest ankle SBP by the highest arm SBP **(Figs. 2A and B)**.

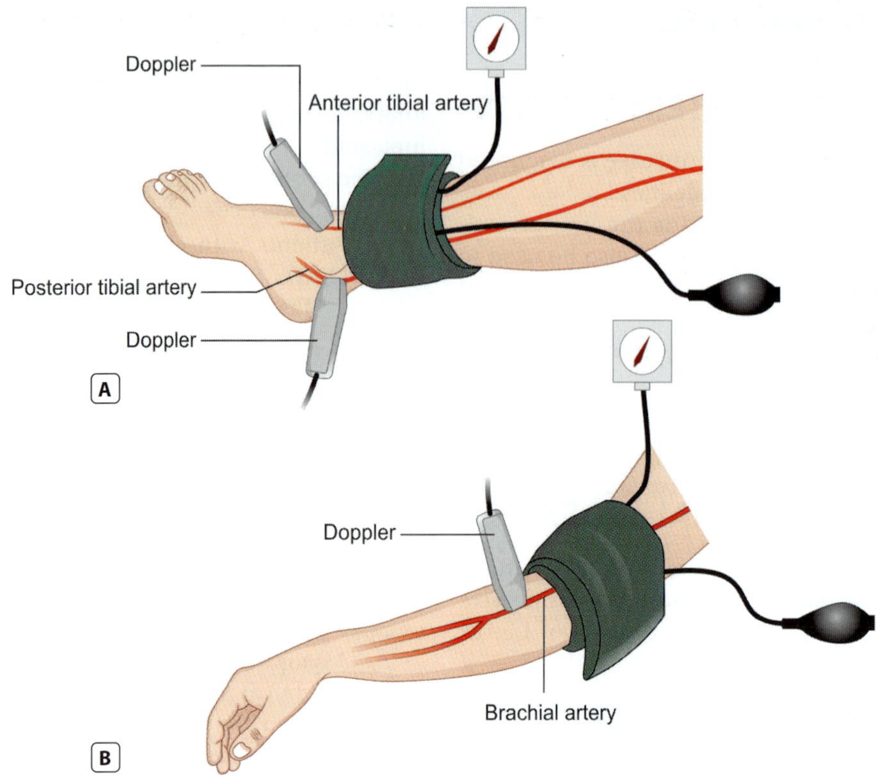


**FIGS. 2A AND B:** Method of measuring systolic blood pressure for ankle-brachial index (ABI) assessment.

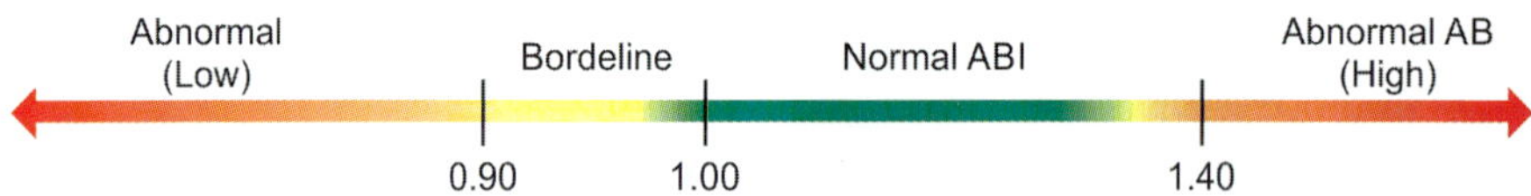


**FIG. 3:** Interpretation of ankle-brachial index (ABI) result.

- How to interpret the ABI?
  - For the diagnosis of LEAD, interpret each leg separately (one ABI per leg).
  - For the CV risk stratification, take the lowest ABI between the two legs.
  - Interpretation (see **Fig. 3**)

## ASSESSMENT OF CHRONIC LIMB THREATENING ISCHEMIA

Progressive untreated LEAD will culminate into chronic limb threatening ischemia

(CLTI). Early recognition of tissue loss and/or infection and referral to the vascular team are mandatory to improve limb salvage. For limb salvage, revascularization is indicated whenever feasible. In patients with CLTI, assessment of the risk of amputation is indicated by the WIFI (wound, ischemia, and foot infection) scoring system **(Tables 2 and 3)**.

## ASSESSMENT OF ASSOCIATED CARDIOVASCULAR MORBIDITY IN LOWER EXTREMITY ARTERY DISEASE

Lower extremity artery disease is often associated with CAD, heart failure, degenerative aortic valve diseases, and atrial fibrillation predominantly due to common

**Table 2: WIFI (wound, ischemia, and foot infection) scoring system.**

| ***Component*** | ***Score*** | ***Description*** | | |
|---|---|---|---|---|
| *W* (wound) | 0 | No ulcer (ischemic rest pain) | | |
| | 1 | Small, shallow ulcer on distal leg or foot without gangrene | | |
| | 2 | Deeper ulcer (exposed bone), joint or tendon ± gangrenous changes limited to toes | | |
| | 3 | Extensive deep ulcer, full thickness heel ulcer ± calcaneal involvement ± extensive gangrene | | |
| *I* (ischemia) | | *ABI* | *Ankle pressure (mm Hg)* | *Toe pressure or $TcPO_2$* |
| | 0 | ≥0.80 | >100 | ≥0.60 |
| | 1 | 0.60–0.79 | 70–100 | 40–59 |
| | 2 | 0.40–0.59 | 50–70 | 30–39 |
| | 3 | <0.40 | <50 | <30 |
| FI (foot infection) | 0 | No symptoms/signs of infection | | |
| | 1 | Local infection involving only skin and subcutaneous tissue | | |
| | 2 | Local infection involving deeper than skin/subcutaneous tissue | | |
| | 3 | Systemic inflammatory response syndrome | | |

(ABI: ankle-brachial index; $TcPO_2$: transcutaneous oxygen pressure)

**Table 3: Estimate risk of amputation at 1 year for each combination.**

| | ***Ischemia–0*** | | | | ***Ischemia–1*** | | | | ***Ischemia–2*** | | | | ***Ischemia–3*** | | | |
|---|---|---|---|---|---|---|---|---|---|---|---|---|---|---|---|---|
| W-0 | VL | VL | L | M | VL | L | M | H | L | L | M | M | L | M | M | H |
| W-1 | VL | VL | L | M | VL | L | M | H | L | M | H | H | M | M | H | H |
| W-2 | L | L | M | H | M | M | H | H | M | H | H | H | H | H | H | H |
| W-3 | M | M | H | H | H | H | H | H | H | H | H | H | H | H | H | H |
| | fl-0 | f1-1 | fl-2 | fl-3 | fl-0 | f1-1 | f1-2 | fl-3 | f1-0 | f1-1 | fl-2 | fl-3 | f1-0 | f1-1 | fl-2 | fl-3 |

(fl: foot infection; H: high risk; L: low risk; M: moderate risk; VL: very low risk; W: wound)

etiology. Hence, it is logical to screen for these comorbidities with relevant investigations.

## CONCLUSION

A thorough systematic clinical approach will help us diagnose the LEAD and triage patients for early vascular team referral for timely revascularization.

## CLINICAL PEARLS

- Functional classification is essential in PAD.
- Measurement of ABI is the cornerstone in bedside evaluation.
- Risk of amputation is assessed by WIFI scoring system.

## FURTHER READINGS

1. Libby P, Bonow RO, Mann DL, Tomaselli GF, Bhatt DL, Solomon SD, et al. Braunwald's heart disease a textbook of Cardiovascular Medicine. Philadelphia, PA: Elsevier; 2022.
2. Fuster V, Narula,Jagat, Vaishnava P, Leon MB, Callans DJ, Rumsfeld JS, et al. Fuster and Hurst's the heart: 15th edition. New York: Mc Graw Hill; 2022.
3. Loscalzo J, Kasper DL, Longo DL, Fauci AS, Hauser SL, Jameson JL, et al. Harrison's principles of Internal Medicine, twenty-First edition vol 1 & 2, New York: McGraw Hill; 2022.
4. Aboyans V, Ricco JB, Bartelink MEL, Björck M, Brodmann M, Cohnert T, et al. 2017 ESC Guidelines on the Diagnosis and Treatment of Peripheral Arterial Diseases. Eur Heart J. 2018;39(9):763–816.

CHAPTER 6

# Heart Sounds

*Mainak Mukhopadhyay*

## INTRODUCTION

Heart sound evaluation is a very important component of the clinical cardiac examination. It is generated because of the vibrations created by the various cardiac structures and turbulent flows in the heart.

Auscultation should be started from the apical area, then "inching" toward the left lower sternum, then along the left sternal border upward, then to the right upper sternal border and downward to complete the process. The base of the heart is auscultated in sitting posture, and various maneuvers are followed, including various postures and respiratory phases for dynamic auscultation. All right-sided cardiac events are increased in inspiration except for the pulmonary ejection click, which decreases on inspiration.

High-pitch sounds such as opening snap (OS) are evaluated using the diaphragm of the stethoscope, whereas the bell is used to pick up low-pitch sounds such as the third heart sound ($S_3$). Bell if compressed tightly on the chest wall acts as a diaphragm.

*Cardiac sounds of our concern are:*

- First heart sound ($S_1$)
- Second heart sound ($S_2$)
- Third heart sound ($S_3$)
- Fourth heart sound ($S_4$)
- Click
- OS
- Pericardial knock
- Tumor plop
- Prosthetic valve sounds
- Pericardial friction rub

## FIRST HEART SOUND

- *It has got two components*: Mitral closure ($M_1$) and tricuspid closure ($T_1$); the $M_1$–$T_1$ interval is 20–30 ms.
- $M_1$ is best heard in the apical area.
- $T_1$ is mainly appreciable in the fourth and fifth left intercostal space - parasternal area.
- $S_1$ is generated during isovolumetric contraction and precedes the carotid upstroke.
- The interval between $S_1$ and $S_2$ is systole, whereas the interval between $S_2$ and $S_1$ is diastole.
- *Accentuated $S_1$*: The intensity of $S_1$ is more than the intensity of $S_2$ in the second left intercostal space—parasternal area. Causes include rheumatic mitral stenosis (MS) (early stage), hyperdynamic state, PR interval <120 ms, and increased flow through the mitral valve (ventricular septal defect, patent ductus arteriosus).
- *Causes of attenuated $S_1$*: Calcified MS (grossly restricted and calcified valve in

advanced stage); systolic dysfunction; PR interval >200 ms; acute aortic regurgitation (AR)

- *Variable intensity of $S_1$*: Atrial fibrillation; atrioventricular dissociation; tamponade. Spilt $S_1$ (split sound in the fifth left intercostal space): Right bundle branch block; atrial septal defect (delayed $T_1$): Tricuspid stenosis (delayed $T_1$); Ebstein's anomaly

## SECOND HEART SOUND

- $S_2$ is "the key to the auscultation of heart"!
- $S_2$ occurs due to the closure of the semilunar valves at the end of the systole during isovolumetric relaxation time.
- *$S_2$ is composed of two components*: Aortic ($A_2$) and pulmonary ($P_2$).
- It is best heard at the base of the heart.
- *Normal physiological splitting* **(Fig. 1)** (normal $A_2$-$P_2$ gap) occurs during inspiration. It is conspicuous in the second left intercostal space; the normal interval is 20–60 ms.
- Respiratory variation in splitting is because of the time variation of $P_2$.
- *Narrow inspiratory splitting* is found in pulmonary hypertension (associated with accentuated $P_2$).
- Causes of *widened splitting* are right bundle branch block (RBBB) due to delayed $P_2$, severe mitral regurgitation (early $A_2$), ventricular septal defect (early $A_2$), and right ventricular outflow tract (RVOT) obstruction (late $P_2$).
- *Fixed splitting* ($A_2$-$P_2$ variation <20 ms) is found in atrial septal defect (fixed and wide split) and right heart failure.
- In the *paradoxical splitting* **(Fig. 2)**, $A_2$-$P_2$ widens during expiration but shortens during inspiration. It may happen in the left bundle branch block (LBBB), right ventricular paced rhythm, aortic stenosis (prolonged ejection), hypertrophic cardiomyopathy, and left ventricular systolic dysfunction.
- *Accentuated aortic component of $S_2$ ($A_2$) causes*: Hypertension, coarctation of aorta, ascending aortic aneurysm
- *Attenuated aortic component of $S_2$ ($A_2$) causes*: Valvular aortic stenosis, aortic regurgitation
- *Accentuated pulmonary component of $S_2$ ($P_2$) causes*: Pulmonary hypertension
- *Loud $P_2$* means it is louder than $A_2$ in the left second intercostal space or $P_2$ is audible in the same intensity in the lower left parasternal region or at the apical area or palpable $P_2$.
- *Attenuated pulmonary component of $S_2$ ($P_2$) causes*: Valvular pulmonary stenosis, pulmonary regurgitation unless secondary to pulmonary hypertension

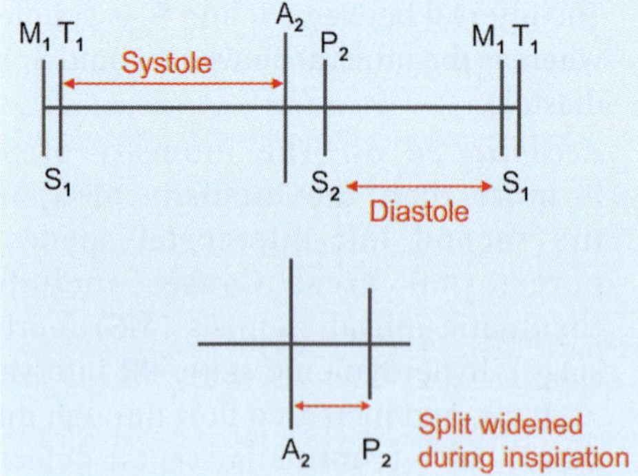


**FIG. 1:** Normal physiological $S_2$ split.

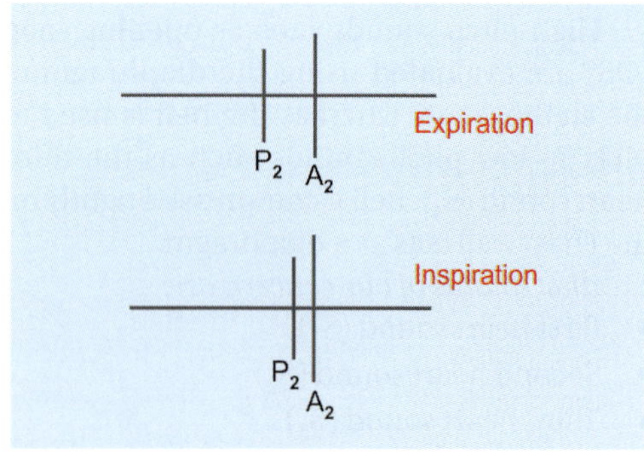


**FIG. 2:** Paradoxical $S_2$ split.

- *Causes of single $S_2$*: Reduced $A_2$, reduced $P_2$, Fallot's tetralogy

## THIRD HEART SOUND

- Left ventricular $S_3$ ($LVS_3$) is best heard in the left lateral supine position with a stethoscope bell at the apex.
- It comes 140–160 ms after $S_2$.
- $LVS_3$ appears during rapid ventricular filling (at the end of the y descent).
- It is associated with left ventricular volume overload—dilated cardiomyopathy, LV failure, mitral regurgitation, aortic regurgitation, ventricular septal defect, patent ductus arteriosus: young subjects in good health, normal pregnancy
- Right ventricular $S_3$ ($RVS_3$) is best heard in the lower left parasternal.
- $RVS_3$ increases on inspiration.
- *It is found in tricuspid regurgitation*: Right heart failure.

## FOURTH HEART SOUND

- Left ventricular $S_4$ ($LVS_4$) is best heard in the left lateral supine position using a stethoscope bell at the apex.
- It occurs during atrial systole (after the P wave).
- It is associated with noncompliant ventricle and increased filling pressure and is heard in left ventricular hypertrophy due to any cause (e.g., hypertension, aortic stenosis, hypertrophic cardiomyopathy), ischemia, acute aortic regurgitation, acute mitral regurgitation, and elderly age.
- Causes of right-sided $S_4$ are right ventricular hypertrophy and pulmonary hypertension.
- Right ventricular $S_4$ ($RVS_4$) is best heard in the lower left parasternal region in inspiration.
- Summation gallop is the fusion of $S_3$ and $S_4$ during tachycardia.

## CLICK

- *Valvular ejection click* coincides with a carotid upstroke (120–140 ms after QRS).
- It is a high-pitched sound with diffuse radiation.
- It is heard in bicuspid aortic valve or valvular pulmonary stenosis (PS).
- Click is lost when the valve is no longer pliable.
- Pulmonary valvular click intensity gets reduced during inspiration.
- With progressive severity, the click of PS merges with the $S_1$.
- *Vascular ejection* click is heard mostly because of vessel dilatation.
- Common examples are aortic root dilatation and pulmonary artery dilatation.
- Mid-systolic click of mitral valve prolapse is known as a *nonejection click*.
- It is a high-pitched sound and comes after the carotid pulsation.
- It comes earlier if the patient stands up or with strain phase of Valsalva (preload reducing maneuvers).
- There may be an associated mitral regurgitation murmur.

## OPENING SNAP

- In MS, mitral OS is a high-pitched diastolic sound that comes 40–120 ms after $S_2$.
- It is best heard with diaphragm of stethoscope just medial to the apical area
- $A_2$-OS interval is inversely proportional to the severity of MS
- Intensity of OS decreases when the valve is calcified and immobile.

## PERICARDIAL KNOCK

- It is found in constrictive pericarditis.
- An early diastolic sound (at the end of the y descent in JVP) comes 100–120 ms after $S_2$.
- It happens because of the sudden halting of the diastolic filling.

## TUMOR PLOP

- It is heard due to the prolapse of the tumor through the atrioventricular valve.
- It is posture dependent. One must never try to elicit it, as it may cause sudden cardiac death.

## PROSTHETIC VALVE SOUNDS

- Prosthetic valves can be metallic or bioprosthetic. Modern-day bioprosthetic valve sounds are often indistinguishable from normal native heart sounds.
- Valves used in transcatheter aortic valve replacement (TAVR)/transcatheter aortic valve implantation (TAVI) are bioprosthetic valves.
- Metallic heart valves produce an opening click and metallic closure sound.
- There may be thrombotic occlusion of the prosthetic valve or degeneration or endocarditis or pannus growth or patient prosthetic mismatch.
- Suspect pathological prosthetic valve if there is any significant diastolic murmur in the prosthetic semilunar valve, any grade 4 or above ejection systolic murmur in the prosthetic semilunar valve, any systolic murmur in the prosthetic atrioventricular valve, absence of the metallic opening clicks, or absence of metallic closure sound.

## PERICARDIAL FRICTION RUB

- It may have up to three components in the following phases of the cardiac cycle—(i) rapid ventricular filling, (ii) atrial contraction, and (iii) ventricular systole.
- It is heard best with the diaphragm in the left parasternal region with forced expiration while leaning forward.
- With pericardial effusion, the rub goes away.

## CONCLUSION

Readily available advanced technologies are challenging bedside clinical examinations nowadays. In the western world, the practical significance of using a stethoscope is under the microscope. Bedside clinical examination is an art that helps us not only to diagnose and triage our patients but also to justify further relevant investigations, and it also strengthens the bond between physician and patient. It requires great practice to acquire that level of clinical skill. Hence, the clinical evaluation of cardiac sounds is a time-tested acumen that will always remain relevant in the future world too.

## CLINICAL PEARLS

- The intensity of $S_1 > S_2$ in the second left intercostal space is an accentuated $S_1$.
- In the paradoxical splitting $A_2$–$P_2$ widens during expiration but shortens during inspiration.
- $S_3$ is associated with ventricular volume overload.
- $S_4$ is related to ventricular noncompliance.

## FURTHER READINGS

1. Libby P, Bonow RO, Mann DL, Tomaselli GF, Bhatt DL, Solomon SD, et al. Braunwald's heart disease a textbook of Cardiovascular Medicine. Philadelphia, PA: Elsevier; 2022.
2. Fuster V, Narula,Jagat, Vaishnava P, Leon MB, Callans DJ, Rumsfeld JS, et al. Fuster and Hurst's the heart: 15th edition. New York: Mc Graw Hill; 2022.
3. Loscalzo J, Kasper DL, Longo DL, Fauci AS, Hauser SL, Jameson JL, et al. Harrison's principles of Internal Medicine, twenty-First edition vol 1 & 2, New York: McGraw Hill; 2022.

CHAPTER 7

# Cardiac Murmur

*Mainak Mukhopadhyay*

## INTRODUCTION

Bedside proper identification of the cardiac murmur has fascinated clinicians since long past the lane of history of medicine. It requires astute clinical skills that can only be acquired through grueling practice. But with the advent of advanced cardiac imaging modalities, these bedside provisional clinical soft data must be confirmed with an echo Doppler study with proper correlation with the patient's symptoms and other clinical parameters.

## BEDSIDE CLINIC AND PATHOPHYSIOLOGY OF CARDIAC MURMUR

Auscultation should be started from the apical area, then "inching" toward the left lower sternum, then along the left sternal border upward, then to the right upper sternal border, and downward to complete the process. The base of the heart is auscultated in sitting posture, and various maneuvers are followed including various postures and respiratory phases for dynamic auscultation. All right-sided cardiac events are increased in inspiration except pulmonary ejection click, which decreases on inspiration.

High-pitch murmurs [outflow stenotic murmur, e.g., aortic stenosis (AS)] are evaluated using the diaphragm of the stethoscope, whereas the bell is used to pick up low-pitch murmurs [murmur of mitral stenosis (MS)]. The bell if compressed tightly on the chest wall acts as a diaphragm.

Description of a cardiac murmur is done under the following headings:

- *Timing*—reflects the relationship of the pathophysiological hemodynamic with the cardiac cycle
- *Location where best heard*—reflects the location of the pathology
- *Intensity or grade* **(Box 1)**—depends upon the pressure gradient

**BOX 1: Grading of murmur.**

- Grade 1/6: Very faint, barely perceptible
- Grade 2/6: Faint but readily perceptible
- Grade 3/6: Moderate-intensity murmur, no thrill
- Grade 4/6: Associated with thrill
- Grade 5/6: Very loud—can be auscultated even when only a part of the stethoscope touches the chest wall
- Grade 6/6: Very loud—can be auscultated even when the stethoscope is not in contact with the chest wall

- *Character*—complex interplay in between the rate of change of pressure gradient and flow pathway anatomy
- *Dynamic auscultation*—various maneuvers interfering with the murmur character
- *Radiation*—reflects the predominant flow direction

Normal blood flow is silent. Turbulent flow causes auscultatory vibrations, i.e., murmur, and sometimes palpable vibrations, i.e., thrill. A peripheral arterial equivalent feature of murmur is arterial bruit; for venous, it is hum. The eight mechanisms by which flow turbulence comes into play are as follows:

1. Blood flow through a stenotic valve (inadequate opening)
2. Blood flow through a regurgitant valve (improper closing)
3. Increased blood flow through a normal valve (functional stenosis) or vessel
4. Intracardiac shunt
5. Extracardiac shunt or arteriovenous fistula
6. Narrowing of the artery
7. Abnormal structure in the flow pathway (e.g., chordal tear)
8. Forward flow through a normal valve into a distal dilated vessel

## INNOCENT MURMUR

Sometimes, murmur is found even in a healthy individual without any cardiovascular disease with normal blood pressure (BP), chest X-ray, and electrocardiogram (ECG). These are innocent murmurs. They are flow ejection systolic murmur (ESM) or may be continuous too. The murmur intensity is mostly 2/6 or maybe rarely 3/6. A few such examples are:

- Pulmonary flow murmur in adolescence
- Venous hum in the cervical area that disappears on lying down or rotation of head or compression of the ipsilateral lower neck
- Innocent murmur of the neonate
- Mammary souffle of pregnancy due to engorged breasts

**BOX 2: Classification of cardiac murmur.**

- *Systolic murmur*:
  - Holosystolic murmur
  - Ejection systolic murmur
  - Early systolic murmur
  - Late systolic murmur
- *Diastolic murmur*:
  - Early diastolic murmur
  - Mid-diastolic murmur
  - Late diastolic murmur
- Continuous murmur

## CLASSIFICATION OF CARDIAC MURMUR

The classification of cardiac murmur is given in **Box 2**.

## EJECTION SYSTOLIC MURMUR

*Terminology*: ESM is also known as mid-systolic murmur (MSM).

*Causes*: AS, pulmonary stenosis (PS), hypertrophic obstructive cardiomyopathy (HOCM), high output flow status

*Pathogenesis*: ESM represents outflow tract or semilunar valve obstruction (organic or functional).

*Characteristics*: In ESM, there is a *characteristic gap between the first heart sound ($S_1$) and the onset of the murmur*. The murmur ends at the second heart sound, i.e., $S_2$. The intensity of the murmur gradually increases and then decreases (*diamond-shaped or crescendo-decrescendo murmur*). They are high-pitch murmurs; hence, they are auscultated with the diaphragm of the stethoscope **(Fig. 1)**.

*Aortic stenosis*: Harsh ESM of AS is best heard in the right upper parasternal area in sitting posture with the diaphragm of the stethoscope. The murmur radiates toward the carotids. With severity, the duration of

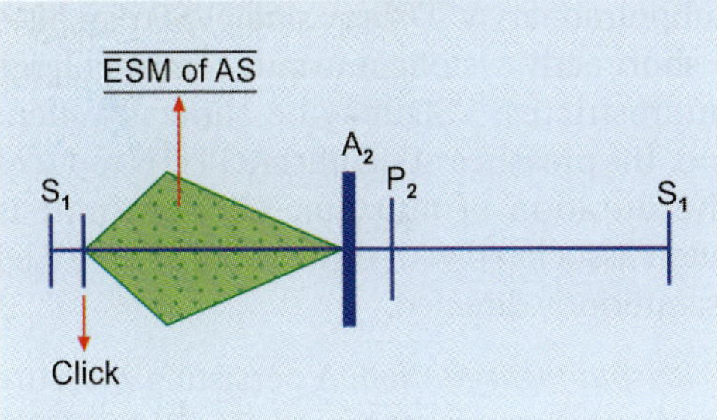


**FIG. 1:** Ejection systolic murmur (ESM) of aortic stenosis (AS).

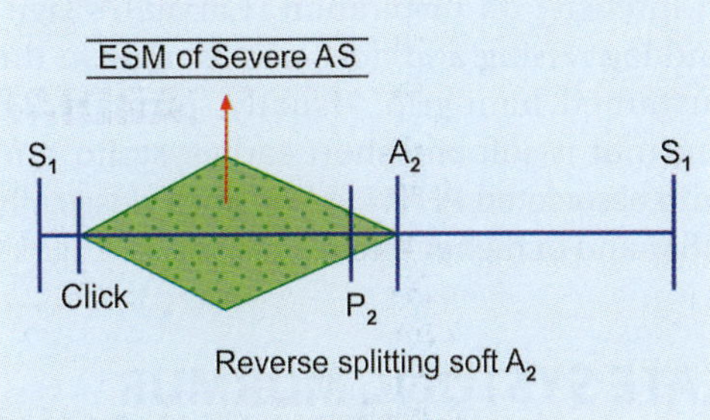


**FIG. 2:** Ejection systolic murmur (ESM) of severe aortic stenosis (AS).

murmur increases with delayed peaking and is often associated with thrill. Severe AS is associated with a delayed aortic component of second heart sound ($A_2$) and paradoxical splitting **(Fig. 2)**. AS can be valvular, subvalvular, or supravalvular. Valvular AS is having valvular click, supravalvular AS is often characterized by differential limb BP, and subvalvular AS is often associated with aortic regurgitation (AR). Often, degenerative AS murmur is quite conspicuous in the apical area; it is called the Gallavardin effect and may mimic mitral regurgitation (MR) murmur.

*Pulmonary stenosis*: ESM of PS is best heard in a left upper parasternal area with radiation toward the back. Valvular PS murmur is often associated with valvular click. Although the PS murmur increases with inspiration, the click decreases with inspiration. With progressive severity, the click tends toward the first heart sound and finally merges with $S_1$ **(Fig. 3)**. In such a situation, the intensity of $S_1$ will vary with respiration.

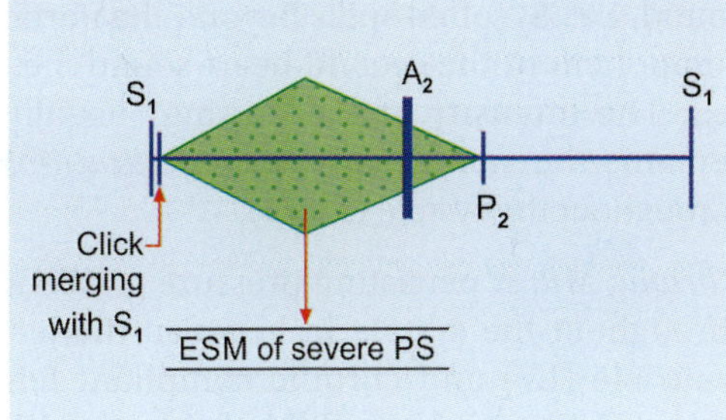


**FIG. 3:** Ejection systolic murmur (ESM) of severe pulmonary stenosis (PS).

*Hypertrophic obstructive cardiomyopathy*: ESM of HOCM is best heard in the mid precordium, and the murmur increases on standing from squatting and in the Valsalva strain phase. HOCM is often associated with MR.

*High output flow status*: Sometimes, even with a normal valve, owing to high flow status [e.g., anemia, thyrotoxicosis, fever, ventricular septal defect (VSD), patent ductus arteriosus (PDA), and atrial septal defect], outflow tract ESM may be audible. But hardly the intensity ever crosses beyond grade 3, and they are never associated with any ejection click.

## HOLOSYSTOLIC MURMUR

*Terminology*: Holosystolic murmur (HSM) is also known as pansystolic murmur (PSM) or regurgitant systolic murmur (RSM).

*Causes*: Chronic MR, VSD, tricuspid regurgitation (TR)

*Pathogenesis*: A significant pressure gradient persisting throughout the systole in between the two participating chambers is the main pathology of HSM. HSMs are high-pitch murmurs; hence, they are auscultated with the diaphragm of the stethoscope. HSM represents atrioventricular valve regurgitation or interventricular restrictive shunt.

*Characteristics*: In HSM, there is no gap between the $S_1$ and the onset of the murmur. The murmur ends at the second heart sound, i.e., $S_2$ (often spills beyond the aortic component of the second heart sound, i.e., $A_2$). The intensity of the murmur usually remains the same (*plateau configuration*) throughout the systole **(Fig. 4)**.

*Chronic MR*: A persisting pressure gradient throughout the systole in between the left ventricle (LV) and chronic compliant left atrium (LA) causes the HSM of chronic MR. The murmur is best heard in the apical area, "blowing" in nature, and increases in intensity on sustained handgrip (afterload increasing maneuver). It radiates toward the left axilla when the pathology involves the anterior mitral leaflets, whereas the HSM radiates to the base of the heart when it is due to the posterior leaflet prolapse or flail. In that case, it may be confused with the long ESM of severe AS and is often impossible to differentiate clinically. In the subsequent normal beat of ventricular premature contraction (VPC), the murmur of AS increases in intensity, whereas the murmur of MR remains the same. Acute severe MR presents with a short early systolic murmur in the apical area.

*Ventricular septal defect*: A persisting pressure gradient throughout the systole in between the LV and right ventricle (RV) causes the HSM in restrictive VSD without significant pulmonary hypertension (PHTN). The murmur is harsh in nature and is best heard in the mid-left parasternal area (murmur of VSD can be heard all over the precordium) and may be best heard in the base if it is subpulmonary VSD. Very small VSD can have a short early systolic murmur, whereas large nonrestrictive VSD may be clinically silent too. The presence of significant PHTN reduces the duration of murmur. VSD murmur is often associated with thrill as the LV to RV jet is anteriorly directed.

*Tricuspid regurgitation*: A persisting pressure gradient throughout the systole in between LV and RV causes the HSM of TR with PHTN (secondary TR). The murmur is best heard in the left lower parasternal area and increases in intensity on inspiration (Carvallo's sign) and leg raising and does not change on the sustained handgrip. Usually, primary TR murmur is soft and short early systolic, and with associated PHTN, it becomes classically HSM and of higher pitch.

## LATE SYSTOLIC MURMUR

*Terminology*: Late systolic murmur (LSM) is also known as end systolic murmur.

*Causes*: Mitral valve prolapse (MVP), ischemic/functional MR, tricuspid valve prolapse (TVP)

*Characteristics*: The murmur of MVP starts in late systole, may be with nonejection click, and ends at $S_2$ **(Fig. 5)**. It is best heard in the apical area. Click murmur complex moves toward $S_1$ (duration increases) during the strain phase of Valsalva and also from squatting to standing (preload reducing maneuvers).

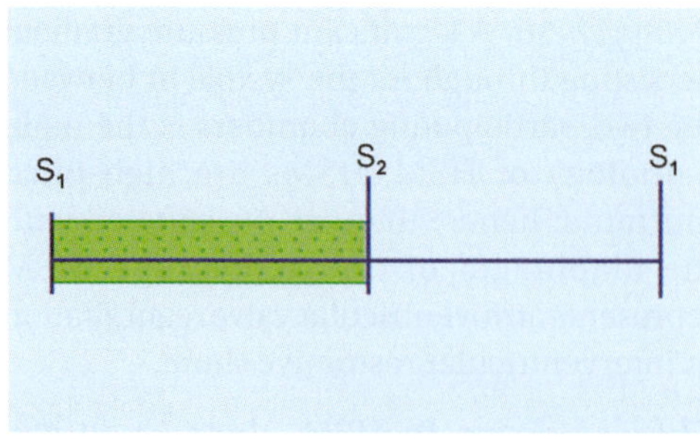


**FIG. 4:** Holosystolic murmur/pansystolic murmur.

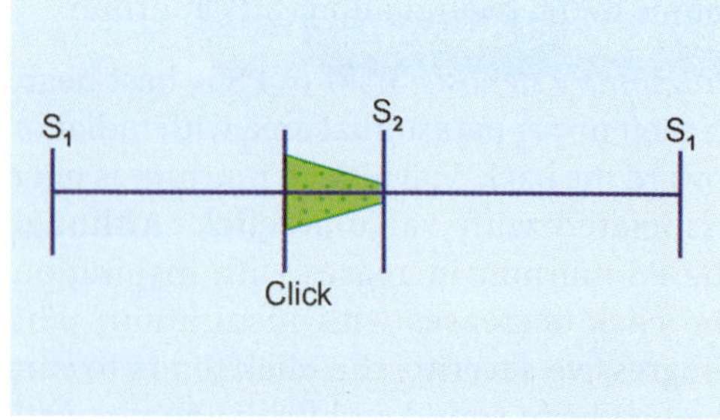


**FIG. 5:** Late systolic murmur of mitral valve prolapse.

## EARLY SYSTOLIC MURMUR

*Causes*: Acute MR, small muscular VSD or VSD with PHTN, primary TR

*Pathogenesis*: Pressure gradient in the initial phase of the systole in between the two participating chambers is the main pathology of early systolic murmur. Hence, it is decrescendo murmur.

*Characteristics*: In an early systolic murmur, there is no gap between the $S_1$ and the onset of the murmur. The murmur ends well before $S_2$. The intensity of the murmur gradually decreases (decrescendo) **(Fig. 6)**.

*Acute MR*: In acute MR, there is rapid equalization of pressure in between the LV and acute noncompliant LA. The patient is usually very unstable.

*Ventricular septal defect*: Small muscular VSD gets closed during systole; hence, VSDs have a short early systolic murmur. The presence of significant PHTN even with restrictive VSD reduces the duration of murmur.

*Tricuspid regurgitation*: Usually, the primary TR murmur is soft and short early systolic, and with associated PHTN, becomes classically HSM and of higher pitch.

## EARLY DIASTOLIC MURMUR

*Causes*: AR, pulmonary regurgitation (PR)

*Pathogenesis*: Pathology lies within the semilunar valves. A pressure gradient in the initial phase of the diastole in between the great vessel and the concerned ventricle is the main pathology of early diastolic murmur (EDM). Hence, it is decrescendo murmur.

*Characteristics*: In EDM, the murmur starts with $A_2$ or $P_2$. The murmur ends before $S_1$. The intensity of the murmur gradually decreases (decrescendo) **(Fig. 7)**.

*Aortic regurgitation*: In acute AR, there is rapid equalization of pressure in between the aorta and LV; hence, the duration of the murmur is short. The patient is usually very unstable. In chronic AR, with progressive severity, the duration of the murmur exceeds >50% of the diastole. AR murmur (due to primary valve pathology) is best heard in the mid-left parasternal area (neo-aortic area) and may radiate toward the apical area. AR when occurs due to annular pathology, usually the murmur radiates along the right parasternal area. A sustained handgrip increases the AR murmur but does not alter the PR murmur. Vasodilators decrease the AR murmur. Chronic severe AR is always associated with distal aortic runoff signs. There is often associated aortic ESM (usually up to grade 2 or grade 3 unless associated with AS) with severe AR because of excessive flow during ejection.

*Pulmonary regurgitation*: Murmur of PR when associated with significant PHTN (GrahamSteell murmur) is well audible in the left upper parasternal area and accompanied by other signs of PHTN and pulmonary vascular ejection click. A sustained handgrip increases the AR murmur but does not alter

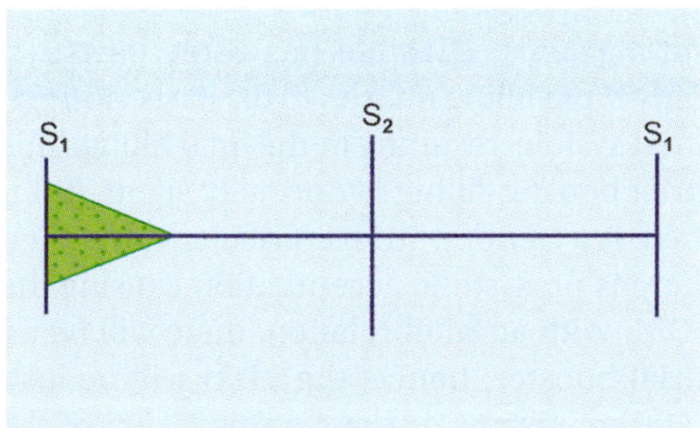


**FIG. 6:** Early systolic murmur.

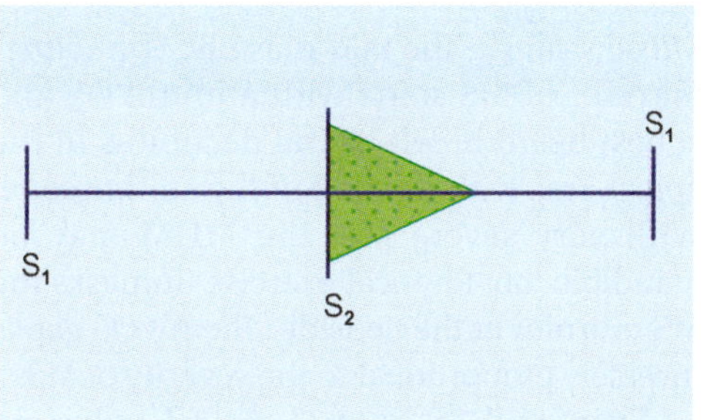


**FIG. 7:** Early diastolic murmur.

the PR murmur. The murmur of acute PR unless associated with PHTN is soft.

## MID-DIASTOLIC MURMUR

*Causes*: MS, tricuspid stenosis (TS), Austin Flint murmur (AFM), left atrial myxoma, Carey Coombs murmur, functional mitral stenosis (fMS), functional tricuspid stenosis (fTS)

*Pathogenesis*: Atrioventricular valve is pathological, causing a significant pressure gradient in between LA and LV or right atrium (RA) and RV in diastole, resulting in the mid-diastolic murmur (MDM). In sinus rhythm, it may be associated with late diastolic accentuation due to the atrial systole. Sometimes valves may remain normal, but because of excessive blood flow, there can be functional MS or functional TS murmur, although they are never associated with presystolic accentuation.

In active rheumatic carditis, there may be a diastolic murmur due to valvulitis, i.e., Carey Coombs murmur.

In left atrial myxoma, MDM can be posture dependent and may be associated with tumor plop. LA myxoma patients must never undergo repeated posture changes for academic interest only as sudden obstruction of the MV orifice with the mass can lead to sudden cardiac death.

*Characteristics*: In MDM, the "*rumbling*" murmur starts with an opening snap (OS) and ends with $S_1$. With progressive severity, the murmur's duration increases. OS is lost in a fixed nonpliable valve **(Fig. 8)**.

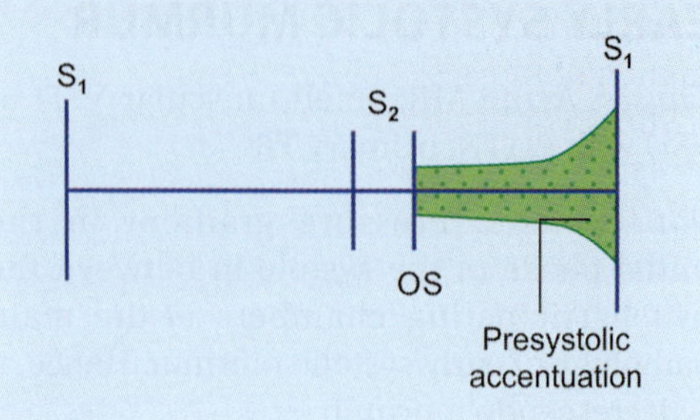


**FIG. 8:** Mid-diastolic murmur of mitral stenosis.

*Mitral stenosis*: The mid-diastolic "*rumbling*" murmur of MS starts with a mitral OS and is best heard in left lateral decubitus in the apical area with the bell of the stethoscope. With very severe MS, the MDM may be inaudible too. Physical exercise unmasks the MS murmur at the bedside. The $A_2$–OS gap is inversely proportional to the severity of MS.

Even with a normal mitral valve, in PDA and VSD, there is excessive blood flow through the valve, generating a soft MDM of functional MS.

*Tricuspid stenosis*: Murmur of TS is similar to MS murmur but is well audible in the left lower parasternal area and increases with inspiration.

Even with a normal tricuspid valve, in atrial septal defect (ASD), there is excessive blood flow through the valve, generating a soft MDM of functional TS.

*Austin Flint murmur*: With severe AR, the jet impinges upon the anterior mitral leaflet and causes AFM. AFM increases with handgrip and decreases with vasodilators. It is always associated with the AR murmur and peripheral signs of aortic runoff. There will be no OS, and $S_1$ will not be accentuated in AFM.

## LATE DIASTOLIC MURMUR

*Terminology*: Late diastolic murmur (LDM) is also known as a presystolic murmur.

*Causes*: MS in sinus rhythm, TS in sinus rhythm

*Pathogenesis*: Diastole has three parts: (i) Early rapid filling phase, (ii) diastasis, and (iii) atrial systole, resulting in the final filling. This atrial booster filling is normally silent, but if there is a stenotic atrioventricular valve, then there is presystolic accentuation causing the LDM. With atrial fibrillation, there will be no atrial booster; hence, the LDM will be lost. LDM represents a true organic lesion of the atrioventricular valve.

*Characteristics*: LDM is the presystolic accentuation of the MDM of the MS or TS in sinus rhythm. For MS, it is heard in the apical area, preferably in left lateral decubitus, and in TS, it is heard in the left lower parasternal area in the supine position, although TS is often associated with other valve diseases; hence, the audible sounds are often buried under the other valve pathology sounds **(Fig. 8)**.

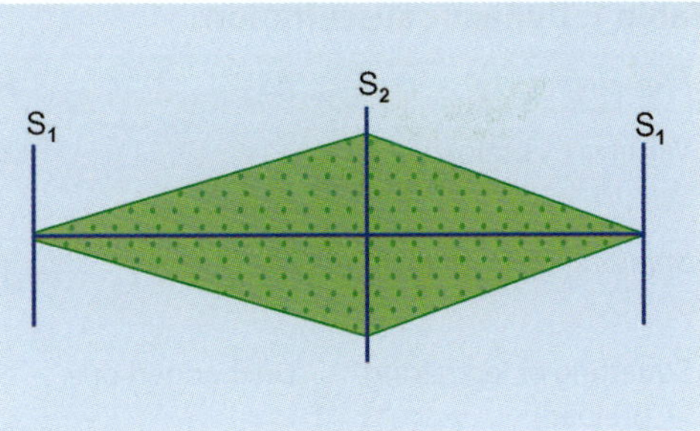


**FIG. 9:** Continuous murmur—patent ductus arteriosus.

## CONTINUOUS MURMUR

In a continuous murmur, there is no gap between the systolic and the diastolic phases of the murmur. If there is any gap, then it is a "*to and fro murmur*" and not a continuous murmur. A classic example of such continuous murmur is PDA murmur in the left second intercostal space or infraclavicular area and continuous bruit over the arteriovenous fistula of hemodialysis access **(Fig. 9)**. Identification of continuous murmur is important as it has got only a few differential diagnoses.

The causes of continuous murmur are given in **Box 3**.

**BOX 3: Causes of continuous murmur.**

- *Continuous murmur in an acyanotic patient*:
  - PDA
  - Aortopulmonary window
  - Peripheral pulmonary artery stenosis
  - Coronary arteriovenous fistula
  - Systemic arteriovenous fistula
  - Ruptured sinus of Valsalva (RSOV)
  - Coarctation of aorta
  - Anomalous left coronary artery from the pulmonary artery (ALCAPA)
  - MS with small ASD
  - Venous hum
  - Mammary souffle of pregnancy
- *Continuous murmur in a cyanotic patient*:
  - Bronchial collaterals in Fallot's physiology
  - PDA in Fallot's physiology
  - Pulmonary arteriovenous fistula
  - Persistent truncus arteriosus
  - Total anomalous pulmonary venous connection (TAPVC)
  - Surgically created shunts

(ASD: atrial septal defect; MS: mitral stenosis; PDA: patent ductus arteriosus)

## DYNAMIC AUSCULTATION

Various maneuvers are often used at the bedside to augment the murmur concerned and to narrow down the differential diagnosis. **Table 1** illustrates the dynamic auscultation.

## CONCLUSION

We are in the time of artificial intelligence (AI). Nowadays, high-definition stethoscopes are equipped with app-based phonocardiographs. Very soon, an AI algorithm will be added to it so that bedside murmur identification will provides more information. With a click of a button, we can completely evaluate any cardiac valvular pathology by advanced 4D echocardiography. Technologies have engulfed cardiovascular science in such a way that the sagacity of even using a stethoscope is being questioned nowadays. Albeit so many technical humming, the importance of bedside identification of murmur by clinical acumen is extremely necessary in the resource-limited developing world. With astounding clinical ability, clinicians can not only identify a murmur but also pick up any change in the character

**Table 1: Dynamic auscultation.**

| *Maneuvers* | *AS* | *HOCM* | *MVP* | *MR* | *Other* |
|---|---|---|---|---|---|
| Valsalva (↘ preload) | ↘ | ↗ | ↗ Duration of murmur | ↘ | ↘ AR |
| Standing up (↘ preload) | ↘ | ↗ | ↗ Duration of murmur | ↘ | |
| Squatting or leg raising (↗ preload) | Unchanged or ↗ | ↘ | ↘ Duration of murmur | ↗ | ↗ AR–↗ VSD |
| Handgrip (↗ afterload) | Unchanged or ↘ | ↘ | ↘ Duration of murmur | ↗ | ↗ AR–↗ VSD<br>↗ MS (↗ HR) |
| Amyl nitrate (↘ afterload) | ↗ | ↗ | ↗ Duration of murmur | ↘ | ↗ MS (↗ HR)<br>↘AR–↘ VSD<br>↘Austin Flint |
| Post-PVC (↗ contractility) | ↗ | ↗ | ↘ Duration of murmur (↗ LV volume) | Unchanged | |

(AR: aortic regurgitation; AS: aortic stenosis; HOCM: hypertrophic obstructive cardiomyopathy; HR: heart rate; LV: left ventricle; MR: mitral regurgitation; MS: mitral stenosis; MVP: mitral valve prolapse; PVC: premature ventricular contraction; VSD: ventricular septal defect)

of the murmur (e.g., infective endocarditis in bicuspid aortic valve or VSD or prosthetic heart valves) in a long-term follow-up that can be often rewarding as well as lifesaving for the patient.

## CLINICAL PEARLS

- Murmur must be described under the following points—timing, location, intensity, radiation, character, and dynamic auscultation.
- Systolic murmur can be holosystolic or ejection systolic or early systolic or late systolic.
- Diastolic murmur can be early diastolic or mid-diastolic or late diastolic.
- Continuous murmur narrows down the differential diagnosis.

## FURTHER READINGS

1. Libby P, Bonow RO, Mann DL, Tomaselli GF, Bhatt DL, Solomon SD, et al. Braunwald's heart disease a textbook of Cardiovascular Medicine. Philadelphia, PA: Elsevier; 2022.
2. Fuster V, Narula,Jagat, Vaishnava P, Leon MB, Callans DJ, Rumsfeld JS, et al. Fuster and Hurst's the heart: 15th edition. New York: Mc Graw Hill; 2022.
3. Loscalzo J, Kasper DL, Longo DL, Fauci AS, Hauser SL, Jameson JL, et al. Harrison's principles of Internal Medicine, twenty-First edition vol 1 & 2, New York: McGraw Hill; 2022.

CHAPTER 8

# Pulse and Blood Pressure

*Ruchit Shah, BR Bansode*

## PULSE

The pulse begins with opening of the aortic valve and ejection of the blood from the left ventricle into the aorta.

Factors determining the pulse wave:

- Left ventricular stroke volume (SV)
- Ejection velocity
- Antegrade blood flow
- Waves returning from the peripheral circulation
- Compliance, distensibility, and capacity of the vessels

Phases of the pulse:

- *Early systolic (percussion wave)*: It is due to rapid ejection of blood stored in central aorta. This is the only palpable part of the pulse.
- *Mid and late systolic (anacrotic notch and shoulder)*: It is due to propagation of blood from aorta to periphery and reflection of waves from upper extremity.
- *Diastole (dicrotic notch)*: The nadir coincides with closure of the aortic valve (A2 part of S2).

### Examination

We use three fingers (trisection method) to determine the upstroke, systolic peak, and diastole. We measure the following parameters:

- *Rate and rhythm*: We count the radial pulse for 15 seconds and multiply by 4 to get the rate. The normal pulse rate is 60–100 bpm. We check the rhythm, whether regular or irregular. We compare this with the apical impulse. Apex pulse deficit > 6 bpm is suggestive of atrial fibrillation and <6 bpm is suggestive of premature ventricular contractions **(Tables 1 and 2)**.
- *Character and volume of the pulse*: Since the carotid artery is close to the aorta, it is used to determine the volume of the pulse.
  - *Hyperkinetic (bounding) pulse*: It is a pulse with a large amplitude due to increased left ventricular ejection and SV. It is seen in high output states, decreased sympathetic activity, and decreased arterial compliance.
    - Anemia
    - Thyrotoxicosis
    - Anxiety
    - Exercise
    - Aortic regurgitation (AR)
    - Patent ductus arteriosus
    - Arteriovenous fistula
    - Paget's disease
    - Alcohol intake
  - *Hypokinetic pulse*: It is a low volume pulse due to low cardiac output (CO),

decreased left ventricular SV, and decreased ejection time.
- Heart failure
- Left ventricular dysfunction
- Left ventricular outflow tract obstruction
- Hypotension

- *Pulsus parvus et tardus*: It is a slow rising pulse with a delayed systolic peak.
  - Aortic stenosis
- *Water hammer or collapsing pulse (Corrigan's sign)*: It consists of an early swift peak due to rapid ejection of SV. This is followed by a brief descent without a dicrotic notch due to diastolic runoff. The diastolic runoff is caused due to backflow in the left ventricle, rapid runoff to the periphery due to decreased systemic vascular resistance, and systemic vasodilation. Clinically, the examiner holds the wrist of the patient with his palm facing the supinated forearm and suddenly lifts the forearm above the head and feels the collapsing pulse.
  - AR
  - Patent ductus arteriosus
  - Aortopulmonary window
  - Rupture of sinus of Valsalva into the right heart
  - Tetralogy of Fallot with broncho-pulmonary collaterals
- *Double beating pulse*: Simultaneous auscultation at the apex and palpation

**Table 1: Clinical conditions manifesting as tachycardia and bradycardia.**

| ***Tachycardia (>100 bpm)*** | ***Bradycardia (<60 bpm)*** |
|---|---|
| *Physiological*: Infancy and childhood, anxiety, excitement, exercise, pregnancy | *Physiological*: Athlete, sleep |
| *Pharmacological*: Nicotine, alcohol, amyl nitrate, atropine | *Pharmacological*: Beta blockers, verapamil, diltiazem |
| *Pathological*:<br>• *Cardiac*: Heart failure, acute myocardial infarction (MI), pulmonary embolism, shock, myocarditis<br>• *Noncardiac*: Fever, thyrotoxicosis, anemia, bleeding, hypotension | *Pathological*:<br>• *Cardiac*: Acute inferior wall MI, sinoatrial block, vasovagal syncope<br>• *Noncardiac*: Myxedema, hypothyroidism, hypothermia, enteric fever, obstructive jaundice, raised intracranial pressure |
| *Tachyarrhythmias*: Atrial fibrillation, atrial tachycardia, supraventricular tachycardia, ventricular tachycardia | *Bradyarrhythmias*: High-grade atrioventricular (AV) block, complete heart block |

**Table 2: Causes of irregular pulse.**

| ***Regularly irregular pulse*** | ***Irregularly irregular pulse*** |
|---|---|
| • Sinus arrhythmia<br>• Pulsus bigeminus<br>• Pulsus alternans<br>• First- and second-degree atrioventricular block | • Atrial fibrillation<br>• Multifocal atrial tachycardia<br>• Premature ventricular contractions |

at the carotid artery help to determine the timing of the double impulse.

- Bisferiens pulse: The double peaked pulse occurs in systole. For example, AR, severe AR, and mild/moderate aortic stenosis
- Bifid pulse: It consists of a bifid or spike and dome pattern. For example, hypertrophic obstructive cardiomyopathy
- Dicrotic pulse: It consists of one wave in systole and another wave in diastole. The two waves are separated by S2 on auscultation. For example, cardiomyopathy with severe left ventricular dysfunction, low CO, low blood pressure (BP), during inspiration in cardiac tamponade, fever in young

○ *Pulsus alternans*: It occurs due to beat to beat variation in CO. It can be detected by slow decompression of the sphygmomanometer cuff and auscultating the brachial artery. When the variation is >20 mm Hg, it can be palpated with breath held in deep expiration. For example, congestive cardiac failure with S3 gallop in patients with severe left ventricular dysfunction

○ *Pulsus paradoxus*: This was coined by Kussmaul. The word paradoxus is a misnomer. During inspiration, systolic BP falls by 4–6 mm Hg. Clinically, the sphygmomanometer cuff is inflated above the peak systolic BP. If the difference between the first appearance of Korotkoff sounds on expiration and sounds well heard during both phases of respiration during quiet breathing is >10 mm Hg, it is pulsus paradoxus. For example, cardiac tamponade, constrictive pericarditis, severe congestive cardiac failure, severe asthma, and emphysema.

- *Condition of the arterial wall*: The examiner tries to feel the artery between the index and middle finger while trying to examine for tortuosity and arteriosclerosis.
- All pulses should be palpated and compared bilaterally
  ○ *Superficial temporal artery*: It is palpated at the zygomatic process anterior to the tragus.
  ○ *Common carotid artery*: It bifurcates at the C4 level at the upper border of the thyroid cartilage. It is palpated at the lower half of the neck with the neck rotated slightly toward the examiner to relax the sternocleidomastoid. Never palpate both carotids simultaneously as it can precipitate carotid sinus hypersensitivity syncope.
  ○ *Subclavian artery*: It can be palpated against the first rib in the angle between the sternocleidomastoid and the clavicle.
  ○ *Axillary artery*: It is palpated in the middle of the humerus.
  ○ *Brachial artery*: It is palpated in the antecubital fossa medial to the biceps tendon.
  ○ *Radial artery*: It is palpated at the head of the radius with the forearm slightly pronated and wrist slightly flexed.
  ○ *Femoral artery*: It is palpated at the head of the femur just below the inguinal ligament midway between the iliac crest and pubic rami.
  ○ *Popliteal artery*: The patient lies supine with knees flexed at 120°. The thumbs are placed on the patella, and the fingers palpate the popliteal artery in the popliteal fossa.
  ○ *Posterior tibial artery*: The foot is placed in a relaxed position, and the popliteal artery can be palpated 1 cm behind the medial malleolus.
  ○ *Dorsalis pedis artery*: It is palpated on the first metatarsal between the first and second toes (between the tendons of extensor hallucis longus and extensor digitorum).

Conditions with unequal/absent pulses:

- Takayasu arteritis
- Thoracic outlet syndrome
- Dissection of aorta

- Coarctation of aorta
- Subclavian steal syndrome
- Acute microembolism
- Atherosclerosis of innominate, left subclavian artery

*Radiofemoral delay*: The central aortic pulse reaches the radial artery at 80 ms and femoral artery at 75 ms. Place the patient's palm beside the femoral artery and try to appreciate the difference in the pulsations. In coarctation of aorta, the brachial pulse is bounding whereas the femoral pulse has a slow rise, late peak, and low pulse pressure. Radiofemoral delay can also be seen in atherosclerotic diseases of the descending aorta, diseases of aortic bifurcation, and common iliac and external iliac arteries.

## BLOOD PRESSURE

Blood pressure is a measure of potential energy or lateral force per unit area. Systolic BP is the maximum pressure exerted by the heart during systole. It depends on SV, velocity of left ventricular ejection, distensibility of vessels, and volume of blood at end diastole. Diastolic BP is the minimum pressure exerted by the heart during diastole. It depends on peripheral arteriolar resistance, cardiac cycle length, and compliance of the arterial tree.

- CO = heart rate (HR) × SV
- BP = CO × peripheral vascular resistance (PVR)
- Pulse pressure = (systolic) – (diastolic) BP (approximately 40 mm Hg)
- Mean BP = diastolic + 1/3 pulse pressure (approximately 95–100 mm Hg)

### Measurement of Blood Pressure

The BP is measured with a mercury or aneroid apparatus. The cuff length:width should be 80:40% (2:1) of arm circumference. The cuff should be tightly wrapped around the arm, leaving 1–2 inches to place the diaphragm. There should be no intervening clothing between the arm and the cuff. The patient should be seated comfortably with arms at the level of the heart, back supported, legs uncrossed, and should not be talking. He should not have consumed alcohol, cigarettes, tobacco, tea, coffee, or aerated beverages. The radial pulse is palpated and the sphygmomanometer is inflated 20 mm Hg above the point of disappearance of the radial pulse. The cuff is deflated at 2–3 mm Hg/s. The systolic pressure is the point where two consecutive Korotkoff sounds are heard, and the diastolic pressure is the point where there is complete disappearance of the Korotkoff sounds. Korotkoff sounds arise because of oscillation of blood with every cardiac impulse in the partially distended arterial wall.

Five phases of Korotkoff sounds:

- *Phase I*: Onset of auscultatory sound suggestive of peak systole
- *Phase II*: It is a swishing sound which occurs 10–15 mm Hg below the peak systole.
- *Phase III*: It is crisp, easily heard, and 10–15 mm Hg below phase II.
- *Phase IV*: Abrupt damping, muffling, or tapping sound
- *Phase V*: Disappearance of sound is suggestive of diastolic pressure.

After phase V, the clinician must deflate the cuff completely and wait for complete venous return before the next reading is taken. In AR, the diastolic reading should be taken in phases IV and V. In atrial fibrillation, since there is beat to beat variation, an average of three readings should be taken.

For measurement of BP in the lower limbs, a thigh cuff should be used and pressure should be measured at the popliteal artery. If thigh cuff is unavailable, the same arm cuff can be tied just above the ankle and posterior tibial or dorsalis pedis pulsations can be used to measure the BP.

Sources of error during BP measurement:

- *Insufficient inflation, rapid inflation*: Failure to detect correct systolic pressure
- *Failure to detect auscultatory gap*: Always palpate the radial artery and inflate 20 mm Hg above the point of occlusion of the radial artery

- *Loose cuff*: Falsely elevated readings
- Intervening clothing
- *Fat arm with small cuff*: Pseudo hypertension
- *Thin arm with large cuff*: Pseudo hypotension
- *Excessive venous congestion in arm*: Decreased intensity of Korotkoff sound
- *Arm above the level of the heart*: Underestimation of BP
- *Arm below the level of the heart*: Overestimation of BP

### Orthostatic Hypotension

In normal individuals, systolic BP drops by 10–12 mm Hg on standing and diastolic BP remains same or increases. When there is >20/10 mm Hg drop in BP from supine to standing position within 3 minutes of standing, it is suggestive of postural hypotension. There may or may not be compensatory tachycardia. The patient may have postural giddiness or syncope.

Differential diagnoses of orthostatic hypotension:

- *Drugs*: Diuretics, angiotensin converting enzyme inhibitors, angiotensin receptor blockers, alpha blockers, nitrates, vasodilators
- Diabetics
- Elderly
- Hypovolemia
- Baroreflex dysfunction
- Autonomic insufficiency

At every clinical visit, the above group of patients should be carefully checked for postural hypotension. Postural hypotension is an important preventable cause of falls and fractures in the elderly.

### Ambulatory Blood Pressure Monitoring

It consists of a BP cuff tied to the patient's arm with a portable device. The cuff is inflated at every 15–30-minute intervals for a period of 24 hours. In a normal individual, there is 10–20% dip in BP during sleep and a surge during early morning, stress and mental activity. Patients who have persistently elevated nighttime BP above 135/85 mm Hg and failure to dip at night are at a high risk of cardiovascular events. Ambulatory BP monitoring should be done in:

- White coat hypertension
- Drug resistant hypertension
- Drug induced hypotension
- Autonomic dysfunction
- Episodic hypertension
- Titrating the dose and timing of the antihypertensive agents

### Ankle Brachial Index

Ankle brachial index is the ratio of the systolic BP in the ankle to the higher of the systolic BP of both the arms.

- *More than 0.9*: Normal
- *Less than 0.9*: Peripheral vascular disease
- *Less than 0.3*: Critical limb ischemia and rest pain

Causes of differential BP in upper limbs (>10 mm Hg):

- *Arterial occlusion*: Embolism, postcardiac catheterization, atherosclerosis, Takayasu arteritis
- Dissection of aorta, dissecting aortic aneurysm
- Subclavian steal syndrome
- Thoracic outlet syndrome
- Supravalvular aortic stenosis

Causes of differential BP in upper and lower limbs (>20 mm Hg):

- Severe AR (Hill's sign)
- Dissection of aorta
- Coarctation of aorta
- Aortic arch syndrome
- Subclavian steal syndrome

*Causes of wide pulse pressure*: A wide pulse pressure arises due to increased SV and decreased PVR.

- *Hyperkinetic circulation*: Pregnancy, exercise, anemia, hyperthyroidism, arteriovenous fistula, hot weather

- AR
- Patent ductus arteriosus
- Truncus arteriosus
- Complete heart block

*Causes of narrow pulse pressure*: A narrow pulse pressure arises due to decreased SV and increased PVR.
- Heart failure
- Severe aortic stenosis
- Diabetic ketoacidosis

## Cardiovascular Subsets

*Aortic stenosis*: The classical pulse in severe aortic stenosis is pulsus parvus et tardus or anacrotic pulse. It is described as slow rising, delayed peak, delayed drop off, small volume pulse. There may be a palpable thrill and anacrotic notch due to blood passing through a narrowed orifice. A bisferiens pulse is seen in severe aortic stenosis and moderate AR with preserved left ventricular function. Pulsus alternans may be seen with severe aortic stenosis and left ventricular dysfunction.

As the severity of aortic stenosis increases, the pulse pressure narrows. In patients with hypertension, there may be high BP. If there is associated AR, diastolic BP reduces and pulse pressure widens.

*Supravalvular aortic stenosis*: The patient has selective streaming of blood in the right innominate vessels causing higher amplitude in carotid, subclavian, and brachial vessels. The left carotid has features of aortic valve obstruction. The BP in the right arm is 10–20 mm Hg higher than the left arm.

*Aortic regurgitation*: There is a collapsing pulse. The large SV ejected causes an increase in force and amplitude of the pulse followed by a rapid diastolic runoff due to decreased PVR and early diastolic reflux of blood in the left ventricle.

As the severity increases, the diastolic pressure decreases and the pulse pressure widens.

*Peripheral signs of AR*:
- *Bisferiens pulse*: Palpate the brachial artery to feel it.
- *Water hammer pulse*: Palpate it at the radial artery in the forearm.
- *Hill's sign*: It is used to grade the severity of AR. If the difference in systolic BP between the brachial and popliteal arteries is:
  - *20–40 mm Hg*: Angiographic 2+ AR
  - *40–60 mm Hg*: Angiographic 3+ AR
  - *>60 mm Hg*: Angiographic 4+ AR
- *Palmar click*: It is a palpable, abrupt flushing of the palms in systole.

*Eyes*
- *Landolfi's sign*: It is the alternate contraction and dilation of pupils in systole and diastole, respectively.
- *Becker's sign*: Prominence of the retinal artery pulsations

*Head and neck*
- *De Musset's sign*: Bobbing of the head with each heartbeat
- *Corrigan's sign (dancing carotids)*: Visible pulsations of the carotid artery
- *Müller's sign*: Visible pulsations of the uvula
- *Minerva's sign*: Strong lingual pulsations cause the tongue depressor to move up and down
- *Logue's sign*: If AR is associated with aortic dissection, there would be a pulsatile sternoclavicular joint.

*Upper limb*
- *Locomotor brachialis*: Brachial artery pulsations
- *Quincke's pulse*: Apply light pressure to the tip of the finger nail or press a glass slide against the lips to observe exaggerated sequential reddening and blanching.
- *Palfrey's sign*: Pistol shot sound heard over the radial artery

*Lower limb*
- Pistol shot sound of Traube on the femoral artery
- *Duroziez's sign*: A diastolic bruit caused by pressing the femoral artery distal to the edge of the stethoscope. A systolic murmur can be appreciated by pressing

the femoral artery proximal to the stethoscope.

*Abdomen*

- *Rosenbach's sign*: Pulsatile liver
- *Gerhardt's sign*: Pulsatile spleen
- *Dennison's sign*: Pulsatile cervix

*Acute AR*: There will be sinus tachycardia, low systolic BP with a near normal diastolic BP, and pulsus alternans. Peripheral signs are absent.

*Hypertrophic cardiomyopathy*: The carotid pulse is rapid, jerky, with a sharp upstroke, followed by a midsystolic dip or collapse. This is followed by a second late diastolic wave (spike and dome or pointed finger pulse). In obstructive hypertrophic cardiomyopathy, after an extrasystolic pulse, there is Starling effect which causes increased contractility and increased obstruction, so the pulse remains same or reduces. This is called *Brockenbrough phenomenon*.

*Mitral stenosis*: There is decreased pulse volume and normal contour.

When it is associated with atrial fibrillation, the pulse is irregularly irregular with variable pulse volume.

When there is associated mitral or AR, there is an increase in the carotid pulse amplitude and rate of rise.

*Mitral regurgitation*: Decreased forward SV causes a brisk, jerky pulse with reduced volume. It may be quick rising, poorly sustained with low amplitude.

*Mitral valve prolapse*: The pulse is normal.

If there is severe mitral regurgitation, the arterial pulse is brisk and collapsing. A retraction notch coincident with midsystolic click has been recorded but is not palpable.

*Tricuspid regurgitation*: There is low amplitude pulse. It may be associated with atrial fibrillation.

## CLINICAL PEARLS

While examining the pulse, the clinician should focus on the rate, rhythm, character, volume, condition of arterial wall, bilateral equality, and radiofemoral delay. BP should be measured in both arms and one lower limb. Postural BP should be measured to look for orthostatic hypotension.

## FURTHER READINGS

1. Abrams J. Essentials of Cardiac Physical Diagnosis, Philadelphia: Lea and Febiger; 1987. pp. 13-54.
2. Narasimhan R, Vahe S, Franklin S. The Art and Science of Cardiac Physical Examination with Heart Sounds, Jugular and Precordial Pulsations, 2nd edition. New Delhi: Jaypee Brothers Medical Publishers; 2015. pp. 20-140.
3. Constant J. Essentials of Bedside Cardiology, 2nd edition. Totowa: Humana Press Inc.; 2003. pp. 29-88.
4. Mann DL, Zipes DP, Libby P, Bonow RO. Braunwald's Heart Disease: A Textbook of Cardiovascular Medicine, 10th edition. Philadelphia: Elsevier Saunders; 2015. pp. 98-102.
5. Loscalzo J, Fauci A, Kasper D, Hauser S, Longo D, Jameson JL. Harrison's Principles of Internal Medicine, 21st edition. New York: McGraw Hill; 2022.
6. Glynn M, Drake W. Hutchison's Clinical Methods, 23rd edition. Philadelphia: Elsevier Saunders; 2012.
7. Houghton AR, Gray D. Chamberlain's Symptoms and Signs in Clinical Medicine, 13th edition. London: Hodder Arnold; 2010.

CHAPTER 9

# Cyanosis

Saumitra Ray

## DEFINITION

Cyanosis is a bluish discoloration of skin and/or mucous membrane due to increased amount of deoxygenated hemoglobin (5 g/dL or more) in the underlying capillaries. The oxygen saturation is usually below 85%. (The word cyan means a blue-green color.)

## TYPES

Cyanosis is classified as central or peripheral, depending on whether the increased amount of deoxygenated hemoglobin is produced centrally due to impaired oxygenation in the lungs or mixing up of venous and arterial blood (central cyanosis) or whether there is more deoxygenation of hemoglobin in the peripheral parts due to sluggish circulation, allowing more time for oxygenated hemoglobin to get deoxygenated/reduced in a particular part of the body.

## HOW TO DETECT?

Peripheral cyanosis is evident as a bluish tinge in the nail beds, tip of tongue, ear lobules, palm and sole and, if severe, in the general skin. Usually, the affected part is cold.

Central cyanosis is evident in all the above areas and additionally in the tongue, buccal mucosa, lips, and lower palpebral conjunctiva. The body is generally warm.

## DIFFERENTIAL DIAGNOSIS

- *Methemoglobinemia*: When the capillaries contain 1.5 g/dL or more of methemoglobin, it gives the same bluish hue. It may be an inherited or a congenital condition or more commonly due to exposure to certain drugs and toxins such as nitrites, dapsone, and benzocaine.
- *Sulfhemoglobinemia*: When the capillaries contain 0.5 g/dL or more of sulfhemoglobin, it causes cyanosis. It may occur with sulfur-containing drugs such as phenacetin, dapsone, and sulfonamides.
- *Pseudocyanosis*: This may occur due to exposure to drugs such as amiodarone, gold salts, and silver salts. This is primarily due to pigmentation of the skin.
- *External pigmentation*: This may come from fruits such as blueberry or from artificial colors as used during festivals. Sometimes, skin pigmentation in certain ethnic populations may mimic cyanosis, and at other times, it may mask true cyanosis.

## CAUSES

- *Central cyanosis*: The usual causes of central cyanosis are either—

- Cardiac, e.g., congenital cyanotic heart disease, Eisenmenger's syndrome, valvular heart disease, and advanced heart failure
- Pulmonary, e.g., pulmonary embolism, asthma and chronic obstructive airway disease, pneumonia, bronchiectasis, lung fibrosis, massive pleural effusion, arteriovenous shunts, and pulmonary hypertension
- Sometimes, it may occur due to hypoventilation states such as intracranial hemorrhage, tonic-clonic convulsion, obstructive sleep apnea, or heroin overdose.

- *Peripheral cyanosis*: It may occur due to—
    - Reduced cardiac output (heart failure or shock)
    - Local vasoconstriction (cold exposure, Raynaud phenomenon)
    - Vasomotor instability
    - Venous or arterial obstruction (deep vein thrombosis, Buerger disease, arterial embolism)
    - Hyperviscosity syndrome (polycythemia, multiple myeloma)

## DIFFERENTIAL CYANOSIS

This condition occurs in the presence of patent ductus arteriosus with reversal of shunt, where the venous blood mixes with the arterial blood at the level of the ductus, thus causing cyanosis only at the lower part of the body. The accompanying clubbing also develops in the toes and not in the fingers.

Just the reverse occurs in transposition of great arteries with patent ductus arteriosus where the upper part of the body is more cyanosed than the lower part.

## ANEMIA VERSUS POLYCYTHEMIA

As the color of cyanosis depends on the absolute amount of deoxygenated hemoglobin and not on the percentage of total hemoglobin, it is very difficult to see cyanosis in anemic people, as even with 50% of hemoglobin being deoxygenated, if the total hemoglobin is low, it will not cross the 5 g/dL threshold. On the other hand, in the presence of very high hemoglobin, for example, 20 g/dL, even a normal 25% oxygen extraction will give a tinge of cyanosis.

## DIAGNOSTIC WORK-UP

The diagnosis of cyanosis is clinical. A thorough history and physical examination usually give away the diagnosis, type, and cause of cyanosis.

An oxygen saturation meter shows <85% value, but it may be falsely negative in the presence of methemoglobinemia or sulfhemoglobinemia. Here, CO-Oximetry is useful along with hemoglobin electrophoresis.

Depending on the initial suspicion of the cause, further investigations are warranted.

## CLINICAL PEARLS

- Cyanosis is an important clinical sign indicating hypoxemia
- Major causes are cardiac and pulmonary
- Peripheral cyanosis is detectable in skin only, whereas central cyanosis is seen in mucosa as well
- A thorough history taking and clinical examination is mandatory to detect important diseases and to proceed with appropriate investigations and treatment.

## FURTHER READINGS

1. Innes JA, Dover AR, Fairhurst K. Macleod's Clinical Examination, 14th edition. Amsterdam: Elsevier; 2018.
2. Glynn M, Drake WM. Hutchison's Clinical Methods, 25th edition. Amsterdam: Elsevier; 2022.

# CHAPTER 10

# Edema

*Saumitra Ray*

## DEFINITION

Edema is a clinical condition of excess subcutaneous fluid accumulation due to extravasation of fluid from the capillaries, resulting from an imbalance between the intravascular hydrostatic pressure and osmotic pressure, or sometimes due to capillary damage.

## TYPES

Edema may be pitting or solid.

Pitting edema produces a dimple on the skin when pressed firmly but gently with the thumb for at least 5 seconds against a bony surface. Solid edema is noncompressible.

## MECHANISM AND CAUSES

When intravascular hydrostatic pressure exceeds the osmotic pressure, plasma tends to seep out into the interstitial space. As the gravitational force adds to the hydrostatic force in dependent areas, edema tends to be more prominent in the lower limbs of mobile patients and in the sacral area of bedridden patients.

Increased hydrostatic pressure is commonly caused by heart failure, with reduced, mildly reduced or preserved left ventricular ejection fraction, pericardial effusion, or constrictive pericarditis. Expansion of plasma volume occurs because of salt and water retention by the kidneys due to either reduced salt delivery to the nephrons by vasoconstriction due to sympathetic or rennin activity, or due to excess salt reabsorption by the kidneys by the renin–angiotensin–aldosterone system as occurs in heart failure.

On the other hand, low osmotic pressure occurs due to hypoalbuminemia due to nephritic syndrome, chronic liver disease, or protein–energy malnutrition.

Nonpitting edema occurs in conditions such as myxedema or Graves' disease (pretibial myxedema) due to deposition of myxomatous tissue in the subcutaneous areas.

Lymphatic edema occurs due to blockage of the local lymphatic system as occurs in filariasis, and this is a solid edema.

Local inflammation of skin, subcutaneous tissue, or blood vessels may cause local leakage of plasma causing urticaria and other edematous swellings. Deep vein thrombosis may also raise hydrostatic pressure in the veins causing edema.

Certain drugs such as amlodipine causes ankle edema due to selective dilatation of precapillary arterioles causing increased intracapillary pressure.

## DIURNAL VARIATION

In people with heart failure, often the edema appears in the ankles after mid-day when the person is mobile for a few hours, whereas during sleeping hours, the ankle edema disappears and fluid accumulates in the periorbital areas. Edema due to renal causes is usually fixed topographically.

## CLINICAL RELEVANCE

Edema is an important sign of heart failure and alerts the physician to assess the cardiovascular system thoroughly. It may disclose an underlying hypoalbuminemic state as mentioned above and warrants appropriate investigations. Usually, the later variety of edema is associated with anasarca, where ascites, pleural effusion, pericardial effusion, and scrotal edema are present.

Progression and regression of edema indicate the disease state and dictate the diuretic doses.

In edema due to heart failure, diuretics are the mainstay to treat edema along with medicines to improve left ventricular ejection function. Thiazide-like diuretics do not work in reduced glomerular filtration rate, whereas loop diuretics are needed. Sometimes, sequential diuretic is warranted in a combination of loop diuretic, metolazone, and mineralocorticoid receptor antagonist, which work on different parts of the nephron simultaneously. Recent interest has been generated on acetazolamide as an effective diuretic.

Edema associated with amlodipine-like drugs may be safely ignored and patient reassured, but if not acceptable by patients, it may be reduced by the addition of an angiotensin-converting-enzyme inhibitor or angiotensin receptor blocker. In some cases, the drug may have to be withdrawn.

Edema associated with allergic or inflammatory conditions is treated with steroids and anti-allergic drugs along with the treatment of the underlying cause.

Deep vein thrombosis is treated with oral anticoagulants and/or thrombectomy.

## CLINICAL PEARLS

- Edema is an important clinical sign
- Edema is classified in various ways depending on its character, distribution or underlying pathology
- Disease of major organs like heart, lung, liver, kidney, all can cause edema
- Various local conditions may cause regional edema
- A thorough history taking and clinical examination is mandatory to detect important diseases and to proceed with appropriate investigations and treatment.

## FURTHER READINGS

1. Innes JA, Dover AR, Fairhurst K. Macleod's Clinical Examination, 14th edition. Amsterdam: Elsevier; 2018.
2. Glynn M, Drake WM. Hutchison's Clinical Methods, 25th edition. Amsterdam: Elsevier; 2022.

CHAPTER 11

# Neck Veins

*Saumitra Ray*

## INTRODUCTION

Examination of the neck veins forms an essential part of clinical medicine as it gives a host of useful information about the cardiovascular system along with some very important noncardiovascular conditions.

## WHAT ARE NECK VEINS?

There are four clinically relevant neck veins: The internal and external jugular veins (EJV) of right and left sides.

Generally, the right-sided veins are examined as they directly drain into the right atrium (RA) and reflect the hemodynamics of the RA. In some situations such as congenital anomaly, surgical or traumatic damage, or local distortion by tumors, the left-sided veins are examined. Also, as it is customary to examine a patient from the right side, it is more convenient to see the right-sided veins.

Internal jugular vein (IJV) is seen preferentially to the EJV because of the following factors:

- The latter is more likely to have congenital anomaly
- More liable to be damaged by trauma, surgery, or radiation
- As it has to penetrate the deep fascia of the neck or may have valves, the RA pressure may not be truly reflected in the EJV.

## HOW TO EXAMINE NECK VEINS?

Conventionally, the neck veins are examined when:

- The patient is reclining with a 45° angle at pelvis
- Neck and body remain in same plane
- Neck is relaxed with adequate support
- Neck is fully exposed without any external pressure
- Examiner's eyes are parallel to the neck level

If the IJV is not seen in that position, then the patient needs to be positioned more horizontally. A firm steady pressure on the right upper quadrant of the abdomen by the flat of the hand may make the vein visible (hepatojugular reflux). This is significant if there is 3 cm or more rise of jugular venous pressure (JVP) sustained even after release of pressure. This may be seen in right-sided heart failure.

On the other hand, if the pressure is too high, the patient needs to be seated at a 90° angle on the bed to make the upper level visible, which gives a clearer view of the venous waves.

## HOW TO DIFFERENTIATE BETWEEN INTERNAL JUGULAR VEIN AND CAROTID ARTERY?

As both the IJV and the common carotid artery (CCA) run parallel to each other in close proximity, one may be confused with the other. The following points may help differentiating between the two:

- The CCA is medial to the sternal head of the sternocleidomastoid muscle, whereas the IJV is lateral to it.
- The pulsation of the CCA is more palpable than visible, whereas the pulsation of the IJV is more visible than palpable.
- The pulsation of the CCA is more outward and jerky, whereas that of the IJV is more inward and wavy.
- The pulsation of the IJV is compressible at the root of the neck and can be obliterated, whereas that of the CCA is noncompressible.
- There is a definite upper level of the IJV, whereas the CCA has no upper level.
- The level and nature of the pulsation of the IJV vary with body position and respiration, whereas those of the CCA do not.
- Hepatojugular reflux is present in the IJV but not in CCA.
- The CCA disappears at the angle of the mandible, whereas the IJV may be visible up to the back of the ear lobe if the pressure is sufficiently high.
- A bruit may be audible on the CCA, whereas the IJV does not produce any bruit.

## WHAT TO SEE IN THE NECK VEINS?

Neck veins are examined for two primary objectives:

1. To assess the JVP
2. To analyze the pulse waves

### Jugular Venous Pressure

Jugular venous pressure is measured as the vertical distance between the sternal angle and the top level of the IJV pulsation. A ruler is placed vertically on the sternal angle and a piece of paper is held horizontally at the top level of venous pulsation to meet the ruler and the reading is taken.

The normal RA pressure is 5-6 mm Hg, which means (13.6 × 5-6) mm of water (or blood), that is, about 7-8 cm. In a normally built adult person, the standard distance between the center of the RA and the sternal angle at all body positions is 5 cm. At 45° recline, the vertical height from the sternal angle to the root of the neck is approximately 3 cm. So, any venous pulsation seen beyond the root of the neck at 45° recline position tells immediately that the JVP is raised.

All the conditions that increase the RA pressure cause a raised JVP. JVP is also raised in constrictive pericarditis. In these situations, the vein is pulsatile. But in certain situations such as cardiac tamponade or superior mediastinal syndrome, the JVP is raised but nonpulsatile. Here, it does not reflect the RA pressure.

Normally, the JVP falls with deep inspiration as there is negative suction of blood into the thoracic cavity as intrathoracic pressure falls. But in certain conditions such as constrictive pericarditis, cardiac tamponade, severe right heart failure, right ventricle (RV) infarct, restrictive cardiomyopathy, and pulmonary hypertension, there is paradoxical rise of JVP during inspiration (Kussmaul's sign).

### Jugular Venous Pulse

Typically, JV pulse is a sequence of four waves: Two outward and two inward. They reflect different phases of the cardiac cycle and are thus affected by various clinical conditions, giving important clues to the diagnosis.

- *"a" wave*: "*a*" wave is the first wave of the cycle and is an outward wave. It represents RA contraction/systole to push blood from RA to RV. The RA pressure rises above the RV pressure, and this raised pressure is reflected back into the IJV. In atrial fibrillation, "*a*" wave is absent.
- *"x" descent*: This is the first inward or suction wave after "*a*" wave and represents the fall of RA pressure as the tricuspid ring is drawn toward the RV with RV having isometric contraction period. This inward suction may be interrupted by a small positive "*c*" wave coinciding with the closure of the tricuspid valve at the end of RV diastole.
- *"v" wave*: "*v*" wave is a positive wave coinciding with the RV systole. As the tricuspid valve is closed, the continuous venous return to the RA raises the RA pressure.
- *"y" descent*: This prominent negative wave corresponds to the opening of the tricuspid valve with sudden fall in RA pressure as blood rushes from RA to the RV.

### Abnormalities of the Jugular Venous Waveforms

As it is evident that the different JV waveforms are closely linked to the different intracardiac events, it is useful to study the abnormalities in the waveforms in different clinical conditions.

- *"a" wave*: "*a*" wave becomes very prominent ("giant *a* wave") when RA has to produce extra pressure to push blood into the RV. This situation may arise either in tricuspid valve stenosis or when RV pressure is supranormal as in conditions causing RV hypertrophy.

  "Cannon *a* wave" is an extraordinarily large "*a*" wave produced when RA contracts against a closed tricuspid valve. This occurs regularly in junctional rhythm when RA and RV contract together in every cycle or irregularly in complete heart block and ventricular tachycardia when in some beats the RA and RV contract together.
- *"x" descent*: This may be prominent in constrictive pericarditis or uncommonly in cardiac tamponade.
- *"v" wave*: "Giant *v* wave" is produced by tricuspid regurgitation. Along with passive venous return, RA gets the extra blood from the RV and the JV pressure as well as the "*v*" wave rises.
- *"y" descent*: A prominent "y" descent is an important feature of constrictive pericarditis (Friedreich's sign) and distinguishes constrictive pericarditis from restrictive cardiomyopathy and cardiac tamponade.

## CLINICAL PEARLS

- Examination of neck veins requires sophisticated clinical skills and a thorough clinical approach
- There are interesting differences in detection and significance of internal versus external jugular veins, and right sided versus left sided veins
- Both the venous pressure and the wave form have immense clinical values
- An astute clinician can diagnose a lot of diseases by examining neck veins properly

## FURTHER READINGS

1. Innes JA, Dover AR, Fairhurst K. Macleod's Clinical Examination, 14th edition. Amsterdam: Elsevier; 2018.
2. Glynn M, Drake WM. Hutchison's Clinical Methods, 25th edition. Amsterdam: Elsevier; 2022.

# PART 2

# Dermatology

CHAPTER 12

# Pigmentation

*Arunima Dhabal, Indrashis Podder, Nilay Kanti Das*

## WHAT IS PIGMENTATION?

Pigmentation refers to the color of the skin or its appendages. Normal human skin color is primarily attributable to melanin, along with other chromophores such as hemoglobin and carotenoids. Racial and ethnic differences in skin color occur due to varying number, size, shape, and distribution of melanin-containing organelles called melanosomes, produced by melanocytes. Two types of melanin pigmentation occur in humans—constitutive skin color, which refers to the genetically determined pigmentation, in the absence of environmental or other influences, and facultative (inducible) skin color or "tan," which primarily results from sun exposure.

## HOW DOES PIGMENTATION OCCUR?

The process of formation and distribution of melanin pigment in the skin is called melanogenesis. It grossly involves the steps shown in **Flowchart 1**.

## WHAT ARE THE DISORDERS OF PIGMENTATION?

Pigmentary disorders can be grouped under the following heads:

- *Hyperpigmentation*: Increased pigment deposition causing darkening of skin color
- *Hypopigmentation*: Decreased pigment deposition causing lightening of skin color (complete loss of pigment is called depigmentation)
- *Dyspigmentation/dyschromatosis*: Any abnormality in skin color leading to a combination of hyper- and hypopigmentation.

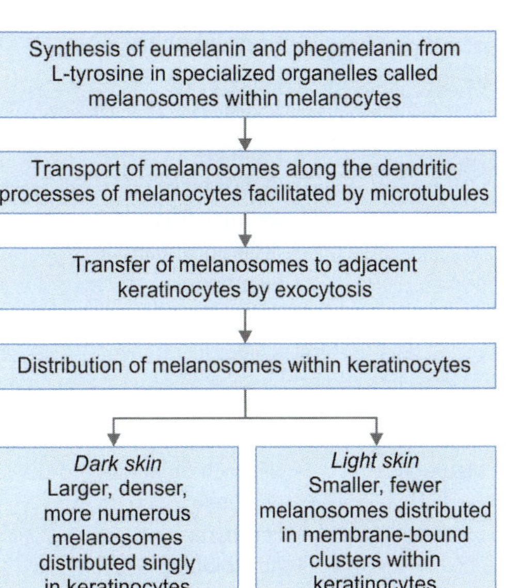


**FLOWCHART 1:** Steps in the process of formation and distribution of melanin pigment in the skin.

## WHAT ARE THE CAUSES OF DIFFERENT TYPES OF PIGMENTATION?

The common causes of hyperpigmentation and hypo- or depigmentation are enumerated in **Tables 1 and 2**, respectively.

**Table 1: Causes of hyperpigmentation.**

| *Etiology* | *Selected examples* |
|---|---|
| Congenital | • Café-au-lait macule<br>• Melanocytic nevus—nevus of Ota, Hori nevus |
| *Acquired* | |
| Infective | • Pityriasis versicolor (hyperpigmented variety)<br>• Chikungunya |
| Inflammatory | • Lichen planus pigmentosus<br>• Fixed drug eruption<br>• Pigmented contact dermatitis (Riehl's melanosis)<br>• Postinflammatory hyperpigmentation |
| Physical agents | • Sun exposure (tanning, freckles, lentigines)<br>• Radiation<br>• Friction/trauma |
| Chemicals and drugs | • Arsenic<br>• Oral contraceptives<br>• Psoralen<br>• Clofazimine<br>• Antimalarials<br>• Cyclophosphamide<br>• Bleomycin<br>• Zidovudine |
| Nutritional | • Pellagra<br>• Kwashiorkor<br>• Marasmus |
| Metabolic | • Hemochromatosis (bronze diabetes)<br>• Porphyria<br>• Amyloidosis<br>• Wilson's disease<br>• Alkaptonuria |
| Endocrine | • Acanthosis nigricans<br>• Addison's disease<br>• Hyperthyroidism<br>• Pheochromocytoma |
| Systemic disease-associated | • Chronic kidney disease<br>• Chronic liver disease<br>• Connective tissue diseases |
| Neoplastic | • Melanoma<br>• Mastocytosis |
| Multifactorial | Melasma |

**Table 2: Causes of hypopigmentation/ depigmentation.**

| *Etiology* | *Selected examples* |
|---|---|
| Congenital | • Albinism<br>• Piebaldism<br>• Waardenburg syndrome<br>• Nevus depigmentosus<br>• Ash-leaf macules (tuberous sclerosis) |
| *Acquired* | |
| Infective | • Pityriasis versicolor<br>• Leprosy<br>Post kala-azar dermal leishmaniasis |
| Inflammatory or immune-mediated | • Vitiligo<br>• Pityriasis alba<br>• Seborrheic dermatitis<br>• Morphea<br>• Lichen sclerosus<br>• Postinflammatory hypopigmentation (following psoriasis, pityriasis rosea, pityriasis lichenoides chronica, etc.) |
| Physical agents | • Thermal injury/burns<br>• Radiation<br>• Mechanical injury |

Continued

*Continued*

| *Etiology* | *Selected examples* |
|---|---|
| Chemicals and drugs (chemical leukoderma) | • Sulfhydryls<br>• Phenolic compounds<br>• Arsenic<br>• Para-phenylene diamine (dyes)<br>• Thiouracil, mercaptobenzothiazole (rubber products)<br>• Corticosteroids—topical and intradermal |
| Nutritional | • Kwashiorkor<br>• Micronutrient deficiencies—copper, selenium |
| Metabolic | Phenylketonuria |
| Endocrine | Hypopituitarism |
| Idiopathic | Idiopathic guttate hypomelanosis |

Dyspigmentation is primarily seen in:

- Genetic disorders—xeroderma pigmentosum, dyschromatosis universalis hereditaria, Dowling-Degos disease, etc.
- Acquired disorders—chronic arsenicosis (leukomelanosis) **(Box 1)**.

## HOW WOULD YOU APPROACH A PATIENT PRESENTING WITH HYPERPIGMENTATION?

As with other medical disorders, patient history is of paramount importance, followed by relevant clinical examination and investigations. The approach is detailed in the following text.

### History

- *Age of onset*:
  - At birth or early childhood—genetic and nevoid conditions, nutritional deficiencies
  - Middle age—melasma
  - Old age—melanoma
- *Gender*: Melasma has a significant female predilection.
- *Residence*: Chronic arsenicosis is commonly found in the districts alongside the river Ganges in West Bengal and in other states in the Ganga/Brahmaputra plains such as the North-Eastern states, Bihar, Jharkhand, and Uttar Pradesh.
- *Duration and progression*:
  - Infective conditions generally have a shorter duration, while inflammatory disorders have a chronic relapsing course.
  - Sudden change in the appearance or size of a mole—melanoma
- *Occupation*:
  - Jewelry makers are prone to develop argyria and chrysiasis due to chronic exposure to silver and gold, respectively.
  - Diffuse hyperpigmentation is common in factory workers using dye, tar, and chromium, as well as among coal miners.
  - Farmers using rodenticides and fungicides and dye industry workers may develop chronic arsenicosis.
  - Occupational exposure to physical agents may be contributory.
- *Personal history*:
  - Outdoor activities—tanning, freckles, lentigines, melasma
  - Use of hair dye—pigmented contact dermatitis
- *Family history:* Contributory factor in genetic and metabolic disorders.
- *Drug history*:
  - Nonsteroidal anti-inflammatory drugs (NSAIDs), tetracyclines, fluoroquinolones, nitroimidazoles—fixed drug eruption
  - Oral contraceptives—melasma
  - Antimalarials—bluish-gray pigmentation
  - Clofazimine—red-brown discoloration

**BOX 1: Four basic patterns of pigmentation in chronic arsenicosis.**

1. Spotty raindrop pigmentation over presternal area, back, and limbs
2. Diffuse hyperpigmentation of the trunk, especially on skin folds
3. Leukomelanosis—hypo- or depigmented macules in a background of normal or hyperpigmentation on chest, back, and arms, sparing the face
4. Blotchy mucosal pigmentation involving the tongue, gums, or buccal mucosa

## Clinical Examination

General examination may reveal features associated with systemic diseases such as icterus in chronic liver disease, pallor in chronic kidney disease, edema in kwashiorkor, and bradycardia in Addison's disease.

Relevant findings in cutaneous examination include the following:

- *Color of pigmentation*:
  - Brown color indicates epidermal pigmentation—freckles, melasma (epidermal), Addison's disease, pellagra.
  - Bluish-gray color is seen in dermal pigmentation due to Tyndall effect—dermal melanocytic nevus, fixed drug eruption, macular amyloidosis, lichen planus pigmentosus, melasma (dermal).
- *Site and pattern of involvement*:
  - Face—melasma **(Fig. 1)**, freckles, nevus of Ota **(Fig. 2)**, Hori nevus, pigmented contact dermatitis
  - Sun-exposed sites—lentigines, pellagra, porphyria
  - Freckle-like pigmentation on centrofacial area, especially tip of the nose—chikungunya
  - Diffuse palmoplantar involvement, raindrop pigmentation on chest, back, and limbs, or oral mucosal involvement—chronic arsenicosis
  - Symmetric involvement of neck, axillae, groins, knuckles with formation of velvety plaques—acanthosis nigricans
  - Lower back and buttocks (in infants)—Mongolian spots

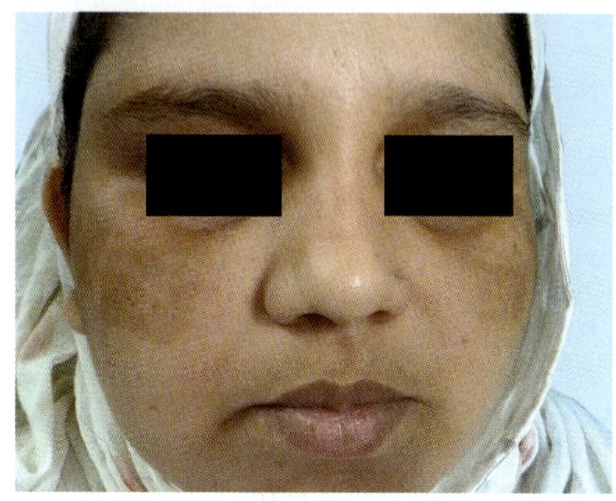

**FIG. 1:** Melasma. Bilaterally symmetrical brown pigmentation (epidermal) over the malar area in a middle-aged female.

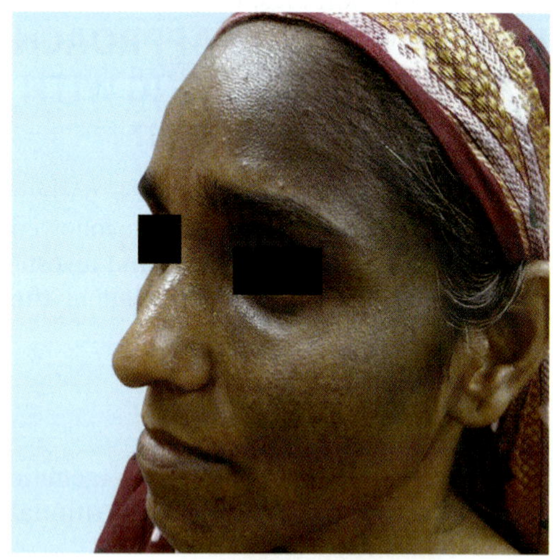

**FIG. 2:** Nevus of Ota. Unilateral bluish-gray pigmentation in the distribution of ophthalmic and maxillary divisions of trigeminal nerve with scleral involvement.

- Preauricular region and temple, progressing to upper back, trunk, and upper extremities—lichen planus pigmentosus
- Rippled hyperpigmentation over upper back and arms—macular amyloidosis
- Frictional areas, nipple, areola, palmar creases, scars, sun-exposed sites, and mucosa—Addison's disease
- Linear involvement along Blaschko's lines—nevoid disorders
- Pigmented macule on palm, sole, subungual or sun-exposed area with variegated pigmentation, induration, or ulceration—melanoma

- *Associated cutaneous, hair and nail findings*:
  - Branny scales over lesions that become prominent with scratching—pityriasis versicolor (hyperpigmented variety) **(Fig. 3A)**.
  - Palmoplantar keratotic pits or keratoderma, oral mucosal pigmentation, Bowen's disease, basal cell carcinoma, squamous cell carcinoma—chronic arsenicosis
  - Acne, skin tags, hirsutism, obesity—acanthosis nigricans
  - Photosensitivity, skin fragility, milia, scarring—porphyria cutanea tarda
  - Dry crackled skin over dorsa of hands, Casal's necklace, photosensitivity—pellagra
  - Dry skin with flaky paint dermatosis, dry lusterless hair with flag sign—kwashiorkor
  - Photosensitivity, blindness, poikiloderma (triad of dyspigmentation, atrophy, and telangiectasia), basal cell carcinoma, squamous cell carcinoma—xeroderma pigmentosum
  - Palmar erythema, spider angioma—chronic liver disease
  - Azure lunulae, Kayser-Fleischer rings in the eye—Wilson's disease
  - Muehrcke's lines (transverse white bands in pairs on nails) and half and half nails (whitish proximal half and reddish-brown distal half)—chronic kidney disease

## Investigations

- *Wood's lamp examination*:
  - To differentiate between epidermal (accentuation of light) and dermal (no accentuation) pigmentation
  - Yellowish-white or copper-orange fluorescence—pityriasis versicolor
  - Red-pink fluorescence of urine and feces—porphyria cutanea tarda

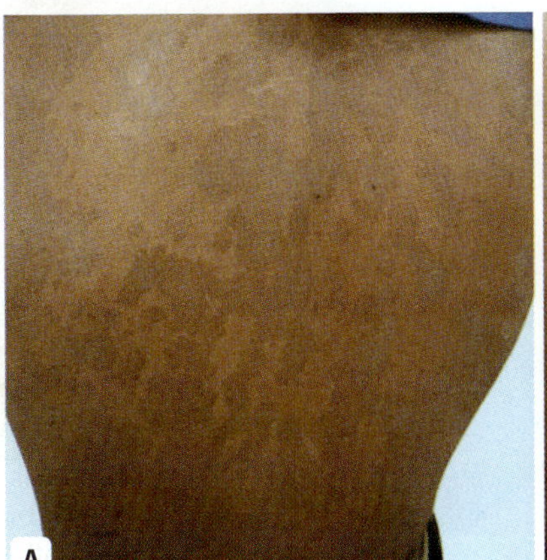


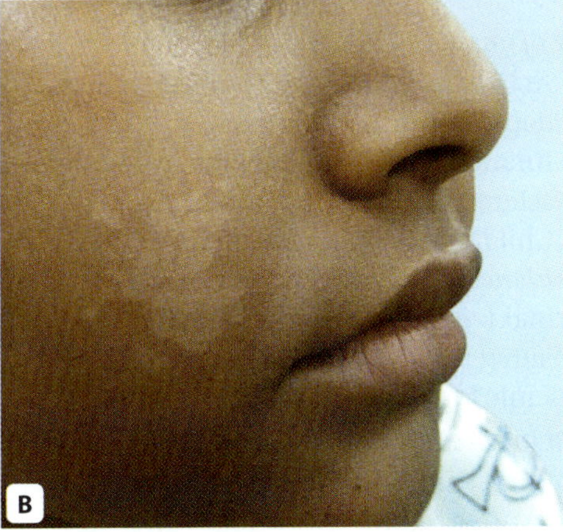


**FIGS. 3A AND B:** Pityriasis versicolor. (A) Hyperpigmented variant; (B) Hypopigmented variant.

- Complete blood count, liver and renal function tests, thyroid profile, blood sugar—to evaluate for systemic, metabolic, and endocrine causes
- *Arsenic levels* in hair, nail, and drinking water—chronic arsenicosis
- *Potassium hydroxide (KOH) mount* of skin scraping—pityriasis versicolor (spaghetti and meatball appearance)
- *Dermoscopy* may help to identify inflammatory and infective conditions, melanocytic nevi, and melanoma.
- *Histopathology* helps to confirm diagnosis by indicating the following:
  - Nature of pigment (melanin, non-melanin, mixed, or undetermined)
  - Localization of pigment (epidermal or dermal)
  - Concomitant increase in the number of melanocytes (present or absent)

## HOW WOULD YOU APPROACH A PATIENT PRESENTING WITH HYPOPIGMENTATION?

Approach to a patient with hypopigmentation involves a detailed history, along with relevant clinical examination and investigations, as detailed below.

### History

- *Age of onset*:
  - At birth—albinism, piebaldism, nevus depigmentosus
  - Infancy—ash-leaf macules (tuberous sclerosis)
  - Childhood—pityriasis alba
- *Residence*: Leprosy and post kala-azar dermal leishmaniasis (PKDL) should be considered in persons hailing from areas endemic for these diseases.
- *Past history*:
  - Burns/mechanical injury/radiation
  - Exposure to chemical agents—chemical leukoderma
  - History of inflammatory skin disease, e.g., psoriasis, pityriasis rosea, pityriasis lichenoides chronica—postinflammatory hypopigmentation
  - History of kala-azar—PKDL
  - History of atopy, asthma, allergic rhinitis—pityriasis alba
- *Family history*—relevant in vitiligo, genetic and metabolic disorders

### Clinical Examination

- *Degree of hypopigmentation*:
  - Depigmented—albinism, piebaldism, vitiligo **(Fig. 4)**, lichen sclerosus, chemical leukoderma, burns
  - Hypopigmented—nevus depigmentosus, pityriasis alba, seborrheic dermatitis, pityriasis versicolor **(Fig. 3B)**, leprosy, PKDL
- *Distribution*:
  - Generalized—albinism, vitiligo universalis, metabolic and nutritional disorders
  - Localized—pityriasis versicolor, leprosy, morphea, lichen sclerosus, focal vitiligo, idiopathic guttate hypomelanosis
- *Site of involvement*:
  - Face—pityriasis alba, seborrheic dermatitis

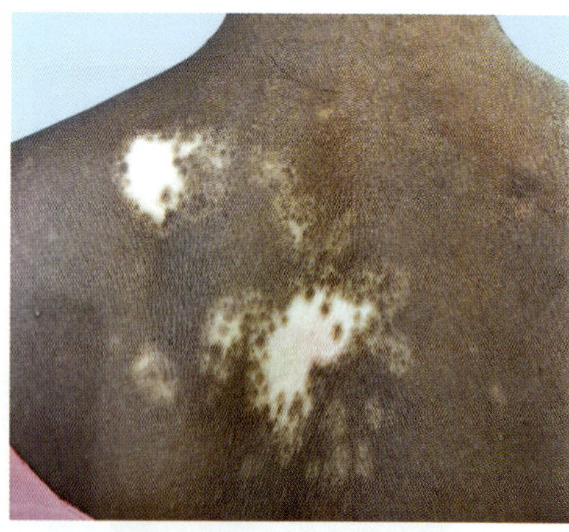

**FIG. 4:** Vitiligo. Well-defined depigmented patches with repigmentation in few areas following treatment.

 - Forehead—piebaldism
 - Acral and periorificial areas—acrofacial vitiligo
 - Chest, axillae, and upper back—pityriasis versicolor
 - Hypo- or depigmented macules in a background of normal or hyperpigmentation on chest, back, and arms, sparing the face (leukomelanosis)—chronic arsenicosis
 - Sun-exposed areas of extremities—idiopathic guttate hypomelanosis
- *Associated cutaneous, hair and nail findings*:
 - White forelock—piebaldism
 - Heterochromia iridis, dystopia canthorum (lateral displacement of medial canthus of the eye)—Waardenburg syndrome
 - Ocular nystagmus—albinism
 - Angiofibromas (adenoma sebaceum), shagreen patch, periungual fibromas—tuberous sclerosis
 - Branny scales over lesions that become prominent with scratching—pityriasis versicolor.
 - Loss of sensation, hair and sweating over lesion, peripheral nerve thickening and tenderness—leprosy
 - Skin-colored, yellow or pink papulonodular lesions over centrofacial area, oral mucosa or genitalia—PKDL
 - Whitening of hair over lesions (leukotrichia)—vitiligo
 - Scaling on scalp with seborrhea—seborrheic dermatitis
 - Tightening and induration of lesional skin—morphea
 - Atrophy, telangiectasia on involved skin—lichen sclerosus

## Investigations

- *Wood's lamp examination*—bluish-white fluorescence with accentuated borders in vitiligo
- *Arsenic levels* in hair, nail, and drinking water—chronic arsenicosis
- *rk39 antigen test*—PKDL
- *Slit skin smear*:
 - Acid-fast bacilli—leprosy
 - Leishman-Donovan bodies—PKDL
- *KOH mount* of skin scraping—pityriasis versicolor (spaghetti and meatball appearance)
- *Histopathology*—confirmatory for specific disorders

## ENUMERATE THE VARIOUS THERAPEUTIC OPTIONS FOR PIGMENTARY DISORDERS

The therapeutic options in hyper- and hypopigmentation are enumerated in **Table 3**.

**Table 3: Therapeutic options in hyperpigmentation and hypopigmentation.**

| | *Hyperpigmentation* | *Hypopigmentation* |
|---|---|---|
| General measures | • Photoprotection, broad-spectrum sunscreens<br>• Avoidance of known triggers<br>• Treatment of underlying infective, systemic, metabolic, endocrine, or nutritional disorder | • Avoidance of offending agent in chemical leukoderma<br>• Treatment of underlying infective, metabolic, endocrine, or nutritional disorder<br>• Cosmetic camouflage |

*Continued*

*Continued*

| | **Hyperpigmentation** | **Hypopigmentation** |
|---|---|---|
| ***Specific measures*** | | |
| Topical | • Depigmenting agents—hydroquinone, kojic aid, tretinoin, glycolic acid, azelaic acid, vitamin C<br>• Corticosteroids<br>• Chemical peels | • Corticosteroids in inflammatory and autoimmune disorders<br>• Tacrolimus<br>• Calcipotriol<br>• Placental extract preparations |
| Systemic | Corticosteroids in inflammatory disorders | Corticosteroids and nonsteroidal immunosuppressants in immune-mediated disorders |
| Physical | Q-switched Nd:YAG laser in melasma, LPP, nevi | • Phototherapy with PUVA or UV-B radiation<br>• Excimer laser in vitiligo |
| Surgical | Excision in melanocytic nevus, melanoma | Skin grafting and melanocyte transfer techniques |

(LPP: lichen planus pigmentosus; PUVA: psoralen plus ultraviolet A; UV-B: ultraviolet B)

## CLINICAL PEARLS

- Pigmentary disorders are a common cause for dermatologic consultation.
- There can be 3 types of pigmentary disorder —hyper or hypo or dyspigmentation.
- There are several causes of pigmentation disorders ranging from local to systemic causes.
- A proper history with clinical examination is essential for correct diagnosis.

## FURTHER READINGS

1. Ghosh P, Roy C, Das NK, Sengupta SR. Epidemiology and prevention of chronic arsenicosis: an Indian perspective. Indian J Dermatol Venereol Leprol. 2008;74(6):582-93.
2. Meys R. Skin pigmentation. Medicine. 2017;45 (7):438-43.

CHAPTER 13

# Pruritus

*Arunima Dhabal, Indrashis Podder, Nilay Kanti Das*

## WHAT IS PRURITUS?

Pruritus indicates an unpleasant sensation, provoking an irresistible desire or urge to scratch. It is often an extremely distressing symptom and considerably affects the patient's quality of life.

## HOW IS PRURITUS CAUSED?

Pruritus can be stimulated by a variety of exogenous stimuli such as mechanical, thermal, electrical, and chemical pruritogens. Keratinocytes, mast cells, and other inflammatory cells also release various endogenous mediators such as histamine, bradykinin, substance P, prostaglandins, and neuropeptides. These mediators bind to receptors on free nerve endings in the skin, which transmit the impulse further via unmyelinated C nerve fibers. The pruritus pathway is shown in **Flowchart 1**.

## WHAT ARE THE COMMON TYPES OF PRURITUS?

Pruritus may be classified on the basis of etiology as follows:

- Dermatological pruritus—arising from skin disease
- Systemic pruritus—arising from internal organ disease
- Neurological pruritus—arising from disorders in the central or peripheral nervous system
- Psychogenic/psychosomatic pruritus—associated with psychiatric or psychosomatic illnesses
- Mixed—coexistence of multiple factors
- Others—unknown origin

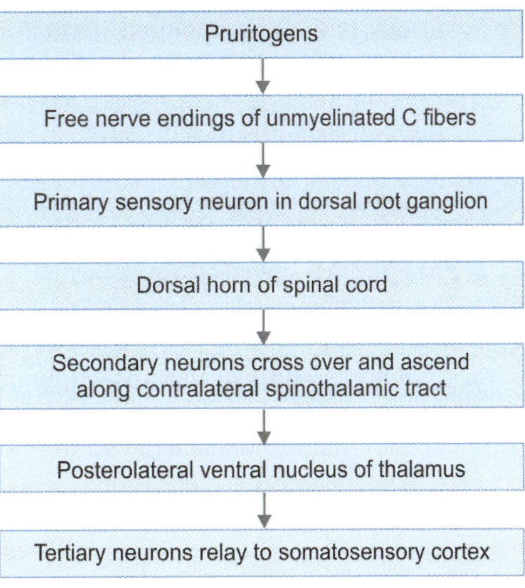


**FLOWCHART 1:** Pruritus pathway.

According to the International Forum for the Study of Itch (IFSI), pruritus can be classified under three heads:

- *Type 1*: Pruritus associated with dermatoses (itching associated with skin disorders)
- *Type 2*: Pruritus associated with normal skin (systemic, neurological, and psychogenic causes)
- *Type 3*: Pruritus associated with chronic scratch lesions (e.g., prurigo)

## ENUMERATE THE COMMON CAUSES OF PRURITUS

Some of the important causes of pruritus are given below.

- *Dermatological causes*:
    - Infections—dermatophytosis, scabies, pediculosis, arthropod reactions, folliculitis, chickenpox
    - Inflammation—atopic dermatitis, contact dermatitis, pompholyx, drug reactions, urticaria, polymorphous light eruption, psoriasis, lichen planus, lichen simplex chronicus
    - Autoimmune—dermatitis herpetiformis, bullous pemphigoid, dermatomyositis, discoid lupus erythematosus
    - Genodermatoses—ichthyosis, Darier's disease, Hailey-Hailey disease
    - Dermatoses of pregnancy—polymorphic eruption of pregnancy, gestational pemphigoid, prurigo gestationis
    - Neoplasms—mycosis fungoides
    - Miscellaneous—xerosis/dry skin
- *Systemic causes*:
    - Infections and infestations—human immunodeficiency virus (HIV)/acquired immunodeficiency syndrome (AIDS), helminthic infestations
    - Metabolic—chronic kidney disease, chronic liver disease with or without cholestasis, malabsorption
    - Endocrine—hyperthyroidism, diabetes
    - Hematological—polycythemia vera, iron deficiency, Hodgkin and nonHodgkin lymphoma
    - Solid organ tumors—tumors of cervix, prostate, colon; carcinoid syndrome
- *Neurological causes*: Multiple sclerosis, postherpetic neuralgia, notalgia paresthetica, brachioradial pruritus, neoplasms, abscesses
- *Psychogenic causes*: Prurigo simplex, prurigo nodularis, anxiety disorders, obsessive-compulsive disorder, delusion of parasitosis, schizophrenia

## HOW WILL YOU APPROACH A PATIENT PRESENTING WITH PRURITUS?

A suitable approach to a patient presenting with pruritus involves detailed history, clinical examination, and relevant investigations, when necessary.

### History

- *Age*:
    - Childhood—atopic dermatitis, scabies
    - Old age—mycosis fungoides, systemic and psychogenic causes
- *Site*:
    - Localized—notalgia paresthetica (scapular area), postherpetic neuralgia (dermatomal), pompholyx (palms and soles), polymorphous light eruption (forearms, neck)
    - Generalized—systemic and psychogenic causes
- *Aggravating factors/triggers*—contact dermatitis, inducible urticaria, aquagenic pruritus, polymorphous light eruption (sun exposure)
- *Past history*:
    - Preexisting skin disease
    - Allergic or atopic diathesis
    - Underlying systemic disease
    - Emotional stress or known psychiatric illness
- *Family history*—genodermatoses, infective diseases (especially scabies) which are contagious
- *Drug history*—opioids, chemotherapeutic drugs, chloroquine

## Clinical Examination

- *General examination*:
  - Icterus—chronic liver disease
  - Pallor, edema—chronic kidney disease
  - Plethora—polycythemia vera
  - Lymphadenopathy—Hodgkin/non-Hodgkin lymphoma, HIV/AIDS
  - Severe weight loss—malignancies, HIV/AIDS
- *Cutaneous examination* for primary and secondary skin lesions
  - Annular polycyclic plaques with central clearing in intertriginous areas—dermatophytosis
  - Papules and excoriations in finger webs, wrists, axillae, areola, periumbilical and genital areas—scabies
  - Dry skin with flexural eczema (or facial and extensor surface involvement in infants)—atopic dermatitis
  - Vesicular lesions on palms and soles—pompholyx
  - Evanescent erythematous, edematous lesions (wheals/hives)—urticaria
  - Well-defined plaques with silvery-white micaceous scales on extensor surfaces and scalp—psoriasis
  - Violaceous, polygonal papules or plaques in flexural distribution—lichen planus
  - Hyperpigmentation, skin thickening, and accentuation of skin markings (lichenification) over frictional areas, ankle, neck, etc.—lichen simplex chronicus
  - Vesicobullous lesions in generalized distribution—bullous pemphigoid
  - Vesicobullous lesions in the periumbilical area in pregnancy—gestational pemphigoid
  - Violaceous papules on dorsal interphalangeal and metacarpophalangeal joints (Gottron's papules), violaceous erythema over the dorsal aspect of fingers (Gottron's sign), around eyelids (heliotrope rash), over deltoids, posterior shoulders and nape of the neck (shawl sign)—dermatomyositis
  - Excoriations and/or hyperpigmented nodular lesions on accessible areas of the body—prurigo simplex/nodularis
- *Systemic examination* to evaluate for an underlying systemic, neurological, or psychological disorder

## Investigations

- *Baseline screening* to evaluate for systemic diseases—complete hemogram, liver and renal function tests, fasting blood sugar, thyroid profile
- *Specific investigations*:
  - Potassium hydroxide (KOH) mount—dermatophytosis
  - Serum immunoglobulin E (IgE)—urticaria, atopic dermatitis
  - Patch test—contact dermatitis
  - Antinuclear antibodies, electromyography (EMG), muscle biopsy—dermatomyositis
  - Skin biopsy—psoriasis, lichen planus, dermatitis herpetiformis, bullous pemphigoid, mycosis fungoides
  - HIV antibodies
  - Stool examination for ova—helminthic infestations
  - Nerve conduction studies, magnetic resonance imaging (MRI)—neurological diseases
  - Chest X-ray, abdominal ultrasound, computed tomography (CT) scan—solid organ tumors

# HOW WILL YOU TREAT A PATIENT PRESENTING WITH PRURITUS?

The treatment strategy would vary depending on the extent of pruritus. A broad overview of the various treatment options is mentioned below.

- *General measures*:
  - Avoidance of aggravating factors such as dry climate, heat, and specific allergens

  - Use of mild soaps, moisturizers, and soft clothing
  - Treatment of underlying conditions
- *Specific measures*:
  - *Topical*:
    - Calamine or other soothing lotions containing menthol, camphor, zinc, etc.
    - Capsaicin—notalgia paresthetica
    - Pramoxine
    - Tacrolimus
    - Corticosteroids—should be used judiciously; potency of the corticosteroid to be used should be based on the diagnosis, patient's age, and site of involvement (e.g., hydrocortisone for atopic dermatitis on face in infancy, clobetasol propionate for pompholyx on palms and soles in adults).
  - *Systemic*:
    - Antihistamines (hydroxyzine, cetirizine, levocetirizine, desloratadine, fexofenadine, bilastine)—second-generation antihistamines are preferred to first-generation antihistamines to avoid adverse effects associated with the latter (e.g., anticholinergic adverse effects, somnolence).
    - Antidepressants (amitriptyline, doxepin, paroxetine, mirtazapine)
    - Ursodeoxycholic acid—chronic liver disease
    - Naltrexone—chronic kidney disease
    - Gabapentin, pregabalin—neurological disorders
    - Corticosteroids—prurigo, eruptive lichen planus
  - *Physical*: Ultraviolet B (UV-B) phototherapy—chronic kidney disease

## CLINICAL PEARLS

- Pruritus is a common presenting symptom in dermatology associated with a myriad of cutaneous, systemic, and neuropsychological conditions.
- Evaluation of pruritus involves detailed history-taking, examination and investigations for assessment of possible causes.
- Treatment of the underlying cause, if present, along with topical, systemic and/or physical agents for symptomatic relief are essential for the management of pruritus.

## FURTHER READINGS

1. Tamargo K, Funovits A, Nguyen TH, Manudhane A, Montanez-Wiscovich ME. Evaluation and Management of the Patient with Pruritus. SN Compr Clin Med. 2019;1:797-805.
2. Rajagopalan M, Saraswat A, Godse K, Shankar DS, Kandhari S, Shenoi SD, et al. Diagnosis and management of chronic pruritus: an expert consensus review. Indian J Dermatol. 2017;62: 7-17.
3. Ständer S. Classification of itch. Curr Probl Dermatol. 2016;50:1-4.

CHAPTER 14

# Erythema

*SK Shahriar Ahmed, Nilay Kanti Das*

## WHAT IS ERYTHEMA?

Erythema derives from the Greek word erythros, which means red. It defines as redness of the skin or mucosa caused due to increased blood flow in superficial capillaries.

## WHAT CAUSES ERYTHEMA?

Erythema occurs due to a cutaneous response toward any infection or inflammation. There is augmented flow of blood through dilated superficial capillaries. Any antigen or immunogen on the skin that is presented by antigen-presenting cells (APC) to the local lymph node causes proliferation of cytotoxic T cells. Then, it releases certain cytokine, chemokine, and inflammatory mediators which cause dilatation of superficial blood vessels. It is the oxygenated hemoglobin that causes erythema and the deoxygenated one produces a bluish hue (cyanosis).

Erythema is blanchable and disappears on finger pressure, while purpura or ecchymosis in the skin does not.

Flushing is a subjective sensation of warmth accompanied by reddening of skin mainly over the face and upper torso. It occurs in certain benign conditions, such as rosacea, fever, and alcohol intake, and in certain serious conditions, such as carcinoid syndrome, pheochromocytoma, anaphylaxis, mastocytosis, and neuroendocrine tumor. Blushing has a close physiological relation to flushing, which occurs in response to some emotional stress, such as embarrassment, anger, romantic stimulation.

## WHAT ARE THE POSSIBILITIES?

- *Physiological cause*: Erythema ab igne, erythema toxicum neonatorum
- *Infectious cause*: Erysipelas, erysipeloid, erythema induratum, erythema infectiosum, erythema chronicum migrans, viral exanthem
- *Congenital diseases*: Erythrokeratoderma variabilis, salmon patch, port-wine stain
- *Immunological diseases*: Erythema multiforme, erythema nodosum, erythroderma, erythema nodosum leprosum, lupus erythematosus, erythromelalgia, rosacea
- *Neutrophilic dermatosis*: Erythema elevatum diutinum
- *Neoplastic manifestation*: Erythema gyratum repens, erythroplasia of Queyrat
- *Drug reaction*: Topical steroid damaged/dependent face (TSDF), drug causing flushing (e.g., vasodilators, calcium channel blocker, nicotinic acid, cholinergic drug, systemic steroid), exanthematous drug reactions

## WHAT ARE THE PHYSIOLOGICAL CONDITIONS THAT CAUSE ERYTHEMA?

### Erythema Ab Igne

Erythema ab igne is a cutaneous rash which presents as erythema followed by hyperpigmentation in a reticulated pattern. It is caused by repeated occupational exposure of the skin to direct heat or infrared radiation. The condition is mostly benign. Livedo reticularis also presents in similar fashion consisting of a reticulated purplish discoloration of the skin mostly involving the lower limb. The discoloration is caused by reduction in blood flow through the arterioles, resulting in accumulation of deoxygenated blood. The condition is pathological and may be associated with several autoimmune diseases, lymphoma, pancreatitis, cryoglobulinemia, antiphospholipid syndrome, etc.

### Erythema (Toxicum) Neonatorum

Erythema (toxicum) neonatorum is a benign absolutely nontoxic dermatosis which presents within the first week of life and usually resolves within 7–14 days. There are self-limited, transient, evanescent tiny eruptions of yellowish pustules and papules with an erythematous background that occurs in 48–72% of infants. They are usually found over the trunk and proximal extremities, sparing the palms and soles. No treatment is generally required.

## WHAT ARE THE INFECTIVE CAUSES OF ERYTHEMA?

### Erysipelas

Erysipelas is a bacterial infection, caused by group A streptococci, involving the dermis and characteristically extends into the superficial cutaneous lymphatics. It presents as a tender, erythematous, indurated plaque with a sharply demarcated border and is associated with high fever and lymphadenopathy. The well-defined margin can help differentiate it from cellulitis, which is also a bacterial infection involving the dermis and subcutaneous tissues. Lower extremity is the most common site of involvement followed by the face. Antistreptococci antibiotics should be initiated when erysipelas is suspected, and penicillin as monotherapy remains the antibiotic of choice.

### Erysipeloid

Erysipeloid is an occupational dermatosis caused by a gram-positive bacillus called *Erysipelothrix rhusiopathiae*. Humans acquire erysipeloid through traumatized skin after direct contact with infected animals. Homemakers, farmers, butchers, and anglers are more prone to get infected. It presents as an erythematous edema with well-defined and raised borders. The back of the hand and fingers are most commonly involved. Rapid remission occurs after treatment with penicillin or cephalosporin group of drugs.

### Erythema Induratum

Erythema induratum is a type of panniculitis which presents as chronic and recurrent tender subcutaneous nodules, sometimes ulcerate, and heals with atrophic scarring. It occurs mainly in women, and calves are the most common site of involvement. There are two types of erythema induratum, one is related to tuberculosis (erythema induratum of Bazin) and other is of nontubercular origin (erythema induratum of Whitfield). Other causes could be infection with *Nocardia, Pseudomonas, chlamydia, Fusarium,* hepatitis C and hepatitis B, etc., autoimmune disease, Crohn's disease, and propylthiouracil therapy.

### Erythema Infectiosum

Erythema infectiosum is caused by infection with parvovirus B19, also known as the fifth disease or slapped cheek syndrome. It typically presents as an erythematous rash over bilateral cheeks and exanthem and occurs more commonly in children of 5–15 years age group. Only 2 out of 10 individuals will present with physical symptoms. The route of transmission is primarily via droplets from respiratory secretions. Treatment is mostly supportive.

### Viral Exanthem

Viral exanthem is a maculopapular rash which appears first over the face and then involves the whole body with a cephalocaudal distribution. It is generally associated with fever and enanthem. The most common viruses include nonpolio enteroviruses, dengue, Epstein–Barr virus, human herpes viruses 6 and 7, parvovirus B19, measles, rubella, mumps, hepatitis viruses, human immunodeficiency virus (HIV) (seroconversion), corona, Zika, etc. Drug rash can also present with a similar type of eruption, but it generally starts from the axilla and groin and then spreads to the limb and trunk. Itching is prominent in drug rash.

## WHAT IS FIGURATE ERYTHEMA? WHAT ARE THE CAUSES?

Figurate erythema (FE) is a heterogeneous group of dermatoses which classically presents as annular, concentric, polycyclic, or arciform erythematous lesions with a tendency to spread centrifugally. Four classic FE are erythema annulare centrifugum, erythema gyratum repens, erythema migrans, and erythema marginatum.

### Erythema Annulare Centrifugum

Erythema annulare centrifugum is a chronic, reactive phenomenon of the skin which presents as an annular, erythematous lesion which enlarges centrifugally and clears centrally. A fine scale appears inside the advancing edge known as a trailing of scale. It has been associated with various underlying conditions, such as fungal infection (dermatophytes and *Candida)*, viruses (Epstein-Barr virus, poxvirus, HIV, etc.), parasites, ectoparasites (*Phthirus pubis*), and bacteria (*Pseudomonas, Escherichia coli*). Some food and drugs [cimetidine, salicylate, diuretics, nonsteroidal anti-inflammatory drugs (NSAIDs), antimalarials, amitriptyline, etc.], autoimmune disease, and malignancy have also been implicated.

### Erythema Gyratum Repens

Erythema gyratum repens is a rare paraneoplastic syndrome which presents as concentric erythematous rings forming a wood-grain appearance. The rings migrate in waves, with the leading edge progressing about 1 cm/day. There is nearly 80% association with an underlying malignancy, and among them, lung cancer is the most common one (33–47%), followed by esophageal, breast, and stomach cancer. It usually resolves once the malignancy has been removed.

### Erythema (Chronicum) Migrans

Erythema (chronicum) migrans appears 7–14 days after tick detachment and typically presents as an expanding erythematous annular macule, usually ≥5 cm in diameter with central clearing forming a bull's eye pattern. The most common sites include the thigh, back, shoulder, and calf. It frequently appears as one of the first and most common symptoms of Lyme disease, caused by the bacteria *Borrelia burgdorferi*. The bacteria are transmitted to humans through infected deer ticks, and the bite mark can sometimes be identified at or near the center of the lesion. Systemic symptoms such as malaise, headache, fatigue, migratory arthralgia, and fever may be present. Treatment includes various antibiotics such as doxycycline and synthetic penicillins.

### Erythema Marginatum

Erythema marginatum is reactive inflammatory erythema commonly associated with acute rheumatic fever. Although a rare cutaneous manifestation, it has got the utmost diagnostic value for acute rheumatic fever and is considered as a major Jones criterion. It presents as an evanescent, blanchable, nonpruritic macular rash distributed generally over the trunk and extremities usually sparing the face. However, the treatment of an underlying condition may not always eliminate the clinical course of the dermatoses.

## WHAT COULD BE THE CAUSES OF FACIAL ERYTHEMA?

### Topical Steroid Damaged/Dependent Face

Topical steroid damaged/dependent face (TSDF) occurs due to severe cutaneous damage on prolonged misuse/abuse/overuse of topical corticosteroid of any potency over the face. This results in the development of erythema, monomorphic acne, atrophy, telangiectasia, and hirsutism.

### Rosacea

Rosacea is characterized by eruptions of pimples and pustules over the face along with flushing, erythema, and telangiectasia. There are four subtypes: Erythematotelangiectatic, papulopustular, phymatous, and ocular. The triggering factors are hot spicy food, caffeine, alcohol, sunlight, stress, exercise, certain cosmetics, etc. Sunscreen, topical brimonidine, oxymetazoline, azelaic acid, ivermectin, metronidazole, and systemic macrolides or retinoids are advisable.

### Malar Rash

Malar rash is characterized by a flat fixed erythematous rash which presents over the bridge of the nose and cheeks, sparing nasolabial folds. It is present in approximately 46–65% of people with systemic lupus erythematosus (SLE). It may appear long before other symptoms of SLE are seen. Investigations should be made thoroughly considering SLE and its complication.

## WHAT ARE THE GENITAL DERMATOSES WHICH PRESENT WITH ERYTHEMA?

### Erythroplasia of Queyrat

Erythroplasia of Queyrat is an in situ squamous cell carcinoma of the penis which mostly occurs in uncircumcised men. It presents as well-marginated erythematous velvety shiny plaques generally involving glans and prepuce. In 30% of cases, it could turn into an invasive carcinoma, and spontaneous regression is unlikely. Treatment includes topical therapy with 5-fluorouracil or 5% imiquimod cream, laser therapy, photodynamic therapy, and local resection.

On the other hand, *Zoon balanitis* (ZB) is a benign, nonvenereal chronic inflammatory mucositis, which presents as a single, well-defined, shiny, persistent, orange-red, glistening macular to slightly raised plaque usually over the glans. Multiple pinpoints and brighter red spots may be seen called "cayenne pepper spots." In histology, dense band-like infiltrates of plasma cells are seen at the papillary dermis. Topical treatment options are corticosteroid, tacrolimus, imiquimod 5%, etc., but circumcision is the most definite treatment of ZB.

### What is the Most Severe Form of Erythema?

### Erythroderma

Erythroderma is a form of generalized inflammatory dermatoses, where erythema and scaling involve >90% of the skin surface. Mostly, it is associated with an underlying inflammatory skin condition, which can result in a variety of systemic symptoms and life-threatening complications. Causes can be psoriasis, atopic dermatitis, allergic contact dermatitis, cutaneous T-cell lymphoma, drug reaction, seborrheic dermatitis, pityriasis rubra pilaris, sarcoidosis, connective tissue diseases like systemic lupus/dermatomyositis, pemphigus foliaceus, infections (e.g., dermatophytosis, Norwegian scabies, staphylococcal scalded skin syndrome), and idiopathic. Complications are temperature dysregulation, fluid-electrolyte and acid-base imbalance, secondary bacterial infections, high-output cardiac failure, hypoalbuminemia, acute respiratory distress syndrome (ARDS), etc. It is a dermatologic emergency where immediate hospitalization is advisable. Maintaining the skin barrier through the application of plenty of moisturizer is the most important part of management. Nutritional support, adequate hydration, maintaining electrolyte and acid-base balance, and antibiotics for secondary infection are also required. Once the underlying diagnosis is established, targeted therapy should be introduced promptly.

## DISCUSS ERYTHEMA NODOSUM AND ERYTHEMA NODOSUM LEPROSUM

### Erythema Nodosum

Erythema nodosum is the most common clinical form of septal panniculitis without vasculitis. It appears as erythematous, firm, tender deep nodules, usually located symmetrically over the shin, but can also be present over thighs, arms, and neck. Females are affected three to six times more. They do not have a tendency to necrosis and resolve spontaneously without sequelae within 2–8 weeks. Systemic symptoms such as fever, malaise, and arthralgia can be associated. The most common underlying cause is infection (e.g., *Streptococcus*, *Mycoplasma*, *Yersinia* species, *Histoplasma*, psittacosis, *chlamydia*, and *Mycobacterium*). Other causes could be sarcoidosis, drugs [oral contraceptive pills (OCP), iodides, bromides, sulfonamides, tumor necrosis factor (TNF)-alpha inhibitor, etc.], pregnancy, malignancy (leukemia, lymphoma, etc.), enteropathies, and idiopathic. Treatment of the underlying etiology is most important along with bed rest, NSAIDs, and a saturated solution of potassium iodide is recommended.

### Erythema Nodosum Leprosum

Erythema nodosum leprosum is a form of type III hypersensitivity reaction which occurs mostly in lepromatous poles of leprosy. It presents with crops of painful, evanescent, erythematous nodules with systemic symptoms of fever and malaise. It affects multiple systems, and manifestations include iritis, arthritis, lymphadenitis, orchitis, neuritis, etc. Lobular panniculitis with vasculitis is a classical finding in histopathology. High-dose oral corticosteroids or thalidomide is the treatment of choice.

## WHAT IS ERYTHEMA ELEVATUM DIUTINUM?

Erythema elevatum diutinum is a form of cutaneous small-vessel vasculitis consisting of violaceous or red-brown papules and plaques distributed mainly over the extensors. They appear mainly over the dorsal hands and feet, knees, and elbows. They first appear as a soft pseudovesicular type of eruptions, eventually turn into fibrotic plaque or nodule, and heal with atrophic scarring. Mostly, lesions are asymptomatic, but sometimes they present with pain or burning sensation. They sometimes can be associated with some infections, hematologic abnormalities, or autoimmune diseases. Early histopathological features are leukocytoclastic vasculitis with some fibrin deposition and eosinophilic infiltrate; gradually histiocytic infiltrates and fibrosis are formed. Dapsone is the treatment of choice at early stages.

## WHAT IS A TARGET LESION AND WHERE IS IT FOUND?

Target lesion over the skin consists of central dusky erythema/necrosis/vesicle, surrounded by pallor and followed by an erythematous ring. It is seen in erythema multiforme. It is a type IV hypersensitivity reaction that involves both skin and mucosa; it classically presents with a target lesion. It is generally preceded by viral infections, most commonly herpes simplex virus (HSV) and *Mycoplasma pneumonia*. The other association could be infections with Epstein–Barr virus, cytomegalovirus, HIV, hepatitis C virus, influenza virus, tuberculosis, *Streptococcus*, and certain drugs such as sulfonamides, antiepileptics, NSAIDs, penicillins, and cephalosporins. It is divided into two broad categories: EM minor (mucosa not involved) and EM major (mucosa involved). Treatment is generally conservative as the lesions typically resolve over the course of several weeks.

## WHAT IS ERYTHROKERATODERMA VARIABILIS?

Erythrokeratoderma variabilis is an autosomal dominant type keratinization disorder, first described by Mendes da Costa, and presents with migratory transient erythema and fixed hyperkeratotic plaques. It commonly appears in the early stage of life. The lesions are usually distributed on the extensor surface of extremities, buttocks, and face. There is a mutation in gap junction proteins including connexin 31 and connexin 30.3. Genetic counseling and systemic retinoid are the mainstay of management.

## WHAT IS ERYTHROMELALGIA?

Erythromelalgia is a rare entity which classically presents with a triad of episodic appearance of severe erythema, warmth, and recurrent intense burning pain, mostly affecting the extremities (hands and feet). The episodes are typically precipitated by exercise or exposure to heat and relieved by cold. Although it typically affects bilaterally, it may sometimes involve unilaterally, especially in secondary cases. Primary erythromelalgia is an autosomal dominant condition where mutation occurs in the *SCN9A*, *SCN10A*, and *SCN11A* genes. Secondary erythromelalgia is associated with hematological conditions such as myeloproliferative disorders, including essential thrombocytosis, polycythemia vera, myelofibrosis, etc., and with certain drugs (e.g., bromocriptine, nifedipine, nicardipine), peripheral neuropathy, and autoimmune disease. Oral medications such as calcium antagonists, selective serotonin reuptake inhibitors (SSRIs), tricyclic antidepressants, gabapentin, or carbamazepine may help in the improvement of symptoms.

## CLINICAL PEARLS

- Erythema is an important cutaneous sign, which gives clue to diagnose various dermatoses.
- Emotional flushing is called blushing
- Various infections give rise to certain classical cutaneous erythema like Erysipelas, erysipeloid, erythema induratum, erythema infectiosum, erythema chronicum migrans which we should not miss.
- Figurate eythema comprises some of the very important dermatoses
- Facial erythema can be a mirror of underlying culprit
- We should be very cautious in a case where patient presents with generalized erythema.

## FURTHER READINGS

1. Britannica T. Editors of Encyclopaedia (2023, December 15). erythema. Encyclopedia Britannica. https://www.britannica.com/science/erythema.
2. Boehner A, Neuhauser R, Zink A, Ring J. Figurate erythemas - update and diagnostic approach. J Dtsch Dermatol Ges. 2021;19(7): 963-72.
3. Khandpur S, Sethy PK, Sharma VK, Das P. An atypical presentation of erythema induratum. Indian J Dermatol Venereol Leprol. 2008;74: 505-6.
4. Sharma V, Mahajan VK, Mehta KS, Chauhan PS, Chander B. Erythema elevatum diutinum. Indian J Dermatol Venereol Leprol. 2013;79: 238-9.
5. Brahma D, Jain VK, Aggarwal K. Erythrokeratoderma variabilis. Indian J Dermatol Venereol Leprol. 2003;69:5-6.
6. Okoduwa C, Lambert WC, Schwartz RA, Kubeyinje E, Eitokpah A, Sinha S, Chen W. Erythroderma: Review of a potentially life-threatening dermatosis. Indian J Dermatol. 2009; 54:1-6.
7. Afra T, Daroach M, Mahajan R, De D, Handa S. Pustular lesions in the neonate: Focused diagnostic approach based on clinical clues. Indian J Dermatol Venereol Leprol. 2022;88: 708-16.
8. Veraldi S, Girgenti V, Dassoni F, Gianotti R. Erysipeloid: a review. Clin Exp Dermatol. 2009; 34(8):859-62.

# CHAPTER 15

# Urticarial Rash

*Rupsa Mukhopadhyay, Chandan Chatterjee*

## WHAT IS URTICARIA?

*Definition*: Urticaria (also known as urticarial rash or hives) is raised, well-circumscribed areas of erythema (redness) and edema (swelling) involving the dermis and epidermis that are very pruritic (itchy), ranging in size from few millimeters to several centimeters in diameter, lasting few hours or days before disappearing, and can appear in one part of the body or be spread across large areas.

## WHAT ARE THE DIFFERENT TYPES?

Urticaria may be: (1) *acute*—if the rash clears completely within 6 weeks, (2) *chronic*—if the rash persists or comes and goes for >6 weeks, often over years, (3) *rarer type*—urticaria vasculitis that can cause blood vessels inside the skin to be inflamed, wheals lasting longer than 24 hours, more painful and can leave a bruise, and (4) *physical or inducible urticaria* which might pop up when in cold, heat, sun, vibrations, pressure, exercising, and sweating.

## WHAT ARE THE COMMON SYMPTOMS?

Common symptoms are itchy skin with raised bumps, reddish colored, blanch on pressure with swelling under the skin causing puffiness (angioedema), sometimes even painful swelling of lips, eyes, and inner throat.

*Pathophysiology*: Urticaria is caused by an immune response triggered by the release of histamine and other chemical mediators from mast cells and basophils in the skin. These chemicals cause blood vessels to dilate, leading to swelling and redness of the skin.

## WHAT ARE THE COMMON CAUSES?

*Etiology*: Common causes include allergic reactions to food, medications, insect bites, and exposure to environmental factors such as pollen or pet dander. It can also be triggered by stress, infection, or autoimmune disorders. Sometimes, the cause is unknown, known as idiopathic urticaria.

*Path to diagnosis*: Diagnosis is made by clinical examination of the skin, asking the patient's medical history, including any recent exposure to potential allergens.

*Tests*: Allergy tests can help in identifying what is triggering the reaction such as follows: (1) *Skin prick tests or scratch tests*—here, different allergens are tested on the skin. If the skin turns red or swells, it means the allergic reaction to the substance is positive. (2) *Blood tests*—checking for specific antibodies in the blood.

## HOW DO YOU TREAT THIS CASE?

Treatment of this case involves lifestyle changes such as avoiding certain foods, environmental triggers, wearing loose clothes, and identifying and avoiding any triggers that may cause such chemical reactions. Pharmacological management includes antihistaminics (loratadine, cetirizine, etc.), corticosteroids, or immunomodulating agents. Stress management techniques such as relaxation exercises or counseling may be helpful in reducing the frequency and severity of outbreaks. Nowadays, allergic shots in the form of monthly injections of drugs are given that block allergic reactions.

## WHAT ARE THE COMMON COMPLICATIONS (RED FLAG SIGN)?

Angioedema (swelling in deeper layers of the skin, often severe caused by buildup fluid), anaphylaxis, and emotional impact such as stress, anxiety, and depression are common complications.

## WHAT IS THE PROGNOSIS?

For most people, it does not cause any serious problem. Children often outgrow allergies that cause hives. In the fewest cases, swelling of airways and lungs occurs in which injectable epinephrines are administered.

## CLINICAL PEARLS

Thus, urticarial rash is a common skin condition that is caused by an immune response triggered by the release of histamine and other chemical mediators. Diagnosis is made by clinical examination and history; treatment involves identifying and avoiding triggers as well as medications to relieve symptoms. With proper management, most cases of urticaria can be effectively controlled and patients can enjoy a good quality of life.

## FURTHER READINGS

1. McSweeney SM, Christou EAA, Maurer M, Grattan CE, Tziotzios C, McGrath JA. Physical urticaria: Clinical features, pathogenesis, diagnostic work-up, and management. J Am Acad Dermatol. 2023. doi: 10.1016/j.jaad.2023.02.062.
2. Bernstein JA, Lang DM, Khan DA, Craig T, Dreyfus D, Hsieh F, et al. The diagnosis and management of acute and chronic urticaria: 2014 update. J Allergy Clin Immunol. 2014; 133(5):1270-7.

# CHAPTER 16

# Macular Rash

*Chandan Chatterjee*

## WHAT IS A MACULAR RASH?

A macular rash is a skin condition characterized by the appearance of flat, discolored spots on the skin. These spots are often reddish or brownish in color and may appear as single spots or in groups. Macular rashes can be caused by a variety of factors, including viral infections, autoimmune disorders, and allergic reactions.

## WHAT IS THE PATHOPHYSIOLOGY?

The pathophysiology of a macular rash depends on the underlying cause of the rash. In some cases, the rash may be caused by an inflammatory response triggered by the immune system. In other cases, it may be caused by a viral or bacterial infection that affects the skin. In all cases, the appearance of the rash is due to changes in the skin's blood vessels, which may become dilated or leaky.

## WHAT ARE THE CAUSES?

There are many different factors that can cause a macular rash. Some of the most common causes include viral infections such as measles or rubella, bacterial infections such as Lyme disease or Rocky Mountain spotted fever, autoimmune disorders such as lupus or psoriasis, and allergic reactions to medications or other substances. In some cases, the cause of the rash may be unknown.

## HOW WILL YOU APPROACH THE PATIENT?

The approach to a patient with a macular rash will depend on the underlying cause of the rash. In most cases, a diagnosis can be made based on a physical examination of the skin and a review of the patient's medical history. Additional tests may be needed in some cases to confirm the diagnosis or rule out other possible causes.

## WHAT IS THE TREATMENT FOR A MACULAR RASH?

The treatment for a macular rash will depend on the underlying cause of the rash. In many cases, the rash will go away on its own without treatment. In other cases, medications may be needed to treat the underlying condition causing the rash. For example, antihistamines may be used to treat an allergic reaction, while antibiotics may be used to treat a bacterial infection.

## CLINICAL PEARLS

A macular rash is a skin condition characterized by the appearance of flat, discolored spots on the skin. The underlying cause of the rash can vary but may include viral or bacterial infections, autoimmune disorders, or allergic reactions. Treatment for a macular rash will depend on the underlying cause of the rash and may include medications or other treatments to address the underlying condition.

## FURTHER READINGS

1. Biesbroeck L, Sidbury R. Viral exanthems: an update. Dermatol Ther. 2013;26(6):433-8.
2. Hogan DJ, Noll KC. Common bacterial skin infections. Am Fam Physician. 2012;85(8):863-8.

CHAPTER 17

# Papular Rash

*Chandan Chatterjee*

## WHAT IS PAPULAR RASH?

A papular rash is a skin condition characterized by small, raised bumps on the skin that are often red or pink in color. These bumps, called papules, can appear in various sizes and can be clustered together or spread out over a large area. A papular rash can be caused by a wide range of conditions and may be a symptom of an underlying illness.

## WHAT IS THE PATHOPHYSIOLOGY?

The pathophysiology of a papular rash depends on the underlying cause. Papules are typically caused by inflammation of the skin due to an immune response to an irritant, infection, or allergic reaction. The papules can also form as a result of a buildup of cells or substances in the skin, such as keratin or oil. In some cases, the cause of a papular rash may be unknown.

## WHAT ARE THE CAUSES?

The etiology of a papular rash is varied and can include a range of underlying conditions.

Common causes of a papular rash include:

- Allergic reactions to medications, foods, or other substances
- Infectious diseases such as chickenpox, shingles, or scabies
- Autoimmune disorders such as lupus or dermatomyositis
- Skin conditions such as eczema or psoriasis
- Reaction to environmental irritants such as poison ivy or insect bites
- Genetic or hereditary conditions such as neurofibromatosis or tuberous sclerosis

## WHAT ARE THE SYMPTOMS AND SIGNS?

Symptoms of a papular rash may vary depending on the underlying cause. In general, the papules may be itchy or painful and can appear anywhere on the body. The rash may also be accompanied by other symptoms such as fever, fatigue, or joint pain. Some conditions that cause papular rashes, such as chickenpox, may also cause other symptoms such as headache or sore throat.

## HOW WILL YOU APPROACH A PATIENT?

The approach to treating a papular rash will depend on the underlying cause. In some cases, the rash may resolve on its own without treatment. In other cases, treatment may be necessary to alleviate symptoms and prevent complications.

If a patient presents with a papular rash, the healthcare provider will likely perform a physical examination and take a medical history to identify any potential underlying conditions. The provider may also order diagnostic tests such as blood tests or skin biopsies to help identify the cause of the rash.

Treatment for a papular rash may include:

- Topical or oral medications to reduce inflammation or itching
- Antibiotics or antiviral medications to treat underlying infections
- Allergy medications or immunotherapy to treat allergic reactions
- Moisturizers or emollients to soothe dry or irritated skin
- Lifestyle changes to avoid environmental triggers or irritants

## CLINICAL PEARLS

A papular rash is a common skin condition characterized by small, raised bumps on the skin that can be caused by a wide range of underlying conditions.

The pathophysiology of a papular rash is typically related to inflammation or buildup of cells or substances in the skin.

Treatment will depend on the underlying cause and may include medications, lifestyle changes, or other interventions to alleviate symptoms and prevent complications.

## FURTHER READINGS

1. Adhicari P, Das S. A hospital-based study on the pattern of papulosquamous disorders in children in a tertiary care center of northeast India. Int Organ Sci Res J Dent Med Sci. 2016;15:10-4.
2. Ramdurg RP, Dogra S. Approach to Papulo-squamous Eruptions. Indian Journal of Dermatology. 2013;58(4):255-8.

# CHAPTER 18

# Scaly Rash

*Sramana Palit, Chandan Chatterjee*

## WHAT ARE SCALY RASHES?

Scaly rashes are defined as abnormal growth or accumulation of dead skin cells on the surface of the skin, resulting in a rough, scaly texture. These lesions can occur due to a variety of underlying medical conditions and may be classified as either primary or secondary lesions.

## WHAT ARE THE COMMON CAUSES?

The causes of scaly lesions are numerous and can include a variety of factors such as:

- *Skin conditions*: These include psoriasis, eczema, seborrheic dermatitis, and lichen planus.
- *Fungal infections*: Fungal infections such as ringworm, candidiasis, and tinea versicolor can lead to scaly lesions.
- *Allergic reactions*: Allergic reactions to drugs, food, or other environmental factors can cause scaly lesions.
- *Autoimmune disorders*: Autoimmune disorders such as lupus and scleroderma can also cause scaly lesions.

## PATHOPHYSIOLOGY

The pathophysiology of scaly lesions is complex and varies depending on the underlying condition. However, the most common pathway involves the hyperproliferation of skin cells, leading to the buildup of dead skin cells on the surface of the skin. This can result in inflammation, itching, and flaking of the affected area.

## HOW WILL YOU APPROACH A PATIENT?

When a patient presents with scaly lesions, a thorough medical history and physical examination are essential to identify any underlying medical conditions that may be contributing to the development of the lesions. The physician may also perform a skin biopsy to confirm the diagnosis.

## WHAT ARE THE RED FLAG SIGNS?

In some cases, scaly lesions may be a sign of a more serious underlying medical condition. Red flag signs that warrant further evaluation include:

- Rapidly growing or changing lesions
- Lesions that bleed or ooze
- Lesions that are painful or itchy
- Lesions that are associated with other symptoms such as fever, weight loss, or fatigue

## HOW WILL YOU TREAT SUCH CASES?

The treatment of scaly lesions depends on the underlying medical condition. For example, topical corticosteroids may be used to treat psoriasis, while antifungal medications may be prescribed for fungal infections. Moisturizers and emollients can be used to relieve itching and reduce dryness in the affected area.

## CLINICAL PEARLS

Scaly lesions are a common dermatological problem that can be caused by a variety of underlying medical conditions. A thorough medical history and physical examination are essential to identify any underlying conditions, and red flag signs should be evaluated further. Treatment depends on the underlying condition, and moisturizers and emollients can be used to relieve itching and dryness in the affected area.

## FURTHER READINGS

1. Siegfried EC, Hebert AA. Diagnosis of Atopic Dermatitis: Mimics, Overlaps, and Complications. J Clin Med. 2015;4(5):884-917.
2. Kantor R, Thyssen JP, Paller AS, Silverberg JI. Atopic dermatitis, atopic eczema, or eczema? A systematic review, meta-analysis, and recommendation for uniform use of 'atopic dermatitis'. Allergy. 2016;71(10):1480-5.

CHAPTER 19

# Vesicular Rash

*Dippyoman Ghosh, Chandan Chatterjee*

## WHAT IS VESICULAR RASH?

A vesicular rash is characterized by the presence of vesicles, which are small, fluid-filled blisters or sacs that can appear on the skin. Vesicles typically have a size of less than 5 millimeters (mm) in diameter. These blisters contain clear or sometimes cloudy fluid and can be surrounded by redness and inflammation. This type of rash can be caused by a variety of factors and may be accompanied by other symptoms, such as itching or pain.

## WHAT IS THE PATHOPHYSIOLOGY?

The pathophysiology of a vesicular rash varies depending on the underlying cause. In general, a vesicular rash occurs when there is an abnormal accumulation of fluid between the layers of the skin. This can be caused by a variety of factors such as infection, allergic reaction, or physical injury.

## WHAT ARE THE CAUSES?

A vesicular rash can be caused by a variety of factors, including:

- *Viral infections*: Viral infections, such as herpes simplex or chickenpox, can cause vesicular rash.
- *Allergic reactions*: Allergic reactions to certain foods, medications, or environmental factors can cause vesicular rash.
- *Autoimmune disorders*: Autoimmune disorders, such as lupus or pemphigus, can cause vesicular rash.
- *Contact dermatitis*: Contact dermatitis is a skin condition caused by exposure to irritants or allergens, which can lead to vesicular rash.
- *Insect bites or stings*: Insect bites or stings can cause vesicular rash as an allergic reaction.

## HOW WILL YOU APPROACH THE DIAGNOSIS?

The diagnosis of vesicular rash usually involves a physical examination of the affected area and a review of the patient's medical history. The doctor may also perform tests, such as skin biopsies or blood tests, to help identify the underlying cause of the rash.

## RED FLAG SIGN

A vesicular rash is characterized by fluid-filled blisters on the skin. A red flag sign is when the rash is accompanied by fever, pain, or a burning sensation, which may indicate an underlying infection or a serious medical condition. Additionally, if the rash appears suddenly or spreads rapidly, it may warrant medical attention.

## HOW WILL YOU TREAT SUCH CASES?

The treatment of a vesicular rash depends on the underlying cause. In general, treatment may include the following:

- *Antiviral medications*: These can be used to treat vesicular rash caused by viral infections such as herpes simplex or chickenpox.
- *Topical medications*: Topical medications, such as corticosteroids or antihistamines, can be used to reduce inflammation and itching associated with vesicular rash.
- *Systemic medications*: In some cases, systemic medications, such as oral steroids or immunosuppressants, may be necessary to treat the underlying condition.
- *Moisturizers*: Moisturizers can help to soothe dry or irritated skin associated with vesicular rash.
- *Lifestyle changes*: Certain lifestyle changes, such as avoiding irritants or allergens, can help to prevent a vesicular rash from occurring.

## CLINICAL PEARLS

A vesicular rash is a skin condition characterized by the presence of small, fluid-filled blisters on the skin surface.

It can be caused by a variety of factors and may be accompanied by other symptoms, such as itching or pain.

Diagnosis usually involves a physical examination and review of medical history, and treatment depends on the underlying cause.

With proper management, most causes of vesicular rash can be effectively controlled, and patients can enjoy a good quality of life.

## FURTHER READINGS

1. Kimberlin DW, Whitley RJ. Herpes Simplex Virus Infections. N Engl J Med. 2013;369(3): 254-65.
2. Gershon AA. Varicella-Zoster Virus Infections: Varicella (Chickenpox) and Herpes Zoster (Shingles). In Harrison's Principles of Internal Medicine, 20th Edition. 2018.

CHAPTER 20

# Oral Ulcers

*Komal Aggarwal*

## WHAT ARE ORAL ULCERS?

Ulceration or breaks in the continuity of the mucosa of the oral cavity is known as an oral ulcer. Common sites of involvement are:

- Oral mucosa (lips and inner side of cheeks)
- Gingivae
- Floor of mouth
- Uvula and palate
- Tongue

## WHAT ARE THE TYPES?

Oral ulcers can be broadly classified into acute and chronic according to their presentation and progression. Usually, if an ulcer lasts for >2 weeks, it is considered chronic.

## WHAT ARE THE COMMON CAUSES?

The common causes are mentioned in **Box 1**.

## WHICH ARE THE DRUGS REPORTED TO CAUSE ORAL ULCERS?

The common drugs reported to cause oral ulcers are:

- Beta-blockers
- Mycophenolate mofetil
- Bisphosphonates such as alendronate
- Nonsteroidal anti-inflammatory drugs (NSAIDs)
- Vasodilators such as nicorandil
- Antihypertensives such as enalapril or captopril

**BOX 1: Causes of oral ulcers.**

*Acute oral ulcers*:
- Aphthous stomatitis
- Traumatic
- Behçet's disease
- Viral infections
- Bacterial infections—Vincent's angina, syphilis
- Erythema multiforme
- Allergic reactions

*Chronic oral ulcers*:
- Drug induced
- Erosive lichen planus
- Pemphigus vulgaris
- Lupus erythematosus
- Reiter's disease
- Tuberculosis
- Fungal infections
- Squamous cell carcinoma (SCC)

## WHAT ARE THE VIRUSES THAT COMMONLY CAUSE ORAL ULCERS?

- Herpes simplex virus (HSV)
- Varicella/herpes zoster
- Human immunodeficiency virus (HIV) infection
- Coxsackie virus—herpangina and hand-foot-and-mouth disease
- Epstein–Barr virus
- *Human herpes virus 8*: Oral Kaposi sarcoma
- Measles virus
- Cytomegalovirus

## WHAT ARE THE FUNGAL INFECTIONS THAT CAN CAUSE ORAL ULCERS?

- *Oral candidiasis*: It is the most common oral fungal infection. It may have various clinical presentations, such as—
    - Oral thrush/acute pseudomembranous candidiasis
    - Chronic pseudomembranous candidiasis
    - Acute atrophic candidiasis
    - Chronic atrophic/erythematosus candidiasis
    - Angular cheilitis
    - Median rhomboid glossitis
    - Chronic multifocal candidiasis
    - Hyperplastic candidiasis
- Histoplasmosis
- Cryptococcosis
- Coccidioidomycosis

## WHAT IS RECURRENT APHTHOUS STOMATITIS?

Recurrent aphthous stomatitis (RAS) is also known as aphthae or canker sores and is characterized by multiple, recurrent, painful, round, or ovoid ulcers with circumscribed margins with an erythematous halo.

## WHAT IS THE PATHOGENESIS BEHIND RECURRENT APHTHOUS STOMATITIS?

Recurrent aphthous stomatitis occurs because of T lymphocyte-mediated localized destruction of oral mucosa.

## WHAT ARE THE PREDISPOSING FACTORS OR ETIOLOGY OF RECURRENT APHTHOUS STOMATITIS?

- Family history [association with human leukocyte antigen (HLA)]
- Autoimmune factors
- Hormonal changes
- Stress
- Zinc deficiency
- Local trauma
- Infectious agents

## WHAT ARE THE TYPES OF APHTHOUS ULCERS?

- *Minor or Mikulicz ulcer*: Ulcers are 2–4 mm in size and heal without scarring.
- *Major or Sutton's ulcer*: Ulcers are >10 mm in size and heal with scar.
- *Herpetiform aphthae*: Multiple ulcers of 2 mm all through the oral cavity and heal without scar.

## WHAT IS HERPES SIMPLEX STOMATITIS?

Herpes simplex stomatitis is caused commonly by HSV-1 and very rarely by HSV-2. The incubation period is usually 3–7 days. It may be a primary or secondary infection.

- *Primary herpes gingivostomatitis*: It presents as diffuse purple boggy gingivitis followed by the formation of vesicles. The vesicles rupture and coalesce to form ulcers covered with yellowish membrane. It is commonly seen on the tongue, lips, pharynx, lips, and palate.
- Secondary infection presents as herpes labialis, which affects the mucocutaneous junction of the lips. It heals in 7–10 days leaving scabs.

# HOW WILL YOU APPROACH A CASE OF ORAL ULCERS?

- History
- Clinical examination
- Investigations

## History

Oral ulcers are mostly diagnosed clinically and rarely require the help of investigations. Important points to be considered in history are as follows:

- Duration of ulcers so as to classify them into acute and chronic
- Association of pain **(Box 2)**
- History of dentures (traumatic ulcers)
- History of drug intake
- Any recent infections
- Signs of immunosuppression

**BOX 2: Classification of oral ulcers on the basis of pain.**

*Painless oral ulcers*:
- Systemic lupus erythematosus
- Discoid lupus erythematosus
- Syphilis
- Malignancy

*Painful oral ulcers*:
- Traumatic
- Aphthous ulcers
- Infections like HSV, VZV
- Erythema multiforme
- Pemphigus vulgaris
- Erosive lichen planus

(HSV: herpes simplex virus; VZV: varicella zoster virus)

## Clinical Examination

On inspection, it is important to examine the number, size, and site of ulcers. The site of ulcers gives a clue about the cause, for example:

- *Hard palate*: Systemic lupus erythematosus (SLE), discoid lupus erythematosus (DLE), pemphigus vulgaris
- *Buccal mucosa*: Aphthous ulcer, pemphigus vulgaris, erosive lichen planus (LP)
- *Tongue*: Squamous cell carcinoma (SCC), erosive LP, nutritional deficiencies

On palpation, the ulcers may be soft or indurated. Common causes of ulcers with induration are syphilitic chancre, fungal infections, and malignancy.

## Investigations

As mentioned earlier, oral ulcers are a clinical diagnosis and investigations are rarely needed. Common investigations that may help are:

- Complete blood count
- Serum ferritin, B12, iron level
- Serology for HIV and venereal disease research laboratory (VDRL)
- Blood for antinuclear antibody (ANA)
- Tzanck smear
- Pathergy test
- Oral mucosal biopsy followed by suitable staining

# WHAT ARE THE TREATMENT OPTIONS FOR ORAL ULCERS?

- It is important to remove any artificial dentures or address causes of trauma in the oral cavity.
- In case of drug-induced oral ulcers, offending drugs should be stopped immediately.
- *Good oral hygiene is vital*: Warm saline gargles or chlorhexidine mouthwash should be used after meals.

- Triggers such as hot spicy food and citrus fruits must be avoided.
- To address nutritional deficiencies, if any.
- Supportive care in the form of analgesics and hydration should be added.
- In case of painful ulcers, topical lidocaine can be used to alleviate the pain.
- In addition to the above general measures, specific measures are to be taken where oral ulcers are associated with an underlying dermatological or autoimmune condition.

## CLINICAL PEARLS

- Mouth ulcers can be broadly classified into acute and chronic according to their presentation and progression. Usually, if an ulcer lasts for >2 weeks, it is considered chronic.
- Drug-induced oral ulcers are commonly seen with beta-blockers, mycophenolate mofetil, bisphosphonates, and NSAIDs.
- Oral ulcers due to SLE, DLE, syphilis, and carcinoma are usually painless.
- Painful oral ulcers are seen in erosive LP, aphthous ulcers, pemphigus vulgaris, erythema multiforme, and trauma.
- Common causes of ulcers with induration are syphilitic chancre, fungal infections, and malignancy.
- Oral ulcers are mostly diagnosed clinically and rarely require help of investigations.

## FURTHER READINGS

1. Mortazavi H, Safi Y, Baharvand M, Rahmani S. Diagnostic features of common oral ulcerative lesions: an updated decision tree. Int J Dent. 2016;2016:7278925.
2. Muñoz-Corcuera M, Esparza-Gómez G, González-Moles MA, Bascones-Martínez A. Oral ulcers: clinical aspects. A tool for dermatologists. Part I. Acute ulcers. Clin Exp Dermatol. 2009;34(3):289-94.
3. Muñoz-Corcuera M, Esparza-Gómez G, González-Moles MA, Bascones-Martínez A. Oral ulcers: clinical aspects. A tool for dermatologists. Part II. Chronic ulcers. Clin Exp Dermatol. 2009; 34(4):456-61.
4. Bruce AJ, Dabade TS, Burkemper NM. Diagnosing oral ulcers. JAAPA. 2015;28:1-10.

# CHAPTER 21

# Excessive Loss of Hair

*Dishari Haldar, Disha Chakraborty*

## WHAT IS HAIR LOSS?

### Definition

Hair is an important cosmetic asset. Excessive loss of hair is also known as alopecia. It is one of the most common complaints to the doctors and is sometimes very difficult to treat. It is a multifactorial phenomenon. Telogen effluvium (TE) is the most common cause, followed by androgenetic alopecia (AGA) and chronic telogen effluvium (CTE); the rest of the causes are not so common. The problem arises in differentiating between TE, AGA, and CTE, which account for the majority of diffuse alopecia.

### Causes

The causes of excessive hair loss are mentioned in **Box 1**.

**BOX 1: Causes of excessive hair loss.**

- Telogen effluvium (TE)
- Androgenetic alopecia and pattern hair loss
- Chronic telogen effluvium (CTE)
- Anagen effluvium
- Loose anagen hair syndrome
- Diffuse type of alopecia areata
- Congenital atrichia, congenital hypotrichosis, and hair shaft abnormalities (hair breakage, unruly hairs)

### Differential Diagnosis

#### *Telogen Effluvium*

Telogen effluvium is characterized by an abrupt onset and rapid, diffuse, self-limited, excessive shedding of normal club hairs, usually seen 2–3 months after a triggering event. It occurs due to premature termination of anagen into catagen and telogen hair follicle. Among the various causes, the most common ones are severe febrile illness, postpartum (telogen gravidarum), accidental trauma, major surgery, emotional stress, chronic systemic illness, large hemorrhage, and crash diet. Acute TE or classical TE is a self-limiting condition which lasts for about 3–6 months. CTE is chronic diffuse loss persisting beyond 6 months. The causes of chronic diffuse TE are iron deficiency anemia, hypo/hyperthyroidism, malnutrition, acrodermatitis enteropathica, and acquired zinc deficiency **(Box 2)**.

#### *Androgenetic Alopecia and Pattern Hair Loss*

It is a gradual onset, slowly progressive non-scarring alopecia most commonly seen in the age group of 20–40 years. It results from a progressive reduction of successive hair cycle time leading to miniaturization of hair follicles. These changes are mediated through interaction between androgens,

**BOX 2: Causes of telogen effluvium (TE).**

- *Physiologic conditions*: Postpartum effluvium (telogen gravidarum), physiologic effluvium of newborn, early stage of androgenetic alopecia
- *Physical or emotional stress*: Severe febrile illness, severe infection, crash diet, starvation, malnutrition, kwashiorkor, marasmus, malabsorption, iron deficiency, hypo- or hyperthyroidism, acrodermatitis enteropathica, acquired zinc deficiency, major surgery, traumatic accident, chronic illness [systemic lupus erythematosus (SLE), syphilis, hepatic and renal failure], advanced malignancy, chronic telogen effluvium (idiopathic), severe psychological stress
- *Drugs*: Oral retinoids, especially etretinate and acitretin, high-dose contraceptive pills (OCP) or hormone replacement therapy (HRT), antithyroids, anticoagulants (especially heparin), and anticonvulsants, hypolipidemic drugs, heavy metals, beta-blockers

their respective receptors, and enzymes such as 5α-reductase and p450 aromatase. As the pattern of hair loss differs between men and women, the terms "male pattern hair loss" and "female pattern hair loss" (FPHL) are also used although the "male" pattern may occur in women and vice versa. Pattern hair loss in men is predominantly due to a combination of genetic predisposition and the effect of androgens; hence, the term AGA is often applied. Pattern hair loss in women has also long been referred to as female AGA.

#### Male Pattern Hair Loss

The age of onset of male balding is highly variable. The Hamilton–Norwood scale is used for grading male pattern hair loss. The posterior and lateral scalp margins are relatively spared and only affected in the most advanced cases and with old age **(Fig. 1)**.

#### Female Pattern Hair Loss

The clinical presentation of pattern hair loss in women differs from men. Women may present with either an episodic or a continuous increase in hair shedding without any noticeable reduction in hair volume, increased hair shedding with loss of hair volume over the crown, or diffuse thinning over the crown with no history of hair shedding. The pattern of hair loss in women was first defined by Ludwig. FPHL presents with diffuse thinning (loss of hair volume) over the midfrontal scalp with minimal or no bitemporal recession. Vertex baldness is rare.

Three types of FPHL patterns have been described.

1. *Diffuse central thinning (Ludwig type)*: The diffuse hair loss is concentrated over the frontoparietal region leading to thinning/rarefaction over the central scalp with intact frontal hairline **(Fig. 1)**. Ludwig graded it into three stages depending upon whether the central thinning is mild (stage I), moderate (stage II), or severe, that is, near-complete baldness of the crown (stage III).
2. *Frontal accentuation (Olsen type)*: It leads to the widening of the central parting line and thereafter to a Christmas-tree pattern.
3. *Frontotemporal recession/vertex loss (male pattern/Hamilton type)*: It leads to the recession of frontotemporal hairline or bitemporal recession and/or thinning at the vertex.

The first two types are common and the third type is seen infrequently. The first type is often confused with CTE.

### Chronic Telogen Effluvium

Chronic telogen effluvium is characterized by an excessive alarming diffuse shedding of hairs in females aged 30–60 years, with a prolonged fluctuating course and near-normal histology. It is hypothesized that it is due to reduction in the duration of the anagen growth phase without miniaturization of hair follicles. The exact etiology is unknown.

#### Path to Diagnosis

- *History*:
  - *Presenting complaints*: Most patients may present with complaints of

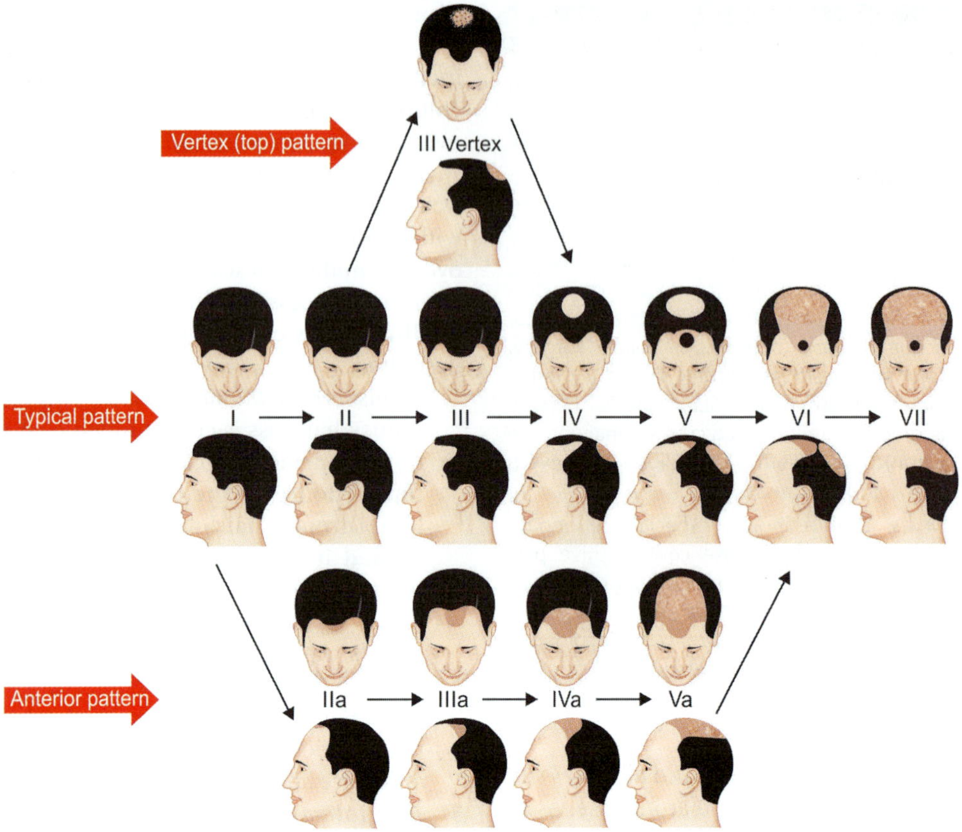

FIG. 1: Hamilton scale for male androgenetic alopecia.

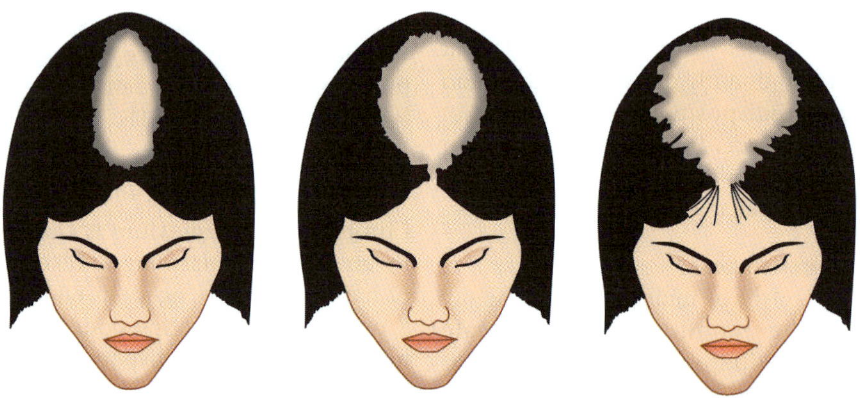

FIG. 2: Ludwig scale for female patterned hair loss classification.

gradual thinning of hair in a pattern. Patients should be asked if the hair is found on the pillows, carpets, in the shower, or while brushing. Family history should be taken in case of genetic hair loss. History of itching, burning, and pain should be included as it may be associated with inflammation, which will lead to scarring. Female patients should be asked about their menstrual cycle and the presence of hair on the face as hair shedding can be due to hormonal imbalances. Contraceptive history should be recorded. Other factors such as physical illness, psychological stress, new medications, diet restriction, and loss of weight may aggravate hair loss.

- *Clinical examination*: This should include visual assessment of the hair loss pattern. It may be diffuse or patchy. The pattern of the hair loss should be seen as it may be male pattern hair loss or FPHL. Hair color, shine, and texture can also be changed due to hair shedding for a prolonged period.
    - *Hair pull test*: This test has high interoperator variability. It is performed to assess hair shedding in generalized hair loss and disease activity in focal alopecia. Approximately 60 hairs are grasped between the thumb and the index and middle fingers and gently pulled. A negative test (≤6 hairs obtained) indicates normal shedding, whereas a positive test (>6 hairs obtained) indicates active hair shedding. The extracted hair gives a clue to the diagnosis.
    - *TE*: Sudden-onset, rapid diffuse generalized shedding of hairs, usually seen 2–3 months after a triggering event. Nearly 100–1,000 hairs/day may be lost. Hair pull test is found to be strongly positive. Usually, >10% of the total hairs pulled are easily extracted from any part of the scalp in the acute phase of TE.
    - *AGA*: Gradual-onset, slowly progressive hair loss, which is often diffuse, and predominantly affects the frontoparietal region leading to central thinning with intact frontal hairline or widening of central parting line. Presence of miniaturized or vellus hairs (short thin hairs <3 cm and a shaft diameter ≤0.03 mm) at the frontoparietal region is an important diagnostic feature of AGA. Vellus hairs along with bald scalp are more commonly seen in males than in females. However, absolute bald area is not a feature of FPHL. Hair pull test is usually negative. Shedding may or may not be present, and if present, it is mild.
    - *CTE*: Chunks of hair are seen in the bathroom, pillow, brush, and comb. History of abrupt, excessive, alarming, diffuse, and generalized shedding of hair is the main feature of CTE. Moderate-to-severe bitemporal recession may also be seen. A positive hair pull test at all sites of the scalp (vertex, occiput, and sides) is seen in an active phase. There is no underlying cause of CTE.
- *Investigation*:
    - *TE*: Videodermoscopy will show a large number of short-tip pointed regrowing hairs in the absence of hair diameter variability.

      Biopsy shows normal histology except for an increase in the telogen follicles. The proportion of normal telogen follicles in excess of 15% is considered suggestive of TE and 25% or more is definite TE. Though biopsy is not absolutely necessary, it helps to differentiate TE from diffuse alopecia areata.

      History and examination will generally suggest the cause of TE, and if not, then a minimum battery of laboratory tests, which includes complete blood count (CBC), routine urine, serum ferritin, triiodothyronine (T3), thyroxine (T4), and thyroid-stimulating hormone (TSH) should be performed Iron deficiency anemia and thyroid hormone disorders are the two common conditions associated with TE.
    - *AGA*: On dermoscopy, hair shaft diameter diversity is a key feature of

AGA. Peripilar halos and peripilar atrophy can also be seen during dermoscopy in a few patients of androgenetic hair loss.
Hair pull test is usually negative.
Histopathological examination shows miniaturization of hair follicles, which is the histological hallmark of FPHL and leads to a significant reduction of the terminal to vellus hair ratio. If the ratio becomes <4:1, it is diagnostic of AGA.
    - *CTE*: A positive hair pull test at all sites of the scalp (vertex, occiput, and sides) is seen in an active phase.
    On dermoscopy, there is no significant variation or miniaturization. The ratio of terminal and vellus hair is normal (8:1).
- *Therapy*:
    - *General measures*: Identification and treatment of the underlying cause.
    *Reassurance to the patients*: All the hair lost would be replaced by regrowth and does not lead to baldness. TE generally ceases within 3–6 months if the stimulus is removed, while CTE may take 3–10 years.
    *Treatment of iron deficiency and thyroid disorder*: Oral iron sulfate 300 mg (60 mg elemental iron) thrice daily may be given till a concentration of 70 μg/mL of serum ferritin is achieved. Screening for T3, T4, and TSH is also recommended.
    Proper dietary intake, vitamin A, vitamin A containing preparations such as antioxidants, etretinate, acitretin, and high-dose contraceptive pills (OCP)/hormone replacement therapy (HRT), etc., should be stopped or replaced with suitable substitutes.
    - *Specific treatment*:
        - *TE*: TE does not require specific drugs as the condition is self-limiting and usually resolves in 3–6 months if the trigger is removed. Complete recovery may take 1 year.
        - *AGA or pattern hair loss*: Female pattern hair loss—minoxidil topical solution 2% for mild-to-moderate FPHL (Ludwig stages I and II) without hyperandrogenism.
        Minoxidil 2% plus antiandrogens/finasteride for mild-to-moderate FPHL (Ludwig stages I and II) with hyperandrogenism.
        Male pattern hair loss—minoxidil topical solution 5% twice daily for mild-to-moderate hair loss.
        Topical minoxidil has been shown to arrest hair loss and/or induce mild-to-moderate growth. Minoxidil increases the duration of anagen and enlarges miniaturized hair follicles. It is applied as 1 mL twice daily to dry scalp, preferably through a dropper. Efficacy of minoxidil should not be judged before 6–12 months.
        Adverse effects of minoxidil are not so common. These include irritation, hypertrichosis over the forehead and cheeks (avoid manual spread of minoxidil to sites other than the scalp), which disappears within 4 months of stopping the treatment, allergic contact dermatitis, and temporary self-limited shedding (TE) of hair which begins at 2–8 weeks after treatment and subsides shortly with continued treatment. Minoxidil should not be used in pregnant and nursing mothers.
        *Antiandrogens*: Antiandrogens are beneficial, especially in cases of FPHL with hyperandrogenism. Systemic antiandrogens, spironolactone (100–300 mg/day), flutamide (250–500 mg twice or thrice a day), and cyproterone acetate are effective.

Finasteride (1-1.25 mg/day) is a potent 5α-reductase (type II) inhibitor which blocks the conversion of testosterone to dehydrotestosterone (DTH). It has shown positive results in AGA with hyperandrogonism.
    - *CTE*: There are no specific drugs for CTE. Empiric use of topical minoxidil 2% has been suggested in anticipation that it will prolong anagen growth. It is said that CTE is a self-limiting process, which may resolve spontaneously in 3–10 years.
  - Hair prosthesis (wig, hair extension, hairpiece) and hair cosmetics (tinted powders, lotions, sprays) for severe FPHL (Ludwig stage III).
  - *Hair transplantation*: Ideal candidates for hair transplantation are moderate cases of FPHL (Ludwig stage II) who have high-density donor hair (>40 follicular unit/cm$^2$) in some areas and extensive loss or thinning at frontal or midfrontal scalp only.

**Poor Prognostic Indicators**

- Grade > 4
- Old age
- Immunosuppression
- Genetic predisposition

## CLINICAL PEARLS

1. *Patient History is Key*:
    - Take a detailed patient history, including family history of hair loss, recent life events, diet, and any significant changes in medication or lifestyle.
2. *Pattern Recognition*:
    - Recognize the different patterns of hair loss, such as androgenetic alopecia (male/female pattern baldness), alopecia areata, telogen effluvium, and scarring alopecias.
3. *Scalp Examination*:
    - Thoroughly examine the scalp for signs of inflammation, scarring, or infections. A scalp biopsy may be necessary in certain cases.
4. *Laboratory Investigations*:
    - Conduct appropriate laboratory tests, including complete blood count, thyroid function tests, iron studies, and hormonal assessments to rule out systemic causes of hair loss.
5. *Nutritional Considerations*:
    - Emphasize the importance of a balanced diet rich in vitamins and minerals, particularly iron, zinc, and biotin, for maintaining healthy hair.
6. *Topical Minoxidil*:
    - Discuss the use of topical minoxidil as a common and effective treatment option for androgenetic alopecia. Emphasize patient compliance and realistic expectations.
7. *Hormonal Therapies*:
    - Consider hormonal therapies, such as finasteride for men or spironolactone for women, in cases of androgenetic alopecia under appropriate clinical supervision.
8. *Alopecia Areata Management*:
    - Highlight the unpredictable nature of alopecia areata and the various treatment modalities, including intralesional corticosteroid injections, topical immunotherapy, and systemic immunosuppressive agents.
9. *Telogen Effluvium Management*:
    - Address underlying causes of telogen effluvium, such as stress, nutritional deficiencies, or hormonal imbalances. Educate patients on the transient nature of this condition.
10. *Patient Education*:
    - Provide comprehensive patient education on the natural hair growth cycle, the importance of early intervention, and the realistic expectations of treatment outcomes.

11. *Psychosocial Impact*:
    - Acknowledge and address the psychological impact of hair loss on patients. Consider collaborating with mental health professionals when necessary.
12. *Follow-up and Monitoring*:
    - Stress the importance of regular follow-up appointments to monitor treatment progress and adjust therapeutic approaches as needed.

## FURTHER READINGS

1. Kligman AM. Pathologic dynamics of hair loss. I. Telogen effluvium. Arch Dermatol. 1961;83: 175-98.
2. Headington JT. Telogen effluvium. New concepts and views. Arch Dermatol. 1993;129: 356-63.
3. Fiedler VC, Hafeez A. Diffuse alopecia: telogen hair loss. In: Olsen EA (Ed). Disorders of Hair Growth. Diagnosis and Treatment, 2nd edition. New York: McGraw Hill; 2003. pp. 301-21.
4. Bordin MB. Drug-related alopecia. Dermatol Clin. 1987;5:571-9.
5. Shapiro J, Wiseman M, Lui H. Practical management of hair loss. Can Fam Physician. 2000;46:1469-77.
6. Thiedke CC. Alopecia in women. Am Fam Physician. 2003;67:1007-14.
7. Chong AH, Wade M, Sinclarer RD. The hair pull test and hair pluck for analysis of hair abnormalities. Modern Med Australia. 1999;42: 105-18.
8. Shapiro J, Lui H. Common hair loss disorders. In: Hordiwnsky MK, Sawaya ME, Scher RK (Eds). Atlas of Hair and Nails. London Churchill Livingston; 2000. pp. 91-103.
9. Saitoh M, Uzuka M, Sakamoto M. Human hair cycle. J Invest Dermatol. 1970;54:65-81.
10. Dhurat R. Phototrichogram. Indian J Dermatol Venereol Leprol. 2006;72:242-4.
11. Hoffman R. TrichoScan: combining epiluminescence microscopy with digital image analysis for the measurement of hair growth in vivo. Eur J Dermatol. 2001;11:362-8.
12. Tosti A, Piraccini BM. Telogen effluvium. In: Tosti A, Piraccini BM (Eds). Diagnosis and Treatment of Hair Disorders. UK: Taylor and France; 2006. pp. 57-61.
13. Ross EK, Vincenzi C, Tosti A. Videodermoscopy in the evaluation of hair and scalp disorders. J Am Acad Dermatol. 2006;55:799-806.
14. de Lacharriere O, Deloche C, Miscicali C, Piraccini BM, Vincenzi C, Bastein P, et al. Hair diameter diversity: a clinical sign reflecting the follicle miniaturization. Arch Dermatol. 2001; 137:641-6.
15. Lacarruba F, Dall'Oglio F, Rita Nasca M, Micali G. Videodermatoscopy enhances diagnostic capability in some forms of hair loss. Am J Clin Dermatol. 2004;5:205-8.
16. Whiting D, Howsden F. Colour Atlas of Differential Diagnosis of Hair Loss. Cedar Grove, NJ: Carnfield Publishing; 1996.
17. Sperling L. Evaluation of hair loss. Curr Probl Dermatol. 1996;8:99-136.
18. Loffrede M. Inflammatory diseases of hair follicles, sweat glands and cartilage. In: Elder D, Elenitsas R, Johnson BL, Murphy GF (Eds). Lever's Histopathology of the Skin, 9th edition. Philadelphia: Lippincott Williams and Wilkins; 2005. pp. 483-5.
19. Trost LB, Bergfeld WF, Calogeras E. The diagnosis and treatment of iron deficiency and its potential relationship to hair loss. J Am Acad Dermatol. 2006;54:824-44.
20. Ross EK, Shapiro J. Management of hair loss. Dermatol Clin. 2005;23:227-43.
21. Chartier MB, Hoss DM, Grant-Kels JM. Approach to the adult female patient with diffuse nonscarring alopecia. J Am Acad Dermatol. 2002;47:809-18.
22. Sinclair R. Diffuse hair loss. Int J Dermatol. 1999;38:8-18.
23. Pringle T. The relationship between thyroxine, oestradiol, and postnatal alopecia, with relevance to women's health in general. Med Hypotheses. 2000;55:44-9.
24. Dallob AL, Sadick NS, Unger W, Lipert S, Geissler LA, Gregoire SL, et al. The effect of finasteride, a 5 alpha-reductase inhibitor, on scalp skin testosterone and dihydrotestosterone

concentrations in patients with male pattern baldness. J Clin Endocrinol Metab. 1994;79:703-6.
25. Sawaya MF, Price VH. Different levels of 5 alpha-reductase type I and II, aromatase, and androgen receptor in hair follicles of women and men with androgenetic alopecia. J Invest Dermatol. 1997;109:296-300.
26. Olsen EA. Hair. In: Freedberg IM, Eisen AZ, Wolff K, Austen KF, Goldsmith LA, Katz SI (Eds). Fitzpatrick's Dermatology in General Medicine, 6th edition. New York: McGraw Hill Publishing; 2003. pp. 643-4.
27. Futterweit MD, Dunaif A, Yeh HC, Kingslay P. The prevalence of hyperandrogenism in 109 consecutive female patients with diffuse alopecia. J Am Acad Dermatol. 1988;19:831-6.
28. Pitaway DE. Neoplastic causes of hyperandrogenism. Infertil Reprod Med Clin North Am. 1991;2:479-94.
29. Whiting DA. Scalp biopsy as a diagnostic and prognostic tool in androgenetic alopecia. Dermatol Ther. 1998;3:24-33.
30. Whiting DA. Diagnostic and predictive value of horizontal sections of scalp biopsy specimens in male pattern androgenetic alopecia. J Am Acad Dermatol. 1993;28:755-63.
31. Whiting DA. Chronic telogen effluvium: increased scalp hair shedding in middle-aged women. J Am Acad Dermatol. 1996;35:899-906.
32. Rebora A, Guarrera M, Baldari M, Vechhio F. Distinguishing androgenetic alopecia from chronic telogen effluvium when associated in the same patient: a simple noninvasive method. Arch Dermatol. 2005;141:1243-5.
33. Sinclair R, Jolley D, Mallari R, Maqee J. The reliability of horizontally sectioned scalp biopsies in the diagnosis of chronic diffuse telogen hair loss in women. J Am Acad Dermatol. 2004;51:189-99.
34. Kantor J, Kessier LJ, Brooks DG, Cotsarelis G. Decreased serum ferritin is associated with alopecia in women. J Invest Dermatol. 2003;121:985-8.
35. Sinclair R. There is no clear association between low serum ferritin and chronic diffuse telogen hair loss. Br J Dermatol. 2002;147:982-4.
36. Aydingöz IE, Ferhanoğlu B, Güney O. Does tissue iron status have a role in female alopecia? J Eur Acad Dermatol Venereol. 1999;13:65-7.
37. Rushton DH. Management of hair loss in women. Dermatol Clin. 1993;11:47-53.
38. White MI, Currie J, Williams MP. A study of tissue iron status of patients with alopecia areata. Br J Dermatol. 1994;130:261-3.
39. Rushton DH. Nutritional factors and hair loss. Clin Exp Dermatol. 2002;27:396-404.
40. Boffa MJ, Wood P, Griffiths CE. Iron status of patients with alopecia areata. Br J Dermatol. 1995;132:662-4.
41. Rushton DH, Ramsay ID, James KC, Norris MJ, Gillkis JJ. Biomedical and trichological characterization of diffuse alopecia in women. Br J Dermatol. 1990;123:187-97.
42. Olsen EA. Iron deficiency and hair loss: the jury is still out. J Am Acad Dermatol. 2006;54:903-6.
43. Goddard AF, McIntyre AS, Scott BB. Guidelines for the management of iron deficiency anaemia. British Society of Gastroenterology. Gut. 2000;46:IV1-5.
44. Sinclair R. Chronic telogen effluvium: a study of 5 patients over 7 years. J Am Acad Dermatol. 2005;52:12-6.
45. Olsen EA, Messenger AG, Shapiro J, Bergfled WF, Hordinsky MK, Robert JL, et al. Evaluation and treatment of male and female pattern hair loss. J Am Acad Dermatol. 2005;52:301-11.
46. DeVillez R, Jacobs JP, Szpunar CA, Warner ML. Androgenetic alopecia in the female. Treatment with 2% topical minoxidil solution. Arch Dermatol. 1994;130:303-7.
47. Lucky AW, Piacquadio DJ, Ditre CM, Dunlap F, Kantor I, Pandya AG, et al. A randomized, placebo-controlled trial of 5% and 2% topical minoxidil solutions in the treatment of female pattern hair loss. J Am Acad Dermatol. 2004;50:541-53.
48. Vexian P, Chaspoux C, Boudon P, Fiet J, Jaun-anique C, Hardy N, et al. Effects of minoxidil 2% vs. cyproterone acetate treatment on female androgenetic alopecia: a controlled, 12-month randomized trial. Br J Dermatol. 2002;146:992-9.
49. Dawber RP, Rundegren J. Hypertrichosis in females applying minoxidil topical solution and in normal controls. J Eur Acad Dermatol Venereol. 2003;17:271-5.
50. Shapiro J. Safety of topical minoxidil solution: a one-year, prospective, observational study. J Cutan Med Surg. 2003;7:322-9.
51. Diamanti-Kandarakis E. Current aspect of antiandrogens therapy in women. Curr Pharm Des. 1999;5:707-23.
52. Adamopoulos DA, Karamerlzanis M, Ncckopoulou S, Gregoriou A. A beneficial effect

of spironolactone on androgenetic alopecia. Clin Endocrinol (Oxf). 1997;47:759-60.

53. Rushton DH. Quantitative assessment of spironolactone treatment in women with diffuse androgen-dependent alopecia. J Soc Cosmet Chem. 1991;42:317.
54. Shapiro J. Hair Loss: Principles of Diagnosis and Management of Alopecia. London: Martin Dunitz; 2002. pp. 83-121.
55. Carmina E, Lobo RA. Treatment of hyper-androgenic alopecia in women. Fertil Steril. 2003;79:91-5.
56. Peereboom-Wniya JD, van der Willigen AH, van Jost T, Stolz E. The effect of cyproterone acetate on hair roots and hair shaft diameter in androgenetic alopecia in females. Acta Derm Venereol. 1989;69:395-8.
57. Barth H, Cherry CA, Wofnazowska F, Dawber RP. Cyproterone acetate for severe hirsutism: results of a double-blind dose-ranging study. Clin Endocrinol (Oxf). 1991;35:5-10.
58. Shum KW, Cullen DR, Messenger AG. Hair loss in women with hyperandrogenism: four cases responding to finasteride. J Am Acad Dermatol. 2002;47:733-9.
59. Price VH, Roberts JL, Hordinskym, Olsen EA, Savin R, Bergfed W, et al. Lack of efficiency of finasteride in postmenopausal women with androgenetic alopecia. J Am Acad Dermatol. 2000;43:768-76.
60. Thai KE, Sinclair RD. Finasteride for female andro-genetic alopecia. Br J Dermatol. 2002;147:812-3.
61. Shrivastava SB. Diffuse hair loss in an adult female: approach to diagnosis and management. Indian J Dermatol Venereol Leprol. 2009;75(1):20-7.

# PART 3

# Endocrinology

# CHAPTER 22

# Goiter

*Sumit Chakraborty*

## WHAT IS GOITER?

Goiter or thyromegaly suggests the enlargement of the thyroid gland. It may be visible, palpable, or both. Roughly, it can be stated that goiter is present when the size of the lateral lobes of the gland exceeds the size of the terminal phalanx of the thumb of the concerned subject. According to World Health Organization (WHO), goiter is classified into three grades **(Figs. 1 and 2)**:

- *Grade 0*: No goiter is visible or palpable.
- *Grade 1*: Palpable goiter, not visible when the neck is held in normal position.
- *Grade 2*: Clearly swollen neck, visible in the normal neck position as well as palpable.

Goiter may be because of diffuse enlargement of the gland or the presence of one or more nodules in it. It can be symmetric or asymmetric.

## WHAT ARE THE COMMON ETIOLOGIES?

Worldwide, the most common cause of goiter is iodine deficiency.

The causes may be classified as below:

- *Deficiency disorder*: Iodine deficiency. Can occur at any age.
- *Autoimmune mechanism*: Hashimoto's thyroiditis and Graves' disease. Can occur at any age but are more commonly seen in young adults with a female preponderance.
- *Exposure to goitrogens*: Some vegetables, such as cassava root, cabbage, and cauliflower, may impair the synthesis of thyroid hormones and may produce goiter.
- *Inflammatory causes*: Acute/subacute/viral thyroiditis.
- *Dyshormonogenesis*: Deficiency of enzymes of thyroid hormone synthesis, often resulting in congenital hypothyroidism. Commonly present in infants and children.
- *Thyroid nodular disease*: Single or multiple nodules in the gland. Common in the adult population.
- *Thyroid malignancy*: It usually occurs in adults as well as the elderly population.
- *Idiopathic/simple goiter or colloid goiter*: Can occur at all ages, more often seen in young adults.

## WHAT IS THE PATHOGENESIS?

The enlargement of the thyroid gland is generally considered an adaptive response of thyroid follicular cells to low thyroid hormones. Thyroid-stimulating hormone

(TSH) acts as the trophic factor, resulting in the enlargement of the gland. Iodine deficiency alone is unable to explain all goiters. The presence of genetic susceptibility and environmental factors is also relevant. Mutations in genes encoding thyroglobulin (Tg), thyroid peroxidase (TPO), dual oxidase 2 (DUOX2), sodium iodide symporter (NIS), and TSH receptor often play important roles in the development of goiter.

During puberty, thyroid glands may enlarge in size, resulting in puberty goiter. This is not pathological. It is because of an appropriate response of the gland in response to the increased demand of thyroid hormones during puberty.

## HOW TO EVALUATE A CASE OF GOITER?

While examining a case of goiter, it needs to be approached from two directions. One is the *examination of the gland proper* and the other is *peripheral examination to assess the functional status* of the patient. Only then relevant investigations can be advised to reach a proper diagnosis.

### How is the Clinical Examination to be Conducted?

*Thyroid gland proper*: The patient is to be seated comfortably in a well-lit room. On inspection, the gland moves up on deglutition, which may be made easier for the patient by sipping a gulp of water. The neck may be slightly extended. If the swelling does not move up on deglutition, it is not thyroid swelling; it may be a dermoid cyst. Next, ask the patient to protrude the tongue. A goiter does not move up on tongue protrusion; if it moves up, it can be a thyroglossal cyst.

Palpation may be done from both front and back. Palpate with the pulp of the fingers. Look if the goiter is symmetrical or asymmetrical. Palpate the consistency. Soft goiter may be because of increased vascularity as in Graves' disease. Firm goiter may be found in long-standing Graves' disease and Hashimoto's thyroiditis. Hard-to-feel goiter suggests malignancy. Next, check if one can get below the goiter. If is not possible, it suggests retrosternal prolongation of the goiter. Raising both arms above the head will result in facial congestion and engorgement of neck veins. Respiratory distress can also occur. This is known as Pemberton's sign and suggests retrosternal extension of the goiter. Look for any pain or tenderness while palpation. Pain may be seen in acute or subacute thyroiditis.

Palpate carefully for any nodules. Try to ascertain size, shape, number, consistency, fixity on palpation, and any tenderness. Always palpate for neck lymph nodes, which may be a clue to the presence of thyroid malignancy.

Careful auscultation over the thyroid may reveal a bruit because of increased vascularity. It may be seen in Graves' disease early in the course and over a large goiter.

*Peripheral examination*: It gives an idea about the functional status of the gland. A patient with a goiter may be in euthyroid, hypothyroid, or thyrotoxic state. Investigations are planned accordingly.

#### *What are the Features Suggestive of a Hypothyroid State?*

The features that suggest a hypothyroid state include a listless and fatigued appearance, slowed mentation, puffy face, dry and falling hair, loss of eyebrows over lateral half (madarosis), cold extremities, cold and dry nonpitting edematous skin, bradycardia, diastolic hypertension, delayed relaxation of the ankle jerk, ataxia, and proximal muscle weakness.

#### *What are the Features Suggestive of a Thyrotoxic State?*

The features that suggest a thyrotoxic state include a fidgety appearance, irritability, restlessness, increased sweating, tremor of hands, palmar erythema, loss of weight despite increased appetite, increased stool frequency, insomnia, palpitation, tachycardia, irregularly irregular rhythm or collapsing pulse, brisk deep tendon reflexes, proximal muscle weakness, onycholysis, clubbing, exophthalmos, and red congested painful eyes.

Patients may not have any of the abovementioned features but still may have a goiter. They are said to have nontoxic goiter.

## How to Proceed with Investigations?

To begin with, for the anatomic evaluation of goiter, the best is to do an ultrasonography (USG) of the neck.

*Ultrasonography of the neck*: It gives a clear idea about the size, echotexture, and vascularity of the lobes. Most importantly, it detects thyroid nodule/nodules. The presence of a nodular goiter is always a concern for malignancy. USG neck can delineate the characteristics of a nodule, namely size, shape, margin, echogenicity, microcalcification, vascularity, etc. The larger the nodule (>4 cm), the more the chance of malignancy.

### *What are the USG Features Suggestive of Malignancy?*

Hypoechogenicity, irregular margin, presence of punctate calcification, and increased vascularity increase the detection risk of malignancy. Purely cystic nodules are more often benign in nature.

Nowadays, thyroid USG is reported in a TIRADS (Thyroid Imaging Reporting and Data Systems) format. It provides a score of TIRADS 1 to TIRADS 5. The higher the score, the higher the risk of malignancy.

### *When to Perform Fine Needle Aspiration Cytology?*

If the nodule is a solid or solid-cystic one, size is >1 cm, and shows hypoechogenicity, microcalcification, and increased vascularity, then the next step should be a USG-guided fine needle aspiration cytology (FNAC) test. Purely cystic nodules may be observed without FNAC. FNAC may find characteristic nuclear changes in the thyroid follicular cell and detect thyroid malignancy. But at times, it remains inconclusive and may come up with findings such as follicular lesion of unknown significance (FLUS) or atypia of unknown significance (AUS).

In these gray situations, the present day has witnessed the development of molecular tests to detect genetic mutations known to be associated with thyroid malignancy. Tests such as gene expression classifier (GEC) and gene sequencing classifier (GSC) can detect mutation in *RET/PTC*, *RAS*, *BRAF*, and *PPAR-γ* genes from FNAC samples of indeterminate thyroid nodules.

### *What is Thyroid Function Test?*

*Thyroid function test*: Estimation of serum T3, Total/free T4 and TSH constitute thyroid function tests. For that we need to send fasting blood sample for thyroid function test (TFT). Serum T3, T4/free T4, and TSH are the tests advised. When clinically it appears to be hypothyroid, serum free T4 and TSH should be sent for. Serum T3, T4/free T4, and TSH should be sent for in thyrotoxic subjects. Anti-TPO antibody and anti-Tg antibody should be tested to detect thyroid autoimmunity. Special tests, such as anti-TSH receptor antibody, may be needed to establish Graves' disease or for the evaluation of orbitopathy.

### *What is the Radionuclide Uptake Study?*

Technitium 99m pertechnetate thyroid scan is a very useful tool to detect the functional status of the gland. Clinically detection of a nodular goiter with some thyrotoxic features can be better investigated by this test to find out whether there is increased uptake in a single area (suggestive of toxic adenoma) or multiple areas [suggestive of toxic multinodular goiter (MNG)] or increased uptake bilaterally in a diffuse way (suggestive of Graves' disease). Poor uptake of radionuclide suggests subacute thyroiditis.

### *What is the Usefulness of Computed Tomography Scan?*

The computed tomography (CT) scan of the neck and chest can define the anatomic extent of thyroid enlargement, particularly intrathoracic extension. It cannot differentiate benign from malignant lesions of the thyroid.

### What Other Investigations are Relevant?

Patients should be advised to do a complete blood count [at least Hb%, total and differential count, erythrocyte sedimentation rate (ESR)], liver function test (bilirubin and liver enzymes are a must), fasting blood sugar, and renal function test.

## HOW TO MANAGE A CASE OF GOITER?

It mainly depends on the underlying cause and functional status of the gland.

### How to Treat if the Patient is Hypothyroid?

If the patient with goiter clinically appears hypothyroid and TFT confirms it, the treatment is to start levothyroxine (LT4) replacement. The usual replacement dose is about 1.6–1.8 μg/kg/day. The tablet is ideally to be taken in the morning on an empty stomach, and patients should be advised to remain so for about 30 minutes as the intake of food or other medication might hamper the absorption of LT4. A lower starting dose is considered in elderly patients and in subjects with coronary artery disease or heart failure. Initial monitoring is recommended after 2–3 months. Monitoring is done with FT4, TSH, or TSH test only.

### How to Treat a Thyrotoxic Patient?

For patients with goiter who are thyrotoxic, treatment depends on the underlying cause. For Graves' disease, the treatment options are antithyroid drugs, radioiodine ablation, or thyroidectomy.

### What are the Antithyroid Drugs?

Methimazole, carbimazole, and propylthiouracil are the three drugs available. The first two drugs are commonly used. Propylthiouracil is used in limited situations because of its fatal liver toxicity.

Major side effects of antithyroid drugs include neutropenia, altered liver function, and skin rash, and the appearance of these side effects warrants discontinuation of the drug.

Thyroid status should be monitored after 6–8 weeks, and FT4 is the preferred tool.

### What are the Treatment Options for Toxic Adenoma/MNG?

For goitrous and thyrotoxic patients, when the diagnosis comes to be toxic adenoma or toxic MNG, treatment options are radioiodine ablation or surgery. Antithyroid drugs cannot cure these conditions but may have to be used initially to reduce the thyrotoxic state and make them fit to receive radioiodine or to undergo surgery.

### What to do if Thyroid Malignancy is Diagnosed?

If nodular goiter on evaluation reveals malignancy, the therapy is total thyroidectomy followed by radioiodine ablative therapy.

### What to do for Euthyroid Patients with Goiter?

For patients with goiter who are clinically and biochemically euthyroid, management is debatable. Theoretically, giving LT4 to any

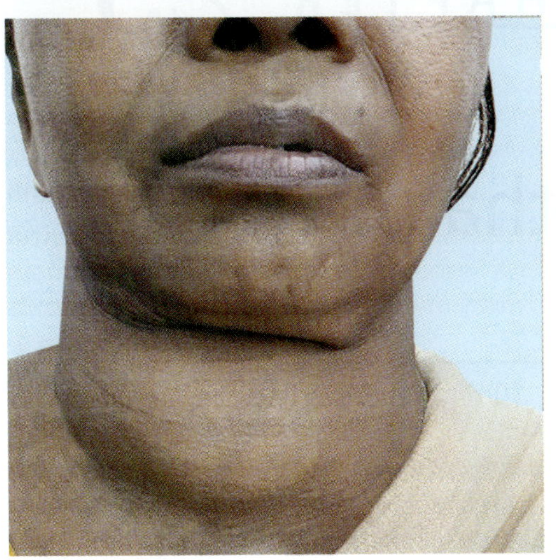

**FIG. 1:** Diffuse goiter.

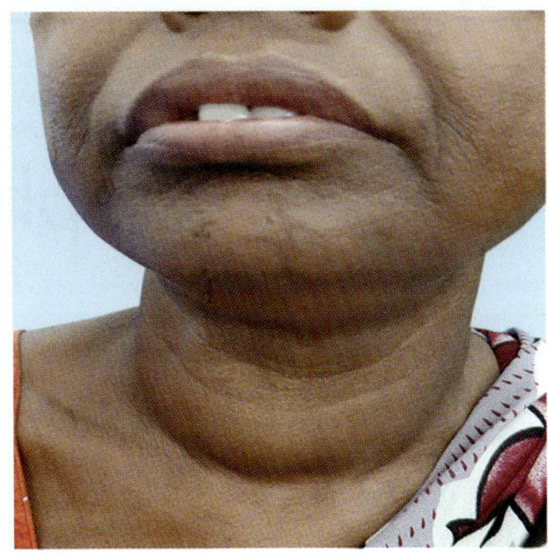

**FIG. 2:** Asymmetric goiter.

subject will suppress TSH and may therefore reduce the trophic factor for the thyroid gland and hence may reduce the goiter size, but this is controversial. Giving LT4 to reduce goiter size may render the patient thyrotoxic and prone to adverse effects on the cardiovascular system and bone health, especially in the elderly. So, this is not recommended.

Patients are to be counseled and followed up. If the goiter is large enough to cause compressive symptoms or is cosmetically challenging for the patient, surgery may remain the only option left.

## CLINICAL PEARLS

Goiter is a common clinical observation and worrisome to the patient, so it needs evaluation.

It may be diffuse (symmetric/asymmetric) or nodular.

Assessment of functional status is crucial.

Relevant investigations should be done to reach a specific diagnosis, so that appropriate therapy may be properly chosen.

Counseling and follow-up are crucial if the patient with goiter appears to be euthyroid. Unnecessary therapy with LT4 may cause harm to the patient.

## FURTHER READINGS

1. Jameson JL. Harrison's principles of internal medicine. 20th edition. Vol. 1. New York Mcgraw-Hill Education; 2018.
2. Melmed S, Koenig R, Rosen C, Auchus R, Goldfine A. Williams Textbook of Endocrinology, 14 Edition: South Asia Edition, 2 Vol Set - E-Book. Elsevier India; 2020.
3. American Thyroid Association. ATA guideline and statements. [online] Available from https://www.thyroid.org/professionals/ata-professional-guidelines/ [Last accessed August, 2023].
4. Desai MP. Hypothyroidism, goitre and thyroid neoplasia. Paediatric Endocrine Disorders. Hyderabad: University Press; 2012.
5. Khardori R, Prasanna Kumar KM. Disorders of Thyroid. New Delhi: Jaypee Brothers Medical Publishers; 2018.

CHAPTER 23

# Exophthalmos

Sumit Chakraborty

## WHAT IS THE DEFINITION OF EXOPHTHALMOS?

Exophthalmos means the forward protrusion of one or both eyeballs beyond the margin of the orbit. The eyeball on the affected side appears more prominent. It is also designated as proptosis as the two terms are often loosely used synonymously.

In unilateral proptosis, the globes appear asymmetric, but it is to be decided first which eye is abnormal because an eyeball recessed into the orbit (enophthalmos) in one eye may result in apparent prominence of the other eye.

However, some authorities have stressed that the two terms are slightly different in a stricter sense. Exophthalmos denotes an active or a dynamic process that leads to protrusion of the eyeball beyond its socket as classically seen in Graves' disease causing thyroid-associated orbitopathy (TAO). Proptosis is a passive process produced by space-occupying lesion or a tumor in the orbit.

## WHAT ARE THE TYPES OF EXOPHTHALMOS?

Exophthalmos may be:

- Unilateral—acute/chronic
- Bilateral—acute/chronic

## WHAT ARE THE ETIOLOGIES?

### Unilateral Proptosis

Etiology may be classified as:

- *Inflammatory*:
  - Orbital cellulitis
  - Panophthalmitis
- *Neoplastic*:
  - *Benign*: Hemangioma, neurofibroma, dermoid, glioma of the optic nerve, lacrimal gland tumor, etc.
  - *Malignant*: Retinoblastoma, lymphosarcoma, maxillary antral carcinoma, metastatic deposits into orbit (usually from carcinoma of the lung or breast).
- *Vascular*: Retrobulbar hemorrhage, cavernous sinus thrombosis, caroticocavernous fistula.
- *Systemic diseases*:
  - Leukemia [acute myeloid leukemia (AML)/acute lymphoblastic leukemia (ALL)], lymphoma.
  - Graves' disease with TAO may present unilaterally at least in the initial part of the disease course.

Usually, inflammatory and vascular causes present as acute proptosis that is often rapidly growing. Tumors and thyroid disease present with slow-growing course.

A caroticocavernous fistula may present with pulsating exophthalmos.

### Bilateral Proptosis/Exophthalmos

Its causes are:
- Congenital—craniosynostosis
- Endocrine—Graves' disease resulting in TAO
- Malignancy—metastatic deposits, leukemia, lymphoma, neuroblastoma

## HOW TO PERFORM CLINICAL EXAMINATION?

The degree of protrusion of the eyeballs can be assessed clinically by standing behind the patient, observing the eyes from above, and looking down upon the orbit.

*Measurement of proptosis*: It measures the distance between the corneal apex and the deepest portion of the lateral orbital margin. Hertel's exophthalmometer is the instrument used for precise measurement. The normal value is <20 mm. A value of 21 mm or more suggests proptosis.

## WHAT ARE THE DIFFERENT EYE SIGNS?

A few eye signs are observed in the thyrotoxic state. They are as follows:
- *Dalrymple's sign*—visibility of upper sclera. It is because of spasm of the upper eyelid.
- *Von Graefe's sign*—presence of lid lag. The lid lags behind the globe when the patient is asked to look down suddenly.
- *Joffroy's sign*—loss of wrinkling of the forehead on looking upward.
- *Mobius sign*—failure of convergence on accommodation while looking at a near object.
- *Stellwag's sign*—staring look with infrequent blinking.

These features may be observed in any thyrotoxic state irrespective of the cause and occur because of the hyperadrenergic state.

## WHAT ARE THE SPECIFIC FEATURES OF TAO?

Specific features of TAO are observed in Graves' disease. Proptosis is often asymmetric or may be unilateral to begin with. The eye signs may precede or follow the appearance of other thyrotoxic features. In addition to exophthalmos, other observed features are:
- Pain in the eyes at rest and/or on movement of the eyes
- Edema of the lids; that of the upper eyelid is more specific.
- Congestion of the lids
- Edema of conjunctiva
- Congestion of conjunctiva
- Congestion of the caruncle
- Paresis of extraocular muscles resulting in restricted eye movement. Squint is observed, and the patient complains of diplopia.
- Visual loss from optic nerve compression in advanced/untreated cases

## WHEN TO SUSPECT THYROID-RELATED EYE DISEASE?

Thyroid evaluation is a must. Thyrotoxic manifestations must be sought by detailed clinical examination **(Fig. 1)**. These include a history of weight loss despite increased appetite, increased sweating, tremor of hands and/or eyelids, palpitation, etc. The presence of a goiter along with above-mentioned features suggestive of thyrotoxicosis, if present, strongly points to a thyroid-associated eye disease **(Fig. 2)**.

Examination of paranasal sinuses is important.

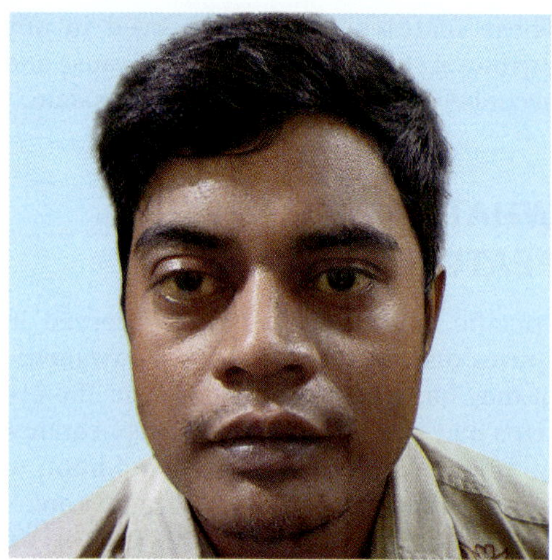

**FIG. 1:** A case of Graves' disease showing thyroid-associated orbitopathy (TAO) (asymmetric exophthalmos, visibility of lower sclera, right upper eyelid edema).

*Courtesy*: Dr Sumit Chakraborty.

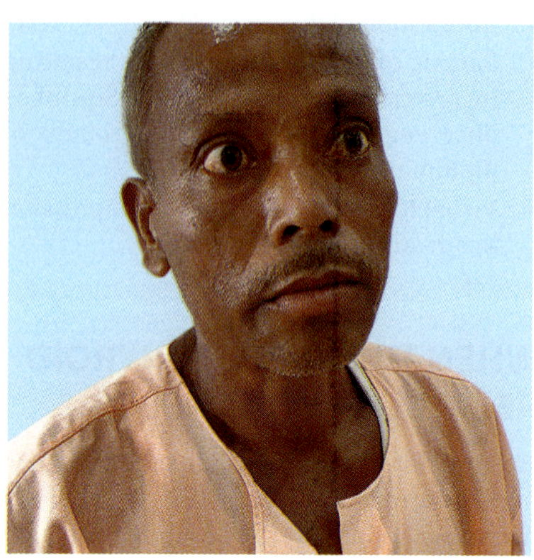

**FIG. 2:** A case of Graves' disease showing bilateral proptosis along with a goiter.

*Courtesy*: Dr Sumit Chakraborty.

Possible primary sites of malignancy must be examined carefully. These include the breast, lungs, stomach, etc.

The presence of anemia, purpuric spots, bony tenderness, hepatosplenomegaly, and lymphadenopathy may indicate toward leukemia or lymphoma.

## WHAT ARE THE LABORATORY INVESTIGATIONS?

- Blood for complete hemogram can provide a clue to inflammatory lesions and hematological malignancy.
- Thyroid function tests include T3, T4, and thyroid-stimulating hormone (TSH). Antithyroid peroxidase antibody and anti-TSH receptor antibody may also be needed to confirm the etiological association with Graves' disease.
- Plain X-ray of the orbits is important for a composite view of the orbital bones and can compare between the two orbits.
- Ultrasonography (USG) of the orbits is easily available and a noninvasive effective method of investigation.
- *Computed tomography (CT) scan of the orbit*: This is the most important noninvasive method of investigation. Structures of eyeballs, optic nerve, and extraocular muscles can be viewed clearly.
- *Magnetic resonance imaging (MRI) of the orbit*: It is a major recent advance in imaging modality.
- Fine needle aspiration cytology (FNAC) or biopsy is the final invasive investigation for tissue diagnosis. These are done under USG or CT guidance.

## WHAT ARE THE TREATMENT APPROACHES?

*Medical*: For inflammatory lesions, such as orbital cellulitis and panophthalmitis, antibiotics and anti-inflammatory therapy are effective. Intravenous (IV) antibiotics may be preferred in severe cases. Third-generation cephalosporins and quinolones are often the initial choice.

For Graves' disease, antithyroid drugs prove to be helpful. These include methimazole or carbimazole. In the clinically active stage of TAO, weekly IV methylprednisolone is advised for about 6 weeks. Radioactive iodine ablation therapy, if planned to be used for Graves' disease, may exacerbate orbitopathy. Concomitant therapy with oral prednisolone may reduce the worsening of symptoms.

For leukemia or lymphoma, specific chemotherapy is to be used.

*Radiotherapy*: For rapidly growing malignant tumors and secondary deposits, radiotherapy may be palliative.

*Surgical approach*: Different types of orbitotomy or decompression surgery are available. Orbital decompression may prove sight saving in optic nerve compression.

## CLINICAL PEARLS

- Exophthalmos can occur because of local causes of orbit.
- Presence of exophthalmos may be but never only because of Graves' disease.
- Graves' disease can present with unilateral/asymmetric eye involvement at least in the beginning.
- Eye involvement can precede, follow or occur simultaneously with other features of Graves' disease.
- Opinion of an ophthalmologist can be very important in diagnosis and management.

## FURTHER READINGS

1. Jameson JL. Harrison's principles of internal medicine. 20th edition. Vol. 1. New York Mcgraw-Hill Education; 2018.
2. Melmed S, Koenig R, Rosen C, Auchus R, Goldfine A. Williams Textbook of Endocrinology, 14 Edition: South Asia Edition, 2 Vol Set - E-Book. Elsevier India; 2020.
3. Saha ML. Bedside Clinics in Surgery. New Delhi: Jaypee Brothers Medical Publishers; 2018.
4. Basak SK. Essentials of Ophthalmology. New Delhi: Jaypee Brothers Medical Publishers; 2019.

# CHAPTER 24

# Hirsutism

*Parinita Ranjit*

## INTRODUCTION

Hirsutism is a clinical diagnosis defined as the presence of excess terminal (long, coarse, and pigmented) hair growth on the body and face, in androgen-sensitive areas of the skin in a female **(Figs. 1A and B)**.

Approximately 5–10% of reproductive women suffer from hirsutism.

## MECHANISM OF HIRSUTISM

- Due to an increased level of androgenic hormones such as testosterone (most important), androstenedione, dehydroepiandrosterone (DHEA), and its sulfated form (DHEAS), either from increased peripheral binding (idiopathic) or from increased production from ovaries, adrenals, and body fat.
- In the peripheral tissue, testosterone is converted to the more potent dihydrotestosterone (DHT) by 5-alpha reductase present in the pilosebaceous unit (PSU). This DHT serves as the primary mediator of androgen action at the level of PSU. The fraction of testosterone that is not bound to sex hormone-binding globulin (SHBG) is available for conversion to DHT.

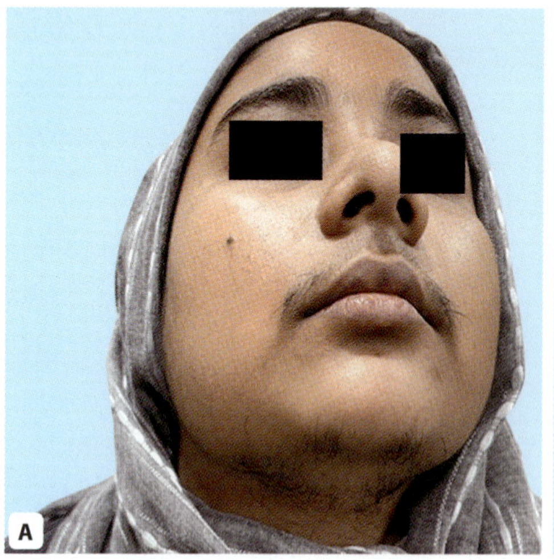


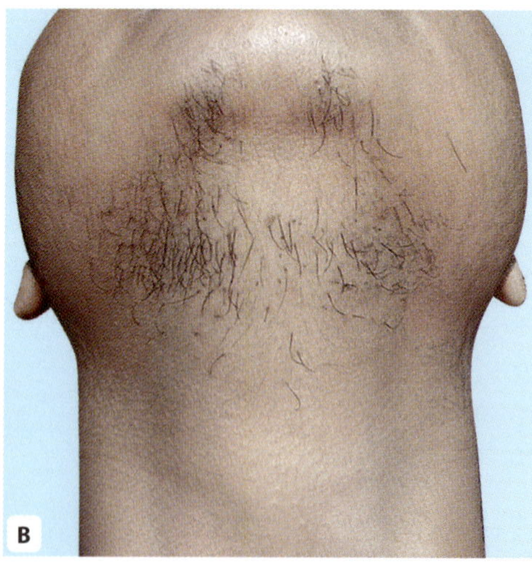


**FIGS. 1A AND B:** Women with hirsutism.

- In hyperinsulinemia and/or androgen excess, decreased hepatic production of SHBG results in an increased free testosterone level.
- In postmenopausal women, although there is decreased ovarian testosterone production, greater reduction in ovarian estrogen production causes a decrease in SHBG. Consequently, there is an increase in the relative proportion of unbound testosterone, and it may exacerbate hirsutism after menopause.
- In idiopathic hirsutism, although the androgen level is normal, there is increased 5-alpha reductase activity and polymorphism of androgenic receptors resulting in increased DHT and its peripheral binding, causing hirsutism.

## What are the Possibilities?

- *Generalized hyperandrogenism*:
  - Polycystic ovary syndrome (PCOS) (most common, 90%)
  - Ovarian neoplasm
  - Hyperthecosis
- *Adrenal hyperandrogenism*:
  - Congenital adrenal hyperplasia (CAH) (nonclassic)
  - Abnormal cortisol action/metabolism
  - Adrenal neoplasm
- *Other endocrine disorders*:
  - Cushing's syndrome
  - Hyperprolactinemia
  - Acromegaly
- *Peripheral androgen overproduction*:
  - Obesity
  - Idiopathic
- *Pregnancy-related hyperandrogenism*:
  - Hyperreactio luteinalis
  - Thecoma of pregnancy
- *Drugs*:
  - Androgen
  - Androgenic progestin
  - Minoxidil
  - Phenytoin
  - Cyclosporine
  - Valproic acid

# PATH TO DIAGNOSIS

## History

- Age at onset and rate of progression of hair growth
- Weight
- Associated symptoms such as menstrual irregularities and acne
- Age of menarche and pattern of menstrual cycle (irregular cycles point more toward ovarian rather than adrenal androgen excess)
- Fertility history
- Presence of galactorrhea points toward hyperprolactinemia or possibly hypothyroidism.
- Hypertension, easy bruising, centripetal weight gain, and weakness suggest hypercortisolism.
- Presence of virilization (deepening of voice, breast atrophy, increased muscle bulk, clitoromegaly) may be due to hyperthecosis or ovarian or adrenal neoplasm.
- Family history of infertility and/or hirsutism may indicate nonclassic CAH.
- Medication history also from partners (such as topical androgen use).

## Physical Examination

- Measurement of height and weight and calculation of body mass index (BMI). BMI > 25 kg/m$^2$ or, more commonly, >30 kg/m$^2$ is often seen in hyperinsulinemia and insulin resistance syndrome (IRS).
- Other cutaneous features such as acanthosis nigricans and acne are also seen in IRS.
- Presence of hypertension may indicate adrenal causes.
- The presence of virilization—gradual onset in ovarian hyperthecosis, rapid onset in ovarian, and adrenal neoplasm.
- Objective clinical assessment done by the *modified scale of Ferriman and*

*Gallwey*, where hair growth is rated in nine androgen-sensitive areas from 0 (no hair growth) to 4 (hair growth typically seen in adult males). A score >8 suggests positivity in the case of non-Hispanic white and moderate and >25 suggests severe hirsutism.

The limitations of this score are as follows:

- It varies in different racial groups. For Asians and Native Americans, a score >2 is considered abnormal as pustular acne and thinning of scalp hair may be the only cutaneous evidence of androgen excess for them.
- It can be altered by the use of previous cosmetic measurements so baseline measurement may not be an accurate reflection of the severity and distribution of hair growth.
- It underrates patient perception of hirsutism.

## DIFFERENTIAL DIAGNOSIS

*Polycystic ovary syndrome* (72–82%): Oligomenorrhea, anovulation (defined as an ovulatory cycle >35 days), clinical or biochemical evidence of hyperandrogenism, polycystic ovaries on ultrasound (two out of three required for diagnosis as per Rotterdam criteria).

*Idiopathic hyperandrogenemia* (6–15%): Hirsutism with a normal menstrual cycle, normal ovaries on ultrasound with an elevated androgen level with no other explainable cause.

*Idiopathic hirsutism* (4–7%): Hirsutism with a normal menstrual cycle, normal ultrasonography (USG), normal androgen level with no other explainable cause.

*Late-onset CAH* (4–7%): It is mostly due to a defect in 21-hydroxylase deficiency leading to deficient cortisol production. This causes increased adrenocorticotropic hormone (ACTH) secretion, in turn leading to increased adrenal steroid production upstream of the defective enzyme. More severe and earlier onset hirsutism is present in adolescence in amenorrheic or oligomenorrheic women. They may also have features of virilization.

*Androgen-secreting tumor* (0.2%): Ovarian neoplasms are more common in causing hirsutism than adrenal tumors. Sertoli–Leydig cell tumor more commonly occurs in the reproductive age group, while hilus cell tumor is more common in the postmenopausal group.

Adrenocortical carcinomas, though rare, can present with features of hirsutism and virilizations. Usually, the onset is very rapid, and they have very high levels of DHEAS and testosterone. Prognosis is very poor.

*Ovarian hyperthecosis*: Increase in testosterone by ovarian theca cell, gradual onset hirsutism, frank virilization, mostly affect postmenopausal women.

*Cushing's syndrome*: Occurs due to excessive production of cortisol, either due to increased secretion of ACTH from the pituitary or due to direct increased cortisol secretion from the adrenals. Women may present with oligomenorrhea, hirsutism, central obesity, stria, proximal muscle weakness, and development of diabetes, hypertension, and osteoporosis. Diagnosis can be done by the overnight dexamethasone suppression test.

*Acromegaly*: Patients with acromegaly have high levels of insulin-like growth factor-1 (IGF1), which stimulates adrenal androgen synthesis and inhibits hepatic SHBG production. Patients have typical features of prognathism, which include spade-like hands, along with hirsutism and acne.

*Hypothyroidism*: This may decrease the SHBG binding and thus may lead to increased levels of bioavailable testosterone. Usually, it is associated with hyperprolactinemia.

## DIAGNOSTIC TESTS

### Initial Investigations (Flowchart 1)

- Assess androgen levels in all women with significant hirsutism along with thyroid screen (TSH).
- A total serum testosterone level should be assessed. The normal upper limit in adults is 1.4–2.1 nmol/L. Marked elevation >12 nmol/L indicates a virilizing tumor, whereas that >7 nmol/L is suggestive of a tumor but may seen in women with hyperthecosis.
- If total testosterone is normal but features are consistent with PCOS, early morning serum free testosterone should be assessed. A morning free testosterone is 50% more sensitive.

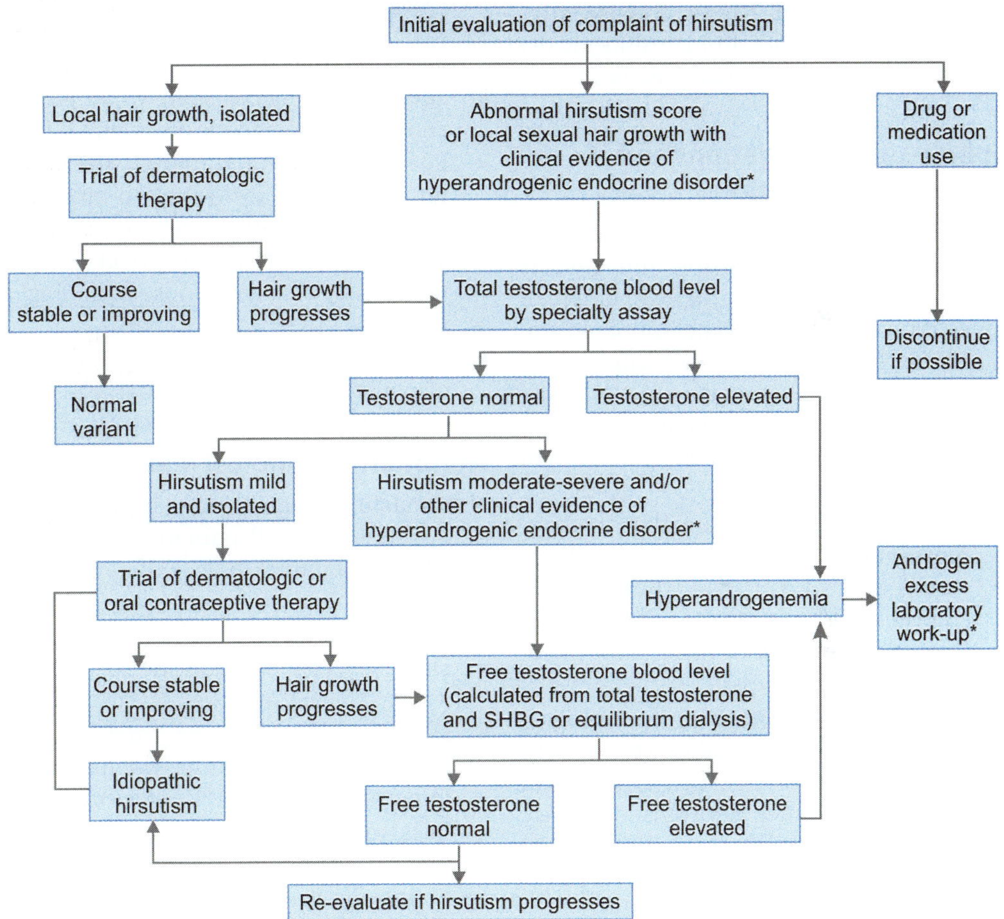


**FLOWCHART 1:** Algorithm for evaluation of hirsutism.

(SHBG: sex hormone-binding globulin)

- If PCOS is suspected, luteinizing hormone (LH), follicle-stimulating hormone (FSH), and prolactin should be sent. LH/FSH ratio > 2 suggests PCOS.
- USG lower abdomen needs to be done to show polycystic ovaries in PCOS.
- The workup for PCOS recommended by the American College of Obstetricians and Gynecologists includes the above plus screening for metabolic syndrome with fasting and 2-hour glucose after 75 g glucose load, lipid profile, waist circumference, and blood pressure.

## Follow-up Investigations and Special Considerations

- If testosterone is markedly elevated, dexamethasone suppression test is done to broadly distinguish between ovarian and adrenal hyperandrogenism. Adrenal androgen is readily suppressed by low-dose glucocorticoids (0.5 mg dexamethasone every 6 hours for 4 days). Incomplete suppression suggests ovarian androgen excess.
- An overnight 1 mg dexamethasone suppression test, with measurement of 8 AM serum cortisol, is useful when there is clinical suspicion of Cushing's syndrome (hypertension, easy bruising, centripetal weight gain, weakness).
- Measurement of 8 AM 17-hydroxyprogesterone level is suggested in women with suspected nonclassic CAH. It should be done in women with onset in early adolescence, having family history, or high-risk group (Mediterranean, Hispanic, Ashkenazi Jewish).

  A level >200 ng/dL in the early follicular phase strongly suggests the diagnosis. Further confirmation is done by a high-dose (250 mg) corticotropin (ACTH) stimulation test. In most patients, values exceed 1,500 ng/dL 60 minutes after administration.
- DHEAS should be checked in virilization. Values >700 may indicate adrenal tumor.
- Computed tomography (CT) or magnetic resonance imaging (MRI) should be done to localize adrenal mass.
- MRI of the pituitary should be done in case of a very high prolactin level without a history of intake of any offending drugs.

# TREATMENT

*Goals of therapy*:

- Treatment depends on patient preference and psychosocial effect.
- The goal is to decrease new hair growth and improve metabolic disorder.
- For all pharmacological therapies for hirsutism, according to the 2018 Endocrine Society guidelines, a trial of at least 6 months is necessary before making any changes in dose or adding or switching to a new medication.
- If a patient desires pregnancy, induction of ovulation may be necessary.

## Nonpharmacological Measures

Nonpharmacological measures should be considered in all patients, either only treatment or adjunct to drug therapy. These include:

- Bleaching
- Depilatory (removal from the skin surface) such as shaving and chemical treatments.
- Depilator (removal of hair including the root) such as plucking, waxing, laser, intense pulsed light (IPL), electrolysis.
- Laser and IPL are used to treat large areas of pigmented terminal hair. Light of specific wavelength and duration is absorbed by the melanin in the hair shaft and follicle, leading to photosynthesis. If properly delivered, it delays hair regrowth and causes permanent hair removal in many patients.

## Pharmacological Measures

Pharmacological measures are mainly directed at interrupting one or more steps in the pathway of androgen synthesis and action.

- Suppression of adrenal/ovarian androgen production
- Enhancement of androgen binding to plasma-binding protein, particularly SHBG
- Impairment of peripheral conversion of androgen precursors to active androgens
- Inhibition of androgen action at the target level

## Combined Oral Contraceptives

Combined oral contraceptives (COCs) are the first-line endocrine treatment for hirsutism and acne, after or adjunct to cosmetic and dermatological treatment. The combined estrogen-progestin therapy reduces hyperparathyroidism and hirsutism by the following mechanisms:

- Inhibition of ovarian androgen production through the suppression of LH secretion and also, to a lesser extent, FSH secretion.
- Stimulation of hepatic production of SHBG, thereby increasing androgen binding in serum and reducing free androgen concentration. Mainly estrogen causes a dose-dependent increase in SHBG over 3–4 weeks in hyperandrogenic women. This increase is smaller in women treated with a COC containing a progestin that has significant androgenic properties (such as levonorgestrel).
- Reduction in total and free testosterone concentration, approximately 50% in hyperandrogenic woman.
- *Secondary mechanisms*: It also reduces adrenal androgen secretion, but to a lesser extent, by inhibiting peripheral conversion of testosterone to DHT and also by inhibiting the binding of DHT to androgen receptors.
- *Choice of pills*: Typically, a pill that contains a progestin with low or neutral androgenicity, such as norethindrone or norgestimate, is chosen. Some clinicians prefer to start with a COC containing antiandrogenic progestin such as drospirenone or cyproterone acetate (CPA). Limited data shows better clinical advantage for these two new progestins, but there is a concern regarding possible excess risk of venous thromboembolism (VTE) with both these preparations. Generally, pill containing levonorgestrel is avoided for its androgenic property.
- *Dose*: 20–35 µg ethinyl estradiol effectively reduces ovarian androgen production.
- At least a 6-month trial is done before making any changes in the dose or adding or switching to a new medication. This is because the growth phase of a hair follicle is approximately 6 months; a significant reduction of hair growth may not occur before then.
- Oral preparations, compared to vaginal and transdermal, are better at controlling hirsutism.
- In women with a high risk of VTE or an increased risk of breast and endocrine cancers, generally COCs are contraindicated. However, the lowest dose of an ethinyl estradiol-based oral contraceptive pill (OCP) may be tried.
- COCs are also recommended over glucocorticoids as the first-line treatment of hirsutism in CAH. If the response is inadequate, glucocorticoids may be used at the lowest effective doses (dexamethasone 0.2–0.5 mg or prednisone 5–10 mg taken at bedtime).

## Antiandrogens

Combination of COC with antiandrogens is only recommended in patients with severe hirsutism causing significant distress or who have not had a good response to COC monotherapy for 6 months. Available antiandrogens are spironolactone, flutamide, and finasteride.

- *Spironolactone*: It is used in relatively high doses (100–200 mg) along with COC. Caution is required for hypotension and hyperkalemia, though rare. Pregnancy should be avoided because of the risk of feminization of male fetus.

- *Finasteride*: 5 mg/day decreases androgen binding as an inhibitor of 5-alpha reductase type 2.
- *Flutamide*: Not recommended because of its potential hepatotoxicity.

### Eflornithine (Vaniqa) HCL Cream

Approved by Food and Drug Administration (FDA) for unwanted facial hair in women, it reduces facial hair in 40% of women. The usual dose is twice-daily application.

*Pregnancy consideration*:

- May cause related infertility.
- Several medications used for treatment are contraindicated in pregnancy.
- If a patient desires pregnancy, induction of ovulation may be needed.

*Follow-up*:

- Patient monitoring should be done for known side effects of medication.
- Low calorie, low glycemic index diet improves fertility in obese PCOS patients with an anovulatory cycle.
- Patient should be educated that hormonal treatment will stop further hair growth but will not reverse the present hair. Cosmetic measures may be needed for the already present hair.

## CLINICAL PEARLS

Polycystic ovary syndrome is the most common cause of hirsutism.

Diagnosis is based on androgen level in all women with an abnormal hirsutism score. Testosterone and TSH are the initial tests.

The presence of virilization with testosterone level > 150 ng/dL and DHEA > 700 is a red flag sign; hence, adrenal and ovarian tumor should be suspected.

Lifestyle modification along with OCP is the first-line therapy for hirsutism in the case of PCOS.

## FURTHER READINGS

1. Ehrmann DA. Hirsutism. In: Loscalzo J, Fauci A, Kasper D, Hauser S, Longo D, Jameson J. eds. Harrison's Principles of Internal Medicine, 21e. McGraw Hill; 2022.
2. Rosenfield RL. Clinical practice. Hirsutism. N Engl J Med. 2005;353(24):2578-88.
3. Azziz R. The evaluation and management of hirsutism. Obstet Gynecol. 2003;101(5 Pt 1): 995-1007.
4. Azarchi S, Bienenfeld A, Lo Sicco K, Marchbein S, Shapiro J, Nagler AR. Androgens in women: Hormone-modulating therapies for skin disease. J Am Acad Dermatol. 2019;80(6):1509-21.
5. Martin KA, Anderson RR, Chang RJ, Ehrmann DA, Lobo RA, Murad MH, et al. Evaluation and Treatment of Hirsutism in Premenopausal Women: An Endocrine Society Clinical Practice Guideline. J Clin Endocrinol Metab. 2018;103(4):1233-57.

# CHAPTER 25

# Gynecomastia

*Parinita Ranjit, Subhankar Naskar*

## WHAT IS GYNECOMASTIA?

Gynecomastia is defined as the presence of palpable breast tissue in a male.

Gynecomastia results from the enlargement of glandular breast tissue and should be distinguished from excess accumulation of adipose tissue (i.e., pseudogynecomastia). True gynecomastia feels firm, mobile, and gritty compared with the surrounding adipose tissue.

Usually, gynecomastia is bilateral, but asymmetry is also common. Unilateral enlargement is present in 5–25% of patients and may be the preliminary stage in the development of bilateral disease. In autopsy, it has been seen that unilateral enlargement is often found to be bilateral gynecomastia histologically.

## PATHOGENESIS

Estrogen stimulates and androgen inhibits the growth and differentiation of the mammary gland. Estradiol binds to estrogen receptors (ERs) and stimulates ductal and glandular cells proliferation in the male breast, whereas testosterone exerts a generalized inhibitory action on the growth and differentiation of breast tissue through a specific antiestrogenic action. So, gynecomastia results from an imbalance between the stimulatory effect of estrogen on ductal proliferation and the inhibitory effect of androgen on breast development. The imbalance of the ratio of estrogen to androgen is most commonly caused by increased production of estrogen, decreased production of testosterone, or increased conversion of androgens to estrogens in peripheral tissue. Thyroxine increases the level of sex hormone binding globulin (SHBG), a protein that binds testosterone more avidly than estradiol (thereby increasing estrogen to androgen ratio) and causes gynecomastia. Disorders associated with androgen receptor binding and function can also result in gynecomastia. Prolactin, growth hormone, insulin, insulin-like growth factor-I (IGF-I), and cortisol are permissive trophic factors that require an imbalance in estrogen and androgen in order to cause gynecomastia. Corticosteroids and prolactin lower circulating testosterone concentration indirectly by suppressing the hypothalamic secretion of gonadotropin-releasing hormone (GnRH). Corticosteroids also directly inhibit testicular steroid excess. These physiologic principles provide a framework for the evaluation of gynecomastia on a physiological basis.

There are two phases of life where gynecomastia is due to normal physiology: Just after birth and at the onset of puberty. Even in adulthood, gynecomastia is so common that a modest amount of gynecomastia (<5 cm) is also considered "physiologic."

## Physiologic Forms of Gynecomastia

### *Newborn Gynecomastia*

A high concentration of estradiol and progesterone produced by the mother during fetal life stimulates newborn breast tissue that may persist for several weeks after birth in boys. Minimal galactorrhea, called Witch milk, can be seen in up to 5% of newborn boys.

### *Pubertal Gynecomastia*

It has been seen that in the early stages of puberty (11–12 years of age), ~30% of boys may develop detectable gynecomastia (i.e., glandular tissue >0.5 cm in diameter). By the age of 14 years, gynecomastia is detectable in ~65% of cases. Usually, it is bilateral, but unilateral can be seen in 20% of cases. Spontaneous regression occurs in most of the cases after 1–2 years. It may persist on a long-term basis in <5% of cases. There are variable hormonal alterations during the stage of puberty in boys. The most likely explanation of pubertal gynecomastia is a relative increase in the ratio of estrogen to androgen concentration in circulation due to highly variable aromatization of testosterone during early puberty. In addition, some recent data suggest that there are relatively higher concentrations of Erβ expression than Erα in stromal cells of breast tissue obtained from gynecomastia **(Fig. 1)**.

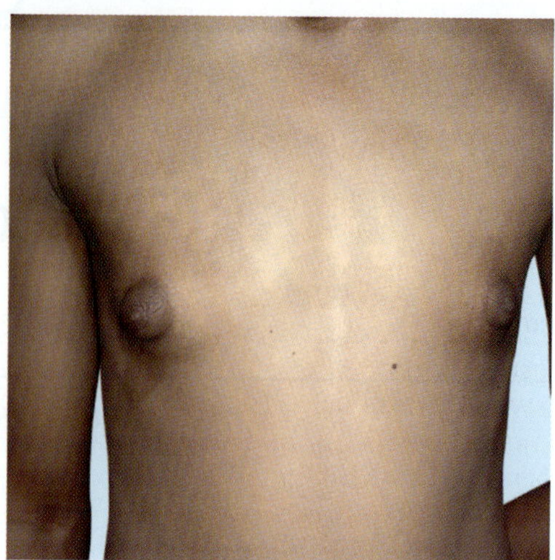

**FIG. 1:** Unilateral pubertal gynecomastia.

### *Adult and Senescent Gynecomastia*

Gynecomastia >2 cm of palpable breast tissue is very common in adults. In most of the cases, these are asymptomatic, and no identifiable causes are found; they are considered normal as a physiologic variant. Usually, it is an incidental finding. It is likely that age-related decline in serum testosterone after 30 years of age, obesity, environmental factors, systemic illness, and medications that lower circulating or breast tissue testosterone concentrations (or effects) or raise circulating or breast tissue estradiol concentration (or effects) contribute to the high prevalence of physiologic adult gynecomastia.

## Pathologic Forms of Gynecomastia

Pathologic gynecomastia is determined by its size (>4 cm diameter) and symptom (tenderness).

It is defined as tender palpable breast tissue or nontender breast tissue >4 cm in diameter. Documentation of the growth of breast tissue over time is also considered to be a pathologic form of gynecomastia, even when the diameter of the breast tissue is <4 cm in size.

Pathologic gynecomastia can be caused by an elevated level of estrogen (usually estradiol), deficiency of testosterone, or an imbalance in the ratio of estrogen to androgen concentration.

# WHAT ARE THE POSSIBILITIES?

Some causes of gynecomastia are due to elevated estrogen levels rather than androgen deficiency.

As the circulating concentration of estrogens inhibit pituitary gonadotropin secretion, testosterone production is also inhibited (which depends on pulsatile secretion of gonadotropin). Excess estrogen and low testosterone level is responsible for gynecomastia.

### *Tumors*

Testicular tumors of germ, sex cord, and Leydig or Sertoli cell origin can secrete excess amount of estrogen or estradiol precursor. Usually, testicular tumors are large enough to be palpated in 50% of patients, but the remainder required ultrasonography to be detected. Choriocarcinoma may produce human chorionic gonadotropin (hCG), which acts on luteinizing hormone (LH) receptors in the testes to produce estradiol and testosterone. Ectopic production of hCG by lung, kidney, liver, and gastric carcinoma also stimulates testosterone and estradiol production and causes gynecomastia. HCG and LH increase the activity of aromatase and therefore raise estrogen concentration than testosterone concentration.

## Aromatase Excess

Overexpression of aromatase is an important feature of several causes of gynecomastia.

Aromatase-associated causes of gynecomastia:

- ↑ *Amount of aromatase enzyme*
- ↑ *Activity at normal tissue*
  - Obesity
  - Aging
- *Aromatase dysregulation*
- *Aromatase excess syndrome*:
  - Familial
  - Sporadic
- *Neoplasm*:
  - *Gonadal tumors*:
    - Sertoli cell tumors:
      - Isolated
      - Peutz-Jeghers syndrome
      - Carney complex
    - Trophoblastic tumors
  - *Extragonadal tumors*:
    - Feminizing adrenocortical neoplasm
    - Hepatocellular carcinoma
    - Melanoma
- *Hormonal stimulation of aromatase*:
  - Thyrotoxicosis
- *Idiopathic*

## Testosterone Deficiency

Sometimes, gynecomastia is caused by androgen deficiency rather than estrogen excess, though androgen deficiency is associated with a relative excess of estrogen.

### *Hypogonadotropic Hypogonadism*

In secondary hypogonadism due to hypothalamic or pituitary disease, patients present with gynecomastia due to greater relative decline in serum testosterone than estradiol. Cushing's syndrome can cause gynecomastia by two mechanisms. Glucocorticoids suppress hypothalamic secretion of GnRH and directly inhibit testosterone synthesis, resulting in lower circulating testosterone concentration and a decreased testosterone to estrogen radio.

### *Anorchia*

Almost 50% of anorchic patients also have gynecomastia due to the absence of testicular androgen and adrenal secretion of aromatizable precursors of estrogen.

## Imbalance of Estrogen to Testosterone Ratio

Some causes of gynecomastia are driven equally by estrogen excess and androgen deficiency.

### *Hypergonadotropic Hypogonadism*

Primary hypogonadism tends to have more gynecomastia than secondary hypogonadism due to the dual effects of decreased circulating androgen and markedly increased circulating estrogen concentration. The increased aromatization of testosterone to estrone occurs due to high level of LH which occurs in primary hypogonadism. Klinefelter syndrome is the classic example of this hormonal imbalance. Other forms of primary testicular disease, including mumps orchitis, are associated with an increased risk of developing gynecomastia.

### *Partially Compensated Testicular Dysfunction with Aging*

Aging is a low androgen state where free testosterone concentration declines to a greater extent than total testosterone concentration. As men age, circulating follicle-stimulating hormone (FSH) and LH concentrations also tend to increase; as a result, estrogen concentrations decline to a lesser extent than androgens. This effect of aging increases the estrogen to androgen ratio. This finding partially explains the high prevalence of gynecomastia in men older than 50 years of age.

### *Androgen Resistance*

Some disorders and drugs cause decreased tissue responsiveness to androgen. Male patients with complete androgen resistance have female-type breast development, despite being genetically male (XY). Androgen resistance is associated with an increased level of LH and testosterone concentrations, resulting in significantly increased estradiol concentration. Kennedy syndrome is associated with androgen resistance at the androgen receptor level due to variably expanded numbers of CAG repeats in the exon of the androgen receptor gene.

### *Systemic Illness*

Chronic liver disease and human immunodeficiency virus (HIV) infection may cause gynecomastia by additional mechanisms.

Chronic liver disease is a state of an increased estrogen level due to increased hepatic aromatization of androgen to estrogen.

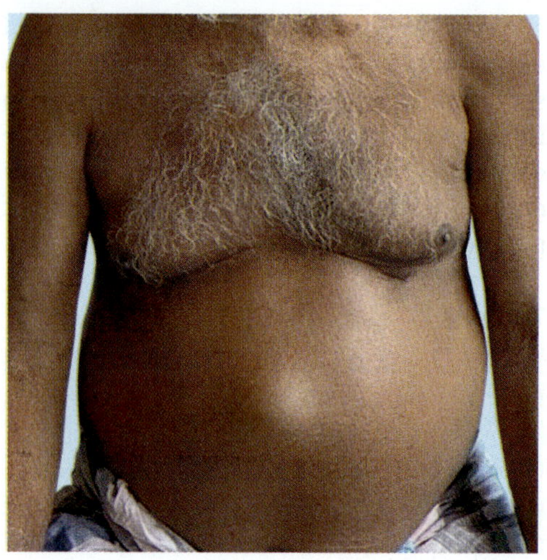

**FIG. 2:** Bilateral gynecomastia in a CLD patient.

Liver disease due to alcohol consumption also damages testicular steroidogenic capacity, and a state of hypergonadotropic hypogonadism can ensue **(Fig. 2)**.

Human immunodeficiency virus infection has a higher prevalence of gynecomastia, which might be due to hypogonadism and the adverse effects of drug therapy. Efavirenz appears to be the main culprit.

## Imbalance to Modulatory Hormones

Prolactin, growth hormone, IGF-I, and thyroxine modulate the action of androgens and estrogens on breast tissue.

Prolactin is a permissive lactotroph that stimulates breast growth, but it is unlikely that prolactin directly causes gynecomastia because men with significant hyperprolactinemia lack this finding. However, hyperprolactinemia reduces GnRH (and therefore LH and testosterone) secretion in many men. So, prolactin can cause gynecomastia by combination of its permissive lactotrophic effect and lowering the testosterone level. So, prolactinoma and antidopaminergic drugs may cause gynecomastia.

Hyperthyroidism is commonly associated with breast tenderness and gynecomastia. Thyroxine stimulates the production of SHBG that binds circulating testosterone more avidly than estradiol. Hyperthyroidism is also associated with increased aromatization of androgens to estrogens.

Growth hormones also have permissive trophic effect on breast tissue growth. In acromegaly, due to large pituitary tumors, there may be hypogonadotropic hypogonadism due to compression of the gonadotropes. So, in this setting of low androgen concentration, excess GH contributes to the development of gynecomastia. It is also hypothesized that GH causes breast growth by increased circulating IGF-I concentration.

### Other Causes

- Drug induced gynecomastia
- *Exogenous estrogen or estrogen substances*:
  - Drug therapy with estrogen
  - Estrogen creams and lotions
- *Drugs that inhibit testosterone synthesis:*
  - Opioids
  - Corticosteroids
  - Alcohol
- *Androgen antagonistic drugs*:
  - Cimetidine
  - Flutamide
  - Cyproterone, spironolactone
- *5α reductase inhibitors:* Finasteride, dutasteride
- *Uncertain mechanism*: Angiotensin-converting enzyme (ACE) inhibitor, atorvastatin, amiodarone, β-blocker, calcium channel blocker (CCB), efavirenz (and other antiretrovirals), fluoxetine, heparin, isoniazid, and metronidazole.

#### *Breast Enlargement due to Malignancy or Infection*

Carcinoma of the breast is very uncommon in men, but Klinefelter syndrome has an increased risk for breast carcinoma. A firm, irregular, unilateral mass is characteristic and suggests a diagnosis.

Certain infectious agents (e.g., Hansen's disease, filariasis) may cause breast enlargement.

## PATH TO DIAGNOSIS

The first important step in diagnosis is to exclude pseudogynecomastia, where adipose tissue is present underneath the nipple. The appropriate technique for physical examination to detect gynecomastia is to pinch the tissue between the thumb and forefinger laterally to the nipple. In the case of breast tissue that feels firm and rubbery with a firm edge, malignancy is suggestive. The ability to feel an edge of tissue at the interface of normal and glandular tissue confirms the presence of gynecomastia.

A careful history taking and physical examination are sufficient to evaluate a case of gynecomastia. It is also unnecessary to perform radiological or biochemical tests to evaluate adult males with chronic stable gynecomastia <5 cm in diameter. It is prudent to perform a more extensive evaluation in the case of new onset of gynecomastia, rapidly progressive hard, irregular masses, or gynecomastia >4 cm in diameter.

### History

The following history is important to evaluate the cause:

- Time of onset, rate of progression, and degree of pain associated with gynecomastia
- Use of medications
- Symptoms of androgen deficiency
- Presence of systemic diseases, such as poorly controlled diabetes mellitus, or severe renal, hepatic, and cardiac disease where the hypothalamic gonadal axis is suppressed.
- Nutritional deficiency due to diet of gut malabsorption
- Symptoms of underlying malignancy, especially testicular

- Symptoms associated with excess of estradiol, thyroxine, prolactin, and growth hormone
- Family history of gynecomastia

### Physical Examination

After using the pinch test to exclude pseudogynecomastia, the following physical examination should be done:

- Assessment for obesity or body mass index
- Skin examination for signs of Cushing's syndrome (striae, ecchymosis), acromegaly, and hyperthyroidism
- Thyroid examination for goiter
- Breast examination for galactorrhea or hard, firm mass
- Axillary lymph node examination
- Genital examination for genital volume and genital mass **(Flowchart 1)**.

### Investigation

The following biochemical tests are necessary in a case of new-onset, rapidly progressive hard irregular mass or gynecomastia >4 cm in diameter:

- Routine test of testosterone, FSH, and LH is a reasonable laboratory assessment.
- Thyroid-stimulating hormone (TSH) measurement should be done to rule out hyperthyroidism.

Many experts recommend measurement of adrenal androgen and estrogen precursors, such as dehydroepiandrosterone (DHEA) or DHEA sulfate, but these are not necessary for routine initial evaluation. Adrenal sex steroid-producing tumors are very rare causes of gynecomastia and are always associated with bulky abdominal mass.

### Imaging

Usually, imaging is not required. If malignancy is suspected, then imaging with mammography or ultrasonography and obtaining tissue by fine needle aspiration or core biopsy should be performed.

## MANAGEMENT

Management depends upon the clinical circumstances, severity, and presence of pain. The first principle is to stop the offending agent and treat the underlying cause if detected.

Boys with pubertal gynecomastia can be reassured that regression usually occurs after 1 year and at most after 3 years, and no treatment is required.

Based on the pathophysiology of gynecomastia, aromatase inhibitors should be expected to be responsive in both pubertal and adult subjects although anecdotal reports suggested that there is no benefit for anastrozole over placebo in the treatment of significant pubertal gynecomastia (>3 cm).

Selective ER modulators (tamoxifen, raloxifene, clomiphene) have been shown to significantly reduce the amount of breast tissue in males.

However, if gynecomastia is of long duration, surgery is the most effective therapy. Indications for surgery include severe psychological and/or cosmetic problems, continued growth or tenderness, and suspected malignancy.

## CLINICAL PEARLS

No treatment and evaluation are required for physiological gynecomastia.

Adult men with new-onset gynecomastia, rapidly enlarging eccentric, hard irregular mass, or gynecomastia >4 cm in diameter should be evaluated properly.

The most important differentiation is between gynecomastia and breast cancer. If doubt remains after physical examination, mammography should be performed.

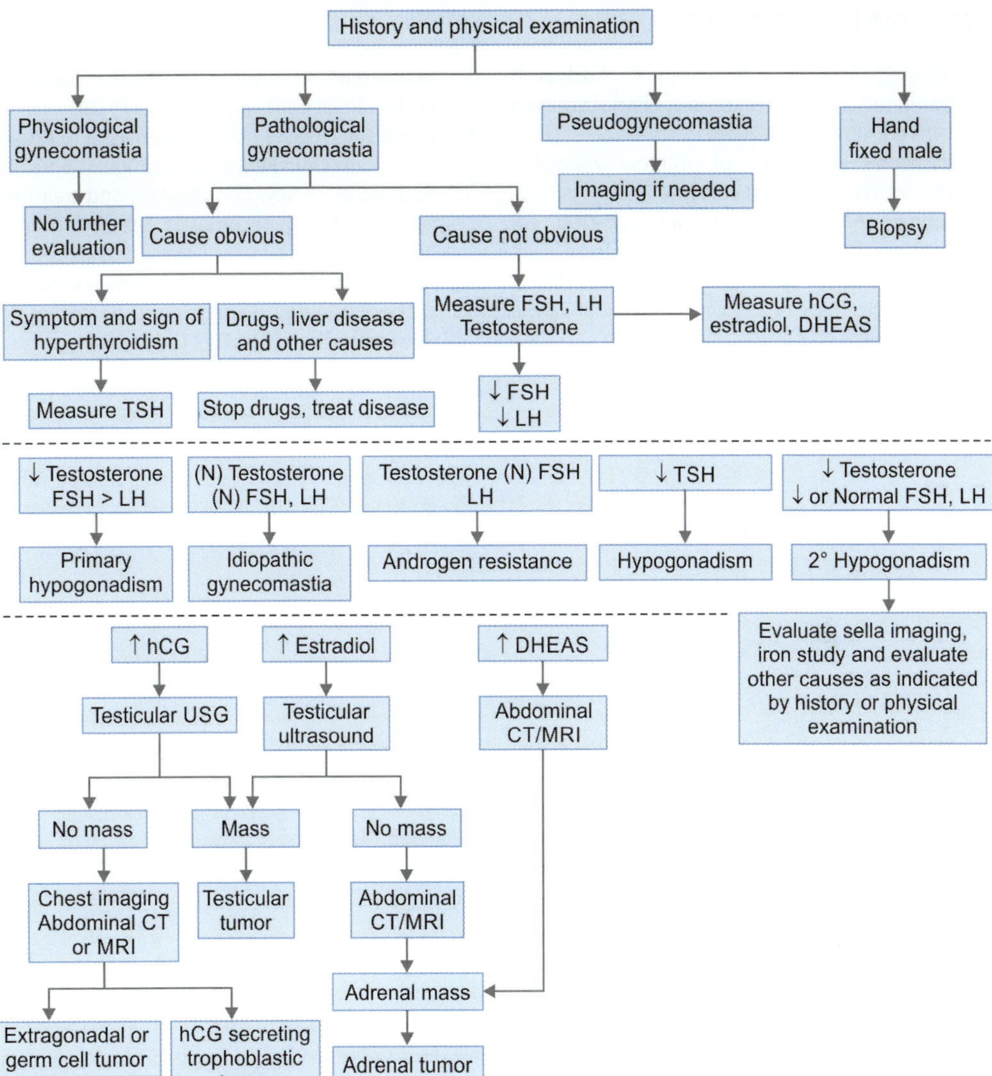


**FLOWCHART 1:** Approach to gynecomastia.

(CT: computed tomography; DHEAS: dehydroepiandrosterone sulfate; FSH: follicle-stimulating hormone; hCG: human chorionic gonadotropin; LH: luteinizing hormone; MRI: magnetic resonance imaging; TSH: thyroid-stimulating hormone; USG: ultrasonography)

## FURTHER READINGS

1. Melmed S, Koenig R, Rosen C, Auchus R, Goldfine A. Williams Textbook of Endocrinology. 14th ed. SL: Elsevier; 2019.
2. Harrison's principles of internal medicine. 21st ed. New York: McGraw Hill; 2022.
3. Labhart A. Clinical Endocrinology. 2nd ed., Springer, 1986.
4. Bannayan GA, Hajdu S1. Gynecomastia: clinicopathologic study of 351 cases. Am J Clin Pathol. 1972;57(4):431-7.
5. Braunstein GD. Aromatase and Gynecomastia. Endocr Relat Cancer. 1999;6(2):315-24.
6. Nordt CA, DiVasta AD. Gynecomastia in Adolescents. Curr Opin Pediatr. 2008;20(4):375-82.
7. Ratnam BV. A new classification and treatment protocol for gynecomastia. Aesthet Surg J. 2009;29(1):26-31.
8. Narula HS, Carlson HE. Gynaecomastia—pathophysiology, diagnosis and treatment. Nat Rev Endocrinol. 2014;10(11):684-98.

CHAPTER 26

# Short Stature

*Sattik Siddhanta*

## INTRODUCTION

A child's growth pattern is a strong indicator of his or her general health. Short stature can be a sign of disease, disability, and social stigma, causing psychological stress. It is important to have early diagnosis and prompt treatment.

## WHAT IS SHORT STATURE?

Short stature is defined as a height that is 2 standard deviations (SD) or more below the mean height for individuals of the same sex and chronological age (CA) in a given population. Alternatively, height >1.5 SD below the midparental height (MPH) or a fall in growth velocity below the 25th percentile over 6–12 months of observation is also termed short stature. Approximately 3% of children in any population will be short, among which half will be physiological (familial or constitutional) and half will be pathological.

## NORMAL GROWTH VELOCITY

Normal postnatal growth is determined by adequate nutrition, growth-promoting hormones, and the genetic potential of the individual. The important hormones are growth hormone (GH), insulin-like growth factor (IGF)-1, thyroid hormones, sex steroids, and other growth factors. Short stature could be due to either intrinsic bone defect or any of the extrinsic factors that are necessary for normal growth and development.

## WHAT ARE CAUSES OF SHORT STATURE?

### Proportionate Short Stature

*Normal variants*:
- Familial

*Prenatal causes*:
- Intrauterine growth restriction (placental, infections, or teratogen)
- Genetic disorders (chromosomal and metabolic disorders), e.g., Turner syndrome, Noonan syndrome, neurofibromatosis type 1, Silver–Russell syndrome, Prader–Willi syndrome, CHARGE syndrome, Bloom syndrome, Fanconi anemia, 3-M syndrome

*Postnatal causes*:
- Undernutrition
- *Chronic systemic illness*:
    - Chronic infections
    - Malabsorption syndromes
    - *Birth defects*: Congenital heart defect (CHD), urinary tract, and nervous system anomalies

  - *Miscellaneous*: Cirrhosis of the liver, bronchiectasis, acquired heart diseases, cardiomyopathies
- Psychosocial short stature (emotional deprivation)

*Endocrine causes*:
- Growth hormone deficiency (GHD)
- GH insensitivity
- Hypothyroidism
- Cushing's syndrome
- Pseudohypoparathyroidism

## Disproportionate Short Stature

*With short limbs*:
- Achondroplasia, hypochondroplasia, chondrodysplasia punctata, chondroectodermal dysplasia, diastrophic dysplasia, metaphyseal chondrodysplasia
- Deformities due to osteogenesis imperfecta, refractory rickets

*With short trunk*:
- Spondyloepiphyseal dysplasia, mucolipidosis, mucopolysaccharidosis
- Caries spine, hemivertebrae

# PATH TO DIAGNOSIS

## History

The following few pointers in the history may provide clues to the etiological diagnosis of short stature:
- History of delayed puberty in parents—constitutional delay in growth
- Low birth weight—small for gestational age
- Neonatal hypoglycemia, jaundice, micropenis—GHD
- Low dietary intake—undernutrition
- Headache, vomiting, visual problem—intracranial space-occupying lesion
- Lethargy, constipation, weight gain—hypothyroidism
- Polyuria—renal disease
- Diarrhea, greasy stools—malabsorption
- Poor social history—psychosocial dwarfism

## Physical Examination

The following clues from physical examination may help to streamline the etiology of short stature:
- Disproportion—skeletal dysplasia, rickets, hypothyroidism
- Dysmorphism—congenital syndromes
- Hypertension—chronic renal failure
- Goiter, coarse skin—hypothyroidism
- Central obesity, purple striae—Cushing's syndrome

### *Accurate Height Measurement*

- *Below 2 years*: Supine length with infantometer
- *For older children*: Stadiometer

### *Assessment of Body Proportion*

Assessment of body proportion helps in differentiating between proportionate and disproportionate short stature.
- Upper segment:lower segment ratio
  - Increased ratio: Rickets, achondroplasia, untreated hypothyroidism
  - Decreased ratio: Spondyloepiphyseal dysplasia, vertebral anomalies
  - Comparison of arm span with height

### *Assessment of Height Velocity*

It is rate of increase in height over a period of time, expressed as cm/year. If it is low, it suggests a pathological cause of short stature.

### *Comparison with Population Norms*

Height plotted on appropriate growth charts **(Fig. 1)** and expressed as centile or SD score.

### *Comparison with Child's Own Genetic Potential*

- MPH for boys = (Mother's height + father's height)/2 + 6.5 cm
- MPH for girls = (Mother's height + father's height)/2 – 6.5 cm

The target height is plotted on the growth chart, and if the child is falling within the target height, the cause could be genetic or constitutional. Otherwise, it is considered abnormal.

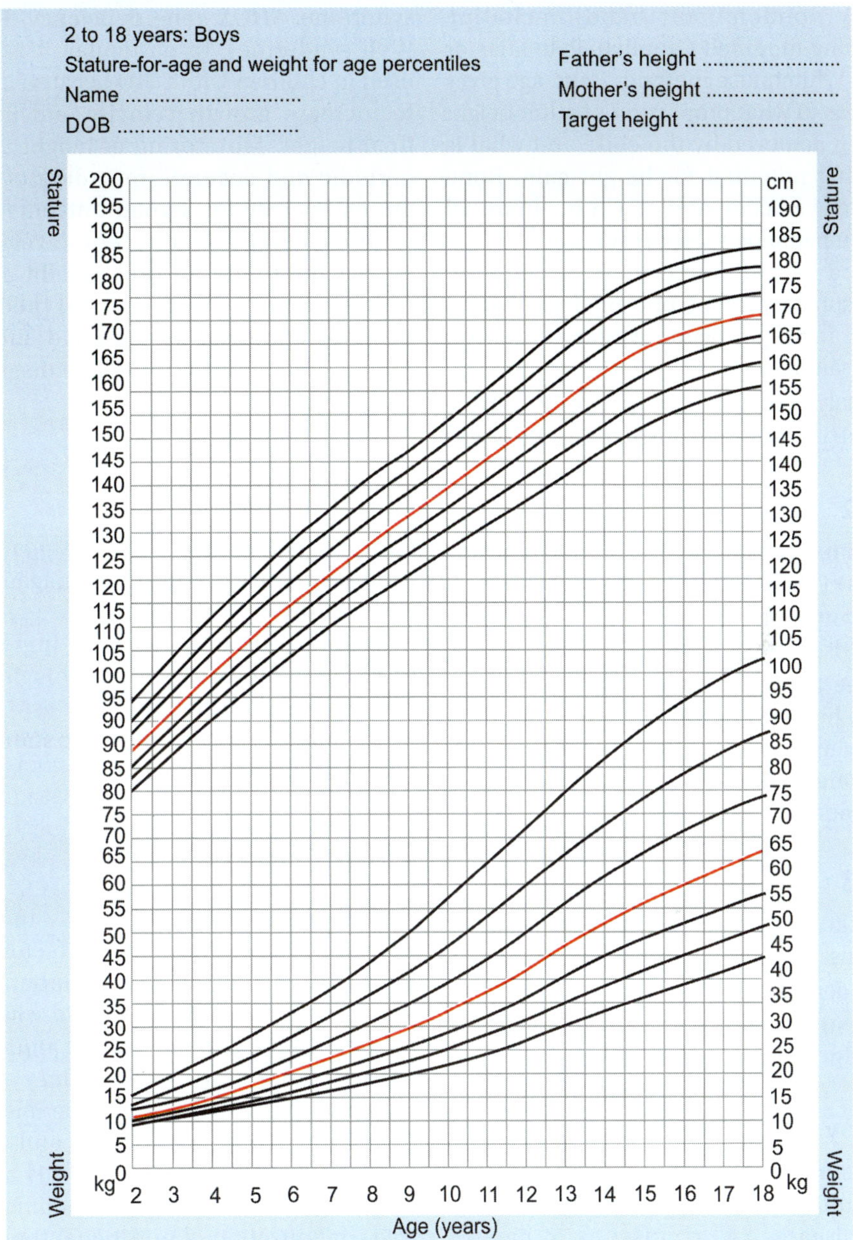


FIG. 1: Growth chart.

# INVESTIGATIONS

## Level 1 (Essential Investigations)

- Complete hemogram with erythrocyte sedimentation rate (ESR)
- Bone age

Assessment of bone age is mandatory for all children with short stature. The appearance of various epiphyseal centers and fusion of epiphyses with metaphyses guide us about the skeletal maturity of the child. It is conventionally read from X-ray of hand (usually nondominant hand) including wrist using modified Greulich-Pyle atlas or Tanner-Whitehouse method. Bone age gives an idea as to what proportion of adult height has been achieved by the child and what is remaining potential for height gain. Bone age is delayed compared to CA in almost all causes of pathological short stature.

- Blood (renal function test, calcium, phosphate, alkaline phosphatase, venous gas, fasting plasma sugar, albumin, transaminases)
- Urinalysis (microscopy, pH, osmolality)
- Stool (parasites, steatorrhea, occult blood)

### Level 2

- Serum thyroxine, thyroid-stimulating hormone (TSH)—juvenile hypothyroidism
- Karyotype to rule out Turner's syndrome in girls

If the above investigations are normal and the height is between 2 and 3 SD, then observe height velocity for 6–12 months.

If height <3 SD, proceed to level 3 investigations.

### Level 3

- Celiac serology (antiendomysial or antitissue transglutaminase antibodies)
- Duodenal biopsy
- GH stimulation test with glucagon or insulin and serum IGF-1 levels

### Therapy

The treatment of short stature depends on the identification of the underlying cause of the disease, e.g., counseling of parents (for physiological causes), dietary advice [undernutrition, celiac disease, renal tubular acidosis (RTA)], and limb lengthening procedures for skeletal dysplasia. GH therapy is recommended as a growth-promoting treatment for many different disorders (e.g., GHD, Turner syndrome, Noonan syndrome, *SHOX* gene deficiency, Prader-Willi syndrome). In particular, it is widely used in children with GHD because it is able to increase growth velocity and improve final height. Monitoring of height velocity periodic and accurate recording of height are mandatory for a good outcome in any form of therapy. One recent development is "Macimorelin," an oral ghrelin agonist, which is a new stimulus for GH production that was approved by the Food and Drug Administration (FDA) in 2017 for diagnosis of GHD in adult patients.

## RED FLAG SIGNS

Early diagnosis and prompt treatment are of utmost importance in the management of short stature.

Auxology is of paramount importance to differentiate between physiological and pathological short stature.

Endocrine causes of short stature are usually associated with obesity.

## CONCLUSION

Growth is a complex process in which nutrition, hormones, genetic factors, and environmental factors play important roles. Management options for a child with short stature would depend on the underlying cause. Short stature secondary to any systemic illness will not reverse unless the underlying cause is evaluated and treated accordingly. Since malnutrition is a major cause of short stature in developing countries, optimization of nutritional status with appropriate dietary advice or nutritional therapy should be included in the management. Diagnosis of genetic syndromes necessitates the need for genetic counseling. Treatment of endocrine causes includes timely and adequate replacement of the deficient hormone.

## CLINICAL PEARLS

- Short stature is a common problem encountered in clinical practice.
- Early diagnosis and prompt treatment is of utmost importance.
- Differentiation between physiological and pathological short stature is the key to allay the anxiety of the patient guardians and care givers.
- A thorough history, meticulous physical examination along with some necessary investigations may guide in streamlining the etiology of short stature and plan therapeutic strategies accordingly.
- Always rule out endocrine causes of short stature if it is associated with obesity.

## FURTHER READINGS

1. Desai MP, Menon PSN, Bhatia V. Pediatric Endocrine Disorders. Chennai, India: Orient Longman; 2001.
2. Sperling MA. Sperling's Textbook of Pediatric Endocrinology, 3rd Edition. Philadelphia: Saunders Elseviers; 2008.

# PART 4

# Gastroenterology

# CHAPTER 27

# Chronic Diarrhea

*Pranab Kumar Maity*

## INTRODUCTION

Chronic diarrhea occurs in 3–5% of the population, and diagnosis sometimes becomes difficult as different types of diagnostic studies may be needed.

## DEFINITION

Diarrhea is defined in adults by abnormal stool weight (>200 g/day), consistency (loose or liquid), and/or frequency (3 times/day). A 4-week symptom duration is generally considered as a cutoff point to distinguish acute (<4 weeks) from chronic (>4 weeks).

Stool outputs as high as 300 g may be normal when a high-fiber diet is consumed.

Urgency and fecal incontinence may drive a patient's perception of the severity of "diarrhea" and often go unvoiced if not specifically asked by the physician. Most of the studies used to define a 4-week cutoff for a diagnosis of chronic diarrhea were done in industrialized countries. Information from less developed parts of the world is needed to evaluate how practical such a cutoff is in those regions.

## CLASSIFICATION

The classification of chronic diarrhea is listed in **Box 1**.

## CLINICAL APPROACH TO CHRONIC DIARRHEA

A detailed history and thorough examination are crucial for evaluating patients with chronic diarrhea.

- *Demographics*: Irritable bowel syndrome (IBS) commonly occurs in the third and fourth decade; acquired immunodeficiency syndrome (AIDS)-related diarrhea is common in younger patients whereas the peak incidence of microscopic colitis is in the seventh and eighth decade of life. Colon cancer should be excluded in a patient with new onset of diarrhea over the age of 50 years.

  IBS and microscopic colitis are more common in females.
- *Mode of onset*: Some causes of chronic diarrhea have been triggered with an acute infectious episode. Postinfectious IBS, giardia, inflammatory bowel disease (IBD), lactose intolerance. Other conditions such as lymphoma, celiac disease, and amyloidosis usually develop insidiously.
- *Pattern of diarrhea*: The Bristol Stool Form Scale (with visual aids if need be) is useful in understanding the patient's symptoms.
  - Fat-laden stools are pale and bulky, often float, and are sticky, typically needing several flushes of the toilet, a useful feature that patients may

**BOX 1: Classification of chronic diarrhea.**

*Osmotic*:
- Medications
  - Laxatives (Mg, $SO_4$, $PO_4$), elixirs
- Undigested sugars
  - Diet foods/drinks/gum (sorbitol, mannitol, others)
  - Enzyme dysfunction (e.g., lactose, fructose)

*Secretory*:
- Medications
  - Nonosmotic laxatives, antibiotics, and many others
- Small intestinal bacterial overgrowth
- Endocrine
  - Tumors: Carcinoid, gastrinoma, medullary thyroid cancer, VIPoma
  - Systemic: Adrenal insufficiency, hyperthyroidism
- Bile salt malabsorption (ileal resection, idiopathic, postcholecystectomy)
- Noninvasive infections: Giardiasis, cryptosporidiosis, steatorrhea
- Maldigestion
  - Decreased bile salts (cirrhosis, bile duct obstruction, ileal resection)
  - Pancreatic dysfunction (chronic pancreatitis, cystic fibrosis, duct obstruction)
- Malabsorption
  - Celiac sprue, tropical sprue, giardiasis, Whipple's disease
  - Chronic mesenteric ischemia
  - Short bowel syndrome
  - Bacterial overgrowth (diabetes mellitus, scleroderma, prior bowel surgery)
  - Lymphatic obstruction

*Inflammatory*:
- Inflammatory bowel disease: Ulcerative colitis, Crohn's disease, microscopic colitis
- Malignancy: Colon cancer, lymphoma
- Radiation colitis/enteritis
- Mastocytosis
- Invasive or inflammatory infections: *Clostridium difficile*, Cytomegalovirus, *Entamoeba histolytica*, tuberculosis
- Ischemia

*Motility*:
- Post-surgical (vagotomy, dumping)
- Scleroderma
- Diabetes mellitus
- Hyperthyroidism

*Miscellaneous*:
- Irritable bowel syndrome
- Functional diarrhea
- Factitious

recognize, as most do not examine their stool minutely. The presence of malabsorption is usually evident by steatorrhea which includes pale, bulky, malodorous stool.
- Erratic and unpredictable bowel movements are typical of IBS patients. It may be useful for the patient to complete a 1-week stool diary. Important in IBS is the periodicity of symptoms with bouts lasting a few days and remitting for a further few days. This short-lived fluctuation would be unusual in most organic diseases.
- Psychiatric symptoms such as anxiety and depression are frequently associated with IBS and may be present in up to 67% of cases.
- Nocturnal diarrhea has been considered to be an "alarm" feature, suggesting the likelihood of an organic process and the need for more extensive investigations. However, more recent studies suggest that nocturnal symptoms occur in similar proportions of patients with IBS and with a typical organic problem like microscopic colitis (40 and 39%, respectively). Nocturnal diarrhea is recognized as common in diarrhea associated with diabetic autonomic neuropathy and is also a feature of postinfectious bile salt malabsorption.
- It is important to differentiate between small and large bowel diarrhea. In small bowel involvement, usually the frequency is less than 4 per day, large volume, bulky, frothy, and greasy. In large bowel involvement, the frequency is more than 4 with small volume. Blood, mucous, and pus may be present.

*Associated symptoms*:
- Rectal bleeding needs endoscopic evaluation for polyp, IBD, hemorrhoid, and malignancy. The presence of blood in stool necessitates further examination, usually by colonoscopy, although minor bleeding because of trauma is common in all diarrheal diseases.
- Weight loss—celiac disease, tuberculosis, malignancy, IBD.
- New-onset diarrhea in elderly (>50 years), family history of colonic carcinoma—need evaluation with colonoscopy.
- Pain may occur in IBD, tuberculosis, and malignancy. Patients of IBS may have crampy abdominal pain, which may be relieved by defecation. Inflammatory diseases affecting the rectum may be associated with tenesmus (painful defecation).
- The presence of lymphadenopathy or significant weight loss could suggest chronic infection or malignancy.

*Comorbidity*: Patients with celiac disease often have had previous iron deficiency anemia or other autoimmune disorders. Systemic diseases, such as diabetes mellitus, hyperthyroidism, hyperparathyroidism, and Addison's disease, may produce chronic diarrhea as a complication.

*Drug history* and its relation to the onset of diarrhea are important because drugs can cause diarrhea through several mechanisms, including direct pharmacological effects (e.g., β-blockers, metformin, magnesium-containing antacids) or indirect effects (e.g., proton-pump inhibitors causing microscopic colitis or antibiotics causing *Clostridium difficile* colitis) **(Box 2)**.

*Family history* is important in cases of IBD, celiac disease, or neoplastic diseases.

*Dietary history*: High fermentable oligosaccharides, disaccharides, monosaccharides, and polyols (FODMAP) diet, high fructose corn syrup used as artificial sweetener, grapes, and stoned fruits, such as plums, mangos, and cherries, can cause diarrhea if ingested in excess.

Diarrhea is likely to be due to lactose intolerance only if the patient ingests >12 g/day (240 mL of milk or its equivalent in other dairy foods). Excessive alcohol intake, particularly beer, impairs intestinal

**BOX 2: Drugs causing diarrhea.**

*More common*:
- Antacids, proton-pump inhibitor (PPI)
- Cephalosporins, clindamycin, ampicillin, amoxycillin, erythromycin
- Colchicine
- Metformin
- Nonsteroidal anti-inflammatory drugs, 5-aminosalicylates
- Cholesterol-lowering agents (clofibrate, gemfibrozil, lovastatin)
- Antineoplastic drugs

*Less common*:
- Angiotensin-converting enzyme inhibitor
- Angiotensin receptor-blocking agents
- Beta-adrenergic receptor antagonists, other-antiarrhythmics
- Carbamazepine
- Lithium
- Vitamin and mineral supplements

water absorption and can cause diarrhea. Caffeine causes jejunal secretion and may be responsible for diarrhea in some patients.

*Physical examination* **(Table 1)**:
- Assessment of hydration and nutritional status (anemia, vitamin deficiency), presence of clubbing, lymphadenopathy.
- Abdominal examination is usually unremarkable apart from vague tenderness. Abdominal masses are rare, but fullness in the right iliac fossa may be felt in ileocolonic Crohn's disease (CD).
- Perineal inspection and rectal examination are useful to exclude any induration or local tenderness that might suggest CD or an anal fissure.
- Assessment of voluntary squeeze is useful in assessing patients with urgency to see if there is any sphincter defect because incontinence may lead to a complaint of diarrhea.

**Table 1: Physical findings of interest in chronic diarrhea.**

| ***Findings*** | ***Potential implications*** |
|---|---|
| Orthostasis | Hypotension, dehydration, neuropathy |
| Muscle wasting, edema | Malnutrition |
| Urticaria pigmentosa, dermatographism | Mast cell disease (mastocytosis) |
| Pinch purpura, macroglossia | Amyloidosis |
| Hyperpigmentation | Addison's disease |
| Migratory necrotizing erythema | Glucagonoma |
| Flushing | Carcinoid syndrome |
| Malignant atrophic papulosis | Kohlmeier–Degos disease |
| Dermatitis herpetiformis | Celiac disease |
| Thyroid nodule, lymphadenopathy | Medullary carcinoma of the thyroid |
| Tremor, lid lag | Hyperthyroidism |
| Right-sided heart murmur, wheezing | Carcinoid syndrome |
| Hepatomegaly, endocrine tumor | Amyloidosis |
| Arthritis, inflammatory bowel disease | Yersiniosis |
| Lymphadenopathy, human immunodeficiency virus (HIV) | Lymphoma, cancer |
| Abdominal bruit | Chronic mesenteric ischemia |
| Anal sphincter weakness | Fecal incontinence |

## LABORATORY WORKUP TO EVALUATE CHRONIC DIARRHEA

### Routine Investigations

Complete blood count, serum albumin, globulin, urea, creatinine, glucose, and electrolytes are routine investigations done to diagnose chronic diarrhea.

### Stool Examination

Fecal electrolytes can help to differentiate between osmotic and secretory diarrhea. It is based on the calculation of the osmotic gap. Stool osmotic gap: Serum osmolarity (typically 290 mOsmol/kg) – [2 × (fecal sodium + potassium concentration)]. A fecal osmotic gap of <50 mOsmol/kg indicates a secretory diarrhea, while a gap of >75 mOsm/kg indicates an osmotic diarrhea. A low fecal pH (<7.0) is suggestive of carbohydrate malabsorption. Leukocyte enzyme, lactoferrin, or calprotectin are used as surrogate markers of fecal leukocytes to diagnose mucosal inflammation. Fecal calprotectin has been found to be more sensitive.

### Imaging Tests (Table 2)

A plain abdominal radiograph showing pancreatic calcifications is diagnostic of chronic pancreatitis. Barium studies have been used extensively in the past in the diagnosis of chronic diarrhea. With the introduction of abdominal computed tomography (CT) scans, the role of barium studies has become limited. A chest X-ray should be done to exclude tuberculosis.

**Table 2: Radiographic findings in chronic diarrhea and malabsorption syndromes.**

| *Condition* | *Classical findings* |
|---|---|
| Celiac disease | Dilated caliber; increased fluid; thin, effaced folds (moulage), segmentation of barium column, painless intussusception |
| Whipple's disease | Normal caliber; thick, wild fold pattern; patchy micronodularity |
| Scleroderma | Dilated, especially duodenum; delayed peristalsis, hypomotility |
| Lymphoma | Variable caliber; coarse folds; wall infiltrated, stiff; extraluminal masses; micronodularity |
| Amyloidosis | Normal caliber; symmetrical fold thickening, no edema; stiff walls; micronodularity |
| Lymphangiectasia | Increased luminal fluid; thick, edematous folds |
| Crohn's disease | Stenotic (string sign); deformed/thickened folds; rigidity/ulceration of walls; sometimes extraluminal mass |
| Dysgammaglobulinemia | Increased luminal fluid; nodular lymphoid hyperplasia |
| Giardiasis | Dilated duodenum; thick duodenal folds; spasm, rapid transit |
| Zollinger–Ellison syndrome | Dilated duodenum; thick duodenal folds; peptic ulcer; reticulated pattern |
| Cystic fibrosis | Thick folds; nodularity in duodenum |
| Abetalipoproteinemia, fine mucosal graininess | Abetalipoproteinemia, fine mucosal graininess |
| Mastocytosis | Thick gut wall; mucosal nodularity |

## Computed Tomography and Magnetic Resonance Enterography

Computed tomography and magnetic resonance (MR) enterography are useful in the diagnosis of chronic diarrhea because of CD and eosinophilic gastroenteritis and in the detection of small bowel tumors, such as carcinoids.

## Nuclear Medicine Imaging

Radioligand scintigraphy is useful in detecting neuroendocrine tumors that express somatostatin receptors, such as gastrinomas and carcinoid tumors. Single photon emission computed tomography (SPECT)-CT provides better localization of these tumors.

## Endoscopy

Colonoscopy with biopsy is helpful for the diagnosis of IBD, neoplasia, and microscopic colitis. Upper gastrointestinal (GI) endoscopy and duodenal biopsy can confirm a diagnosis of celiac disease. Duodenal biopsy may also aid in the diagnosis of giardiasis and other protozoal infections and Whipple's disease. Upper endoscopy also helps in the collection of duodenal aspirate for quantitative diagnosis of small intestinal bacterial overgrowth.

## Colorectal and Terminal Ileal Biopsy

Colonoscopy and biopsy have a significant role in diagnosing conditions such as IBD, microscopic colitis, inflammatory conditions, and neoplasia. Multiple studies have evaluated the role of colonoscopy stating the yield of specific diagnoses of chronic diarrhea in 15–31%.

## Serological Tests

Immunoglobulin A (IgA) anti-tissue transglutaminase (TTG) is the preferred single test for the detection of celiac disease in individuals over the age of 2 years. Total serum IgA should be measured at the same time to rule out IgA deficiency that might cause a falsely negative test. Anti-*Saccharomyces cerevisiae* antibodies are measured to diagnose IBD.

## Breath Tests

*Hydrogen breath tests (HBT)*: The breath tests help in diagnosing carbohydrate malabsorption and small intestinal overgrowth. However, the sensitivity and specificity vary widely.

## Pancreatic Function Tests

The standard secretin stimulation test is rarely used nowadays, whereas the modified endoscopic secretin stimulation test done using endoscopic retrograde cholangiopancreatography (ERCP) has limited diagnostic yield. Various other tests for pancreatic function include serum trypsin, fecal chymotrypsin, and fecal elastase, which again show limited utility in mild insufficiency. Pancreatic imaging using endoscopic ultrasound and magnetic resonance imaging (MRI) is used invariably to detect abnormal anatomy.

## Bacteriology/Microbiology

In developing countries, chronic bacterial, mycobacterial, and parasitic infections are common. Additionally, some clinical situations require an extensive search for a source of infection in case of diarrhea of chronic origin. They include diarrhea in immigrants from endemic areas, immunocompromised subjects, patients with human immunodeficiency virus (HIV)/AIDS infection, men who have sex with men, and individuals with chronic travelers' diarrhea.

Giardiasis, amebiasis, yersiniosis, and *C. difficile* infections are frequent causes of chronic diarrhea in immunocompetent hosts. *Strongyloides* is occasionally seen but is quite unusual. These five pathogens should be sought in such patients.

Giardia is most reliably detected with a stool enzyme-linked immunosorbent assay (ELISA). Ameba and *Strongyloides* are sought with serological tests and stool examination for ova and parasites. Three stool samples should be sent for microscopic examination. *C. difficile* is most reliably detected with a stool deoxyribonucleic acid (DNA) amplification assay.

Patients on immunosuppressant medications or those with HIV/AIDS infection have a greater likelihood of chronic infections. Enteropathogens that can cause acute, self-limited diarrhea in immunologically normal individuals can cause chronic diarrhea in these patients. These pathogens are *Salmonella, Shigella, Campylobacter, Escherichia coli, Yersinia,* and others. Traditionally, these infections are detected with standard stool cultures. However, new molecular techniques may prove to be better in time, making standard stool cultures obsolete.

Patients with HIV/AIDS suffer from potential infectious etiologies related to their degree of immunosuppression. With lesser degrees of immunosuppression (CD4 count > 200 cells/mm$^3$), the usual pathogens predominate. However, if the CD4 count is <200 cells/mm$^3$, the spectrum includes mycobacterial and protozoan infections also along with the enteropathogens. These include *Mycobacterium avium* complex (MAC), cryptosporidium, *Cyclospora, Isospora belli,* and microsporidium. Viral infections, such as cytomegalovirus (CMV) and herpes simplex virus, and fungal infections, such as candidiasis and histoplasmosis.

## MANAGEMENT ISSUES

The etiology of chronic diarrhea should be identified and treated accordingly. Dietary measures include the restriction of unabsorbed carbohydrates and sweets, avoidance of milk and milk products in patients with lactose intolerance, and fat restriction and supplementation of fat-soluble vitamins and calcium in patients with steatorrhea.

Empirical therapy for chronic diarrhea may be used when the diagnostic workup has failed to confirm the diagnosis, when no specific treatment is available, or when the treatment has failed. Opiate antidiarrheal agents such as loperamide are frequently used. They are safe and effective but should not be used in infectious diarrhea or in severe IBD.

Bile acid sequestrates like cholestyramine are useful in diarrhea caused by bile acid malabsorption. Octreotide is used to control diarrhea occurring in carcinoid syndrome, VIPomas, and neuroendocrine tumors.

Alpha2-adrenergic agonist, clonidine, is used to treat diabetic diarrhea. Eluxadoline, a μ opioid receptor agonist, is a new drug approved for use in patients with IBS. Diarrhea in Zollinger–Ellison syndrome responds to treatment with proton-pump inhibitors. Bacterial overgrowth is treated with antibiotics.

## CLINICAL PEARLS

- Changes in stool frequency weight or consistency for more than 4 weeks is chronic diarrhea
- Etiology has a wide spectrum ranging from various infections to IBD and neoplasms
- Diagnosis needs individualized investigations

## FURTHER READINGS

1. Ghoshal UC, Mehrotra M, Kumar S, Ghoshal U, Krishnani N, Misra A, et al. Spectrum of malabsorption syndrome among adults and factors differentiating celiac disease and tropical malabsorption. Indian J Med Res. 2012;136(3):451-9.
2. Yadav P, Das P, Mirdha BR, Gupta SD, Bhatnagar S, Pandey RM, et al. Current spectrum of malabsorption syndrome in adults in India. Indian J Gastroenterol. 2011;30(1):22-8.

CHAPTER 28

# Abdominal Swelling: Localized or Generalized

*Sanjay Bandyopadhyay (Banerjee)*

## INTRODUCTION

An abdominal swelling is defined as enlargement or distention of the abdomen. It can be a generalized swelling or localized to a specific site of the abdomen. A localized abdominal swelling can also be referred to as an abdominal lump/mass.

## PATHOGENESIS

The localized or generalized abdominal swelling can be of the following origin:

- *Inflammatory/infective*:

  *Acute*: A hepatic abscess developing in the right hypochondrium.

  *Chronic*: For example, a hydatid cyst developing in the liver or spleen.
- *Obstructive*: Obstructive abdominal swelling is mostly localized.

  Most obstructive swellings are acute in nature like an intussusception develops over mere days although some obstructive masses can also be a chronic lump like a gastric outlet obstruction.

  Hernial swellings, on the other hand, can be both acute and chronic in nature.
- *Traumatic*: Perforation of hollow viscus can lead to a generalized swelling like peritonitis or a localized swelling due to walling off of the viscera by the omentum and the peritoneum.

  Following trauma, internal hemorrhage can lead to hemorrhagic peritonitis/ascites or a capsulated hemorrhagic swelling within the abdomen.
- *Motility disorder*: Motility disorders are a result of muscles or enteric nervous system not working in a coordinated manner. It can lead to a variety of symptoms among which is abdominal swelling, which is mostly chronic in nature.
- *Vascular*: An abdominal aneurysm could be a medical emergency depending on its size. It generally presents as a pulsatile localized swelling.
- *Malignancy*: Ascites can be the first presenting symptom for many malignant conditions, commonly, hepatocellular carcinoma to rarer malignancies like appendicular carcinoma.
- *Medication*: Narcotics, iron supplements, anticholinergics, and some antihypertensives like calcium channel blockers can cause abdominal swelling of generalized nature due to bloating or constipation.

## DIFFERENTIAL DIAGNOSIS

### Generalized Swelling

Generalized swelling could be due to fat, fetus, flatus, feces, or fluid.

Accumulation of fluid in the abdominal cavity is called ascites (Greek *askos* meaning bag or sac). Ascites can be exudative (where ascitic fluid protein level is >3 g/100 mL) or transudative (ascetic fluid total protein is <3 g/10 mL).

The causes of both types of ascites are given in **Box 1**.

## Localized Swelling

- *Organic causes*:
  - Bowel obstruction
  - Gastroparesis
  - Gastrointestinal diseases like complicated diverticular disease, inflammatory bowel disease
  - Organ enlargement
  - Internal bleeding
- *Functional causes*:
  - Intestinal pseudo-obstruction
  - Constipation
  - Bloating from food intolerance, indigestion, or irritable bowel syndrome
  - Urinary retention
  - Abdominal muscle weakness
- Hernia
- Pelvic masses

**BOX 1: Common causes of exudative and transudative ascites.**

*Exudative ascites*:
- Peritonitis like tubercular, trauma, perforation
- Malignant disease: Hepatic, peritoneal
- Acute pancreatitis
- Lymphatic obstruction
- Hypothyroidism

*Transudative ascites*:
- Cardiac failure
- Cirrhosis of liver
- Hypoproteinemia
- Hepatic venous occlusion
- Meigs syndrome
- Constrictive pericarditis
- Nephrotic syndrome

# PATHWAY TO DIAGNOSIS

*History*
- *Site*: Where did the swelling appear?
- *Duration*: How long has been the swelling present for?
- *Mode of onset*: Whether the swelling developed after trauma or spontaneously.
- *Progression*: Has the size of the swelling been growing (rapidly or slowly) or has it been static?
- Has there been any regression in the size of the swelling?
- Pain over the swelling?
  - *Duration of pain*
  - *Character of pain*
  - *Radiation of pain*
  - *Periodicity of pain*
- Any other swelling?
- Previous history of such swelling, recurrence, and operation done, if any?
- History of fever, loss of appetite, weight loss, hematemesis, hemoptysis, melena, hematochezia, decreased urinary output
- Past history of tuberculosis
- Medication history

*Physical examination*
- General survey
- Local examination

*Inspection*
- *Localized swelling*:
  - Site (with respect to the nine quadrants of the abdomen)
  - Shape
  - Surface
  - Margin
  - Movement with respiration
  - Skin over the swelling:
    - *Venous prominence*
    - *Ulcer*
    - *Discharge*
    - *Pigmentation*
    - *Scar*
  - Visible peristalsis
  - Grey Turner's sign which is bluish discoloration of flanks due to

accumulation of blood (found in diseases like acute hemorrhagic pancreatitis).
    - Cullen's sign which is bluish discoloration of area around the umbilicus due to accumulation of blood.
- *Generalized swelling*:
    - Shape of abdomen
    - Position of umbilicus—everted or inverted?
    - Skin over the abdomen:
        - *Venous prominence*
        - *Ulcer*
        - *Discharge*
        - *Pigmentation*
        - *Scar*

*Palpation*
- *Localized swelling*:
    - Temperature over the swelling
    - Tenderness—present or absent?
    - Size—measurement of size of the swelling with a measuring tape or a caliper
    - Shape—confirmation of inspection findings
    - Surface of swelling
    - Margin of the swelling—extent?
    - Consistency—solid or cystic?
    - Fluctuation test, if the swelling is cystic
    - Transillumination test, if the swelling is cystic
    - Reducibility—reducible or not
    - Compressibility—compressible or not?
    - Ballotability of the swelling?
    - Movement of the swelling with respiration?
      The swelling might move coupled with respiration, but this movement should not be confused with the anteroposterior movement of the abdomen. The movement of the swelling with respiration can be ascertained by placing one's hand over the lower border of the swelling and asking the patient to take a deep breath; with inspiration, the swelling will move up and with expiration it will move down.
    - Is the swelling parietal or intra-abdominal?
      If the swelling becomes more prominent with asking the patient to raise their hands straight while only lifting their torso, then it is a parietal swelling; otherwise, it is an intra-abdominal swelling.
    - Fixity to skin?
    - Fixity to muscle? Trying to move the swelling with muscles contracted and relaxed.
    - Pulsation: If present, transmitted or expansile in nature?
    - Any palpable thrill?
    - Deep palpation of the organ should be done—liver and spleen.
    - If it is a lower abdominal mass—lower end palpable or not?
    - Hernia sites should be examined for hernias can present as localized swelling.
- *Generalized swelling*:
    - Rigidity or guarding—present or not?
    - Tenderness—present or not?
    - Organomegaly by deep palpation.
    - Hepatojugular reflux should be tested.
    - Direction of venous prominence should be ascertained, if present.

*Percussion*
- *Fluid thrill*: It is tested for by putting either an assistant's hand or the patient's in the midline and then percussing the flanks to see if the impulse is being transmitted or not.
- *Shifting dullness*: It is tested for by starting to percuss the abdomen from the flanks till the midline to find the most resonant area. The patient is then turned sideways and the flanks are percussed again. In ascites, there is a change in dullness with a change in position.
- Liver and splenic dullness

*Auscultation*

- Intraperistaltic sounds should be listened for—present or absent? If present—sluggish or not?
- Succussion splash test and auscultopercussion are done for gastric outlet obstruction presenting with swelling (tested when a patient has not eaten/drank in the last 1–3 hours).
- If the swelling is suspected to be of vascular nature, bruit over swelling should be auscultated for.

Per rectal examination and vaginal examination (in parous women only) should be done in all cases of localized abdominal swelling.

## INVESTIGATIONS

- *Blood tests*:
  - Routine blood test like electrolyte level, liver function test, renal function test, complete blood count
  - Amylase and lipase
  - Coagulation profile for generalized swelling
  - Malignancy markers are also tested for if cancer is suspected.
- *Radiological investigation*:
  - Every abdominal swelling should get an ultrasonography (USG) of the whole abdomen done as a preliminary investigation after which, more specialized investigations are done to reach a conclusive diagnosis.
  - A contrast-enhanced computed tomography (CECT) scan of the whole abdomen can be done for better visualization of the swelling with respect to other abdominal structures.
  - An endoscopic-guided USG is done after the above investigations if they do not give us a conclusive diagnosis. Biopsy samples can be taken as well in such a scenario.
  - Upper gastrointestinal endoscopy and colonoscopy are done if deemed necessary for diagnosis based on USG or CECT whole abdomen. A big advantage of these procedures is that biopsies can be performed as well as therapies can be administered.
  - Magnetic resonance cholangiopancreatography is done to look at the biliary and pancreatic system if clinical findings and blood test results point toward the swelling of being biliary or pancreatic in origin.
  - FibroScan of the liver is a noninvasive investigation to determine the median stiffness of the liver.
  - Chest X-ray—high-resolution (HR) CT is done to look for gas under the diaphragm in an acute emergency setting.

## POOR DIAGNOSTIC SIGNS

- A rapidly growing swelling
- Recurrence after therapeutic/surgical management
- Loss of weight or loss of appetite
- Pain in a previously painless swelling
- Changes over the skin of the swelling in the form of ulceration or discharge
- Presence of blood in stool
- Loss of bowel sounds
- Recent complaints of fever, tachycardia, tachypnea, decrease in urinary output, sudden-onset breathlessness, sudden-onset vomiting, obstipation, constipation
- Changes in mentation of the patient

## MANAGEMENT

- Nil per mouth if abdominal pain is present
- Ryle's tube is done for decompression.
- Catheterization is done if low urine output/strict intake output monitoring.
- Intravenous fluid is started.
- Injectable antiemetic if nausea is present.
- Intravenous pain management with injectable analgesics

- Injectable empirical antibiotics started in all cases
- USG-guided therapeutic and diagnostic tapping of ascites

## CLINICAL PEARLS

- Detailed history and step-wise clinical examination clinch the diagnosis in most of the cases of localized or generalized abdominal swelling.
- Remembering the anatomical structure in each of the nine abdominal quadrants will help in shortlisting the causes of localized abdominal swellings.
- Rigidity in a distended abdomen is an ominous sign.
- Sudden increase in the size of a swelling necessitates emergency attention.

## FURTHER READINGS

1. Ferguson CM. Inspection, Auscultation, Palpation, and Percussion of the Abdomen. In: Walker HK, Hall WD, Hurst JW, (Eds). Clinical Methods: The History, Physical, and Laboratory Examinations, 3rd edition. Boston: Butterworths; 1990. Chapter 93. PMID: 21250260.
2. Mealie CA, Ali R, Manthey DE. Abdominal Exam. [Updated 2022 Oct 10]. In: StatPearls [Internet]. Treasure Island (FL): StatPearls Publishing; 2023. PMID: 29083767.
3. Sharma N, Memon A, Sharma AK, Dutt V, Sharma M. Correlation of radiological investigations with clinical findings in cases of abdominal mass in the paediatric age group. Afr J Paediatr Surg. 2014;11(2):132-7.
4. Ballard DH, Mazaheri P, Oppenheimer DC, Lubner MG, Menias CO, Pickhardt PJ, et al. Imaging of Abdominal Wall Masses, Masslike Lesions, and Diffuse Processes. Radiographics. 2020;40(3):684-706.
5. Expert Panel on Gastrointestinal Imaging; Fowler KJ, Garcia EM, Kim DH, Cash BD, Chang KJ, Feig BW, et al. ACR Appropriateness Criteria® Palpable Abdominal Mass-Suspected Neoplasm. J Am Coll Radiol. 2019;16(11S):S384-S391.
6. Kodaganur S, Hosamani IR, Doddamani M, Uday-kumar KV. Mass in the Left Iliac Fossa-a Diagnostic Dilemma. Indian J Surg. 2016;78(1):54-6.
7. Stevenson RJ. Abdominal masses. Surg Clin North Am. 1985;65(6):1481-504.

CHAPTER 29

# Abdominal Pain

*Saikat Datta*

## INTRODUCTION

In the science and art of medical practice, abdominal pain is probably a symptom which encompasses all the domains of medical science, including surgery, gynecology, internal medicine, psychiatry, or dermatology. The symptomatology remains vague, the signs elusive, and the diagnosis tricky. A thorough evaluation, including the history and clinical examination, remains the cornerstone to plan out specific investigations and standard management. The standard history should always include the time and duration of onset of symptoms, the pattern of pain, location and associated symptoms, aggravating and relieving factors, anorexia, nausea or vomiting, any alteration of the bowel habits, menstrual history or, in specific circumstances, any skin rash. The different types of abdominal pain have special characters, and a brief overview of these types will help in assessing the cause of the abdominal pain.

## TYPES

*Parietal pain*: Direct, usually noxious stimulation of the continuous parietal peritoneum causes parietal pain. It is sharp, intense, and localized pain.

*Visceral pain*: The receptors for visceral pain are diffusely located, e.g., in the mesentery, serosa, hollow organ mucosa. Excessive contraction, stretching, tension, or ischemia causes stimulation of these receptors. Visceral pain receptors are located on the serosa surface, in the mesentery, within the intestinal muscle, and mucosa of hollow organs. When the pain is due to bowel distension, the character is poorly localized. Embolism or thrombosis of the superior mesenteric artery causes sudden and severe abdominal pain. An impending aortic aneurysm rupture also causes acute pain. But these symptoms are often nonspecific and cannot be always relied upon.

*Referred pain*: Referred pain from thorax or spine may be referred to the abdomen. This type of pain is located in the cutaneous dermatomes sharing the same spinal cord level as the visceral inputs. They are challenging to diagnose and should always be kept in mind while evaluating a case of abdominal pain.

*Neurogenic pain*: A burning type of pain limited to the distribution of a peripheral nerve indicates injury to a sensory nerve. It may present with allodynia. On the other hand, radicular pain is a characteristic shooting pain which is of a lancinating type.

It has a dermatomal distribution and might have hyperesthesia along the distribution of pain.

*Abdominal wall:* A constant and aching pain is the characteristic of pain arising from the abdominal wall, e.g., hematoma of rectus sheath. Movement aggravates this pain.

*Acute versus chronic*: There is no strict guideline on the basis of which pain can be classified as acute or chronic. But a pain that is of a few days' duration and progressively worsens is definitely due to an acute cause and needs emergent attention. In contrast, a pain that is persisting for months to years is a chronic one. But arbitrarily, few authors like to term any pain persisting for >6 months as chronic pain.

# CAUSES

## Upper Abdominal Pain

### Right Upper Quadrant Pain

Predominantly, the hepatobiliary etiologies contribute to the pain in these locations:

- *Gallstones*: Dull aching discomfort which might be superadded with an intense pain, predominantly located in the right upper quadrant (RUQ) or the epigastrium. It may be associated with nausea and vomiting.
- *Acute cholecystitis*: It presents with prolonged, steady, severe RUQ or epigastric pain, fever, abdominal guarding, a positive Murphy's sign, and leukocytosis.
- *Acute cholangitis*: It results from the impaction of stone in the biliary or hepatic ducts and cause dilatation of the obstructed duct with superinfection. Charcot's triad—fever, jaundice, and abdominal pain—is a classical presentation.
- *Hepatitis*: Acute hepatitis usually presents with anorexia, nausea, jaundice, and fatigue, in association with other constitutional symptoms. There might be a history of significant alcohol consumption.
- *Liver abscess*: Usual presentations include RUQ pain with fever and toxic features.
- *Budd–Chiari syndrome*: It is defined as hepatic venous outflow tract obstruction, independent of the level or mechanism of obstruction, provided the obstruction is not due to cardiac disease, pericardial disease, or sinusoidal obstruction syndrome (veno-occlusive disease). It is usually caused by thrombosis of the hepatic veins and/or the intrahepatic or suprahepatic inferior vena cava. Usual manifestations include congestive hepatopathy, abdominal pain, ascites, edema, gastrointestinal bleeding, and/or hepatic encephalopathy.

### Epigastric Pain

The causes of epigastric pain are usually gastric or pancreatic ones:

- *Pancreatitis*: Both acute and chronic pancreatitis present with epigastric pain. The pain in acute pancreatitis is acute, severe, and radiates to the back. In chronic pancreatitis, the pain is usually dull aching, and associated with pancreatic insufficiency.
- *Peptic ulcer disease (PUD)*: Upper abdominal pain and discomfort are the most common manifestations of PUD.
- *Gastroesophageal reflux disease (GERD)*: Heartburn and regurgitation is the most common presentation of GERD. But few patients may also present with epigastric pain.
- *Gastritis/gastropathy*: Gastritis (inflammation of the stomach lining) usually presents with epigastric pain, discomfort, nausea, vomiting, and heartburn. When there is a gastric mucosal disorder without inflammation [e.g., due to nonsteroidal anti-inflammatory drugs (NSAIDs)], the term gastropathy is used.

- *Functional dyspepsia*: It is one of the most prevalent functional gastrointestinal disorders, usually presenting with dyspeptic symptoms, defined as discomfort or pain in the upper part of the abdomen.
- *Acute myocardial infarction (AMI)*: AMI should always be included in the differential diagnosis of acute epigastric pain. Relevant history, including chest discomfort, breathlessness, radiation of pain, diaphoresis, etc., should be enquired and further evaluated.

### *Left Upper Quadrant Pain*

Splenic causes should be excluded while evaluating left upper quadrant (LUQ) pain. They mostly include the following:

- *Splenomegaly*: Along with the underlying cause of splenomegaly, there is usually a dragging sensation and discomfort involving the left side of the upper part of the abdomen.
- *Splenic infarction*: This presents with acute, severe LUQ pain. The underlying causes such as hypercoagulable state and sickle cell anemia are usually evident.
- *Splenic abscess*: This presents with fever, LUQ pain, and tenderness.
- *Splenic rupture*: An uncommon finding, splenic rupture is usually post-traumatic. Other causes include vascular anomalies in the spleen, infectious mononucleosis, or hematological malignancy. Kher's sign, the referred pain involving the left shoulder, is due to blood adjacent to the left hemidiaphragm, which occurs in cases of splenic rupture.

## Lower Abdominal Pain

The lower abdominal pain can include various causes like the following:

- *Acute appendicitis*: It usually starts in the periumbilical region and then radiates in the right side of the lower part of the abdomen. Associated features include nausea, vomiting, and anorexia.
- *Diverticulitis*: In Western countries, left-sided diverticulitis is more common than right, and the reverse is seen in Asian populations. Continuous pain for few days associated with occasional nausea and vomiting are the usual manifestations.
- *Kidney stones*: Pain is the most common symptom of renal stone, and it occurs when the stone passes from the renal pelvis to the ureter. It is usually a flank pain and radiates from the loin to the groin.
- *Pyelonephritis and cystitis*: Usual presentations include fever, abdominal pain, and renal angle tenderness. Features of cystitis such as dysuria, hematuria, frequency, or urgency may also be associated with pyelonephritis.
- *Infectious colitis*: Diarrhea is the usual presentation of infectious colitis, although abdominal pain may be a presentation of the same.

### *Diffuse Abdominal Pain*

The causes of diffuse abdominal pain can be varied. They are usually nonspecific, and few important ones are enlisted below:

- *Intestinal obstruction*: It is usually associated with nausea, vomiting, and obstipation. Abdominal distension and tympanitic abdomen with absent bowel sounds are other prominent features.
- *Perforation*: Perforation of hollow viscus usually presents acutely with pain and features of peritonitis.
- *Mesenteric ischemia*: Acute mesenteric ischemia presents with the acute and severe onset of diffuse and persistent abdominal pain, often out of proportion to examination. Chronic mesenteric ischemia usually manifests with abdominal pain after eating ("intestinal angina"), weight loss, nausea, vomiting, and diarrhea.

- *Inflammatory bowel disease (IBD)*: The IBDs, ulcerative disease and Crohn's disease, present with various intestinal and extraintestinal manifestations. These include abdominal pain, blood-mixed stool, tenesmus, and frequent bowel movements.
- *Malignancy*: Various malignancies can be associated with abdominal pain. They include, but are not limited to, colorectal cancer, gastric cancer, and pancreatic cancer.

## Other Causes

Apart from the abovementioned causes, there might be various other causes of abdominal pain. They include celiac disease, adrenal insufficiency, ketoacidosis, irritable bowel syndrome, abdominal aortic aneurysm, angioedema, various helminthic infections, herpes zoster, hypercalcemia, acute lead poisoning, sickle cell crisis, etc. In females, additional causes to be kept in the differential diagnosis include pregnancy with its complications, ectopic pregnancy, pelvic inflammatory disease, ovarian torsion, endometriosis, ovarian hyperstimulation, and even ovarian cancer.

# APPROACH TO A PATIENT OF ABDOMINAL PAIN

Approach to a patient with acute and chronic abdominal pain is shown in **Flowcharts 1 and 2**, respectively.

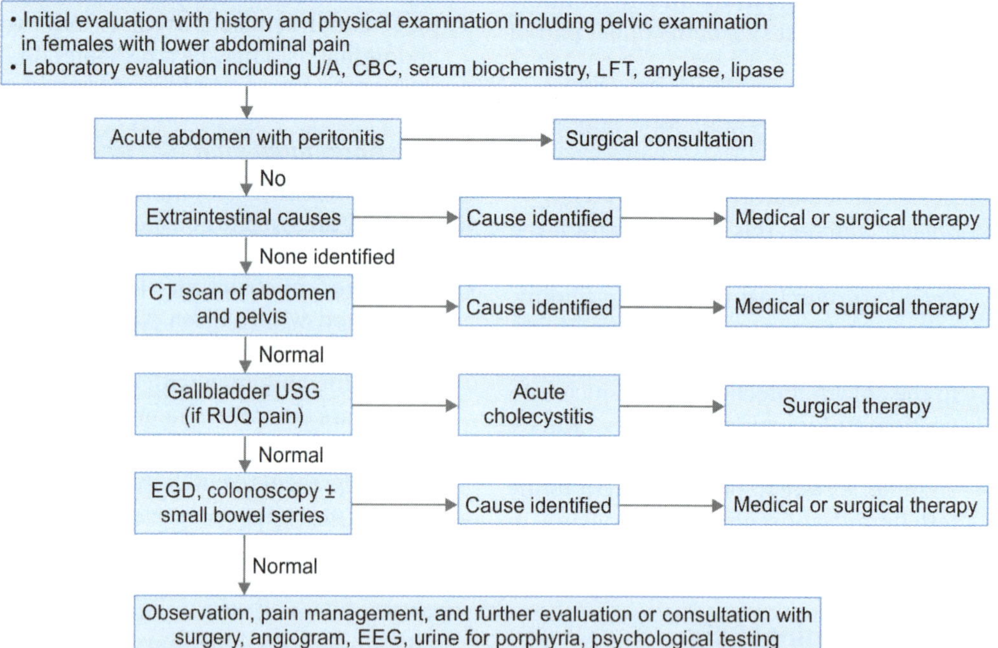


**FLOWCHART 1:** Approach to a patient with acute abdominal pain.

(CBC: complete blood count; CT: computed tomography; EEG: electroencephalography; EGD: esophagogastroduodenoscopy; LFT: liver function tests; RUQ: right upper quadrant; U/A: urinalysis; USG: ultrasonography)

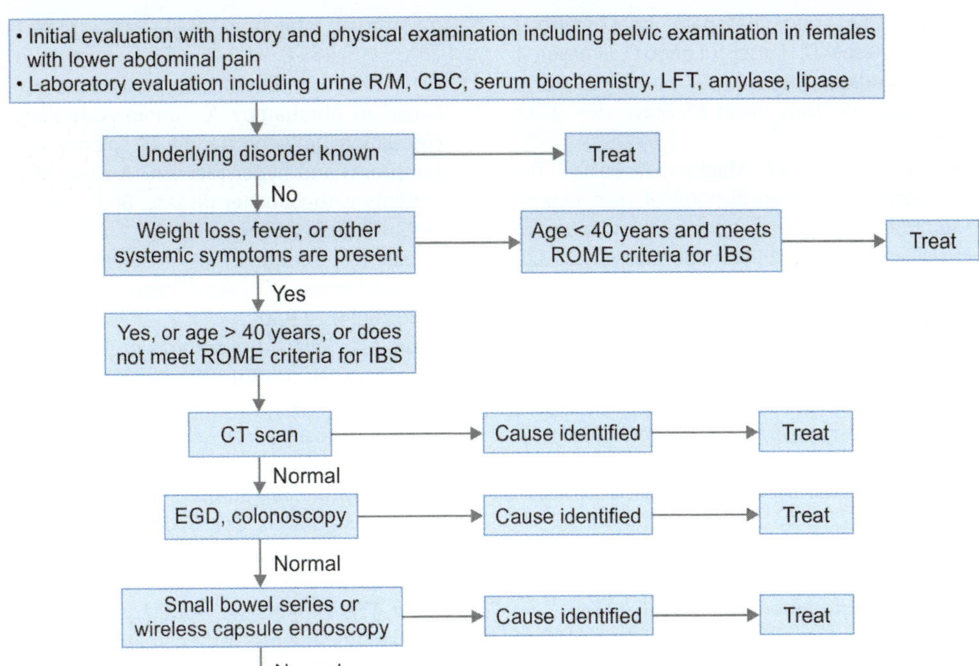


**FLOWCHART 2:** Approach to a patient with chronic abdominal pain ≥6 months.

(CBC: complete blood count; CT: computed tomography; EGD: esophagogastroduodenoscopy; ERCP: endoscopic retrograde cholangiopancreatography; IBS: irritable bowel syndrome; LFT: liver function tests; NSAIDs: nonsteroidal anti-inflammatory drugs; R/M: routine and microscopy)

## CLINICAL PEARLS

- Pain abdomen is an entity that involves various branches of medicine, including surgery, gynecology and obstetrics, medicine, dermatology, etc.
- Evaluation of a case of pain abdomen needs accurate history taking, proper and methodical clinical examination and guided investigations.
- Character of pain, its duration, site, aggravating and relieving factors are all important in evaluation of pain abdomen.
- In acute cases, quick an effective history and evaluation of the patient should be done, and surgical intervention should be advised on an urgent basis if appropriate.
- In chronic cases, proper and detailed history, along with relevant investigations, will help clinch the diagnosis.

## FURTHER READINGS

1. Fleischer AB, Gardner EF, Feldman SR. Are patients' chief complaints generally specific to one organ system? Am J Manag Care. 2001;7(3): 299-305.
2. Miranda A. Abdominal pain. In: Bordini BJ, Toth H, Kliegman RM, Basel D (Eds), Nelson Pediatric Symptom-based Diagnosis. Amsterdam: Elsevier; 2022. p. 222.

3. Jacobs DO. Abdominal pain. In: Loscalzo J, Fauci A, Kasper D, Hauser S, Longo D, Jameson JL (Eds), Harrison's Principles of Internal Medicine, 21st edition. New York: McGraw Hill; 2022. pp. 108-12.
4. Yamamoto W, Kono H, Maekawa M, Fukui T. The relationship between abdominal pain regions and specific diseases: an epidemiologic approach to clinical practice. J Epidemiol. 1997;7(1):27-32.
5. Mcquaid KR. Approach to the patient with gastrointestinal disease. In: Goldman L, Schafer AI (Eds), Goldman-Cecil Medicine, 26th edition. Philadelphia: Elsevier Inc.; 2020. pp. 814-29.
6. Saik RP, Greenburg AG, Farris JM, Peskin GW. Spectrum of cholangitis. Am J Surg. 1975;130(2):143-50.
7. DeLeve LD, Valla DC, Garcia-Tsao G. Vascular disorders of the liver. Hepatology. 2009;49(5): 1729-64.
8. Goodchild G, Chouhan M, Johnson GJ. Practical guide to the management of acute pancreatitis. Frontline Gastroenterol. 2019;10(3):292-9.
9. Ramakrishnan K, Salinas RC. Peptic ulcer disease. Am Fam Physician. 2007;76(7):1005-12.
10. Fujiwara Y, Arakawa T. Epidemiology and clinical characteristics of GERD in the Japanese population. J Gastroenterol. 2009;44(6):518-34.
11. Sipponen P, Maaroos HI. Chronic gastritis. Scand J Gastroenterol. 2015;50(6):657-67.
12. Hawkey CJ. Nonsteroidal anti-inflammatory drug gastropathy. Gastroenterology. 2000;119(2): 521-35.
13. Tack J, Bisschops RA, Sarnelli G. Pathophysiology and treatment of functional dyspepsia. Gastroenterology. 2004;127(4):1239-55.
14. Malik MA, Khan SA, Safdar S. Chest pain as a presenting complaint in patients with acute myocardial infarction (AMI). Pak J Med Sci. 2013;29(2):565-8.
15. Gielchinsky Y, Elstein D, Hadas-Halpern I, Lahad A, Abrahamov A, Zimran A. Is there a correlation between degree of splenomegaly, symptoms and hypersplenism? A study of 218 patients with Gaucher disease. Br J Haematol. 1999;106(3):812-6.
16. Jaroch MT, Broughan TA, Hermann RE. The natural history of splenic infarction. Surgery. 1986;100(4):743-50.
17. Chun CH, Raff MJ, Contreras L, Varghese R, Waterman N, Daffner R, Melo JC. Splenic abscess. Medicine. 1980;59(1):50-65.
18. Renzulli P, Hostettler A, Schoepfer AM, Gloor B, Candinas D. Systematic review of atraumatic splenic rupture. Br J Surg. 2009;96(10):1114-21.
19. Asgari MM, Begos DG. Spontaneous splenic rupture in infectious mononucleosis: a review. Yale J Biol Medicine. 1997;70(2):175-82.
20. Bauer TW, Haskins GE, Armitage JO. Splenic rupture in patients with hematologic malignancies. Cancer. 1981;48(12):2729-33.
21. Miranda HV, Zarazúa RO, Ramírez MA, Briseño JA, Maldonado GE. Spontaneous splenic rupture in a patient with chronic granulocytic leukemia. Int Surg J. 2021;8(9):2786-8.
22. Humes DJ, Simpson J. Acute appendicitis. BMJ. 2006;333(7567):530-4.
23. Young-Fadok TM. Diverticulitis. N Engl J Med. 2018;379(17):1635-42.
24. Sohgaura A, Bigoniya P. A review on epidemiology and etiology of renal stone. Am J Drug Discov Dev. 2017;7(2):54-62.
25. Navaneethan U, Giannella RA. Infectious colitis. Curr Opin Gastroenterol. 2011;27(1):66-71.

CHAPTER 30

# Hematemesis

*Biswajit Banik*

## WHAT IS THE DEFINITION OF HEMATEMESIS?

Hematemesis is defined as vomiting of blood indicative of bleeding from the nasopharynx, esophagus, stomach, and duodenum. Generally, vomiting of bright red blood suggests recent or ongoing bleeding and that of dark material (coffee-ground emesis) suggests bleeding that stopped some time ago. Approximately 50% of gastrointestinal (GI) bleeding results from an upper gastrointestinal (UGI) source. Around 70–80% of UGI bleeding in the general population stops spontaneously.

## WHAT IS SEVERE GASTROINTESTINAL BLEEDING?

Severe gastrointestinal bleeding is documented GI bleeding accompanied by shock or orthostatic hypotension, a decrease in the hematocrit value by at least 6% (or a decrease in the hemoglobin level of 2 g/dL), or transfusion of at least 2 units of packed red blood cells (PRBCs).

## WHAT ARE THE ETIOLOGIES OF HEMATEMESIS?

The most common causes for UGI bleeding with hematemesis are mentioned in **Box 1**. The most common cause of hematemesis is peptic ulcer disease (PUD).

Upper gastrointestinal hemorrhage is the most common complication of peptic ulcers in about 15% of ulcer patients.

Bleeding is self-limited in about 80% of patients with UGI hemorrhage and even without specific therapy for the bleeding. Of the remaining 20% who continue to bleed or rebleed, the mortality rate is 30–40%.

### Risk Stratification for a Hematemesis Patient

Pre-endoscopy scoring for nonvariceal bleeding: Blatchford score, Clinical Rockall score, an artificial neural network score, and the AIMS65 score.

**BOX 1: Common causes of hematemesis.**

- Peptic ulcer
- Esophagitis
- Mallory–Weiss tear
- Dieulafoy lesion
- Esophageal and gastric varix
- Gastroesophageal malignancy
- Hemobilia
- Arteriovenous malformation (AVM) in stomach and duodenum
- Hemosuccus pancreaticus

### *Blatchford Score*

Pre-endoscopy variables: Blood pressure, blood urea nitrogen level, hemoglobin level, heart rate, syncope, melena, liver disease, and heart failure. It assesses a patient's risk for needing clinical interventions to control bleeding.

### *AIMS65 Score*

Five pre-endoscopy variables: Serum albumin 1.5, international normalized ratio (INR) > 1.5, altered mental status, systolic blood pressure ≤ 90 mm Hg, and age > 65 years.

### *Complete Rockall Score*

Postendoscopy scoring system **(Table 1)**: Higher score, higher morbidity and mortality. If the score is <2, the risk of rebleeding is 4% and mortality is <0.1%.

If the score is >5, the risk of rebleeding is >24% and mortality is >11%.

# PATHWAY TO DIAGNOSIS

## History

Assessment of the patient with detailed medical history and vital signs with physical examination is important. Detailed and brief medical history, questions about medications that can cause ulcers or bleeding, and any history regarding GI surgeries are required.

### *History Regarding Source of Bleeding*

Nasopharynx: Recurrent epistaxis/ nasopharyngeal malignancy. Esophageal ulceration: Gastroesophageal reflux disease (GERD)/alcohol abuse/pill ingestion; Esophageal cancer: Dysphagia; Mallory-Weiss tear: Alcohol binge, vomiting; Esophageal/gastric varix: Cirrhosis; Gastric angiodysplasia: Aortic stenosis; chronic kidney disease (CKD); systemic sclerosis; PUD: Epigastric pain; aspirin or nonsteroidal anti-inflammatory drugs (NSAIDs) intake; Gastric cancer: Early satiety; weight loss; and any recent history of pancreatitis, then look for any gastric varix or hematemesis from splenic artery or gastroduodenal artery (GDA) pseudoaneurysm.

## Physical Examination

Start with the patient's vital signs and attention regarding hypovolemia signs such as hypotension, tachycardia, and postural symptoms. Abdominal examination should be conducted to look for any surgical scars, palpable mass, splenomegaly, or epigastric tenderness.

**Table 1: Complete Rockall scoring system.**

| *Variable* | *0* | *1* | *2* | *3* |
|---|---|---|---|---|
| Age (year) | <60 | 60–79 | >/80 | — |
| Pulse (beats/min) | <100 | >/100 | - | — |
| Systolic blood pressure (mm Hg) | Normal | >/100 | <100 | — |
| Comorbidity | None | — | Ischemic heart disease, cardiac failure, other major illnesses | Renal failure, hepatic failure, metastatic cancer |
| Diagnosis | Mallory–Weiss tear or no lesion | All other benign diagnoses | Malignant lesion | — |
| Endoscopic stigmata of recent hemorrhage | No stigmata or dark spot in the ulcer base | - | Blood in UGI tract, adherent clot, visible vessel, active bleeding | — |

Look for signs of chronic liver disease in the form of spider telangiectasias, palmar erythema, gynecomastia, ascites, splenomegaly, caput medusae, and Dupuytren contracture.

The skin, lips, and buccal mucosa for telangiectasias are suggestive of hereditary hemorrhagic telangiectasia (HHT) or Osler-Weber-Rendu disease. Subungual telangiectasias in the fingers indicate scleroderma and are associated with gastric antral vascular ectasia (GAVE) or UGI telangiectasias. Pigmented lip lesions suggest Peutz-Jeghers syndrome. Purpuric skin lesions may suggest Henoch-Schönlein purpura (HSP). Acanthosis nigricans suggest underlying gastric cancer.

## INVESTIGATIONS

Look for standard hematology parameters with urgent hemoglobin level. Hemoglobin level should be monitored 6 hourly in case of UGI bleeding till the bleeding source is secured. Look for urea to estimate hypovolemia. Other routine investigations include liver function test (LFT) and coagulation profile. Thrombocytopenia suggests chronic liver disease.

In case of hematemesis, the main investigation is to look for the source of bleeding by a UGI endoscopy. UGI endoscopy must be done after adequate resuscitation. The ideal time for a UGI endoscopy must be within 12 hours, but urgent UGI endoscopy hampers resuscitation measurement; hence, different endoscopic societies recommend to do a UGI endoscopy within 12 hours. If bleeding is coming from the papilla, then look for a source from any pseudoaneurysm of the hepatic artery, GDA, or splenic artery by a computed tomography (CT) angiography of abdominal vessels.

## TREATMENT

Patients who have an acute GI bleed but are hemodynamically stable can be admitted to a monitored bed (step-down unit) or standard hospital bed, depending on their clinical condition.

Patients should be hospitalized in an intensive care unit (ICU) if they have large amounts of red blood in the nasogastric (NG) tube or per rectum, have unstable vital signs, or have had severe acute blood loss that may exacerbate other underlying medical conditions.

### Resuscitation

At least one large-bore (14- or 16-gauge) catheter should be placed intravenously, and two should be placed when the patient has ongoing bleeding. Normal saline is infused as fast as needed to keep the patient's systolic blood pressure higher than 100 mm Hg and pulse lower than 100/min.

So, for resuscitation purpose, a peripheral large-bore cannula is preferred over the central venous catheter **(Table 2)**.

### Colloid Solutions

Colloid solutions include 3.5% degraded gelatin polypeptides and 4% W/V succinyl gelatin. Initially, 10–20 mL should be infused slowly to look for anaphylactic reactions. Then rapid infusions may be given and up to 25% blood volume, i.e., approximately 1,500 mL, can be replaced by colloids.

### Blood Transfusion

Blood transfusion generally depends on age, hemodynamic status of the patient,

**Table 2: Maximum flow rate in venous catheter.**

| *Venous catheter* | *Maximum flow rate (mL/min)* |
|---|---|
| 14G | 240 |
| 16G | 180 |
| 18G | 90 |
| Triple lumen catheter 18G | 26 |
| Triple lumen catheter 16G | 52 |

hemoglobin level, and more on estimated blood loss and resting and postural hypotension.

Generally, <10% blood loss: No transfusion; 10–20% blood loss: Crystalloids; >20–25%: PRBC transfusion. Even increased lactate indicates decreased tissue oxygenation and consider for blood transfusion.

Restrictive hydration is recommended in case of suspecting variceal bleeding. The patient should be transfused with PRBCs as necessary to keep the hemoglobin level > 7 g/dL; restrictive transfusion strategy is associated with a higher survival rate and a lower rebleeding rate.

*Restrictive transfusion if no cardiovascular (CV) disease*: Transfusion threshold: <7 g/dL and transfusion goal 7–9 g/dL. Acute or chronic CV disease: Transfusion threshold < 8 g/dL and transfusion goal > 10 g/dL.

## Endotracheal Intubation

Endotracheal intubation is considered in patients with active ongoing hematemesis or with altered mental status to prevent aspiration pneumonia.

## Initial Medical Therapy

Administration of a proton-pump inhibitor (PPI) is useful for reducing rebleeding rates in patients with PUD.

Pre-emptive PPI is not mandatory and may be considered according to recent British Society of Gastroenterology (BSG) and European Society of Gastrointestinal Endoscopy (ESGE) guidelines. It generally reduced the need for endoscopic treatment. The need for endoscopic treatment was lower in the omeprazole group than in the placebo group [60 of the 314 patients included in the analysis (19.1%) vs. 90 of 317 patients in the placebo group (28.4%), $p = 0.007$].[5] Give pantoprazole 80 mg intravenous (IV) bolus followed by 8 mg/h continuous infusion or intermittent bolus for 72 hours.

## Need for Nasogastric Tube or Nasogastric Lavage or any Prokinetics

Generally, guidelines do not recommend NG lavage. NG lavage with clean tap water or saline water improves visualization in case of active bleed and NG aspirate of fresh blood indicates active bleeding, but at least 16% of patients with active bleeding UGI lesions have a clear NG aspirate.[6]

High dose before endoscopy accelerates the resolution of endoscopic stigmata of recent hemorrhage (SRH) in ulcers and reduces the need for endoscopic therapy but does not result in improvement in major clinical outcomes.

Patients with a strong suspicion of portal hypertension and variceal bleeding should be started empirically on IV octreotide or IV terlipressin.

## Endoscopic Hemostasis

In earlier days, thermal contact probes have been the mainstay of endoscopic hemostasis but with time, the endoscopic modalities in the view of therapeutic concern revived a lot and in the present scenario, endoscopic hemoclips application and over-the-scope clip (OTSC) have become the main modalities of treatment.

*Thermal contact probes*: Generally, contact probes can physically tamponade a blood vessel to stop bleeding and the mechanism by coaptive coagulation.

A commonly used probe is multipolar electrocoagulation (MPEC) probe.

*Bipolar probes*: Gold probe: 10 and 7 Fr catheters are used. It has a bipolar spiral tip with coagulation at any angle and the central lumen is there for irrigation.

*Endoscopic injection*: Injection therapy is most commonly performed for ulcer disease with a sclerotherapy needle and submucosal injection of epinephrine with a dilution of 1:10,000 or 1:20,000 into or around the bleeding site or stigma of hemorrhage. Mechanisms followed are volume tamponade and local vasoconstriction.

*Endoscopic hemoclips*: These are hemoclips that serve to apply mechanical pressure to a bleeding site. They act by grasp-and-release mechanism.

*Over-the-scope clips*: They may be considered first line in a selectively active bleeding ulcer, especially > 2 cm, and excavated or fibrotic ulcers and large visible vessel and location in high-risk vascular area and for recurrent bleeding.

*Hemospray powder*: It is used as monotherapy or rescue or serves as bridge therapy. Immediate hemostasis in 90% and early rebleeding in 30% of cases. Hemostatic spray is an inorganic powder and also has clotting abilities that can create a mechanical barrier that adheres to and covers a bleeding site. It is used for temporary control of bleeding from peptic ulcers, tumors, and diffusely bleeding lesions.

*Band ligation*: Mucosa with or without submucosal tissue is suctioned into a cap placed at the end of the endoscope and a rubber band is rolled off the cap and over the lesion to compress its base. It is widely used for esophageal variceal bleed and can be used for other bleeding lesions.

## Peptic Ulcer

Most commonly, gastric or duodenal ulcer accounts for most of the UGI bleeds. Peptic ulcers are commonly caused by a decrease in mucosal defense mechanisms attributable to aspirin or NSAIDs or any *Helicobacter pylori* infection or both. The prevalence of *H. pylori* infection is >80% of the population in developing countries and 20–50% in industrialized countries. Generally, *H. pylori* gastritis involves antrum and predisposes the patient to duodenal ulcers and gastric body predominant gastritis associated with gastric ulcers.

Endoscopic stigmata of recent ulcer hemorrhage and rebleeding are mentioned in **Table 3**.

An algorithm of endoscopic and medical management of peptic ulcer-induced UGI bleeding is mentioned in **Table 4**.

## Endoscopic Features Predictive of Adverse Outcomes

FIA; FIB; FIIA; FIIb. Large ulcer size of >2 cm; nonbleeding visible vessel (NBVV) of >2 mm and ulcer located on the posterior duodenal wall or proximal lesser curvature of the stomach.

## Rebleed

Rebleeding rates < 10%. Highest risk within 72 hours and approach to rebleeding is

**Table 3: Endoscopic stigmata of recent ulcer hemorrhage and rebleeding.**

| *Forrest class* | *Endoscopic stigma* | *Frequency* | *Risk of rebleeding* |
|---|---|---|---|
| IA | Active arterial bleeding | 12 | 90% |
| IIA | Nonbleeding visible vessel | 22 | 50% |
| IIB | Adherent clot | 10 | 33% |
| IB | Oozing without stigmata | 14 | 10% |
| IIC | Flat spot | 10 | 10–25% |
| III | Clean base | 32 | 3% |

**Table 4: Management line for the endoscopic and medical management of peptic ulcer-induced UGI bleeding.**

| *Bleeding type* | *Management* |
|---|---|
| Active spurting, oozing | Combined endoscopic therapy (hemoclips and epinephrine injection) |
| NBVV, adherent clot | Hemoclips/epinephrine injection |
| Pigmented base, clean based ulcer | PPI |

(NBVV: nonbleeding visible vessel; PPI: proton pump inhibitor; UGI: upper gastrointestinal)

endoscopic retreatment in first rebleeding. Around 75% will achieve sustained hemostasis with endoscopic retreatment. Generally, after two sessions of endotherapy, angiographic embolization and surgery are advised.

## Esophagitis

Severe erosive esophagitis can present with UGI bleeding. Grade 3 or 4 of the Savary-Miller grading system can cause UGI bleeding. Usually, esophagitis is treated with daily PPI for 8–12 weeks and undergoes repeat endoscopy to exclude Barrett's esophagus.

## Dieulafoy Lesion

Dieulafoy lesion is a large 1-3 mm submucosal artery that generally protrudes through the mucosa without association with an ulcer and can cause massive UGI bleeding. Endoscopic treatment is generally performed with injection therapy, a thermal probe, hemoclipping, or OTSC clips.

## Mallory–Weiss Tear

Mallory–Weiss tear is mucosal or submucosal lacerations that occur at the gastroesophageal (GE) junction and extend distally into hiatal hernia most of the time. Hemoclips are used to stop the bleed and close the tear.

## Cameron Lesions

Cameron lesions are linear erosions or ulcerations in the proximal stomach at the end of the hiatus hernia near diaphragmatic pinch. They occur due to mechanical trauma and local ischemia as the hernia moves against the diaphragm. They commonly causes obscure GI bleed.

## Varices

In compensated cirrhosis, varix is seen in 30–40% of patients, and in case of decompensated cirrhosis, varices are seen in 60% of patients. One-third of patients with varices develop variceal hemorrhage. Vasoconstrictor therapy: This reduces splanchnic blood flow and continues for at least 3 days. Terlipressin or octreotide is generally used.

Esophageal variceal ligation (EVL) or esophageal sclerotherapy is commonly done for esophageal varices. Balloon tamponade of varices can be used to tamponade the active bleeding varices before definite therapy to stabilize the patient. Three types of balloon are used: (1) Sengstaken–Blakemore tube, (2) Minnesota tube, and (3) Linton–Nachlas tube.

## Upper Gastrointestinal Malignancy

Endoscopic hemostasia with thermal probes, laser, injection therapy, or hemoclips can temporarily control acute bleeding.

## Hemobilia

Hemobilia is ongoing bleeding which is treated with endovascular arterial embolization.

### Hemosuccus Pancreaticus

Hemosuccus pancreaticus is treated with endovascular arterial embolization.

## CLINICAL PEARLS

In hematemesis, after admission, look for risk stratification and possibilities of hematemesis and estimate the blood loss and primary treatment according to blood volume loss.

Do UGI endoscopy within 12 hours if possible and target for endoscopic hemostasis.

Most common cause of hematemesis peptic ulcer bleeding and if high-risk stigmata of bleeding are present, use mechanical devices for hemostasis.

Variceal bleeding is mostly managed with vasoconstrictor agents and endoscopic band ligation.

## FURTHER READINGS

1. Van Leerdam ME, Vreeburg EM, Rauws EA, Geraedts AAM, Tijssen JGP, Reitsma JB, et al. Acute upper GI bleeding: did anything change? Time trend analysis of incidence and outcome of acute upper GI bleeding between 1993. Am J Gastroenterol. 2003;98(7):1494-9.
2. Van Leerdam ME. Epidemiology of acute upper gastrointestinal bleeding. Best Pract Res Clin Gastroenterol. 2008;22:209-24.
3. Odutayo A, Desborough MJ, Trivella M, Stanley AJ, Dorée C, Collins GS, et al. Restrictive versus liberal blood transfusion for gastrointestinal bleeding: a systematic review and meta-analysis of randomised controlled trials. Lancet Gastroenterol Hepatol. 2017;2(5):354-60.
4. Fleischer D. Etiology and prevalence of severe persistent upper gastrointestinal bleeding. Gastroenterology. 1983;84:538-43.
5. Lau JY, Leung WK, Wu JC, Chan FK, Wong VW, Chiu PW, et al. Omeprazole before endoscopy in patients with gastrointestinal bleeding. N Engl J Med. 2007;356(16):1631-40.
6. Gilbert DA, Silverstein FE, Tedesco FJ, Buenger NK, Persing J. The national ASGE survey on upper gastrointestinal bleeding. III. Endoscopy in upper gastrointestinal bleeding. Gastrointest Endosc. 1981;27:94-102.
7. Haddara S, Jacques J, Lecleire S, Branche J, Leblanc S, Le Baleur Y, et al. A novel hemostatic powder for upper gastrointestinal bleeding: a multicenter study (the "GRAPHE" registry). Endoscopy. 2016;48:1084-95.
8. Forrest JA, Finlayson ND, Shearman DJ. Endoscopy in gastrointestinal bleeding. Lancet. 1974;2:394-7.
9. Van Loon FHJ, Korsten HHM, Dierick-van Daele ATM, Bouwman ARA. The impact of the catheter to vein ratio on peripheral intravenous cannulation success, a post-hoc analyses. PLoS One. 2021;16(5):e0252166.

# CHAPTER 31

# Melena

*Biswajit Banik*

## WHAT IS THE DEFINITION OF MELENA?

Melena results from the degradation of blood products to hematin and other hemochromes by gut bacteria. It signifies upper gastrointestinal (UGI) bleeding, but usually the source of bleeding can be from UGI, small bowel, or proximal colon.

*Significance*: Generally, 50–100 mL of blood is required in the gastrointestinal (GI) tract with the passage of characteristic melenic stool occurring at least 10–12 hours after the bleeding.

In some cases of melena, UGI endoscopy and colonoscopy do not detect any source of bleeding, and the reasonable source of bleeding is from small bowel unlike hematemesis and hematochezia where the source is usually detected with UGI endoscopy and colonoscopy, respectively.

## WHAT IS THE DEFINITION OF DIFFERENT GI BLEEDING?

*Occult GI bleeding*: GI bleeding that is not clinically visible.

*Obscure GI bleeding (OGIB)*: Bleeding from a site that is not apparent after routine endoscopic evaluation with the performance of standard upper and lower endoscopic examinations, small bowel evaluation with video capsule endoscopy (VCE) and/or enteroscopy, and radiographic testing.

Occult GI bleeding represents 5% of all gastrointestinal bleeding, mostly caused by the small bowel. Small bowel bleeding due to angioectasia, the most common cause, comprises 50% of OGIB, followed by inflammatory conditions and ulcers (27%) and neoplasms (9%).

## WHAT ARE THE CAUSES OF MELENA?

The causes of melena are given in **Table 1**.

## PATHWAY TO DIAGNOSIS

### History and Initial Assessment

Medical history for vital signs and a physical examination are required.

Look for medication that causes ulcers or bleeding prior to GI surgeries.

### Physical Examination

Examination of vital signs, with attention to signs of hypovolemia such as hypotension, tachycardia, and orthostasis, is important.

*Abdomen*: It is examined for surgical scars, tenderness, and masses.

**Table 1: Causes of melena.**

| *Organ* | *Causes* |
|---|---|
| UGI | • Esophageal and gastric varix<br>• Peptic ulcer disease<br>• Portal hypertensive gastropathy<br>• GAVE<br>• Neoplasm |
| Small bowel | • Angioectasia and arteriovenous malformation<br>• Crohn's disease, warm infestation, tuberculosis, and NSAIDs ulcer<br>• GIST and polyp |
| Large bowel | • Crohn's disease, tuberculosis, and malignancy<br>• Polyp, diverticulosis, and angioectasia |

(GAVE: gastric antral vascular ectasia; GIST: gastrointestinal stromal tumor; NSAIDs: nonsteroidal anti-inflammatory drugs; UGI: upper gastrointestinal)

*Chronic liver disease*: Spider telangiectasias, palmar erythema, gynecomastia, ascites, splenomegaly, caput medusa, and Dupuytren contracture.

*Skin, lips, and buccal mucosa*: For telangiectasias, suggestive of hereditary hemorrhagic telangiectasia (HHT), or Osler–Weber–Rendu disease.

# INVESTIGATIONS

The approach to melena is shown in **Flowchart 1**.

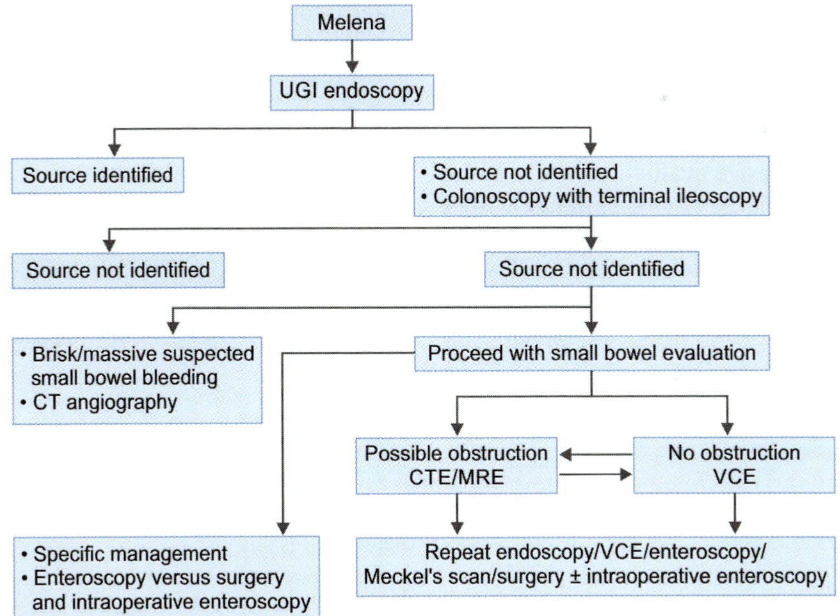


**FLOWCHART 1:** Approach to melena.

(CT: computed tomography; CTE: computed tomography enterography; MRE: magnetic resonance enterography; UGI: upper gastrointestinal; VCE: video capsule endoscopy)

## Endoscopy

### Source Identification

Upper gastrointestinal endoscopy should be followed by colonoscopy, and if no source is identified, then look for small bowel bleeding. A source of small bowel bleeding should be considered overt or occult GI bleeding after the performance of a normal upper and lower endoscopic examination. Patients should be classified as having small bowel bleeding when the source of bleeding is identified distal to the ampulla of Vater and/or proximal to the ileocecal valve.

The common causes of small bowel bleeding are shown in **Table 2**.

Patients undergoing double-balloon enteroscopy (DBE) in Asian countries were likely to have neoplastic findings, whereas angioectasia is more common in Western countries.

## Endoscopic Visualization of the Small Intestine

### Video Capsule Endoscopy

Video capsule endoscopy measures 26 × 11 $mm^2$ and has the capacity to take images at the rate of 2 frames/s over an 8–12-hour period. Capsule endoscopy allows noninvasive evaluation of the entire small bowel in 79–90% of patients, with a diagnostic yield of 38–83% in patients with suspected small bowel bleeding. VCE yield depends on a higher likelihood of positive findings in patients with a hemoglobin < 10 g/dL, more than one episode of bleeding, overt as compared with occult bleeding (60 vs. 46%), and performance of VCE within 2 weeks of the bleeding episode (91 vs. 34%). There is also evidence that VCE within 48–72 hours of overt suspected small bowel bleeding has the greatest yield for lesion detection. Limitations of VCE include a lack of therapeutic capabilities, inability to control its movement through the GI tract, and the difficulty in localizing the lesion. VCE fails to identify the major papilla in the majority of cases and, therefore, may miss important duodenal lesions because of rapid transit through the duodenal loop. VCE does miss clinically important duodenal and proximal jejunal lesions and, thus, cannot be solely relied upon for the exclusion of bleeding lesions in these areas.

### Deep Enteroscopy, Balloon-assisted Enteroscopy

Balloon-assisted enteroscopy uses the principle of push and pull and includes DBE and single-balloon enteroscopy (SBE). The enteroscope in both systems has a working length of 200 cm with an outer diameter of 9.4 mm. The overtube is 140 cm in length.

### Double-balloon Enteroscopy

Double-balloon enteroscopy can be advanced at a distance of ~240–360 cm distal to the pylorus with the oral approach and 102–140 cm proximal to the ileocecal valve with the rectal approach. It has the additional advantage over VCE of both diagnostic and

**Table 2: Common causes of small bowel bleeding.**

| *Under the age of 40 years* | *Over the age of 40 years* |
|---|---|
| Inflammatory bowel disease | Angioectasia |
| Dieulafoy's lesions | Dieulafoy's lesions |
| Neoplasia | Neoplasia |
| Meckel's diverticulum | NSAID ulcers |
| Polyposis syndromes | |

(NSAID: nonsteroidal anti-inflammatory drug)

therapeutic capabilities, including biopsies, tattoo, hemostasis, polypectomy, dilation, and foreign body removal (including retained capsules). The 2.8-mm accessory channel allows the passage of virtually all standard-caliber, through-the-scope diagnostic and therapeutic instruments. The diagnostic yield of DBE ranges from 60 to 80% in patients with suspected small bowel bleeding and other small bowel disorders. Successful performance of endoscopic therapeutic interventions has been reported in 40–73% of patients. Limitations of DBE include its invasive nature, prolonged procedure time, and requirement for additional personnel.

### *Spiral Enteroscopy*

Spiral enteroscopy consists of a unique overtube with an outer raised spiral ridge at its distal end through which an SBE or a DBE can be inserted. The mean (±SD) procedure times for the anterograde approach have been estimated to be 79 ± 15 minutes for DBE (10 studies), 65 ± 16 minutes for SBE (5 studies), and 35 + 6 minutes for spiral enteroscopy (4 trials).

### *Abdominal Imaging*

Cross-sectional imaging techniques optimized for imaging the small bowel have a larger role in small bowel imaging and have shown improved performance over routine computed tomography (CT). Imaging can be performed using either the enterography technique, which requires ingestion of large volumes of contrast medium, or enteroclysis with the direct administration of enteric fluid by a nasoenteric tube. Enteroclysis provides superior small bowel distension; however, it is not as well tolerated or widely used. The fluid administered should be a neutral contrast or near-water density to improve the detection of hyperenhancing abnormalities or bleeding.

### *Computed Tomography Enterography*

In a meta-analysis of 18 studies, computed tomography enterography (CTE) had a pooled yield of 40% compared with 53% for VCE. VCE has higher yields for detecting vascular and inflammatory lesions compared with CTE. An advantage of CTE over VCE is the improved detection of small bowel masses, especially those that are mural-based.

### *Computed Tomography Angiography*

Computed tomography angiography (CTA) has been shown to be able to detect bleeding rates as slow as 0.3 mL/min compared with 0.5–1.0 mL/min for conventional angiography and 0.2 mL/min for 99mTc-tagged RBC scintigraphy. A meta-analysis of nine studies with 198 patients showed that CTA had a pooled sensitivity of 89% and a specificity of 85% in diagnosing acute GI bleeding throughout the GI tract.

### *Scintigraphy: 99mTc-labeled Red Blood Cell Scintigraphy*

The advantages of scintigraphy include the ability to detect lower rates of bleeding and the ability to perform delayed imaging that can improve the detection of intermittent or delayed bleeding. In younger patients with ongoing overt bleeding and negative evaluation with VCE, CTE, or other testing modalities, consideration should be made for testing with a 99mTc-pertechnetate scan for the detection of Meckel's diverticulum.

## TREATMENT

*Resuscitation*: At least one large-bore (14- or 16-gauge) catheter should be placed intravenously and two should be placed when the patient has ongoing GI bleeding. Normal saline is infused as fast as needed to keep the patient's systolic blood pressure higher than 100 mm Hg and pulse lower than 100/min.

*Blood transfusion*: Blood transfusion generally depends on age, hemodynamic status of the patient, hemoglobin level, and more on estimated blood loss, resting hypotension, and postural hypotension.

Generally, <10% blood loss: No transfusion is necessary; 10–20% blood loss: Crystalloids are used; >20–25%: They require packed red blood cells (PRBC) transfusion. Even increased lactate indicates decreased tissue oxygenation and considered for blood transfusion.

Restrictive hydration is recommended in cases of suspecting variceal bleeding. Patients should be transfused with PRBCs as necessary to keep the hemoglobin level > 7 g/dL. The restrictive transfusion strategy is associated with a higher survival rate and lower rebleeding rate.

Restrictive transfusion if no cardiovascular (CV) disease: Transfusion threshold: <7 g/dL and transfusion goal 7–9 g/dL. Acute or chronic CV disease: Transfusion threshold < 8 g/dL and transfusion goal > 10 g/dL.

*Peptic ulcer*: Endoscopic stigmata of recent ulcer hemorrhage and rebleeding is given in Table 3 of Chapter 30.

The algorithm for the endoscopic and medical management of peptic ulcer-induced UGI bleeding is given in Table 4 of Chapter 30.

*Cameron lesions*: These are a common cause of OGIB.

*Gastric antral vascular ectasia (GAVE)*: Endoscopic hemostasis with thermal heat modalities such as laser, multipolar electrocoagulation (MPEC), or argon plasma coagulation has been used successfully.

*Portal hypertensive gastropathy (PHG)*: Severe PHG with diffuse bleeding is treated by measures that decrease portal pressure, usually with β-adrenergic receptor-blocking agents or possibly with the placement of a transjugular intrahepatic portosystemic shunt (TIPS) or surgical portacaval shunt.

*Varices*: Esophageal variceal ligation (EVL) or esophageal sclerotherapy is commonly done for esophageal varices.

*Angioectasia:* Angioectasia, also referred to as angiodysplasia, is the formation of aberrant blood vessels found throughout the GI tract that develop with advancing age. The most common locations are the colon and small intestine. Acquired vascular lesions (angioectasia and telangiectasia) occur in association with various disorders, such as chronic kidney disease, cirrhosis, rheumatologic disorders, and severe heart disease. Angioectasia can be treated endoscopically with various modalities, including epinephrine injection, thermal probe coagulation, argon plasma coagulation, hemoclips, and band ligation.

*Meckel diverticulum*: This has been described by the "rule of 2s": It occurs in 2% of the population, is found within 2 feet of the ileocecal valve, is 2 inches long, results in a complication in 2% of cases, has two types of ectopic tissue (gastric and pancreatic) within the diverticulum, presents clinically most commonly at the age of 2 years (with intestinal obstruction), and has a male-to-female ratio of >2:1. The main treatment is surgical resection.

*Nonsteroidal anti-inflammatory drugs (NSAIDs)-induced small intestinal erosions and ulcers*: Mucosal erosions or ulcers that can be seen on capsule endoscopy develop in 25–55% of patients who take full-dose nonselective NSAIDs.

## CLINICAL PEARLS

Generally, melena signifies UGI bleeding, but the source of bleeding can be from the esophagus to the proximal colon.

If UGI endoscopy and colonoscopy are negative in case of melena, then look for small bowel source by VCE, DBE, or angiography.

In case of overt and brisk GI bleeding, look for any vascular lesions such as aneurysm, arteriovenous malformation (AVM), or vascular tumor by CTA for early diagnosis.

Most of the patients are managed according to their cause and source of bleeding.

# FURTHER READINGS

1. Sey MSL, Yan BM. Optimal management of the patient presenting with small bowel bleeding. Best Pract Res Clin Gastroenterol. 2019;42-43:101611.
2. Liao Z, Gao R, Xu C, Li ZS. Indications and detection, completion, and retention rates of small-bowel capsule endoscopy: a systematic review. Gastrointest Endosc. 2010;71:280-6.
3. Odutayo A, Desborough MJ, Trivella M, Stanley AJ, Dorée C, Collins GS, et al. Restrictive versus liberal blood transfusion for gastrointestinal bleeding: a systematic review and meta-analysis of randomised controlled trials. Lancet Gastroenterol Hepatol. 2017;2(5):354-60.
4. Cangemi DJ, Patel MK, Gomez V, Cangemi JR, Stark ME, Lukens FJ. Small bowel tumors discovered during double-balloon enteroscopy: analysis of a large prospectively collected single-center database. J Clin Gastroenterol. 2013;47:769-72.
5. Rondonotti E, Villa F, Mulder CJ, Jacobs MA, de Franchis R. Small bowel capsule endoscopy in 2007: indications, risks and limitations. World J Gastroenterol. 2007;13:6140-9.
6. May A, Wardak A, Nachbar L, Remke S, Ell C. Influence of patient selection on the outcome of capsule endoscopy in patients with chronic gastrointestinal bleeding. J Clin Gastroenterol. 2005;39:684.
7. Singh A, Marshall C, Chaudhuri B, Okoli C, Foley A, Person SD, et al. Timing of video capsule endoscopy relative to overt obscure GI bleeding: implications from a retrospective study. Gastrointest Endosc. 2013;77:761-6.
8. Teshima CW, Kuipers EJ, van Zanten SV, Mensink PB. Double balloon enteroscopy and capsule endoscopy for obscure gastrointestinal bleeding: an updated meta-analysis. J Gastroenterol Hepatol. 2011;26:796.
9. May A, Manner H, Aschmoneit I, Ell C. Prospective, cross-over, single-center trial comparing oral double-balloon enteroscopy and oral spiral enteroscopy in patients with suspected small-bowel vascular malformations. Endoscopy. 2011;43:477-83.
10. Wiarda BM, Heine DG, Mensink P, Stolk M, Dees J, Hazenberg HJ, et al. Comparison of magnetic resonance enteroclysis and capsule endoscopy with balloon-assisted enteroscopy in patients with obscure gastrointestinal bleeding. Endoscopy. 2012;44:668-73.
11. Wang Z, Chen JQ, Liu JL, Qin XG, Huang Y. CT enterography in obscure gastrointestinal bleeding: a systematic review and meta-analysis. J Med Imaging Radiat Oncol. 2013;57:263-73.
12. Wu LM, Xu JR, Yin Y, Qu XH. Usefulness of CT angiography in diagnosing acute gastrointestinal bleeding: a meta-analysis. World J Gastroenterol. 2010;16:3957-63.
13. Kong MS, Huang SC, Tzen KY, Lin JN. Repeated technetium-99m pertechnetate scanning for children with obscure gastrointestinal bleeding. J Pediatr Gastroenterol Nutr. 1994;18:284-7.
14. Larkai EN, Smith JL, Lidsky MD, Graham DY. Gastroduodenal mucosa and dyspeptic symptoms in arthritic patients during chronic nonsteroidal anti-inflammatory drug use. Am J Gastroenterol. 1987;82:1153-8.

CHAPTER 32

# Bleeding Per Rectum

*Biswajit Banik*

## WHAT IS THE DEFINITION OF BLEEDING PER RECTUM?

Bleeding per rectum usually signifies hematochezia. It usually suggests bright red blood per rectum, which is usually from the colon, rectum, or active upper gastrointestinal (UGI) bleeding, or small bowel bleeding. The rate of hospitalization is lower than for UGI bleeding. The usual cause of lower gastrointestinal (LGI) bleeding causes less significant gastrointestinal (GI) bleeding.

Most of the patients with bleeding per rectum are in old age. If orthostasis is associated with bleeding per rectum, brisk bleeding from the UGI source must be excluded. In approximately 100 cases of hematochezia, 20% are proximal to the ileocecal (IC) valve, 11% are UGI bleeds, and 9% are small bowel bleeds.

*Epidemiology*: LGI hemorrhage accounts for about 20% of all cases of acute GI hemorrhage.

## WHAT ARE THE DIFFERENT ETIOLOGIES OF BLEEDING PER RECTUM?

The different etiologies of bleeding per rectum are shown in **Box 1**.

The most common cause of significant hematochezia is diverticulosis.

*Risk stratification in case of bleeding per rectum*: Look for hemoglobin and hematocrit drop from baseline, the duration of bleeding, and hemodynamic parameters in bleeding per rectum patients.

**BOX 1: Different etiologies of bleeding per rectum.**

- Diverticulosis
- Colon polyps
- Carcinoma of colon
- Inflammatory bowel disease
- Gastrointestinal stromal tumor
- Hemobilia
- Ischemic colitis
- Noninfectious colitis
- Infectious colitis
- Angioectasia
- Aortoenteric fistula
- Rectal varices
- Postpolypectomy ulcer
- Rectal ulcer
- Hemorrhoids
- Radiation colitis
- Esophageal and gastric varices
- Peptic ulcer disease

Calculate shock index (SI) = Heart rate (HR)/systolic blood pressure (SBP). If SI > 1, it signifies unstable GI bleed or suspect active GI bleed. SI < 1 signifies stable GI bleed. Calculate the risk score for GI bleed as either major or minor.

# PATH TO DIAGNOSIS

## History

*Risk factors*: Nonsteroidal anti-inflammatory drugs (NSAIDs), age > 65 years, and intake of antiplatelets and anticoagulants. The following history needs to be asked in case of bleeding per rectum patients: Recent intervention such as endoscopic mucosal resection (EMR)/endoscopic submucosal dissection (ESD)/polypectomy; comorbidities: cardiac disease, aortic disease, peripheral vascular disease, etc.; smoking; antiplatelets and anticoagulants; chronic constipation; and fever.

Colonic or small intestinal angioectasias are suspected if the age is >70 years, there is cardiovascular disease, or there is chronic LGI bleeding/iron deficiency anemia. Hemorrhoids are suspected if there is dripping blood with bowel movements or if there is hematochezia with otherwise normal bowel movements, ischemic colitis if there is cardiovascular disease and hematochezia with or without abdominal pain, ulcerative colitis (UC) if there is bloody diarrhea, and colonic neoplasia if there is a change in bowel habits, chronic bleeding, personal or family history of colon neoplasia, or weight loss.

## Physical Examination

Start with the patient's vital signs and pay attention to signs of hypovolemia such as hypotension, tachycardia, and postural symptoms.

Digital rectal examination is mandatory along with routine abdominal examinations. Look for any scar marks in the abdomen and whether any perianal diseases are present or not.

## Investigations

The algorithm for the management of hematochezia is shown in **Flowchart 1**.

*Colonoscopy*: The overall rate of detecting a presumed or definite cause of LGI bleeding by colonoscopy is 48–90%, with an average of 68%. Usually, it takes 4–6 hours to prepare the patient for early urgent colonoscopy as colonic purge of 6–8 L of polyethylene glycol (PEG) purge orally or via an nasogastric (NG) tube over 4–6 hours to clean all stool and blood clots. In case of severe and active hematochezia, colonoscopy should be done within 12 hours, and in case of mild-to-moderate hematochezia, it should be done within 24 hours.

*Main target of LGI bleed control*: Endoscopic hemostasis in most of the time of colonic bleed.

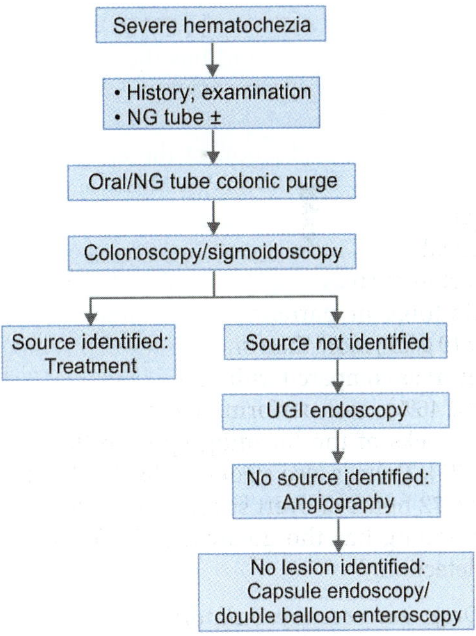


**FLOWCHART 1:** Algorithm for the management of hematochezia.

(NG: nasogastric; UGI: upper gastrointestinal)

*Endotherapy*: Mechanical devices—bands, hemoclip, over-the-scope clip (OTSC), and detachable snare

*Detachable snare*: It is simple and easy to apply. There is no need to remove the scope again.

Mechanical occlusion of the bleeding post polypectomy stalk.

*Angiography*: This has the ability to detect bleeding of >0.5 mL/min. In addition to its diagnostic role, angiography offers therapeutic possibilities via pharmacologic vasoconstriction or superselective embolization.

*Radionuclide scintigraphy*: Two methods are used: One using technetium-99m ($^{99m}$Tc) sulfur colloid and the other using $^{99m}$Tc-labeled red blood cells (RBCs) (tagged RBC scan). This technique detects bleeding at a rate as low as 0.4 mL/min, with a positive diagnostic rate of approximately 45% and an accuracy rate of 78% for localizing the bleeding site.

*Video capsule endoscopy (VCE)*: VCE measures 26 × 11 mm$^2$ and has the capacity to take images at a rate of 2 frames/s over an 8–12-hour period. Capsule endoscopy allows noninvasive evaluation of the entire small bowel in 79–90% of patients, with a diagnostic yield of 38–83% in patients with suspected small bowel bleeding. VCE yield depends on factors such as a higher likelihood of positive findings in patients with a hemoglobin < 10 g/dL, more than one episode of bleeding, overt as compared with occult bleeding (60% vs. 46%), and performance of VCE within 2 weeks of the bleeding episode (91% vs. 34%). There is also evidence that VCE within 48–72 hours of overt suspected small bowel bleeding has the greatest yield for lesion detection.

*Deep enteroscopy balloon-assisted enteroscopy*: Double-balloon enteroscopy—It can be advanced at a distance of approximately 240–360 cm distal to the pylorus with the oral approach and 102–140 cm proximal to the IC valve with the rectal approach. It has the additional advantage over VCE of both diagnostic and therapeutic capabilities, including biopsies, tattoo, hemostasis, polypectomy, dilation, and foreign body removal (including retained capsules).

*Surgery*: The main indications for surgery include malignancy, GI stromal tumor (GIST), diffuse bleeding that fails to cease with medical treatment as seen in ischemic colitis and UC, and recurrent bleeding from a diverticulum.

## MANAGEMENT

*Resuscitation*: Initial resuscitation of any GI bleed will be the same. Initial assessment of blood loss, postural changes, and hemodynamic alterations due to blood loss will always be the priority for initial resuscitation.

At least one large-bore (14- or 16-gauge) catheter should be placed intravenously and two should be placed when the patient has ongoing bleeding. Normal saline is infused as fast as needed to keep the patient's SBP higher than 100 mm Hg and pulse lower than 100 bpm.

### Cause-wise Management

#### *Diverticulosis*

The entry point of vasa recta is a relatively weaker area, and at that point, the mucosa and submucosa can herniate when intraluminal pressure is increased. Bleeding from the base is seen in 52% and from the neck is seen in 48% of cases. Diverticular bleeding is seen in 3–5% of patients with diverticulosis. Right colonic diverticula are more likely to bleed.

#### *Definitive Diverticular Hemorrhage*

Stigmata of recent hemorrhage (SRH) (e.g., active bleeding, visible vessel, adherent clot) on colonoscopy or active bleeding is seen on angiography or radionuclide imaging, with later confirmation of diverticulum in that location by colonoscopy or surgery.

### Presumptive Diverticular Hemorrhage

Colonoscopy reveals diverticulosis without stigmata, and no other significant lesions are seen in colonoscopy, terminal ileum examination, and enteroscopy.

#### Management

In 75% of patients with diverticular bleeding, the bleeding stops spontaneously, and these patients require transfusion of fewer than four units of packed RBCs. For patients in whom bleeding has spontaneously stopped, the rebleeding rate from colonic diverticulosis was reported from 25 to 38% over the next 4 years, with most patients having mild rebleeding.

Endoscopic stigmata include active bleeding, nonbleeding visible vessel (NBVV), and clot. Medically treated active bleeding from a diverticulum 83% rebled and 56% required intervention for hemostasis. In cases of NBVV in a single diverticulum, the rate of rebleeding was 60%, and the rate of intervention for hemostasis was 40%. In an adherent clot treated medically, the rebleeding rate was 43% and the rate of intervention was 29%.

### Endoscopic Hemostasis

Multipolar electrocoagulation (MPEC), epinephrine injection, hemoclips, fibrin glue, rubber band ligation, endoloops, or combinations of epinephrine and MPEC or hemoclips.

### Ischemic Colitis

Ischemic colitis is characterized by painless or painful hematochezia with mild left-sided abdominal discomfort. The painless subtype results due to mucosal hypoxia and is caused by hypoperfusion of the intramural vessels of the intestinal wall.

Watershed area between the superior and inferior mesenteric arteries has the fewest collateral vessels and is at most risk for ischemia. Ischemia is most likely to occur in the watershed area of the splenic flexure, and it can occur anywhere in the colon. Colonoscopic appearance of the mucosa includes erythema, friability, and exudate.

### Infectious Colitis

Infectious colitis are caused by *Campylobacter jejuni*, *Salmonella*, *Shigella*, enterohemorrhagic *Escherichia coli* (O157:H7), *Cytomegalovirus* (CMV), or *Clostridioides difficile*. Treatment is with medical management.

### Inflammatory Bowel Disease

Most of the patients with inflammatory bowel disease (IBD) had Crohn's disease, and most were successfully treated medically.

### Postpolypectomy Bleeding

Clinically relevant bleeding occurs in 1–6% of patients undergoing colonoscopic polypectomy. It is most common 5–7 days after polypectomy but can occur from 1 to 14 days after the procedure. Risk factors for postpolypectomy bleeding include a large polyp size (>2 cm), thick stalk, sessile type, location in the right colon, use of anticoagulants, and use of aspirin or another NSAID. Epinephrine injection, thermal coagulation, hemoclip placement, and combination therapy are recommeded. Most major SRH in postpolypectomy ulcers are treated with hemoclipping.

### Colonic Angioectasia

Overt bleeding from angiodysplasia is typically brisk, painless, and intermittent. Endoscopically, angiodysplasia appears as red, stellate lesions of variable sizes surrounded by a pale mucosal rim. The right colon is preferentially involved, although lesions can occur throughout the intestinal tract and are often multiple.

### Rectal Dieulafoy Lesions

Dieulafoy lesions are large submucosal arteries without overlying mucosal ulceration that can cause massive bleeding.

### Rectal Varices

The treatment of bleeding rectal varices is similar to that for esophageal varices, with sclerotherapy, band ligation, or a portosystemic shunt.

### Radiation Proctitis

Sigmoidoscopy or colonoscopy reveals telangiectasias, friability, and sometimes ulceration in the rectum. Medical therapy with topical or oral 5-aminosalicylic acid (mesalamine), sucralfate, or glucocorticoids may be prescribed but are not generally effective. Thermal therapy is usually successful, but repeated treatments with MPEC or argon plasma coagulation are necessary to achieve good outcomes. Topical formalin applied directly to the rectal mucosa can reduce bleeding.

### Internal Hemorrhoids

Medical therapy consisting of fiber supplementation, stool softeners, lubricant rectal suppositories (with or without glucocorticoids), and warm sitz baths relieve internal hemorrhoids. Anoscopic therapy can also be used and includes injection sclerotherapy, rubber band ligation, cryosurgery, infrared photocoagulation, MPEC, and direct current electrocoagulation.

### Small Bowel Sources

Angiodysplasia is the predominant cause of bleeding from the small intestine, followed by lymphoma, erosions/ulcers, and Crohn's disease. Enteroscopy, barium contrast radiography, and capsule endoscopy are appropriate diagnostic modalities.

A summary of causes and management of bleeding per rectum is shown in **Table 1**.

## CLINICAL PEARLS

In the case of lower GI bleeding, look for possible risk factors and different possibilities of lower GI bleeding.

**Table 1: Summary of causes and management of bleeding per rectum.**

| *Causes of bleed* | *Preferred endoscopic management* |
|---|---|
| Diverticulosis | Mechanical therapy (clips/EBL) |
| Ischemic colitis with ulcerations | Epinephrine/hemoclips/surgery for severe disease/rule out AMI by CTA |
| Post-polypectomy bleed | Hemoclips ± epinephrine |
| Angioectasia | APC |
| Colonic polyps | Polypectomy/surgery for polyposis syndromes |
| Colonic neoplasia | Epinephrine/clips on endoscopically unresectable lesions Surgery indicated for resectable/operable cases |
| Internal hemorrhoids | Medical therapy/sclerotherapy/band ligation |
| Rectal varices | EVL |
| Rectal ulcers (elderly, bedridden patients) | Hemoclips |
| Anal fissure | Medical therapy |
| IBD | Medical therapy/surgical therapy in refractory cases |

(AMI: acute myocardial infarction; APC: argon plasma coagulation; CTA: computed tomography angiography; EBL: endoscopic band ligation; EVL: endoscopic variceal ligation; IBD: inflammatory bowel disease)

In acute lower GI bleeding, do colonoscopy within 12 hours in case of severe bleeding after rapid bowel preparation with PEG 3350 (4–6 L).

Target for endoscopic hemostasis if any diverticulosis, angioectasia, or postpolypectomy bleeding are found and medical therapy is recommended for IBD.

## FURTHER READINGS


1. Zuccaro Jr G. Management of the adult patient with acute lower gastrointestinal bleeding. Am J Gastroenterol. 1998;93:1202-8.
2. Beck KR, Shergill AK. Colonoscopy in acute lower gastrointestinal bleeding: diagnosis, timing, and bowel preparation. Gastrointest Endosc Clin N Am. 2018;28(3):379-90.
3. Brunnler T, Klebl F, Mundorff S, Eilles C, Reng M, von Korn H, et al. Significance of scintigraphy for the localisation of obscure gastrointestinal bleedings. World J Gastroenterol. 2008;14:5015-9.
4. Rondonotti E, Villa F, Mulder CJ, Jacobs MA, de Franchis R. Small bowel capsule endoscopy in 2007: indications, risks and limitations. World J Gastroenterol. 2007;13:6140-9.
5. May A, Wardak A, Nachbar L, Remke S, Ell C. Influence of patient selection on the outcome of capsule endoscopy in patients with chronic gastrointestinal bleeding. J Clin Gastroenterol. 2005;39:684.
6. Singh A, Marshall C, Chaudhuri B, Okoli C, Foley A, Person SD, et al. Timing of video capsule endoscopy relative to overt obscure GI bleeding: implications from a retrospective study. Gastrointest Endosc. 2013;77:761-6.
7. Wong SK, Ho YH, Leong AP, Seow-Choen F. Clinical behavior of complicated right-sided and left-sided diverticulosis. Dis Colon Rectum. 1997;40:344.
8. McGuire Jr HH. Bleeding colonic diverticula. A reappraisal of natural history and management. Ann Surg. 1994;220:653.
9. Bloomfeld RS, Rockey DC, Shetzline MA. Endoscopic therapy of acute diverticular hemorrhage. Am J Gastroenterol. 2001;96: 2367.
10. Sawhney MS, Salfiti N, Nelson DB, Lederle FA, Bond JH. Risk factors for severe delayed postpolypectomy bleeding. Endoscopy. 2008; 40:115.
11. Sorbi D, Norton I, Conio M, Zinsmeister A, Gostout CJ. Postpolypectomy lower GI bleeding: descriptive analysis. Gastrointest Endosc. 2000;51:690.

CHAPTER 33

# Nausea and Vomiting

*Bickram Pradhan*

## WHAT IS NAUSEA AND VOMITING?

- Nausea is the sensation of an urge to vomit and is perceived in the throat or epigastrium.
- Vomiting is the forceful oral ejection of upper gut contents. Vomiting may occur with or without nausea.
- Retching involves no oral discharge of gastric contents.

Nausea and vomiting are distinguished from related symptoms.

## WHAT CAUSES NAUSEA AND VOMITING?

Afferent neural signals for initiating emesis arise from many locations in the body including the pharynx, stomach, and small intestine, as well as from extraintestinal organs such as the heart and the testicle. Pathways from the chemoreceptor trigger zone (CTZ) located in the area postrema activate vomiting. Despite its central location, CTZ serves primarily as a sensitive detection apparatus for circulating endogenous and exogenous molecules that may activate emesis. Pathways arising from other central nervous system (CNS) structures, including the cortex, brainstem, and vestibular system, can also initiate symptoms. Stimulation of brain 5-hydroxytryptamine3 (5-HT3) serotonin receptors provokes the release of dopamine, which in turn stimulates dopamine D2 receptors in the brainstem. Toxins and drugs that act on the gastrointestinal (GI) tract are detected by enteroendocrine cells that release 5-HT and activates 5-HT3 receptors on vagal afferents. Histamine H1 and M1 receptors are abundant in the vestibular center and solitary nucleus that constitute pharmacologic targets for inhibiting motion sickness, vestibular nausea, and pregnancy-related emesis. Cannabinoid CB1 receptors in the dorsal vagal complex inhibit the emetic reflex.

## WHAT ARE THE CAUSES OF NAUSEA AND VOMITING?

*Medications*: Nonsteroidal anti-inflammatory agents/aspirin, opiates; Antibiotics: Macrolides, tetracycline, cardiac antiarrhythmics, metformin, liraglutide, venlafaxine, duloxetine, oral contraceptives

*Infections/Inflammation*: Gastroenteritis, Crohn's disease, pancreatitis, cholecystitis, appendicitis

*Obstruction*: Gastric/small bowel obstruction; superior mesenteric artery syndrome volvulus

*Motility disorders*: Gastroparesis, chronic intestinal pseudo-obstruction

*Functional gastroduodenal disorder*: Cyclic vomiting syndrome (CVS), chronic idiopathic nausea, functional vomiting

*Miscellaneous*: Radiation, chemotherapy induced, cannabis induced, endocrine/ metabolic disease, myocardial infarction, ethanol intoxication, psychiatric disease

# PATH TO DIAGNOSIS

## History

Look for detailed history as it provides useful information that may help to identify the cause of unexplained nausea and emesis. Acute vomiting usually for 1–2 days results from infection, medication or toxin, or endogenous toxic metabolites (uremia, diabetic ketoacidosis). Chronic vomiting (>1 week) results from long-standing medical or psychiatric conditions. History of timing of vomiting and food relation will help to differentiate. Patients with gastric obstruction or gastroparesis report nausea within 5 minutes of eating, and most vomiting occurs >1 hour after a meal. Patients with rumination syndrome regurgitate undigested food within minutes of eating. Nausea and vomiting from cholecystitis and pancreatitis may present in the first hour after eating. Content of vomiting also guides in diagnosis. Undigested food return suggests achalasia, rumination, or Zenker's diverticulum; vomiting of partly digested or old food residue suggests gastric obstruction or gastroparesis. Emesis of bilious material only occurs in conditions in which there is no gastroduodenal obstruction proximal to the ampulla of Vater. Feculent emesis occurs with distal intestine or colon obstruction, bacterial overgrowth, and gastrocolic fistulae.

Central nervous system processes can produce effortless or projectile emesis without nausea. Labyrinthine diseases present with tinnitus or vertigo.

## Physical Examination

Look for the following signs in case of vomiting and nausea:

Tachycardia, orthostatic hypotension, and dry mucous membranes indicate dehydration.

Adenopathy (supraclavicular) raises concern for neoplasm. Absent bowel sounds signify ileus.

High-pitched hyperactive bowel sounds with a distended abdomen are consistent with intestinal obstruction. A succession splash on side-to-side movement is found in gastric outlet obstruction or gastroparesis. Ulcers, cholecystitis, pancreatitis, or peritonitis may produce abdominal tenderness or guarding. Focal neurologic signs, papilledema, neck rigidity, or impaired mentation suggests CNS disorders. Asterixis is present in metabolic disease.

## Investigations

Hypokalemia, alkalosis, or an elevated blood urea nitrogen level reflect dehydration and electrolyte loss from persistent emesis. Endocrine and metabolic causes can be assessed by pregnancy testing, thyroid-stimulating hormone (TSH), serum calcium, and cortisol.

Abdominal radiography by standard X-ray abdomen or computed tomography (CT) enterography can screen for small bowel obstruction, ileus, or pseudo-obstruction (diffuse luminal distention). Upper gastrointestinal (UGI) endoscopy is needed for suspected ulcer disease or gastric outlet obstruction. Finding retained food on endoscopy without obstruction suggests gastroparesis. Pancreaticobiliary disease may be evaluated by CT, magnetic resonance cholangiopancreatography (MRCP), and ultrasound. Finding gastric or duodenal dilation on CT scanning with a diminished distance between the superior mesenteric artery and the aorta is consistent with superior mesenteric artery syndrome.

For gastrointestinal motor function, different investigations are there. Quantification of gastric emptying by gastric scintigraphy, wireless motility capsule, magnetic resonance imaging (MRI), single-photon emission CT, three-dimensional gastric, and the 13C breath test with octanoate acid. Cutaneous electrogastrography is used to identify dysrhythmia of the gastric pacemaker and changes in the frequency of activity in response to feeding. Antroduodenal manometry is recommended for assessing foregut motor disturbances distal to the esophagus. Manometry helps to differentiate myogenic from neurogenic forms of pseudo-obstruction and detects partial small bowel obstruction on the basis of wave pattern analysis.

# TREATMENT

Correction of clinically relevant metabolic complications, pharmacologic therapy, and treatment of the underlying cause comprise treatment **(Table 1)**.

## Correction of Metabolic Complications

If oral hydration is not adequate, intravenous (IV) fluids and electrolytes should be administered. Adequate replacement generally consists of a normal saline solution in volumes sufficient to correct deficits with potassium supplementation (60–80 mEq/24 hours). Patients with long-standing chronic vomiting are at risk of developing malnutrition, so enteral or parenteral feeding should be considered when the patient is unable to resume adequate oral nutrition after 5–8 days.

## Pharmacologic Treatment

*Central antiemetic agents*: Dopamine D2 receptor antagonists: Metoclopramide; domperidone

*Phenothiazines*: Chlorpromazine, perphenazine, prochlorperazine, promethazine: Dopamine D2 antagonist, muscarinic M1 antagonist, histamine H1 antagonist

*Serotonin antagonists*: Serotonin 5-HT3 receptor antagonists (ondansetron, tropisetron) are potent antiemetics that block 5-HT3 receptors in the brainstem and gastric wall receptors that relay afferent emetic impulses through the vagus nerve.

**Table 1: Etiology-wise treatment.**

| *Disease* | *Treatment* |
|---|---|
| Acute gastroenteritis | Symptomatic with 5-HT3 antagonists |
| Chemotherapy- and radiation therapy-induced nausea and vomiting | 5-HT3 antagonist, NK-1 antagonist |
| Gastroparesis | Prokinetics, gastric electrical stimulation |
| Gastric outlet obstruction due to peptic stricture | Endoscopic dilatation, surgery |
| Hyperemesis gravidarum | Pyridoxine and acupressure |
| Superior mesenteric artery syndrome | Surgery |
| Cyclic vomiting syndrome | Tricyclic antidepressants, serotonin reuptake inhibitors |

(5-HT3: 5-hydroxytryptamine3; NK-1: neurokinin-1)

*Cannabinoids*: Nabilone and dronabinol: Used in chemotherapy-induced nausea and vomiting refractory to conventional therapy

*Neurokinin-1 (NK-1) receptor antagonists*: Inhibit substance P and NK-1. Two formulations are available, aprepitant and fosaprepitant; rolapitant

*Gastric prokinetic agents*: 5-HT4 receptor agonists: Cinitapride

*Motilin receptor agonists*: Erythromycin

*Neuromodulators*: Tricyclic antidepressants: Amitriptyline; nortriptyline

## CLINICAL PEARLS

Nausea and vomiting are pathophysiologically different with multiple GI and extra GI causes underlying.

For etiological workup, first, look for any signs of gastric outlet obstruction or any suggestion of intestinal obstruction.

Look for any associated symptoms with nausea and vomiting and start resuscitation if any signs of volume depletion are present.

Initial symptomatic management is usually done with central antiemetic agents and after that treatment is done according to different etiologies.

## FURTHER READINGS

1. Gershon MD. 5-Hydroxytryptamine (serotonin) in the gastrointestinal tract. Curr Opin Endocrinol Diabetes Obes. 2013;20(1):14-21.
2. Takeda N, Morita M, Hasegawa S, Horii A, Kubo T, Matsunaga T. Neuropharmacology of motion sickness and emesis. A review. Acta Otolaryngol Suppl. 1993;501:10-5.
3. Van Sickle MD, Oland LD, Ho W, Hillard CJ, Mackie K, Davison JS, et al. Cannabinoids inhibit emesis through CB1 receptors in the brainstem of the ferret. Gastroenterology. 2001; 121(4):767-74.

# PART 5

# General Signs and Symptoms

# CHAPTER 34

# Facies

Amit Kalwar

## INTRODUCTION

*Facies* is a distinctive facial expression or appearance associated with a specific medical condition.

In the past, the student of medicine did not have all the tools to diagnosis. A man's senses were of utmost demand during that period. As a result of keen observation, Hippocrates describes the change produced in the face by impending death or long illness, excessive defecation, excessive hunger—the Hippocrates facies: "A sharp nose, hollow eyes, collapsed temples, the ears cold, contracted and the lobes turned out; the skin about the forehead being rough, distended and parched; the colour of the whole face being brown, black, livid, or lead-coloured."

The study of the face in health and sickness cannot replace the meticulous, systematic examination of the body as a whole; nevertheless, it is of great importance in clinical medicine because a patient's physiognomy allows for a diagnosis or may guide a clinician's clinical judgment along certain pathological classifications. It can frequently direct the expert observer's attention to the most likely area in which to acquire data for his diagnosis. Both a high level of critical thinking and extensive expertise are necessary.

Some characteristics of the face are so indicative of a particular disease that the diagnosis is implied right away. These are known as diagnostic facies.

*Some of the diagnostic facies associated with specific diseases that we encounter are as follows*:

*Anxious*: Indicates awareness or apprehension of the patient about the disease. It is found in nervous individuals.

*Ashen gray facies*: Pallor or pale skin and grayish or blue skin due to lack of oxygenated blood. It is seen in myocardial infarction.

*Adenoid facies*: Characterized by a long, thin face, persistently open mouth with malar hypoplasia, high-arched palate, narrow maxillary arch, short upper lip, prominent upper teeth, crowded teeth, and narrow upper alveolus. It is found in patients with adenoid hypertrophy. Adenoid facies can be a part of Cowden syndrome.

*Acromegalic facies*: Characterized by large supraorbital ridge and frontal bossing, thickened lips, enlarged tongue, prognathism, and jaw malocclusion. It is seen in acromegaly.

*Amiodarone facies*: Administration of amiodarone may cause phototoxic eruption or a brown or blue-gray discoloration around the malar area and nose.

*Bovine facies*: Characterized by a convex nasal profile, shortened mandible, macroglossia, and defect in the size and shape of the head. It is seen in craniofacial dysostosis or Crouzon syndrome.

*Bird facies*: Characterized by a very small lower jaw, cleft palate, and retroglossoptosis (tongue appears to fall into the throat). It is seen in Pierre Robin syndrome.

*Bell's palsy*: Smoothening of furrows in the forehead, wide palpebral fissure, asymmetry of blinking, watering of eye or epiphora, Bell's phenomenon (eyeball rolls upward and inward during attempted forced eye closure), loss of nasolabial fold, angle of mouth drawn to one side, drooping of the angle of mouth, flapping in and out of the cheek on one side during respiration.

*Bulldog facies*: Seen in congenital syphilis as a result of the local effect of syphilitic rhinitis on the development of adjacent structures. Because the maxilla is small, the normal mandible appears proportionately longer and bigger resulting in a bulldog-like jaw.

*Coarse facies*: Characterized by a large bulging head, prominent scalp veins, "saddle-like, flat bridged nose with a broad, fleshy tip," large lips and tongue, small, widely spaced and/or malformed teeth, hypertrophic alveolar ridges and/or gums. It is present in many inborn errors of metabolism.

*Chipmunk facies*: Combination of expanded globular maxillae and prominent epicanthal folds, characteristic of severe beta-thalassemia. It occurs due to bone marrow expansion secondary to extramedullary hematopoiesis.

*Elfin facies*: The most consistent features are growth deficiency which is predominantly of postnatal onset, mild microcephaly with mental deficiency, and an altered pattern of facial development which includes broad forehead, pointed chin, cupid bow-like upper lips, upturned nose, hypertelorism, and low-set ears. The disorder is a sporadic occurrence of unknown etiology. With associated mental retardation and hypercalcemia, it forms William syndrome.

*Facies of cretinism*: Coarse facial appearance, wrinkling of eyebrows, and thick tongue are characteristics of cretinism. Apathy of hypothyroidism should draw the attention of the clinician.

*Facies of bilateral facial palsy*: Described as a face devoid of any facial expression and loss of nasolabial folds and loss of furrows.

*Flat facies*: Flat appearing face with a small head, flat bridge of the nose, low-set nose, small mouth which causes the tongue to stick out and to appear overly large, upward slanting eyes, epicanthal fold, rounded cheeks, and small ears characteristic of Down syndrome.

*Frog face*: Broadening of the nose and flattening of the face caused by intranasal disease.

*Gargoyle facies*: Head is large and dolichocephalic, with frontal bossing and prominent sagittal and metopic sutures, with midface hypoplasia, depressed nasal bridge, flared nares, prominent lower one-third of the face, thickened facies, widely spaced teeth and attenuated dental enamel, gingival hyperplasia. It is seen in patients with Hurler syndrome.

*Hepatic facies*: Shrunken eyes, hollowed temporal fossa, pinched-up nose, parched lips, muddy complexion, icteric tinge, characteristic of certain chronic liver disorder.

*Hatchet facies*: Characterized by bilateral ptosis, wasting of temporalis and masseter muscles leading to a thin visage referred to as a hatchet face. It is seen in cases of myotonic dystrophy.

*Leonine facies*: Defined as facial features similar to that of a lion with prominent convexities and furrowed creases due to diffuse infiltration of the skin forehead, chin, nose, and ears. It is seen in cases of lepromatous leprosy, leishmaniosis, chronic actinic dermatitis, cutis verticis gyrata, lymphoma, leukemia, sarcoidosis, and scleromyxedema.

*Mongoloid facies (flat facies)*: Dull and vacant look of mentally retarded children. It is characterized by slanting eyes, epicanthic fold, small nose with small oral cavity, Brushfield spot on the iris, low-set ears, saddle nose, narrow, short high arched palate, and smaller teeth, characteristically seen in Down syndrome (trisomy 21).

*Masked facies*: Parkinsonian facies, characterized by an expressionless face with staring eyes, slightly open mouth, and wide palpebral fissures. It is also seen in bilateral facial paralysis, facial myopathies, myasthenia gravis, progressive systemic sclerosis, or scleroderma.

*Moon facies*: Characterized by a bloated appearance of the face with rounding of the facial features. It can be caused by different diseases such as Cushing's syndrome, prolonged steroid therapy, nephrotic syndrome, and myxedema.

*Mitral facies*: Characterized by rosy cheeks and a bluish tinge on the rest of the face. It is seen in severe mitral stenosis.

*Marfanoid facies*: Characterized by widely spaced eyes (hypertelorism), a highly arched palate, an abnormally small jaw (micrognathia) that is recessed farther back than normal (retrognathia), and underdeveloped cheekbones (malar hypoplasia). It is seen in patients with Marfan syndrome.

*Monkey facies*: Characteristic loss of buccal fat, seen in marasmus.

*Mauskopf facies (mouse head)*: Mask-like facies, absence of normal skin wrinkling, pinched-up nose or beaking of the nose, difficulty in opening the mouth fully—small mouth (microstomia), skin over the face appears taut and shiny, pigmentation and depigmentation, telangiectasia over face and lips. It is pathognomonic of systemic sclerosis.

*Malar rash*: Also called butterfly rash, it is characterized by a red or purplish, mildly scaly rash involving the cheeks and bridge of the nose. It is seen in patients with systemic lupus erythematosus.

*Marshal hall facies*: Disproportion of forehead to face seen in hydrocephalus.

*Nephritic facies*: Characterized by a pale and puffy face; swelling is commonly periorbital. It is seen in acute glomerulonephritis

*Plethoric facies*: Erythematous face. It is seen in chronic alcoholism, Cushing's syndrome, polycythemia, superior vena cava (SVC) syndrome, chronic cor pulmonale, and carcinoid syndrome.

*Potter's facies*: Characterized by a flattened nose, recessed chin, prominent epicanthal folds, and low-set abnormal ears. It is seen in babies due to pressure in utero due to oligohydramnios.

*Risus sardonicus*: Characterized by a fixed unmirthful grin due to tonic contraction of the facial muscles drawing the angle of the mouth outward and raising the eyelids. It is seen in tetanus, strychnine poisoning, or Wilson's disease.

*Slapped cheek facies*: In erythema infectiosum, diffuse erythema and edema of the cheeks give a "slapped cheek" facies appearance.

*Snarling facies*: In myasthenia gravis, there may be marked bilateral facial weakness. In some patients, poor retraction and elevation of the corners of the mouth when attempting to smile or grimace may result in a "vertical smile," referred to as a myasthenic snarl or sneer.

*Tabetic facies*: Characterized by persistent wrinkling of the forehead in an attempt to compensate for drooping of eyelids due to pseudoptosis caused by paralysis of Müller's muscle. It is seen in tabes dorsalis.

*Thyrotoxic facies*: Staring look, exophthalmos, and lid lag which results in exposure of the white conjunctiva above the cornea (Von Grafe's sign) are characteristic of Graves' disease.

*Torpid facies*: Characterized by an expressionless face, swelling of the face which can include lips, eyelids, and tongue, pallor, coolness, and dryness of the skin. It is seen in patients with myxedema.

## CLUES TO DISEASE FROM FACIES AND EXPRESSION

*Endocrine disease*: Prognathism of acromegaly; moon facies of Cushing's syndrome; prominent stare of thyrotoxicosis; dull appearance and large tongue of cretinism, loss of lateral eyebrows, puffy face, dry skin, and brittle hair of myxedema; vitiligo and increased freckling in Addison's disease

*Central nervous system (CNS) disease*: Mask-like facies of parkinsonism; drooping eye, sleepy appearance in myasthenia gravis; "coma vigil" in the typhoid state (and any prolonged febrile illness); risus sardonicus in tetanus.

*Cardiovascular disease*: Supravalvular aortic stenosis with elfin facies; mitral facies in mitral stenosis.

*Infections*: Leonine facies of leprosy.

*Renal disease*: Periorbital edema in acute nephritis; earlobe abnormalities in some congenital renal diseases.

*Miscellaneous disorders*: Taut, stretched facies of scleroderma; butterfly rash in lupus erythematosus.

## CLINICAL PEARLS

*"The eyes have been called the windows of the soul, the face the mirror of the mind."*

Reading face is an art, an art which has to be developed through meticulous observation and examination of patients over the years. An expert clinician, by identifying characteristic facies, can diagnose many systemic diseases and syndromes or at least can gather information regarding the mental health of the patient.

## FURTHER READINGS

1. Definition of Facies. [online] Available from: www.merriam-webster.com. [Last accessed August, 2023].
2. Sen SK. Essentials of Clinical Diagnosis, 7th edition. Kolkata: The Standard Book House; 1994.
3. Lloyd 2nd KM, Dennis M. Cowden's disease. A possible new symptom complex with multiple system involvement. Ann Intern Med. 1963;58:136-42.
4. Vorperian VR, Havighurst TC, Miller S, January CT. Adverse effects of low dose amiodarone: a meta-analysis. J Am Coll Cardiol. 1997;30:791-8.
5. Jones K. Pierre Robin Syndrome/Bird Facies—Introduction. Medindia. [online] Available from https://www.medindia.net/patients/patientinfo/pierrerobin.htm. [Last accessed August, 2023].
6. Sanchez M, Luger AF. Syphilis. In: Fitzpatrick TB, Eisen AZ, Wolff K, Freedberg IM, Austen FK (Eds). Dermatology in General Medicine, 4th edition. New York: McGraw Hill; 1993. pp. 2703-43.
7. Sarkany RP, Breathnach SM, Morris AA, Weismann K, Flynn PD. Metabolic and nutritional disorders. In: Burns T, Breathnach S, Cox N, Griffiths C (Eds). Rooks Textbook of Dermatology. 8th edition. Singapore: Wiley Blackwell; 2010. pp. 59.1-103.
8. Bennet FC, LaVeck B, Sells CJ. The Williams elfin facies syndrome: the psychological profile as an aid in syndrome identification. Pediatrics. 1978;61:303-6.
9. Concise Dictionary of Modern Medicine. New York: McGraw Hill; 2002.
10. Miller-Keane Encyclopedia and Dictionary of Medicine, Nursing and Allied Health, 7th edition. Philadelphia, PA: Saunders; 2003.
11. Campbell WW. Augenblickdiagnose. Semin Neurol. 1998;18(2):169-76.

12. Rapini RP. Clinical and pathologic differential diagnosis. In: Bolognia JL, Jorizzo JL, Rapini RP (Eds). Bolognia Dermatology, 2nd edition. USA: British Library Cataloguing in Publication Data; 2008. p. 4.
13. Singh DN. Down's syndrome: a study of clinical features. J Natl Med Assoc. 1976;68:521-4.
14. Kreig T, Scleroderma. In: Burgdorf, Plewig, Wolff, Landthaler (Eds). Braun Falco's Dermatology, 3rd edition. New York: Springer; 2009. p. 707.
15. Sundriyal D, Kumar N, Chandrasekharan A, Gadpayle AK. Mauskopf facies. BMJ Case Rep. 2013;2013:bcr2013200163.
16. Wolff K, Johnson RA (Eds). Fitzpatrick's Color Atlas and Synopsis of Clinical Dermatology, 6th edition. New York: McGraw Hill; 2009. p. 807.
17. Howard JF. The myasthenic facies and snarl. J Clin Neuromuscul Dis. 2000;1:214-5.
18. Sparling PF, Swartz MN, Musher DM, Healy BP. Clinical manifestations of syphilis. In: Holmes KK, Sparling PF, Stamm WE, Piot P, Wasserheit JN, Corey L, et al. (Eds). Sexually Transmitted Diseases, 4th edition. New York: McGraw Hill; 2008. p. 671.

# CHAPTER 35

# Fingers

*Aritra Ray*

## INTRODUCTION

The human hand consists of different bones (carpal bones, metacarpal bones, and phalanges), ligaments, and muscles which allow dexterity and a large range of movements. While each finger consists of three phalanges (proximal, middle, and distal), the thumb consists of two phalanges. The clinical significance of both hands and fingers is enormous and they are used to diagnose a vast array of diseases.

## CLINICAL SIGNIFICANCE OF HANDS AND FINGERS

*Bouchard's nodes*: They are bony hard gelatinous cysts or outgrowths on the proximal interphalangeal (PIP) joints. They may cause pain, stiffness, and restricted movement of the affected joint. Bouchard's nodes may be found in osteoarthritis or after surgery or repetitive trauma to the fingers. Treatments include nonsteroidal anti-inflammatory drugs (NSAIDs), physiotherapy, and rarely surgery.

*Heberden's nodes*: They are bony, hard swelling found in the distal interphalangeal (DIP) joints. Pain, numbness, redness, and swelling are the presenting features. They are seen in osteoarthritis.

*Boutonniere deformity and swan neck deformity*: In Boutonniere deformity, flexion occurs at the PIP joint whereas extension occurs at the DIP joint. This deformity may be seen in cases of rheumatoid arthritis. In swan neck deformity, flexion occurs at the DIP joint whereas hyperextension occurs at the PIP joint, thereby resembling a swan's neck. This deformity is found in rheumatoid arthritis and cerebral palsy or may even occur after trauma.

*Janeway lesions*: These are small, nontender, painless, erythematous, or hemorrhagic lesions seen mostly over palms and soles, particularly at the base of the little finger and thumb. Janeway lesions are seen in infective endocarditis and very rarely in systemic lupus erythematosus, hemolytic anemia, disseminated gonorrhea, and typhoid fever.

*Osler nodes*: They are painful, red lesions found over the hands and feet. They are seen in infective endocarditis and rarely in disseminated gonococcal infection, marantic endocarditis, and systemic lupus erythematosus.

*Holt-Oram syndrome*: Upper limb deformities may be unilateral, bilateral/asymmetric, or bilateral/symmetric and it may range from absent thumb to phocomelia. Upper limb malformations may include abnormal forearm supination and pronation, hypoplasia or aplasia of the radius, anomalous development of the thenar and carpal bones, restricted movement of the shoulder joint, and sloping shoulder.

*Hypermobility of hand joints*: They occur when the structures holding a joint, e.g., joint capsule, muscles, and ligaments, become loose. Conditions include Ehlers-Danlos syndrome, Marfan syndrome, Morquio syndrome, cleidocranial dysostosis, and Down syndrome.

*Tripe palm*: It is a rare skin condition which is characterized by velvety ridged lesions over the palms, thereby resembling the lining of a cow's stomach. It is a paraneoplastic syndrome which is seen in gastric carcinoma. Noncancerous conditions which may be associated with tripe palms include psoriasis, exfoliative dermatitis, and bullous pemphigoid.

*Pallor*: Lower palpebral conjunctiva, nail beds, oral mucosa, tongue, and palm of the hand are the classical sites to look for pallor. Color of nail beds is compared with the normal pink color of healthy nails. To look for pallor, the patient is asked to show the palms. Color of the palm is compared with that of a normal healthy person. Palmar creases are also observed for pallor. Some palmar pallor is said to be present when the creases are darker but the palms remain pale. Severe palmar pallor is said to be present when both the palm and the palmar creases remain pale.

*Cyanosis*: Distal extremities (hands, toes, and fingertips) are examined for peripheral cyanosis, which occurs due to reduced cardiac output, chronic obstructive pulmonary disease (COPD), cold exposure, arterial and venous obstruction, and all factors causing central cyanosis. Asymmetrical bluish discoloration between the lower and upper extremities is called differential cyanosis. It may be found in patent ductus arteriosus associated with pulmonary hypertension.

*Icterus*: Palms and soles, general skin surface, upper bulbar conjunctiva, palate, and undersurface of tongue are observed in natural daylight to look for icterus.

*Palmar erythema*: It is a skin condition in which the palms of both hands turn reddish. It occurs due to dilatation of superficial capillaries. It can be both primary and secondary. Primary palmar erythema may be idiopathic or can be due to pregnancy. Secondary palmar erythema can be due to liver cirrhosis, hemochromatosis, Wilson disease, diabetes, thyrotoxicosis, or autoimmune diseases or can be drug induced.

*Carotenemia*: It is a clinical condition in which yellowish pigmentation of the skin occurs due to increased carotene levels in the blood. It may occur due to consumption of foods rich in carotene. Carotenemia may be rarely associated with diabetes mellitus, hypothyroidism, renal disease, liver disease, and anorexia nervosa.

*Blackened fingers*: This condition may occur due to inflammation, peripheral artery disease (PAD), frostbite, chilblains, and scleroderma. Blackening of fingers is specifically caused by general vasculitis, polyarteritis nodosa (PAN), necrosis, Raynaud's disease, and Buerger's disease.

*Dark knuckles*: Darker pigmentation over knuckles may be associated with conditions such as acanthosis nigricans, prediabetes and diabetes, vitamin B12 deficiency, Addison's disease, dermatomyositis, polycystic ovary syndrome, scleroderma, and autoimmune diseases or due to drug reactions (e.g., estrogen therapy, growth hormone therapy, glucocorticoids, oral contraceptive pills, protease inhibitors).

*Polydactyly*: It is a condition in which a baby is born with extra fingers or toes. It can be radial or preaxial, ulnar or postaxial, and central. Polydactyly may be associated with the following conditions:

- Carpenter syndrome
- Laurence-Moon-Biedl syndrome
- Trisomy 13
- Chondroectodermal dysplasia

- Asphyxiating thoracic dystrophy
- Rubinstein–Taybi syndrome

*Symbrachydactyly*: It is a congenital hand condition where a baby has abnormally short fingers which may be misshaped, webbed, or missing. This condition may be associated with Poland syndrome.

*Clinodactyly*: It is a condition in which a baby is born with an abnormally curved finger. The curved finger may even overlap with other fingers. Clinodactyly may be associated with conditions such as Klinefelter syndrome, Down syndrome, Fanconi anemia, and Turner syndrome.

*Ectrodactyly*: This is a congenital condition which is characterized by deep median cleft over hands and/or foot. Conditions which may be associated with ectrodactyly include craniofacial defects, tibial aplasia, and genitourinary abnormalities.

*Arachnodactyly (achromachia)*: This is a condition which is characterized by abnormally long and slender fingers and toes as compared to the palm of the hands or arch of the foot. It may be associated with conditions such as Ehlers–Danlos syndrome, homocystinuria, Loeys–Dietz syndrome, and Marfan syndrome.

*Sclerodactyly*: It is a localized tightness and thickening of the skin of toes or fingers, which results in a characteristic claw-like appearance of the affected digits, thereby leading to restricted mobility. It may be associated with conditions such as mixed connective tissue disease, autoimmune disorders, and systemic scleroderma. Sclerodactyly is one of the components of the limited cutaneous variant of systemic sclerosis, otherwise known as CREST syndrome.

*Calcinosis*: Fingers may get affected by calcinosis, a condition characterized by the deposition of calcium salts in soft tissues. Calcinosis presents as irregular hard nodules and often it may lead to skin ulcers, contractures, pain, and functional disability.

*Down syndrome*: Broad and small feet and hands are seen in Down syndrome. Palmar crease (single line across the palm of hand) and clinodactyly (incurving of fifth finger) are frequently observed in patients with Down syndrome.

*Froment's sign*: It is a test to detect ulnar nerve palsy, specifically the action of adductor pollicis. The patient is asked to hold a thin piece of paper between her index finger and thumb and an attempt is made to pull it from the grip of the patient. The test is said to be positive if the patient flexes his flexor pollicis longus in order to maintain his grip.

*Phalen's test*: It is a test for carpal tunnel syndrome. The patient is asked to flex both wrist joints maximally while keeping the dorsal aspect of both hands pressed against each other and to remain in that position for 1 minute. The test is said to be positive if the paresthesia gets reproduced in the distribution of the median nerve, namely tingling in the index, middle finger, thumb, and/or the medial aspect of the ring finger.

*Finkelstein test*: This test is used to diagnose De Quervain's syndrome. The patient sits relaxed and comfortable over a table. The patient's hand is examined in the air, while the other hand remains at rest beside the body. The patient is then asked to form a fist around the thumb and do an ulnar deviation. The test is said to be positive if pain occurs over the first extensor compartment of the wrist.

*Claw hand*: It is a hand deformity in which fingers are bent into a claw-like position. In claw hand, flexion at the interphalangeal (IP) joints and hyperextension at the metacarpophalangeal (MCP) joints occur due to weakness of intrinsic muscles of the hands. It may occur following median and ulnar nerve palsy, cubital tunnel syndrome, congenital birth defect, and leprosy.

*Ape hand*: Ape hand deformity is a condition where the patient finds it difficult to oppose or abduct the thumb. This occurs following a deep injury over the forearm, arm, and wrist causing damage of the median nerve leading to impairment of opponens policis and thenar muscles.

*Hand of Benediction (Pope's hand)*: It occurs as a result of injury or prolonged compression of the median nerve at the elbow or forearm. When the patient attempts to make a fist, flexion of the little and ring finger occurs but the middle and the index finger cannot flex at the IP joint.

*Trigger finger*: It is a condition where the thumb or the fingers get locked when the patient tries to bend them. A painful snapping or clicking is noticed when the patient tries to bend or straighten his finger. Forceful and repeated movement of the thumb and fingers may lead to tendon inflammation, thereby causing trigger finger. Gout, rheumatoid arthritis, and diabetes can lead to such condition. It is more common among women, industrial workers, musicians, and farmers who do repeated thumb and finger movements. Rest, splints, stretching exercises, NSAIDs, and steroid injections are the treatment of choice.

*Mallet finger*: It is caused by disruption of the extensor mechanism at the DIP joint of the phalanx.

*Felon finger*: A felon finger is caused by a bacterial infection, namely *Staphylococcus aureus*, which occurs after a penetrating trauma, such as scrape, cut, puncture wound, or splinter. Symptoms of a felon finger include swelling, redness, and throbbing pain. If left untreated, the felon finger may lead to osteomyelitis and pyogenic flexor tenosynovitis.

*Herpetic whitlow*: A herpetic whitlow is a painful lesion on a thumb or a finger which is caused by herpes simplex virus (HSV-1 or HSV-2). Symptoms include reddening, swelling, and tenderness of the affected finger. This may also be associated with fever, lymphadenopathy, and clear small vesicles. Pus formation occurs in bacterial whitlow. Oral or parenteral antiviral drugs, namely acyclovir, is the treatment of choice.

*Rolando fracture*: It is a comminuted Y- or T-shaped intra-articular fracture involving the base of the thumb.

*Bennett's fracture*: It is a two-part intra-articular fracture involving the base of the first metacarpal bone. It results from the forced abduction of the first metacarpal.

*Gamekeeper's thumb*: It is a rupture or an avulsion of the ulnar collateral ligament (UCL) of the MCP joint. It is caused by different activities which involve repetitive or forceful thumb movements like playing sports, skiing or using tools.

*Boxer's fracture*: It is a break in the fifth metacarpal bone near the knuckle. It mostly occurs when a boxer hits their fist on a hard object or on a human face.

*Volkmann contracture*: It is the deformity of fingers, hands, and wrist which occurs following traumatic injuries in the form of crush injuries, fractures, arterial injuries, and burns. Subsequently, deficit in the arteriovenous circulation occurs in the forearm leading to decreased blood flow and damage of nerves, muscles, and vascular endothelium.

*Chilblains*: These are itchy swellings over the skin which occur on exposure to cold temperatures. Body extremities, such as fingers, toes, heels, nose, and ears, usually get affected. These often heal on their own within 1 or 2 weeks without treatment.

*Papillary patterns of human fingers*: Fingerprints afford an invaluable means of identification because the ridge arrangement over every finger of every individual is unique and does not vary with age or growth.

## CLINICAL PEARLS

- Fingers and hands can be used to diagnose a vast array of diseases.
- Meticulous examination of fingers and hands is very essential in clinical medicine as early diagnosis of diseases can have better prognostic significance.

## FURTHER READINGS

1. Osler nodes and Janeway lesions. DermNet NZ. [online] Available from https://dermnetnz.org/topics/osler-nodes-and-janeway-lesions. [Last accessed August, 2023].
2. Rapini RP, Bolognia JL, Jorizzo JL. Dermatology: 2-Volume Set. St. Louis: Mosby; 2007. p. 677.
3. Mullans EA, Cohen PR. Tripe palms: a cutaneous paraneoplastic syndrome. South Med J. 1996;89(6):626-7.
4. Image of Hand of Benediction. Stanford Medicine. [online] Available from: https://stanfordmedicine25.stanford.edu/content/sm/stanfordmedicine25/the25/hand/_jcr_content/main/panel_builder_0/panel_0/panel_builder_3/panel_0/image.img.full.high.jpg/. [Last accessed August, 2023].
5. Radiopaedia. Bennett fracture. [online] Available from: https://radiopaedia.org/articles/bennett-fracture. [Last accessed August, 2023].
6. Dunn JC, Kusnezov N, Orr JD, Paliis M, Mitchell JS. The boxer's fracture: splint immobilization is not necessary. Orthopedics. 2016;39(3):188-92.

# CHAPTER 36

# Nails

*Aritra Ray*

## ANATOMY

- *Nail matrix*: It is the most important structure where new plate cells are formed and older cells get pushed forward leading to the growth of the nail plate.
- *Nail bed*: It is the area on which the nail plate rests.
- *Nail plate*: It is the hard nail area extending from the root of the nail to the free edge and it is made up of hard keratin protein.
- *Nail folds*: It is the area which surrounds the nail plate on three sides (two lateral nail folds and the proximal nail fold).
- *Cuticle*: It is a thin extension of the proximal nail fold skin onto the nail plate.

## DISORDERS

Disorders of nails can be classified as:

- Congenital
- Infections
- Traumatic
- Neoplastic
- Secondary to systemic disease
- Secondary to dermatological disease

### Congenital Disorders of Nails

*Paronychia congenita*: It is an autosomal dominant disorder which is characterized by gross thickening of nail plates. It can be associated with skin thickening and leukoplakia.

### Infections

- *Tinea unguium*: It is a dermatophytic infection of the nails which can be caused by *Trichophyton rubrum*, *Trichophyton mentagrophytes*, and *Epidermophyton floccosum*. Infection starts at the distal end and spreads proximally. Toenails are more frequently involved than fingernails. Nail plate becomes thick and yellow. Nails become ragged, crumbly, dull, and distorted.
- *Paronychia*: It is the inflammation of nail folds and can be both acute and chronic.
    - *Acute paronychia*: It is a staphylococcal infection in which the nail fold becomes red, tender, and swollen. Pus may be visible on the nail bed or under the nail fold. It may be associated with constitutional symptoms and lymphadenopathy. It is treated by systemic antistaphylococcal antibiotics and surgical drainage (if needed).
    - *Chronic paronychia*: Colonization of the space between the nail plate and nail fold by gram-negative bacteria, *Staphylococcus*, and *Candida* leads

to chronic paronychia. Diabetes mellitus, wet work, and associated candidal vulvovaginitis may predispose to chronic paronychia. The nail fold becomes rolled up and swollen, and sometimes pus can be seen under the nail fold. The nail plate becomes discolored and ridged over a period of time. Topical and systemic antibiotics and antifungals remain the mainstay of therapy.

- *Viral nail infection*: Viral warts can lead to changes in both the thickness and the shape of nails. Viruses can lead to the growth of skin below the nails which are known as periungual warts. It is most commonly caused by human papillomavirus (HPV).

## Traumatic

- *Splinter hemorrhages*: These are linear traumatic hemorrhages which are usually seen below the nails of manual workers. They may also be seen in subacute bacterial endocarditis and psoriasis of nails.
- *Subungual hematomas*: Traumatic injury around the nail fold results in accumulation of blood between the nail bed and toenail or fingernail. The patient usually complains of severe pain and dark-colored discoloration of nails (maroon, red, purple-black).
- *Chronic injury*: Injury and pressure from ill-fitting shoes result in different changes—
    - *Ingrowing toenails*: A tiny nail spicule gets embedded into the nail folds and it is caused by improper cutting of the nails.
    - *Onychogryphosis*: It is a nail dystrophy where the nail becomes curved and thickened. Trimming the deformed nails is the treatment of choice.
    - *Onycholysis*: It is a nail disorder in which the nail plate gets separated from the nail bed, resulting in white opaque nails. It may be secondary to nail infections, skin disease, tumors, trauma, or systemic events.
- *Changes due to nervous tics*:
    - *Nail biting*: It is the habit or act of biting the ends of one's fingernails and is frequently encountered in both adults and children. Bitten nails are usually irregular and short with frayed cuticles.
    - *Tic dystrophy*: It is caused due to repeated external trauma to the nail matrix and proximal nail fold resulting in transverse ridges across the entire nail, resembling a ladder. Habit reversal training, behavior therapy, and cyanoacrylate adhesive form the mainstay of treatment.
- *Chemical injury*:
    - *Detergents*: Wet work and detergents cause splitting of the distal portion of the nail plate in a lamellar fashion. It is usually seen in cooks, bakers, housewives, and hairdressers.
    - *Cosmetics*: Nail plate may get damaged by formaldehyde in nail hardeners and adhesives of artificial nails.
- *Nail bed laceration*: An injury with sharp material may cause lacerations, thereby causing bleeding from nail beds.

## Nails in Skin Diseases

- *Psoriasis*: The following nail changes are observed in psoriasis—
    - *Pitting (most frequent change)*: In nail psoriasis, pitting is regular, superficial, and thimble-like. Finer pitting and mottled lunula are found in alopecia areata. Irregular pitting and cross ridges are also seen in dermatitis.
    - *Subungual hyperkeratosis*: It is usually seen in conditions such as psoriasis and tinea unguium. The hyperkeratosis is usually tunneled, friable, and easily removable in subungual hyperkeratosis. Fungal hyphae can also be demonstrated in the debris.

- Other changes in the form of onycholysis, oil spots, and yellowish discoloration of the nail plates are also seen.
- *Lichen planus*: Nail plate thinning, discoloration, irregular longitudinal ridging, and grooving are the most common changes. Other changes may include onychorrhexis, onycholysis, subungual hyperkeratosis, and pterygium. Treatment should be started early to prevent permanent nail dystrophy. Corticosteroids are the first line of treatment. Corticosteroid-sparing immunosuppressants may be required in case of relapse or persistence of the disease.
- *Dermatitis*: When proximal nail fold gets involved in dermatitis, it leads to swelling and inflammation of the nail bed, resulting in different nail abnormalities in the form of Beau's lines, pitting, longitudinal or transverse ridging, twenty-nail dystrophy, onycholysis, and transverse depressions. Fingers and hands may also show signs of dermatitis.

## Nails in Systemic Diseases

- *Clubbing*: It is the soft-tissue swelling of the terminal phalanx resulting in an increase in the angle between the nail fold and nail plate. It is associated with the following conditions:
  - *Lung disease*: Lung cancer, bronchiectasis, empyema, lung abscess, cystic fibrosis, interstitial lung disease (e.g., idiopathic pulmonary fibrosis), sarcoidosis, mesothelioma of pleura, and arteriovenous fistula or malformation
  - *Heart disease*: Subacute bacterial endocarditis, congenital cyanotic heart disease, tetralogy of Fallot, and atrial myxoma
  - *Gastrointestinal and hepatobiliary*: Ulcerative colitis, Crohn's disease, malabsorption, primary biliary cholangitis, cirrhosis, and hepatopulmonary syndrome
  - *Others*: Graves' disease, vascular anomalies (axillary artery aneurysm)
- *Color changes*:
  - *Leukonychia*: Leukonychia or white nails may be seen in conditions associated with hypoalbuminemia (e.g., cirrhosis of the liver). The causes can be as follows:
    - *True leukonychia*: It occurs due to a disease affecting the nail matrix. The most common cause is trauma. Mees' lines are true leukonychia which are characterized by single or multiple, narrow, transverse, white lines running parallel to the lunula and along the width of nails. It may also involve multiple nails. It may be seen in arsenic poisoning, tuberculosis, leprosy, herpes zoster, malaria, chemotherapeutic drugs, cardiac and renal failure, carbon monoxide, and antimony poisoning.
    - *Apparent leukonychia*: It occurs due to a disease affecting the nail bed. It is associated with systemic diseases such as chronic renal disease, liver cirrhosis, systemic chemotherapy, and hypoalbuminemia. *Muehrcke's lines* are apparent leukonychia which is characterized by double transverse line (white in color). *Terry's nails* are also apparent leukonychia which are normal distally but white proximally. It may be associated with adult-onset diabetes mellitus, congestive cardiac failure, hemodialysis, human immunodeficiency virus (HIV), and peripheral vascular disease.
    - *Pseudoleukonychia*: It is caused by conditions affecting the nail plate, e.g., onychomycosis.

Five forms of leukonychia are known: (i) *Leukonychia striata,* (ii) *leukonychia punctata,* (iii) *leukonychia partialis,* (iv) *longitudinal leukonychia,* and (v) *leukonychia totalis.* Leukonychia striata may be hereditary or may be associated with trauma and systemic diseases such as Kawasaki disease, HIV, acitretin, and anticancer drugs. Leukonychia punctata may be seen in persons with normal nails. Leukonychia partialis may be associated with selenium deficiency, nephritis, Hodgkin's disease, metastatic carcinoma, Hansen's disease, chilblains, and complex regional pain syndrome or it may be idiopathic. Longitudinal leukonychia may be seen in oncychopapillomas and Hailey–Hailey disease. Leukonychia totalis may be hereditary in origin.

- *Half and half nails*: This condition may be seen in patients of chronic kidney disease undergoing hemodialysis. It may sometimes be seen in normal individuals.
- *Green nails*: Green nail syndrome or chloronychia occurs due to fungal nail infection. It may also be caused by *Pseudomonas aeruginosa*, which produces green pigments, namely pyocyanin and pyoverdin.
- *Blue nails*: It is seen in conditions such as congestive heart failure, hypothermia, cold exposure, and disease of the peripheral vessels in which supply of the oxygenated blood to the extremities gets hampered resulting in bluish-purple peripheral cyanosis.
- *Black nails*: Blackish brown nails or melanonychia may be found in conditions such as subungual melanoma, nevus, lichen planus, malnutrition, hemochromatosis, smoking, and thyroid disorders or in persons with a dark complexion.
- *Yellow nails*: Yellow nail syndrome may be seen in both adults and children. The nails become yellowish green, thickened, and excessively curved both longitudinally and transversely. Yellow nails may be seen in conditions such as liver disease, bronchiectasis, nephrotic syndrome, rheumatoid arthritis, Raynaud's disease, sinusitis, tuberculosis, and immunodeficiency.

- *Deformities of nail plate*:
  - *Koilonychia*: Spoon-shaped nail or koilonychia may be seen in nutrition deficiency conditions (e.g., iron deficiency anemia), autoimmune conditions (e.g., systemic lupus erythematosus), inflammatory skin conditions (e.g., lichen planus and psoriasis), environmental exposure to petroleum, people living at high altitude, genetic conditions (e.g., hemochromatosis, nail-patella syndrome), nail trauma, celiac disease, vitamin B deficiency, and hypothyroidism.
  - *Beau's lines*: These are transverse ridges or indentations which develop across nails few weeks after acute and severe illness. These may be seen in conditions such as acute kidney failure, thyroid disease, mumps, syphilis, melanoma, endocarditis, pneumonia, diabetes, zinc deficiency, and scarlet fever. They can also develop after traumatic injuries or as a side effect of chemotherapy.
- *Nail fold changes*: Erythema, thrombosed capillaries, and telangiectasia may be seen in connective tissue diseases. Frayed cuticles may be seen in nail biters, connective tissue diseases, and due to excess use of cosmetics.

## SOME TYPES OF NAILS

- *Pincer nails*: When transverse curvature of nails gets increased along the longitudinal axis reaching to its greatest proportion toward the tip, it is called pincer nails.
- *Brachyonychia*: In brachyonychia, the width of the nail plate is smaller than that of the length. It may be found in hyperparathyroidism and psoriatic arthropathy.
- *Parrot beak nail*: It is a condition in which symmetrical overcurvature of the free edge of nails mimics a parrot beak. It may be seen in severe acrosclerosis. The nail plate gets bent around the shortened fingertip.
- *Macronychia*: Nails are too large compared to nails on nearby fingers. It may be seen in local gigantism.
- *Micronychia*: Nails are too small compared to nails on nearby digits. It may be seen in conditions associated with plexiform neuromas.
- *Dolichonychia*: It is a condition in which the length of the nails exceeds the width. It may be associated with Marfan's syndrome and hypopituitarism.

## CLINICAL PEARLS

- Nails can get affected in different congenital, neoplastic and infectious conditions.
- Many dermatological and systemic diseases may show early manifestations through nails.
- Proper examination of nails is of immense value in clinical practice for early diagnosis of diseases.

## FURTHER READINGS

1. Rasi A, Soltani-Arabshahi R, Naraghi ZS. Circumscribed juvenile-onset pityriasis rubra pilaris with hypoparathyroidism and brachyonychia. Cutis. 2006;77:218-22.
2. Nail configuration abnormalities. In: Baran R, Dawber RP, Haneke E, Tosti A, Bristow I (Eds). A Text Atlas of Nail Disorders: Techniques in Investigation and Diagnosis, 3rd edition. London: Routledge; 2005. pp. 18-24.
3. Motswaledi MH, Mayayise MC. Nail changes in systemic diseases. SA Fam Pract. 2010;52:409-13.
4. Cohen PR, Milewicz DM. Dolichonychia in women with Marfan syndrome. South Med J. 2004;97:354-8.

# CHAPTER 37

# Weight Gain and Weight Loss

*Kripasindhu Gantait*

Weight gain and weight loss are nowadays true epidemics and public health crises that both doctors and patients must face. Normal body weight is defined as a body mass index (BMI) of 18.5–24.99 kg/m$^2$; overweight and underweight are defined as BMI ≥25 and <18.5 kg/m$^2$, respectively.

Adipocyte is continuously undergoing remodeling; its average life span is 10 years. It can expand to an average of three times its normal volume because of triacylglycerol (TAG) deposition. With prolonged over-nutrition, preadipocytes within adipose tissue are stimulated to proliferate and differentiate into mature fat cells, thereby increasing the number of adipocytes. So, obesity is due to a combination of increased fat cell size (hypertrophy) and number (hyperplasia). In an obese individual, weight loss is achieved by reduction in the size of the fat cells, although their number remains constant. But the small fat cells have the tendency to reaccumulate fat inside them, hence facilitating weight regain **(Fig. 1)**.

About 80–90% of human body fat is stored in subcutaneous depots in the abdomen (upper body, apple shape, as reflected in waist size) and hips–thighs (lower body, pear shape). The remaining 10–20% is in visceral depots. Excess fat located in the viscera and abdomen is associated with a greater risk for hypertension, insulin resistance, diabetes, dyslipidemia, and coronary heart disease.

## WEIGHT GAIN

The hypothalamus is central to the control of energy balance in the body like the control of hunger via the lateral hypothalamus nucleus which stimulates food intake and satiety via the ventromedial hypothalamus nucleus, which inhibits food intake. Body weight is influenced by the rate of energy expenditure, which is regulated by the secretion of hormones involved in the buildup of energy stores. Ghrelin, an orexigenic hormone, plays a role in the short-term control of appetite while leptin, an adipocyte peptide hormone, controls long-term weight control. Leptin levels decrease in states of starvation **(Flowchart 1)**. Neuropeptide Y is present in the peripheral and central nervous systems and promotes anabolism by stimulating the secretion of insulin. Corticotrophin-releasing hormone has the opposite effect to neuropeptide Y.

The common causes of weight gain are given in **Box 1**.

Overweight and obesity refer to conditions where body fat is in excess and often is expressed as BMI. It is calculated as:

$$\text{BMI} = \frac{\text{Body weight (in kg)}}{\text{Height}^2\text{ (in m)}}$$

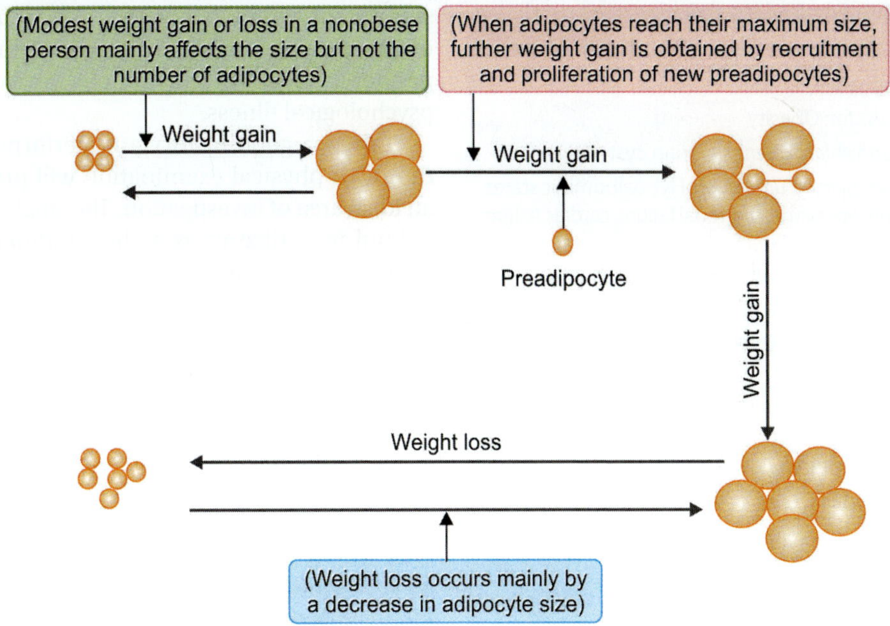


**FIG. 1:** Link between weight and adipocytes.

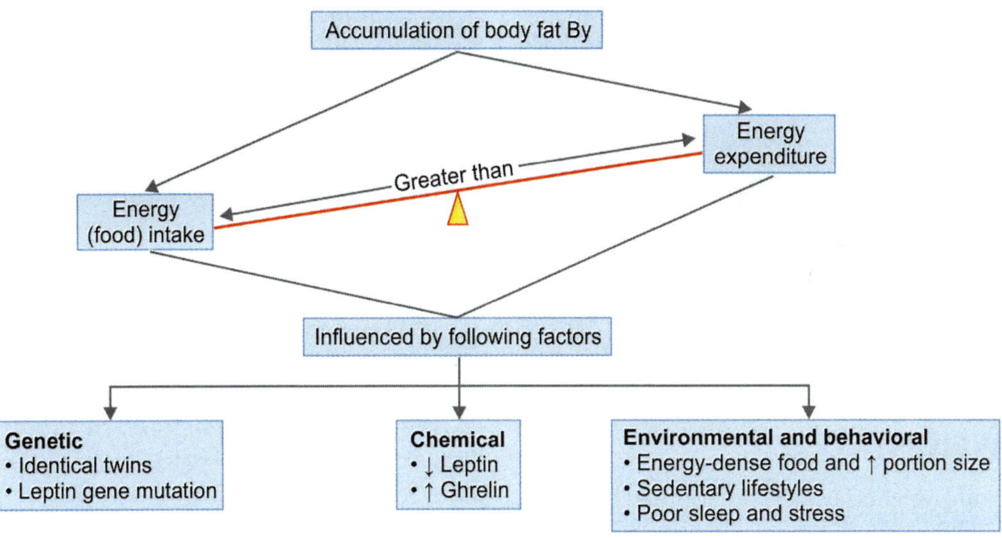


**FLOWCHART 1:** Factors contributing to accumulation of fat in the body.

The World Health Organization (WHO) classification is based primarily on the association between BMI and mortality **(Table 1)**.

Waist circumference over 80 cm in female and 94 cm in male is hazardous to health.

Prevention of weight gain involves increasing physical activity and dietary modification to reduce caloric intake.

**BOX 1: Causes of weight gain.**

- Pregnancy
- *Excess fat*: Obesity
- *Organ enlargement*: Ovarian cyst
- *Excess fluid accumulation*: Hypoalbuminic states, nephrotic syndrome, renal failure, cardiac failure, liver failure
- *Excess muscle bulk*: Athletes, growth hormone, androgenic steroids
- *Lymphatic obstruction*: Filariasis, metastatic cancer
- Hypothyroid/Cushing's syndrome
- *Drugs*: Insulin, corticosteroids, estrogen, alcohol, cyproheptadine
- Idiopathic

**Table 1: Classification of weight status and disease risk.**

| *Classification* | *Body mass index (BMI) (kg/m²)* | *Risk of comorbidities* |
|---|---|---|
| Underweight | <18.5 | Low (but the risk of other clinical problems increased) |
| Normal ranges | 18.5–24.99 | Average |
| Overweight | ≥25 | |
| • Preobese | 25–29.99 | Increased |
| • Obese class I | 30–34.99 | Moderate |
| • Obese class II | 35–39.99 | Severe |
| • Obese class III | ≥40 | Very severe |

## WEIGHT LOSS

Body weight is usually determined by factors such as caloric intake, absorptive capacity, metabolic rate, and energy loss. Body weight reaches peak level physiologically by the fourth or fifth decade and then gradually declines at a rate of 1–2 kg per decade. In postmenopausal women, unintentional weight loss was associated with increased rates of hip and vertebral fractures. Involuntary weight loss is regarded as clinically significant when it exceeds 5% or more of usual body weight over a 6–12-month period. It often indicates serious physical or psychological illness.

Taking a good history and performing a thorough physical examination will provide an ideal area of investigation. The single most helpful investigation is a chest radiograph, which often reveals masses, infiltrates, heart failure, or lymph node enlargement.

### Weight Loss with Normal Appetite

- *Increased utilization*:
  - Pulmonary tuberculosis (TB)
  - Hyperthyroidism
  - Anxiety states
  - *Drug*: Levothyroxine
- *Inadequate absorption*:
  - Intestinal hypermobility states
  - Gluten enteropathy
  - Chronic pancreatitis
  - Postgastrectomy states
  - Chronic liver disease
- *Calorie loss*:
  - Diabetes
  - Intestinal parasites

### Weight Loss with Poor Appetite

- *Gastrointestinal*:
  - Gastric ulcer
  - Malignancy
  - Hepatobiliary disease
- *Malignant states*:
  - Lymphoma
  - Leukemia
  - Carcinoma
  - Sarcoma
- Uremia
- *Chronic states*:
  - Infections
  - Intoxications (alcohol/lead)
  - Cardiac diseases
  - Inflammatory [rheumatoid arthritis (RA)/systemic lupus erythematosus (SLE)]
  - Obstructive lung diseases

- Human immunodeficiency virus (HIV) infection
- Anorexia nervosa

## CLINICAL PEARLS

Obesity is one of the biggest health problems in the world and associated with metabolic syndrome including high blood pressure, elevated blood sugar, lipid abnormality, leading to higher risk of heart disease and type 2 diabetes mellitus, compared to those have healthy weight. The prevalence of obesity and overweight are ~10 to ~35% and ~40% respectively. Therefore, anyone can attempt to maintain healthy weight with four pillers of proper nutrition, adequate sleep, healthy levels of exercise and emotional healthcare.

## FURTHER READINGS

1. Ferrier DR. Lippincott illustrated reviews Biochemistry. South Asian Edition. Wolters Kluwer; 2021. p. 489.
2. Ellis H. French's Index of Differential Diagnosis An A-Z. 16th edition. CRC Press; 2016.

CHAPTER 38

# Hepatosplenomegaly

*Nandini Chatterjee*

## WHAT IS HEPATOSPLENOMEGALY?

Enlargement of the liver, spleen, or both is known as hepatosplenomegaly, which may be associated with a whole gamut of disorders. The clue to etiology lies in careful history taking and clinical correlation with other systemic findings.

## WHAT ARE THE CAUSES?

There is a considerable overlap in the causes of hepatomegaly and splenomegaly, and many diseases cause both hepatomegaly and splenomegaly, which are as follows:

- *Hepatomegaly*:
  - *Infections*:
    - Viral: Hepatitis A–E and other hepatotropic viruses, dengue, human immunodeficiency virus (HIV)
    - Bacterial: Typhoid, tuberculosis (TB), Weil's disease, brucellosis, scrub typhus
    - Protozoal: Malaria, kala-azar
    - Fungal: Histoplasmosis
    - Parasitic: Hydatidosis
  - Liver abscess
  - *Congestive hepatopathy*: Congestive cardiac failure (CCF), constrictive pericarditis, Budd–Chiari syndrome
  - *Autoimmune causes*: Systemic lupus erythematosus (SLE), rheumatoid arthritis (RA), autoimmune hepatitis
  - *Infiltrative disorders*: Lymphoma, leukemia, myeloma
  - *Neoplastic causes*: Secondaries, hepatocellular carcinoma (CA)
  - *Toxic*: Alcohol, arsenic, drugs
- *Splenomegaly*: It is graded as follows—
  - *Mild* (<5 cm below the costal margin):
    - Nutritional anemias
    - Subacute bacterial endocarditis, Epstein–Barr (EB) virus, cytomegalovirus (CMV), enteric fever, leptospirosis, toxoplasmosis, malaria
    - Alcoholic liver disease
    - Collagen vascular disease, Felty syndrome, thyrotoxicosis, congestive heart failure, acute pancreatitis, inflammatory bowel disease
    - Drugs
  - *Moderate* (5–10 cm below costal margin):
    - Infections, e.g., TB, brucellosis, fungal, malaria, kala-azar
    - Cirrhosis, Budd–Chiari syndrome
    - Amyloidosis, sarcoidosis, hemophagocytic syndrome
    - Chronic hemolytic anemia
    - Lymphoma, leukemia, myeloma
    - Hemangioma, hamartoma

- *Massive* (>10 cm below costal margin or weighing >1,000 g):
  - Noncirrhotic portal fibrosis/extrahepatic portal hypertension
  - Hairy cell leukemia
  - Polycythemia rubra vera
  - Chronic myeloid leukemia (CML)
  - Gaucher's disease
  - Myelofibrosis
  - Hyperreactive malarial spleen
  - Non-Hodgkin lymphoma
- *Hepatosplenomegaly*:
  - *Infections*: Malaria, kala-azar, dengue, enteric fever, scrub typhus, leptospirosis, disseminated TB, infectious mononucleosis, histoplasmosis
  - *Hematological disorders*: Leukemia, lymphoma, myeloproliferative disorders, chronic hemolytic anemia
  - *Congestive disorders*: CCF, constrictive pericarditis, Budd-Chiari syndrome
  - *Storage disorders*: Amyloidosis, sarcoidosis

# HOW TO APPROACH CLINICALLY?

## History

- Fever, travel to endemic zones, alcohol intake, jaundice, hematemesis melena
- Exertional dyspnea, skin/gum bleeds, recurrent infections, bony pain
- Joint pain, rashes
- Chest pain, palpitation, shortness of breath

## Examination

- Pallor, lymphadenopathy, sternal tenderness, purpura
- Arthritis, skin rash
- Jaundice, gynecomastia, spider nevi, palmar erythema, tortuous venous prominence over abdomen/back
- Raised jugular venous pressure (JVP), new murmurs
- *Palpation of liver*:
  - *Soft tender liver*: Congestive heart failure, viral hepatitis, liver abscess, Budd-Chiari syndrome
  - *Firm liver*: Cirrhosis, infiltrative disorder, sarcoidosis, amyloidosis, abscess
  - *Hard liver*: Metastasis, hepatocellular CA
- *Nodular surface*: Cirrhosis, metastasis
- *Palpation of spleen*:
  - Soft tender spleen, infective endocarditis
  - Firm nontender spleen

## Investigations

- Complete hemogram including peripheral blood smear, reticulocyte count—for hematological disorders
- *Liver function test*: Hepatitis, chronic hemolytic anemia, chronic liver disease, infiltrative disease
- Malarial parasite (MP), dual antigen, Widal test, RK 39, viral serology—infections
- Antinuclear antibodies (ANA) profile, RA factor—autoimmune diseases
- *Special tests*: Serum angiotensin-converting enzyme (ACE), ferritin, iron, total iron-binding capacity (TIBC), ceruloplasmin, malarial immunoglobulin M (IgM), hemoglobin (Hb) electrophoresis
- Blood culture
- Chest X-ray, ultrasound (USG) abdomen with Doppler study for patency of the splenoportal axis, computed tomography (CT) abdomen, upper gastrointestinal (GI) endoscopy, echocardiography
- *Invasive tests*: Lymph node biopsy, liver biopsy, splenic aspirate, bone marrow biopsy, splenectomy, histopathology

# TREATMENT

Therapy according to the cause.
*Indications of splenectomy*:

- Chronic, severe hypersplenism

**BOX 1: Some of the characteristic etiologies of splenomegaly in the Indian subcontinent.**

- Dengue, typhoid, typhus, melioidosis, histoplasmosis
- Visceral leishmaniasis (VL, kala-azar)—67% of the global burden of VL is from India, Bangladesh, and Nepal. Kala-azar cases were reported from 52 districts (e.g., 4 main states) of India. However, Bihar (31 districts), West Bengal (6 districts), Jharkhand (4 districts), and Uttar Pradesh (11 districts) were highly affected states
- Hyperreactive splenomegaly syndrome—positive malarial immunoglobulin M (IgM) antibody, hypersplenism
- Hemoglobinopathies
- Extrahepatic portal venous obstruction/noncirrhotic portal fibrosis

- Refractory idiopathic thrombocytopenic purpura
- Spontaneous/traumatic rupture of spleen
- Hereditary spherocytosis, thalassemia with hypersplenism
- For diagnosing certain lymphomas
- Certain cases of splenic abscess
- Certain cases of wandering spleen
- Using the splenic artery for kidney revascularization in renovascular hypertension

## SPECIAL MENTION

Some of the characteristic etiologies of splenomegaly in the Indian subcontinent are mentioned in **Box 1**.

## CLINICAL PEARLS

- Clue to etiological diagnosis lies in analysis of associated history and signs
- Infectious etiology predominates in the Indian Subcontinent
- Treatment is individualized.

## FURTHER READINGS

1. Abdullah AYM, Dewan A, Shogib MRI, Rahman MM, Hossain MF. Environmental factors associated with the distribution of visceral leishmaniasis in endemic areas of Bangladesh: modeling the ecological niche. Trop Med Health. 2017;45:13.
2. Bhunia GS, Kesari S, Chatterjee N, Kumar V, Das P. The burden of visceral leishmaniasis in India: challenges in using remote sensing and GIS to understand and control. Int Sch Res Notices. 2013;2013:675846.

CHAPTER 39

# Fever

*Nandini Chatterjee*

## WHAT IS FEVER?

Fever is a rise of body temperature, above the normal circadian variation as a result of a change in the hypothalamic thermoregulatory set point (oral temperature >98.9°F at 6 AM and evening temperature at 4 PM >99.6°F). Rectal temperature is 1°F higher than oral temperature, whereas axillary temperature is 1°F less than oral. Signs and symptoms associated with fever may include chills and shivering, headache, muscle aches, loss of appetite, irritability, sweating, dehydration, and general weakness.

Normal body temperature is typically around 98.6°F (37°C). However, the normal body temperature can vary from person to person. It may also fluctuate at different times of the day. It is lower in the morning and rises slightly in the late afternoon and evening. Other factors, such as menstrual cycle or intense exercise, can also affect body temperature.

*Hyperthermia*: It is an uncontrolled rise of body temperature that exceeds the body's ability to dissipate heat but the hypothalamic set point is unchanged, e.g., heat stroke, neuroleptic malignant syndrome, malignant hyperthermia, and serotonin syndrome. A more common condition in high temperatures though is heat exhaustion characterized by heavy sweating, nausea, vomiting, weak pulses, and cramps.

## WHAT ARE THE CAUSES OF FEVER?

Fever occurs in the presence of pyrogens (Greek pyro, "fire") due to which the hypothalamus shifts the set point of normal body temperature upward. When this happens, neurons in the vasomotor center are activated leading to peripheral vasoconstriction to preserve body heat. The patient starts feeling chill, and shivering (muscle contractions) occurs to generate more body heat. This eventually results in a higher body temperature until it reaches a new thermostat setting.

## WHAT ARE THE POSSIBILITIES? CAUSES OF FEVER

It is important to note that the causes of fever may vary according to geographical distribution, ethnicity, climate, and sociocultural factors. Also, the possibilities vary according to the duration of fever. The current discussion is restricted to more common causes of fever and the list of causes is not

**BOX 1: Common causes of fever.**

- Infections—systemic
- Bacterial
- Viral
- Protozoal
- Fungal
- Localized
- NIID
- Autoimmune, rheumatic
- Autoinflammatory
- Granulomatous
- *Thermoregulatory disorders*: Cerebrovascular accident, brain tumor, hypothalamic dysfunction, hyperthyroididsm, pheochromocytoma
- *Miscellaneous*: Alcoholic liver disease, cirrhosis of liver, pulmonary embolism, aortic dissection, chronic active hepatitis, thyroiditis, chronic pancreatitis, ulcerative colitis, adrenal insufficiency, hemophagocytic syndrome, inherited disorders
- Neoplasms
- Hematological—lymphoma leukemia
- Solid tumors
- Benign tumors

(NIID: noninfectious inflammatory disease)

complete and takes into account possibilities to be considered in daily practice **(Box 1)**.

- *Systemic infections*: Viral, bacterial, rickettsial, protozoal, fungal
- *Localized infection*: Abscesses, empyema
- *Noninfectious immunological disorders*:
    - Systemic autoimmune diseases
    - Granulomatous diseases
    - Vasculitis
    - Autoinflammatory syndromes
- Neoplasms
- Thermoregulatory disorders
- Drug fever
- *Miscellaneous*:
    - Factitious fever/fraudulent fever—artificially induced by a person

# PATH TO DIAGNOSIS

## History Taking

History taking includes duration, type, and intensity of fever, chills, and rigors.

### *Duration of Fever*

*Acute fever*: <7 days—viral, bacterial, parasitic infections

*Acute undifferentiated fever*: Fever undiagnosed for up to 15 days; some prefer 21 days

*Pyrexia of unknown origin*: (1) Fever >38.3°C (101°F) on at least two occasions, (2) illness duration of ≥3 weeks, (3) no known immunocompromised state, and (4) diagnosis that remains uncertain after a thorough history-taking, physical examination, and certain obligatory investigations given below.

Duration of fever gives a clue about etiology as certain febrile illnesses do not exceed 15–20 days or may prove critical beyond that, e.g., dengue, scrub typhus, leptospirosis, chikungunya, and malaria.

### *Types of Fever*

*Intermittent fever*: The temperature which is already elevated touches the baseline in between in intermittent fever. The diurnal variation is extremely large, as occurs in septicemia. Quotidian fever is an intermittent fever occurring daily.

*Continuous fever*: The temperature remains elevated above normal without touching the baseline and fluctuation does not exceed 0.6°C/1°F, e.g., lobar pneumonia.

*Remittent fever*: Fever does not touch baseline, but fluctuation exceeds 1°F.

*Relapsing fever*:

*Quartan fever*: Occurs on the first and fourth day: *Plasmodium malariae*

*Tertian fever*: Occurs on the first and third day: *Plasmodium vivax*

*Saddleback fever*: Fever lasts for 2–3 days followed by a remission for 2 days and the fever reappears and continues for 2–3 days: Dengue fever.

*Pel–Ebstein fever*: Febrile period for 3–10 days and then afebrile period for 3–10 days. It is classically seen in Hodgkin's lymphoma. Borrelia infection and rat bite fever: Both are associated with several days of fever followed by several days of afebrile period.

*Intensity of fever*: Low-grade fever in tuberculosis (TB), brucellosis, pelvic inflammatory disease (PID), and lung abscess

High-grade fever in enteric, malaria, COVID, influenza, and dengue

*Associated history*:

- Rigor—malaria, urinary tract infection, abscess or pus anywhere, bacteremia
- Cough, respiratory distress, expectoration, and hemoptysis—localized respiratory infection, malignancy
- Abdominal pain—cholecystitis, urosepsis, PID abscess
- Jaundice, pale stool, right upper quadrant discomfort—cholangitis, hepatitis
- Headache, vomiting, convulsion—central nervous system (CNS) infection, acute encephalitic syndrome, space-occupying lesion (SOL)-like tuberculoma
- Tenesmus and loose stools, hematochezia—dysentery, inflammatory bowel disease (IBD)
- Chest pain, palpitation, and shortness of breath—myocarditis, endocarditis, pericarditis
- Gum bleeding and purpuric spots—dengue, Weil's disease, hematological malignancy, connective tissue disorder
- Skin rash and joint pain/swelling—connective tissue disorders, chikungunya, dengue
- Drug and addiction history
- Travel to an endemic area
- Sexual exposure
- History of psychiatric disorder—for fraudulent or fictitious fever

## Clinical Examination

Clinical examination is done to look for pallor, jaundice, cyanosis, clubbing, edema, lymphadenopathy, sternal tenderness, tenderness over temporal arteries, skin and mucosa, pulses, blood pressure, and respiratory rate.

It is preferable to have a syndromic approach to fever, which facilitates narrowing down the differential diagnosis according to the pattern of organ involvement.

- *Fever with rash*:
  - *Rash appearing on the first day of fever*: Varicella, vesicular type
  - *Rash appearing on the second day of fever*: Scarlet fever, maculopapular rash
  - *Rash appearing on the third day of fever*: Small pox, vesicular, pustular rash
  - *Rash appearing on the fourth day of fever*: Measles, maculopapular rash
  - *Rash appearing on the fifth day of fever*: Scrub typhus eschar, also macular rashes spreading to arms and legs
  - *Rash appearing on the sixth day of fever*: Dengue, confluent macular rash, generalized erythema with islands of skin sparing, more in trunk and face
  - *Rash appearing on the seventh day of fever*: Enteric fever—rose spots often not recognized in dark complexion
- *Fever with purpura*: Dengue, leptospirosis, malaria, leukemias
- *Fever with palpable purpura*: Systemic vasculitis, thrombotic thrombocytopenic purpura, Henoch–Schönlein purpura

## Systemic Examination

*Respiratory system*: Evidence of consolidation, collapse, and effusion—pneumonia, abscess, pulmonary TB, or malignancy

*Gastrointestinal system*: Hepatosplenomegaly or lump (lymph node mass)

*Cardiovascular system*: New murmur, S3 gallop—infective endocarditis, pericardial rub—pericarditis

*Genitourinary system*: Renal angle tenderness—pyelonephritis, hypogastric tenderness—cystitis

*Central nervous system*: Neck rigidity, papilledema, cranial nerve palsy, weakness of limbs—meningitis, meningoencephalitis

- *Fever with hepatosplenomegaly*:
  - *Infections*: Malaria, kala-azar, dengue, enteric fever, scrub typhus, leptospirosis, disseminated TB, brucellosis, infectious mononucleosis, histoplasmosis
  - *Hematological disorders*: Leukemia, lymphoma, systemic lupus erythematosus (SLE), adult-onset Still's disease (AOSD)
- *Fever with lymphadenopathy*:
  - Human immunodeficiency virus (HIV), infectious mononucleosis, cytomegalovirus (CMV) infection
  - Disseminated TB, brucellosis, secondary syphilis
  - Toxoplasmosis
  - Histoplasmosis coccidioidomycosis
  - Hematological disorders—leukemia, lymphoma
  - SLE, Sjögren's syndrome, rheumatoid arthritis (RA), sarcoidosis
- *Fever with hepatorenal syndromes*: Malaria, leptospirosis, expanded dengue, syndrome, sepsis with multiorgan dysfunction syndrome (MODS)
- *Fever with acute respiratory distress syndrome (ARDS)*: COVID-19, scrub typhus, malaria, dengue, leptospirosis
- *Fever with CNS dysfunction*: Acute encephalitis syndrome (AES), meningitis, acquired immunodeficiency syndrome (AIDS), malaria, dengue, Lyme disease, leptospirosis, neuropsychiatric SLE
- *Fever with arthritis*: SLE, RA, AOSD, temporal arteritis, polyarteritis nodosa (PAN), other vasculitides, dengue, chikungunya, Lyme disease

*Localized infections*: Accumulation of pus anywhere in the body at times may cause prolonged fever difficult to diagnose. In the age of imaging, hepatic abscess, perinephric abscess, appendicular abscess, intracranial, lung abscess, or empyema is easily suspected and diagnosed. However, maxillary/frontal sinus abscesses, prostatic abscesses, ischiorectal abscesses, and pyosalpinx or psoas abscesses are elusive. Thus, the importance of per rectal/per vaginal examination or palpation of sinuses must not be overlooked. Psoas abscesses (often tubercular) are sometimes diagnosed when pus tracks down to produce tender swellings in the groin.

*Drug fever* is characterized by prolonged fever with relative bradycardia and hypotension. It usually begins 1–3 weeks after the beginning of the drug and persists 2–3 days after the drug is withdrawn. It is seen more in the elderly and with polypharmacy. It may be associated with eosinophilia **(Box 2)**.

Once a *potential diagnostic clue (PDC)* has been decided upon from the clinical evaluation, relevant investigations are to be obtained in a focused way. The list given below is a battery of investigations from which the appropriate ones are to be chosen by your clinical acumen.

**BOX 2: Drug-induced fever.**

*Drugs causing fever*:
- Sulfonamide
- Penicillins
- Cephalosporins
- Anti-TB drugs
- Minocycline
- Methyldopa
- Hydralazine
- Hydrochlorothiazide
- Anticonvulsants
- Allopurinol
- Heparin
- Ibuprofen

*Vaccines causing fever*:
- Diphtheria, tetanus, and acellular pertussis (DTaP)
- Pneumococcal vaccine
- COVID vaccine

## Investigations

- Complete blood count with peripheral blood smear
- Erythrocyte sedimentation rate (ESR), C-reactive protein (CRP) level
- Total protein, alkaline phosphatase, alanine aminotransferase, aspartate aminotransferase
- Serum procalcitonin
- Malaria parasite dual antigen (MPDA), Dengue nonstructural protein 1 (NS1) antigen, immunoglobulin M (IgM) for scrub typhus (after fifth day), typhidot IgM, hepatitis profile, HIV serology
- Fasting blood glucose (FBG), postprandial blood glucose (PPBG), glycated hemoglobin (HbA1c)
- Lactate dehydrogenase, creatine kinase, ferritin
- Antinuclear antibodies, rheumatoid factor
- Protein electrophoresis, urinalysis, blood cultures ($n = 3$), urine culture
- Chest X-ray, abdominal ultrasonography, tuberculin skin test (TST)
- Computed tomography (CT)/magnetic resonance imaging (MRI) scan if required for better visualization

If at this juncture the diagnosis is still elusive, we have to go for a fluorodeoxyglucose positron emission tomography (FDG-PET) scan which can reveal hidden inflammatory or malignant foci from where a directed biopsy can be done for histopathology or culture as indicated.

Lymph node biopsy, liver biopsy, bone marrow aspiration, and biopsy from mass lesions if required.

*Infections without fever*: In certain situations, patients having an infection may present without fever.

Those conditions include patients on steroid therapy, chronic renal failure in different stages, and newborn and elderly patients.

# RED FLAG SIGNS

Seek immediate medical attention if any of the following signs or symptoms accompanies a fever:

- Severe headache, confusion, stiff neck, seizures
- Persistent vomiting, abdominal pain
- Difficulty breathing, cough or chest pain, palpitation
- Orthostatic hypotension and dizziness
- Diminished urine output
- Icterus or ascites
- Bleeding in skin, gum, or elsewhere

# THERAPY

Care for a fever depends on its severity. A fever requires adequate fluid intake and rest. Cold sponging and paracetamol are given as symptomatic treatment. Treatment of the cause is warranted.

# CLINICAL PEARLS

Common etiologies of acute undifferentiated fever in the Indian subcontinent are malaria, dengue, scrub typhus, chikungunya fever, enteric fever, bacteremia, and leptospirosis. The clinical association that may give clues are rash, lymphadenopathy, purpura, hypotension, organomegaly, hepatitis, encephalitis, oliguria, and ARDS.

A syndromic approach to the diagnosis of fever is helpful to pinpoint the PDC.

Drug fever is a reality and empiric therapy without diagnosis is to be avoided by all means.

# FURTHER READINGS

1. Kang JH. Febrile illness with skin rashes. Infect Chemother. 2015;47(3):155-66.
2. Antimicrobe. Approach to the patient with fever and rash. Infectious Disease and Antimicrobial Agents. Accessed June 23, 2022.

# PART 6

# Geriatrics

# CHAPTER 40

# Falls in Elderly

*Jyotirmoy Pal*

## INTRODUCTION

Globally, the number of people above the age of 60 years is growing very fast. In India, the number of people aged 60 years and above increased from 76 million in the year 2001 to 104 million in 2011 constituting 8% of the population. The number of older individuals will reach 2 billion forming 21.1% of the world population by 2050.

Globally, injury is the fifth leading cause of death among elderly persons (Rubenstein 2006, Myers et al.1996), of which most of the fatal injuries are related to falls. Falls are one of the four "geriatric syndromes" among the elderly. The others are delirium, urinary incontinence, and frailty (Inouye et al. 2007). Fall among the elderly is a significant health problem globally. Annually, 25–30% of elderly over 65 years living in the society sustain falls (Prudham & Evans 1981; Tinetti et al. 1988; Campbell et al. 1990; Blake et al.1988; WHO 2008). The frequency of falls rises with progressing age and frailty (WHO 2008). Due to the aging process, multiple functions, reactions, and coping mechanisms of the body deteriorate (Injuries among elderly n.d).

## WHAT IS FALL? IS IT SIMPLY AN AGING PHENOMENON OR SOME SERIOUS EVENT?

"A fall is defined as an event which results in a person coming to rest inadvertently on the ground or floor or other lower level" (WHO 2007). All types of falls result from physiological causes, pathological causes, or environmental causes.

### What is Recurrent Fall?

Falls of more than two episodes in 6 months are considered as recurrent falls. Recurrent fall is an issue of concern.

Two falls in the last 1 month are a red flag sign in the elderly and need urgent evaluation.

## CLASSIFICATION OF FALLS

Falls may be precipitated by extrinsic or intrinsic causes. Intrinsic factors are those of physiologic origin or host factors. Extrinsic factors are the environmental or related hazards or falls due to environmental factors or situational factors (Sattin 1992).

Falls are classified in different ways (Davies and Kenny in 1996):

- *Explained fall*: A simple slip, trip, or environmental hazard is the cause.
- *Unexplained fall*: There is no apparent cause of fall (Davies and Kenny 1996)
- *Recurrent fall*: It comprises three or more falls

## FACTORS FOR FALL

- Intrinsic factor
- Extrinsic factor
- Situational factor

### Intrinsic Factors

- *Sensory system*: Vision, vestibular apparatus, sensory system
- *Central nervous system*: Perfusion, attention, reflexes
- *Effector system*: Muscle strength, joint flexibility

#### *Sensory System*

- *Vision*: Decreased acuity, field of vision, macular degeneration
- *Vestibular apparatus*: Benign paroxysmal positional vertigo, Meniere's disease
- *Sensory system*: Peripheral neuropathy

#### *Central Processing*

- *Perfusion*: Orthostatic hypotension, reduced cerebral perfusion
- *Reduced attention*: Acute illness, metabolic abnormality and toxicity, dementia
- *Altered reflexes*: Parkinsonism disease, pyramidal and extrapyramidal disease
- *Psychomotor slowing*: Dementia, medication

#### *Effector System*

*Effector organ*: Muscle strength, assessment of sarcopenia, gait speed, joint, cachexia, osteoarthritis (OA), sarcopenia, foot abnormality

### Extrinsic and Situational Factors

- *Extrinsic factors*: Uneven surface, poor lighting, low-set chair, chair without arm, improper stair, etc.
- *Situational factors*: Walking on slippery surface, walking in darkness, across an obstacle, etc.

## WHAT ARE BALANCE AND GAIT TEST?

- Berg balance test (BBT)
- Performance-oriented mobility assessment (POMA)
- Dynamic gait index (DGI)
- Timed up and go (TUG) test
- Gait speed
- Single-limb stance test
- Functional reach
- *Frailty and injuries*: Cooperative studies of intervention techniques (FICSIT)-4 test
- Four-square step test
- *Static and dynamic balance*:
    - *Dynamic balance*: Dynamic gait index, four-square step test, TUG
    - *Static and dynamic*: POMA, BBT
    - *Static*: Functional reach, single-limb stance, FICSIT-4

### Berg Balance Test

The BBT is a gold standard test for both static and dynamic balance.

The Berg balance scale evaluates the patient's performance on 14 tasks which are common in daily activities. These tasks address the patient's ability to maintain positions of increasing difficulty. Scoring is on a five-point ordinal scale (0—unable to 4—independent). Maximum score to be achieved is 56.

This test takes about 15 minutes to complete and is a sensitive measure as it is able to discriminate between patients with various mobility aids (Berg et al., 1992).

***Components***

- Sitting to standing
- Standing unsupported
- Sitting unsupported
- Standing to sitting
- Transfers
- Standing with eyes closed
- Standing with feet together
- Reaching forward with outstretched arm
- Picking an object from the floor
- Turning to look behind
- Turning 360°
- Placing an alternate foot on the stool
- Standing with one foot in front
- Standing on one foot

*Low risk*: 41–56; medium risk: 21–40; high risk: <20

## Performance-oriented Mobility Assessment

- Designated for elderly persons
- Consist of nine balance items and seven gait items
- Scoring on ordinal scale of 0–2 (0—most impairment, 2—independent)
- Maximum score 28 (balance—16, gait—12)
- Score 19–24, moderate risk; score <19, high risk of fall

Tinetti and Ginter 1988.

## Dynamic Gait Index

The DGI was developed to examine the ability of patients to maintain functional balance during the performance of activities during gait (Shumway-Cook et al., 1997). The DGI integrates rotational head movements (up and down and from side to side) into gait testing. Therefore, the DGI is a very informative test in people with vestibular disorders (Wrisley et al., 2003). The rotational head movements utilized during the test can help to point to specific impairments and potential interventions in people with vestibular disorders. It is a very good predictor of fall in elderly. This test has excellent intrarater, inter-rater, and test-retest reliability. Whitney et al 2000.

***Components***

- Gait at level
- Change in gait speed
- Gait with turning head (R/L)
- Gait with vertical head turn
- Gait-turn-stop
- Step over obstacle
- Step across multiple obstacles
- Step up a stair and come down

  Total score = 24

  A score < 19 signifies the risk of fall.

## Gait Speed: Sixth Vital Sign

Gait speed deterioration is one of the most important indicators of decay in functional ability, with the risk of developing frailty, and later disability. The gait speed is used to measure a person's frailty level.

Gait speed is typically measured by health professionals in hospital or daycare settings, by manually measuring the time the patient takes to walk between two stripes situated on the floor at different distances, depending on the tool used. In the case of the classical short physical performance battery (SPPB) test, the distance is 4 m, but for Fried's criteria, this distance is 4.3 m. Healthcare professionals use a manual chronometer, which has a risk of inaccuracy and discrepancy between different professionals and different sets of measurements (inter- and intraobserver variability).

## Four-square Step Test

The four-square step test is a reliable and valid test to perform multidirectional movement in people with balance disorder.

*Equipment*:

- Stopwatch
- Four canes (laid in a cross pattern)
- Gait belt

*Sequence*:

- Start by standing in square 1, facing square 2 (imagine that direction is facing "north").
- Begin in a clockwise direction, i.e., 2-3-4-1; then immediately move counterclockwise, i.e., to squares 4-3-2-1.

*Instructions*: "Try to complete the sequence as fast as possible without touching the sticks. Both feet must make contact with the floor in each square. If possible, face forward ('north') during the entire sequence."

- Demonstrate
- Allow a practice trial
- Two trials—the best time (in seconds) is taken as the score.
- *Repeat a trial if the subject*:
  - Fails to complete the sequence successfully
  - Loses balance
  - Makes contact with the cane

Subjects who were unable to face forward during the entire sequence and needed to turn before stepping into the next square were still given a score.

*Scoring*: Time in seconds.
*Note*: The stopwatch starts when the first foot contacts the floor in square 2.

"Cutoff score of 15 seconds was identified. Subjects with scores of >15 seconds were considered as multiple fallers and those with scores <15 as non multiple fallers. At 15 seconds, the FSST has a positive predictive value of 86% and a negative predictive value of 94% for the sample tested." (Dite, 2002).

## Timed Up and Go Test

The TUG test is a useful test for dynamic balance. It is easy to perform and is a clinic-based test.

### Intended Population

This test was initially designed for elderly persons but is used for other populations, e.g., those with Parkinson's disease (PD). This tool is validated for a population with PD, multiple sclerosis, hip fracture, Alzheimer's disaese, cerebrovascular accident (CVA), total knee replacement (TKR) or total hip replacement (THR), and Huntington's disease.

It is one of the four tests used in the Balance Outcome Measure for Elder Rehabilitation (BOOMER).

### Materials Needed

- One chair with armrest
- Stopwatch
- Tape (to mark 3 m)

### Method

- The patient wears his regular footwear and can use a walking aid if needed.
- He starts in a seated position.
- He stands up upon the therapist's command, walks 3 m, turns around, walks back to the chair, and sits down.
- The time stops when the patient is seated.
- Be sure to document the assistive device used.

*Note*: A practice trial should be done before the timed trial.

### Observations

Observe the patient's postural stability, gait, stride length, and sway.

- *Note all that apply*: Slow tentative pace, loss of balance, short strides, little or no arm swing, steadying self on walls, shuffling, en bloc turning, not using assistive device properly.
- These changes may signify neurological problems that require further evaluation.

### Cutoff Time for High Risk of Falls

An older adult who takes ≥12 seconds to complete the TUG is at risk for falling.

Cutoff scores indicating risk of falls by population (in seconds) are as follows:

- Community-dwelling adults: 13.5
- Older stroke patients: 14
- Frail elderly: 32.6
- Lower extremity (LE) amputees: 19
- PD: 11.5

- Hip OA: 10
- Vestibular disorders: 11.1

Cutoff times to classify subjects as high risk for falling vary based on the study and participants.

### Interpretations

- TUG (alone): Cutoff 13.5 seconds
- TUG (manual): Cutoff 14.5 seconds
- TUG (cognitive): Cutoff 15.5 seconds

Predictive value > 90%
Shumway-cook, Brawer S, woolacoot M Physical Therapy 2000 80 (9).

## Functional Reach Test

Functional reach test (FRT) is used for testing standing balance.

- In standing, we measure the distance between the length of an outstretched arm in a maximal forward reach while maintaining a fixed base of support. This information is correlated with the risk of falling.
- *Measurement interpretation*:
  - *10"/25 cm or greater*: Low risk of falls
  - *6"/15 to 10"/25 cm*: Risk of falling is two times greater than normal.
  - *6"/15 cm or less*: Risk of falling is four times greater than normal.
  - *Unwilling to reach*: Risk of falling is eight times greater than normal.
- A number of factors exert a major influence on this evaluation: Research revealed that both the movement strategy and reduced spinal flexibility affect the reach distance.

### Intended Population

- FRT was made to predict fall risk in the elderly and frail adult.
- It is one of the four tests used in BOOMER.

### Method of Use

- The patient is instructed to stand next to, but not touching, a wall and position the arm that is closer to the wall at 90° of shoulder flexion with a closed fist.
- The assessor records the starting position at the third metacarpal head on the yardstick.
- Instruct the patient to "Reach as far as you can forward without taking a step."
- The location of the third metacarpal is recorded.
- Scores are determined by assessing the difference between the start and end position which is the reach distance, usually measured in inches.
- Three trials are done and the average of the last two is noted.

### Criteria to Stop the Test

- The patient's feet lifted up from the floor or they fell forward. Most patients fall forward with this test. The therapist should guard from the front as that is the direction that you reach forward.
- Reduced ability to reach has shown increases in future falls with odds ratios of 8.2 if unable to reach at all and 4 if able to reach <15.2 cm.

### Interpretation

- *Eyes open*: 60–69 years: 22.5 ± 8.6 seconds; 70–80 years: 14.2 ± 9.3 seconds
- *Eyes closed*: 60–69 years: 10.2 ± 8.6 seconds; 70–80 years: 4.3 ± 3.0 seconds
- If <5 seconds, the chance of fall and injury is high.

## Prevention and Control of Falls

In a community setting, falls happen frequently, are of high risk, and are cost-intensive (Hester & Wei 2013). With the available evidence, there is an urgent need for prevention programs that address the multiple risk factors of falls among older persons at different levels with an interdisciplinary approach. Fall being a complex event caused by interaction between intrinsic and extrinsic factors, the interventions need to be specific and multidimensional.

As the risk factors are multiple and of different categories, different strategies are warranted for controlling the different risk factors. Prevention and control of comorbidities is one strategy to prevent falls among older persons. Surgical correction of cataract, physical rehabilitation for improving muscle strength, and removing or altering some hazardous features of housing, like removing the door thresholds and eliminating different levels within the house, can reduce the risk of falls. Providing better lighting, fixing railing for stairs, and grab bars inside the toilets and walkways are some of the protective measures for the prevention of falls as mentioned in different studies. Safety equipment such as hip protectors and associated devices such as antiskid mats are also useful in preventing falls.

A randomized trial from Finland showed a risk reduction of fractures by over 60% in 72–74-year-old women with impact exercise (jumping and balance training) for 30 months (Kannus et al. 2005(b)). According to Fairhall, a 12-month multifactorial intervention provided by an interdisciplinary team tailored to each participant could reduce the risk factor for falls with marked progress in mobility, strength, and balance measures (Fairhall 2013).

Physical activity promotion was found effective in reducing falls when implemented alone or as part of multifactorial intervention (Rubenstein & Johnson 2006). According to a review of the interventions by Rubenstein and Johnson, interventions including modification of the house alone did not reduce falls but multifactorial interventions with modification of the house definitely reduced falls (Rubenstein & Josephson 2006). A study which evaluated the effect of an exercise-related fall-prevention program concluded that screening to identify individuals at high risk for falls would be necessary for a successful fall-prevention program. Further research to identify the most accurate, yet easy-to-use, risk assessment instrument would be necessary to move these efforts forward (Hester & Wei 2013).

## Intervention Strategies

*Fall prevention*: Single-intervention strategies

These include studies where only one type of intervention is given to all the participants in the intervention group. Several studies have tried different strategies.

### *Home Hazard Assessment and Modification*

Assessment of home hazards and modification that is professionally prescribed for elderly people with a history of falling may reduce the risk of falling by one-third (Jensen et al. 2002). Environmental hazards in common areas were reduced by rearranging furniture that cause a risk for falling, quickly wiping wet areas on the floor, and clearing snow from the entrance to the facility (Jensen et al. 2002). Adjustments were made in the residents' accommodations such as removal of loose carpets and repair of doorsteps, provision of grip bars, new beds, firm mattresses, furniture changes, and improved lighting in the bedroom and bathroom (WHO 2004).

### *Feet and Footwear Review*

It is suggested to advise older people to wear shoes with a thinner and harder sole to optimize foot position (Menant et al. 2008). To further prevent slips, they should be advised to wear shoes with tread sole and a treaded beveled heel (Menant et al. 2008).

### *Promoting Physical Activity and Balance Training*

In a review of randomized control trials, it was found that physical activity and balance training reduced the risk of falls and fall-related injuries among older people. Studies have confirmed that strength and balance training can reduce the risk of both injurious and noninjurious falls by 15–50% among the older adults in the community in a cost-effective way (Carter et al. 2001; Gillespie et al. 2012; Tinetti 2003; Kannus et al. 2005(b)).

Personalized as well as group exercise programs were found to be effective in the prevention of falls, especially programs targeted to improve balance (Kannus et al. 2005(b)). The different interventions that can be included under this group are gait, balance, and functional training, strength and resistance training, tai chi, square stepping, and general physical activity training (Gillespie et al. 2012). The programs for strength and balance training can improve many risk factors of falling such as muscle strength, flexibility, balance, coordination, proprioception, reaction time, and gait even in very old and frail people (Kannus et al. 2005 (b); Li et al. 2013, Low 2008).

### *Vitamin D and Calcium*

A 50% reduction in the risk of falling was noticed in a randomized controlled trial of elderly women with vitamin D supplementation along with calcium for 12 weeks due to improvement in muscle strength and dynamic musculoskeletal performance (Bischoff et al. 2003; Kannus et al. 2005(b)). It is a single intervention technique which is found to be effective in a community setting (WHO 2007). Apart from the role in calcium and bone absorption, vitamin D has an important role in improving musculoskeletal performance (Kannus et al. 2005(b)).

### *Medication Review*

Use of fall-related drugs like neuroleptics, benzodiazepines, tricyclic antidepressants, selective serotonin reuptake inhibitor (SSRI) antidepressants, and cortisone increases the risk of falling. A randomized trial shows 66% of risk reduction with gradual withdrawal of psychotropic drugs (Kannus et al. 2005(b); Hill & Wee 2012).

### *Expedited Cataract Surgery*

Speeding cataract surgery in patients waiting for surgery has reduced the rate of falling by 34% when compared to those waiting for surgery (Harwood et al. 2005). The pooled data from a systematic review by Desapriya found that there is a seven times increase in visual acuity after expedited cataract surgery when compared to routine cataract surgery (Desapriya et al. 2010).

### *Cardiac Pacing*

Patients suffering from cardioinhibitory carotid sinus hypersensitivity may develop hypotension, bradycardia, paroxysmal asystole, syncope, and subsequent falls. According to Kenny et al., there was almost a two-thirds reduction in the percent of falls and a 70% reduction in injuries following falls among those who underwent cardiac pacing (Kenny 2001).

### *Cognitive or Behavioral Interventions*

Cognitive and behavioral interventions were given as a part of complex interventions and a few studies concentrated on cognitive or behavioral interventions alone which included risk assessments and counseling and a fall prevention education program.

Effectiveness when used alone is unknown but useful if used along with complex interventions (NICE guidelines 2013).

### *Multiple-intervention Strategies*

More than one main type of intervention is implemented in multiple intervention strategies (Gillespie et al. 2012). The potential risk factors of all the participants are assessed independently and they are assigned different strategies of intervention based on the risk factor assessment (Gillespie et al. 2012). Multiple intervention strategies can prevent falls in elderly adults by 20–45% by controlling intrinsic and extrinsic risk factors (Kannus et al. 2005(b); Gillespie et al. 2012; American Geriatric Society et al. 2001; Tinetti et al. 1994). Multiple intervention strategies include components such as strength, balance, and gait training, improving transferring and ambulation with or without the use of aids, footwear improvements, investigation and management of untreated medical problems, medication review and adjustment, vision tests and correction, hip protectors, patient and staff education about fall prevention, fall risk alert cards, postfall assessments, and environmental and home risk assessment and management.

### *Protection of Susceptible Sites*

Frail older people are particularly at risk of falling when getting out of bed. The common cause of hip fracture is a sideways fall with a direct impact on the greater trochanter Kannus (2005(b). Hence, a specially designed device, hip protector, was developed to protect the hips, so that the force and energy of the impact are attenuated and diverted away from the greater trochanter. The safe hip protector developed by Lauritzen and colleagues has been found to be effective in preventing fractures (Lauritzen 1993). A disadvantage of hip protectors is that they only work when worn. The compliance is doubtful as they may be uncomfortable.

## CONCLUSION

Falls should not be viewed as an inevitable part of life but can be a manifestation of serious underline illness.

## CLINICAL PEARLS

- Two falls in last one month in an elderly person needs urgent evaluation
- Falls may be due to intrinsic, extrinsic and situational factors
- Multipronged and multidisciplinary approach to management is required.

## FURTHER READINGS

1. Bánhidy F, Acs N, Horvath-Puhó E, Czeizel AE. Maternal severe migraine and risk of congenital limb deficiencies. Birth Defects Res A Clin Mol Teratol. 2006;76(8):592-601.
2. Chen HM, Chen SF, Chen YH, Lin HC. Increased risk of adverse pregnancy outcomes for women with migraines: a nationwide population-based study. Cephalalgia. 2010;30(4):433-8.
3. Olesen C, Steffensen FH, Sorensen HT, Nielsen GL, Olsen J. Pregnancy outcome following prescription for sumatriptan. Headache. 2000;40(1):20-4.
4. Bánhidy F, Acs N, Horvath-Puho E, Czeizel AE. Pregnancy complications and delivery outcomes in pregnant women with severe migraine. Eur J Obstet Gynecol Reprod Biol. 2007;134(2):157-63.
5. Mogren IM, Pohjanen AI. Low back pain and pelvic pain during pregnancy: prevalence and risk factors. Spine. 2005;30(8):983-91.
6. Ostgaard HC, Andersson GB, Karlsson K. Prevalence of back pain in pregnancy. Spine. 1991;16:549-52.
7. Stapleton DB, MacLennan AH, Kristiansson P. The prevalence of recalled low back pain during and after pregnancy: a South Australian population survey. Aust N Z J Obstet Gynaecol. 2002;42(5):482-5.
8. Ostgaard HC, Andersson GB. Previous back pain and risk of developing back pain in a future pregnancy. Spine (Phila Pa 1976). 1991;16:432-6.
9. Mens JMA, Vleeming A, Stoeckart R, Stam HJ, Snijders CJ. Understanding peripartum pelvic pain. Implications of a patient survey. Spine (Phila Pa 1976). 1996;21(11):1363-70.
10. Mogren IM. Previous physical activity decreases the risk of low back pain and pelvic pain during pregnancy. Scand J Public Health. 2005;33(4):300-6.
11. Kristiansson P, Svärdsudd K, von Schoultz B. Back pain during pregnancy. Spine (Phila Pa 1976). 1996;21:702-9.
12. Sandler SE. The management of low back pain in pregnancy. Manual Ther. 1996;1:178-85.
13. Botsford DJ, Esses SI, Oglivie-Harris DJ. In vivo diurnal variation in intervertebral disc volume and morphology. Spine (Phila Pa 1976). 1994;19:935-40.
14. Rodacki CL, Fowler NE, Rodacki AL, Birch K. Stature loss and recovery in pregnant women with and without low back pain. Arch Phys Med Rehab. 2003;84(4):507-12.

15. Dumas GA, Reid JG, Wolfe LA, Griffin MP, McGrath MJ. Exercise, posture, and back pain during pregnancy: part 1. Exercise and back pain. Clin Biomech. 1995;10(2):104-9.
16. MacLennan AH, Nicolson R, Green RC, Bath M. Serum relaxin and pelvic pain of pregnancy. Lancet. 1986;2:243-5.
17. Harden CL, Meador KJ, Pennell PB, Hauser WA, Gronseth GS, French JA, et al. Management issues for women with epilepsy—focus on pregnancy (an evidence-based review): II. Teratogenesis and perinatal outcomes: report of the Quality Standards Subcommittee and Therapeutics and Technology Subcommittee of the American Academy of Neurology and the American Epilepsy Society. Epilepsia. 2009;50:1237-4.
18. Binks S, Vincent A, Palace J. Myasthenia gravis: a clinical-immunological update. J Neurol. 2016;263:826-34.
19. Roth CK, Dent S, McDevitt K. Myasthenia gravis in pregnancy. Nurs Womens Health. 2015;19(3):248-52.
20. Kalidindi M, Ganpot S, Tahmesebi F, Govind A, Okolo S, Yoong W. Myasthenia gravis and pregnancy. J Obstet Gynaecol. 2007;27(1):30-2.

CHAPTER 41

# Incontinence of Urine

*Jasprabh Karanjit Kaur, Ritu Attri, Saumya Singh, Ashish Goel*

## INTRODUCTION

". . . a patch of urine cannot be readily explained. Its treatment has proved beyond most of us, and as to its significance, it will make the difference between social acceptance and rejection with all that involves in prolonged hospital care and expense."

—*"Old Folks in Wet Beds," British Medical Journal, 1962.*

The above words by JL Newman, said 60 years ago, resonate today with the problem of urinary incontinence (UI) among the elderly. UI remains a major problem in the care of the elderly, with millions of them affected throughout the world. This problem has substantial impact on a person's well-being, on the ability of family or friends to cope with an old person, and on the costs of health care for this population.

Urinary incontinence is one of the priority health issues recognized by the World Health Organization (WHO). It is seen more in elderly females than males. At age above 65 years, approximately one in three women and 15–20% of men have UI in varying degrees. A prevalence of 60–80% is seen in nursing homes. Most of the elderly patients present with stress incontinence followed by mixed and urge incontinence. The causes of UI are heterogeneous, with availability of a dearth of research on its mechanism and management. Knowledge of basic principles on etiology, diagnosis, and treatment can help cope with the burden of this problem.

## DEFINITION

Urinary incontinence is defined by the International Continence Society as "a condition in which the involuntary loss of urine is objectively demonstrable and is a social and hygiene problem."

## PRESENTATION AND THE SYMPTOMS

Most patients experience occasional minor leaks, while others present with small to moderate amounts.

### Risk Factors

- *Age*: Elderly population
- *Gender*: Females more commonly involved, especially post-menopausal
- Obesity
- *Medical disorders*: Diabetes mellitus, hypertension, stroke, Parkinson's disease, acute and chronic pain
- *Psychological conditions*: Depression, delirium, impaired cognition

- *Obstetric and gynecological conditions*: History of difficult childbirth, pelvic surgery, hysterectomy, pelvic floor dysfunction, pelvic organ prolapse
- *Drugs*: Diuretics, psychotropics, narcotics
- *Substance abuse*: Alcohol, smoking, caffeine

## TYPES OF URINARY INCONTINENCE

### Stress Urinary Incontinence

In this type of UI, leakage of small amounts of urine occurs with increases in intra-abdominal pressure. The underlying pathology is usually prolapse of pelvic structures in women, sphincter damage, or uninhibited bladder contractions.

### Urge Incontinence

Urge incontinence presents with leakage of urine due to the inability to delay voiding long enough to reach the toilet after the urge to void is perceived. The underlying pathology is uninhibited bladder contractions, associated especially with central nervous system diseases such as stroke, dementia, Parkinson's disease, multiple sclerosis, prostatic obstruction, and post-prostatectomy.

### Overflow Incontinence

Patients present with the leakage of small amounts of urine without the urge to void. Etiology of this type of incontinence is anatomic obstruction as seen in patients with benign prostatic hyperplasia (BPH) and urethral strictures, patients with hypotonic bladder with underlying conditions such as diabetes, syphilis, spinal cord compression, and elderly patients on anticholinergic drugs.

### Functional Incontinence

A physical or mental impairment keeps the patient from making it to the toilet in time, e.g., in patients of severe arthritis.

### Total Urinary Incontinence

There is complete lack of control over voiding with underlying sphincter damage, nerve damage (peripheral or spinal cord injury), or in patients with severe dementia.

## MAJOR TYPES OF URINARY INCONTINENCE, PATHOLOGY, AND PRESENTATION

The causes of UI are listed in **Box 1**.

**BOX 1: Causes of urinary incontinence.**

- *General causes of incontinence*:
  - Urological
  - Neurological
  - Locomotor
  - Psychological
- *Causes of transient incontinence, reversible after managing the underlying illness*:
  - Urinary tract infection
  - Acute illness, especially when accompanied by:
    - Fatigue
    - Hospital admission
    - Immobilization
    - Confusion
- *Retention with overflow incontinence*:
  - Fecal impaction
  - Anticholinergic drugs
  - Spinal cord compression
  - Drugs affecting the autonomic nervous system
  - Sedatives and tranquilizers
- *Psychological*:
  - Depression
  - Hostility
- *Causes of established incontinence*:
  - Surgeries involving pelvic structures causing damage to sphincters or pelvic innervation
- *Diseases of the cerebral cortex*:
  - Stroke
  - Dementia
  - Parkinson's disease

Continued

*Continued*

- *Diseases of the spinal cord*:
    - Compression by tumor, spondylosis, herniated disc
    - Trauma
    - Demyelination
- *Retention with overflow*:
    - Atonic bladder due to diabetes, alcoholism
    - Prostatic obstruction
    - Urethral stricture
- *Diseases of the bladder*:
    - Chronic cystitis
    - Carcinoma
    - Calculi
    - Uninhibited bladder
- *Stress incontinence*:
    - Associated with increase in intra-abdominal pressure
    - Sneezing, coughing, lifting weights, etc.

## SOCIAL IMPLICATIONS AND THE ASSOCIATED AGEISM

Incontinence of urine is a treatable condition in which the patient continues to suffer psychologically, socially, and physically. It can happen to anyone; however, it is more common in certain groups and at certain stages of life. It is seen more among women and is often related to pregnancy, childbirth, pelvic surgeries, and menopause. Each of these experiences can cause a woman's pelvic support muscles to weaken over time. Many elderly women do not perceive UI as a problem worthy of attention. The reason may lie in its social and cultural construction. The social construction is rooted in the collectivist nature of culture, which makes UI a family problem rather than an individual problem. If incontinence is not managed well, the person with incontinence may experience feelings of rejection, anxiety, frustration, anger, depression, social isolation, dependency, and loss of control.

Because passing urine or feces is regarded as a very private and personal activity in most societies, many people are prone to feeling embarrassed about any accidental leaks and the smell associated with incontinence. As a result, it is understandable that many people with incontinence and their caregivers might become very anxious when thinking about or planning social activities. It is common for people experiencing anxiety to try to avoid the situation they fear the most. They may try to reduce their anxiety by avoiding social activities such as shopping, going out, or having friends over. It is also common for people experiencing incontinence to try to manage their problem by reducing the amount or type of food they eat or fluid they drink. They learn to hide their problem from close friends, family, and even significant others for years. They feel shy to discuss their problem with doctors. Slowly, their isolation and shame may lead to depression and anxiety.

Depression created by personal perception of cognition, negative events, and physiological states may be experienced by patients with UI. Depression occurs when one feels a perceived inefficacy in controlling valued outcomes. This perception impacts the choice of activities one chooses to engage in and the effort and persistence one is willing to invest in the activity.

A person who is incontinent may show their frustration when they are unable to master the incontinence or some aspect of their care or treatment. A key to helping someone who is angry is to listen while you explore the needs that are unmet. Lack of sleep due to frequent toileting at night or from some other reason such as stress, pain, or depression is likely to exhaust the person and their caretakers too. Irritability, impatience, and reduced tolerance can result and place severe strain on the health and relationships of both parties.

Incontinence presents a significant financial burden to the individual and to society. The expenses include costs for things such as absorbent products, medications, doctor visits, and dry cleaning or laundry. Unfortunately, incontinence gets worse with time if left untreated, and costs only go up with the age. Health care costs are classified as direct or indirect. Direct costs are those for delivering treatment and include physician and other health care provider fees, hospital fees, and transportation costs for the purposes of obtaining health care. Indirect costs are those to the individual and ultimately to society from work absenteeism, impaired performance while at work, and changes in job status due to health. It is not just the direct costs that contribute to the financial stress of incontinence. Up to 23% of women take time off work due to incontinence. Thus, the compromised quality of life (QOL) contributes to psychological, physical, and financial burden for both the patients and caregivers.

## APPROACH TO DIAGNOSIS

Urinary incontinence can be classified according to the predominant symptom at presentation by a questionnaire. After categorization, further steps in management vary accordingly.

## RED FLAG SIGNS IN CONDITION

- Associated pain
- Persistent hematuria or proteinuria
- Significant pelvic organ prolapse
- Previous pelvic surgery or radiation
- Suspected fistula
- Elevated postvoid residual

## THERAPY AND MANAGEMENT

A step-wise approach to treatment is directed at the UI category, initiating with conservative management, stepping forward to physical devices and medications, and at last, referring for surgical intervention. First-line treatment with surgical intervention can be considered after appropriate counseling if the patient prefers a surgical approach or if medications are contraindicated. Concurrent behavior and pharmacologic therapy are more effective than pharmacologic therapy alone.

### Conservative Management

Although there is low-quality evidence to suggest that lifestyle interventions improve UI, these interventions are inexpensive and have meager risk of side effects. It is reasonable for physicians to counsel patients on appropriate fluid intake, timed voiding, reduction of caffeinated and carbonated beverages, smoking cessation, regular moderate physical activity, and weight loss in overweight or obese patients. Aggressive fluid restriction should be avoided as there are potential adverse effects of headaches, constipation, and thirst. Optimized prescription of medications and management of comorbidities, especially in geriatric patients, may reverse transient UI or improve chronic UI. Pelvic floor muscle strengthening exercises, such as Kegel exercises, are the mainstay of behavior therapy for stress UI, with cure rates varying from 29 to 59%.

### Stress Urinary Incontinence

No medications are approved by the United States Food and Drug Administration (FDA) for the treatment of stress UI. The American College of Physicians recommends against systemic pharmacotherapy. Alpha-adrenergic agonists (e.g., pseudoephedrine, phenylephrine) have previously been prescribed as an adjunct therapy because they act on receptors in the proximal urethra and bladder neck. Significant adverse effects include palpitations and headache. Behavior therapy has significantly improved outcomes when compared with alpha agonists, and alpha agonists are no longer recommended for stress UI. Mechanical devices for stress UI management include vaginal inserts (cones, pessaries) and urethral plugs. These devices frequently require intravaginal estrogen before use and are most often discontinued because of poor fit; however, they may be effective in patients with predictable, episodic symptoms (e.g., during exercise, pregnancy), in nonsurgical candidates, or in those awaiting surgery. Up to one-third of patients who use urethral plugs develop urinary tract infections in a 2-year period, but patient satisfaction remains high with this device. Urologic surgery for stress UI includes sling procedures and urethropexy to support urethral constriction or to stabilize the bladder neck and urethra.

### Urge Urinary Incontinence

Antimuscarinics and beta-adrenergic agonists are FDA-approved oral medications for urge UI. Antimuscarinics prevent recurrent spasm of the detrusor muscle, but side effects include tachycardia, edema, confusion, constipation, and blurry vision. Selective antimuscarinic agents (darifenacin, solifenacin) are preferred over nonselective agents (oxybutynin, tolterodine) to reduce cognitive side effects. Antimuscarinics are not recommended as first-line pharmacotherapy in the elderly. Mirabegron is a beta-adrenergic agonist that relaxes the detrusor muscle via beta-3 receptors. Adverse effects include gastrointestinal upset, dizziness, headache, and increased blood pressure. If used with antimuscarinics, it increases the risk of urinary retention. Intravaginal estrogen may improve urge UI symptoms but is not approved by the FDA for this indication; systemic estrogen exacerbates incontinence. Percutaneous tibial nerve stimulation requires weekly procedures for the initial 3 months and subsequent monthly maintenance treatments. It has similar effectiveness to antimuscarinic medications. Intravesical onabotulinum toxin A (Botox) injection delivered via cystoscopy is approved by the FDA and results in flaccid paralysis of the detrusor muscle; studies show consistent improvement in UI and QOL. The procedure can be repeated every 6 months as symptoms recur. Sacral, pudendal, and paraurethral nerve stimulators can be surgically implanted; 60–90% of patients with sacral neuromodulators report improvement in symptoms. These devices are expensive and are indicated only for patients with refractory symptoms because of the risk of surgical complications.

### Mixed, Overflow, and Functional Urinary Incontinence

Management of mixed UI should be directed toward treating the predominant symptoms. Reversible causes of overflow UI should be identified. Intermittent or indwelling catheterization is often required if the etiology is irreversible (e.g., neurologic dysfunction because of stroke). Behavior therapies, such as assisted and timed toileting, are the primary treatment for functional incontinence.

## CLINICAL PEARLS

- Urinary incontinence is a major problem in the care of the elderly, affecting their QOL.
- It is more prevalent in elderly females and is underreported and inadequately treated.
- Stress UI is the more common form of UI.
- Red flag signs in the condition need timely recognition and referral.

Lifestyle modifications, behavior therapies, mechanical devices, and pharmacological therapy are the cornerstones to the management of UI.

## FURTHER READINGS

1. Ouslander JG. Urinary incontinence in the elderly. West J Med. 1981;135:482-91.
2. Loscalzo J, Fauci A, Kasper D, Hauser S, Longo D, Jameson J (Eds). Harrison's Principles of Internal Medicine, 21st edition. New York: McGraw Hill; 2022.
3. Charpot V, Sagar V. Prevalence of urinary incontinence among young healthy females in Gujarat—a cross-sectional study. Int J Health Sci Res. 2021;11(6):100-6.
4. Agarwal BK, Agarwal N. Urinary incontinence: prevalence, risk factors, impact on quality of life and treatment seeking behaviour among middle aged women. Int Surg J. 2017;4(6): 1953-8.
5. Abrams P, Cardozo L, Fall M, Griffiths D, Rosier P, Ulmsten U, et al. The standardisation of terminology in lower urinary tract function: report from the standardisation sub-committee of the International Continence Society. Urology. 2003;61(1):37-49.
6. Loh KY, Sivalingam N. Urinary incontinence in the elderly population. Med J Malaysia. 2006;61(4):506-10.
7. Broome BAS. The impact of urinary incontinence on self-efficacy and quality of life. Health Qual Life Outcomes. 2003;1:35.
8. Kang Y, Crogan NL. Social and cultural construction of urinary incontinence among Korean American elderly women. Geriatr Nurs. 2008;29(2):105-11.
9. Park GR, Park S, Kim J. Urinary incontinence and depressive symptoms: the mediating role of physical activity and social engagement. J Gerontol B Psychol Sci Soc Sci. 2022;77(7): 1250-8.
10. Bradley CS, Kennedy CM, Nygaard IE. Pelvic floor symptoms and lifestyle factors in older women. J Womens Health (Larchmt). 2005;14(2):128-36.
11. National Association for Continence. (2002). National Stress Urinary Incontinence Survey. Unpublished Study. Charleston, SC: Author.
12. Bandura A. Self-efficacy mechanisms in human agency. Am Psychol. 1982;37:122-47.
13. Marschall-Kehrel D. Update on nocturia: the best of rest is sleep. Urology. 2004;64:21-4.
14. Miner Jr PB. Economic and personal impact of fecal and urinary incontinence. Gastroenterology. 2004;126(1 Suppl. 1):S8-13.
15. Sinclair AJ, Ramsay IN. The psychosocial impact of urinary incontinence in women. Obstet Gynaecol. 2011;13:143-8.
16. Brown JS, Bradley CS, Subak LL, Richter HE, Kraus SR, Brubaker L, et al. The sensitivity and specificity of a simple test to distinguish between urge and stress urinary incontinence. Ann Intern Med. 2006;144(10):716.
17. Khandelwal C, Kistler C. Diagnosis of urinary incontinence. Am Fam Physician. 2013;87(8):543-50.
18. Hu JS, Pierre EF. Urinary incontinence in women: evaluation and management. Am Fam Physician. 2019;100(6):339-48.
19. Rovner ES, Wein AJ. Treatment options for stress urinary incontinence. Rev Urol. 2004;6(Suppl. 3):S29-47.
20. Cardozo L. Role of estrogens in the treatment of female urinary incontinence. J Am Geriatr Soc. 1990;38:326-8.
21. Balk E, Adam GP, Kimmel H, Rofeberg V, Saeed I, Jeppson P, et al. Nonsurgical Treatments for Urinary Incontinence in Women: A Systematic Review Update. Rockville: Agency for Healthcare Research and Quality; 2018.
22. Willis-Gray MG, Dieter AA, Geller EJ. Evaluation and management of overactive bladder: strategies for optimizing care. Res Rep Urol. 2016;8:113-22.
23. Dumolin C, Hay-Smith J, Habee-Seguin GM, Mercier J. Pelvic floor muscle training vs no treatment, or inactive control treatments, for urinary incontinence in women: a short version Cochrane systemic review with meta-analysis. Neurourol Urodyn. 2015;34:300-8.

CHAPTER 42

# Frequency of Micturition

*Suryasnata Bhowmik, Ashish Jindal, Ashish Goel*

## INTRODUCTION

The adult bladder has a capacity ranging from 400 to 700 mL of urine. The approximate urinary output of an adult is 1,200–1,500 mL daily, with an average daily number of five or six voids and no more than one void after retirement. However, this frequency of normal micturition varies considerably from person to person due to differences in personality traits, bladder capacity, and drinking habits. As a result, a reliable history of the frequency of urination becomes difficult to obtain. A urinary pathology can be suspected if the complaint is accompanied by a recent change in the pattern of frequency or a history of voiding more than once at night after retiring.

## DEFINITION

Increased urinary frequency is when a patient considers that he voids too often during the day or night (nocturia), or both in standard and in subnormal quantities. It is defined as *more than seven voids in 24 hours or more than once during the night*. Increased urinary frequency is a part of the spectrum of lower urinary tract symptoms (LUTS). The definitions of each of the symptoms of LUTS are given in **Table 1**. However, the complaint of increased urinary frequency must not be confused with polyuria, which is an increase in daily total urine output by >3 L.

The prevalence of LUTS is significant in the male population and increases with age as is evident in **Table 2**. Moreover, the *severity* of symptoms *doubles* between the age groups of 40–49 and after 80 years. However, 19% of symptomatic men sought medical advice, and 10.2% received complete treatment.

## CAUSES OF INCREASED URINARY FREQUENCY

The causes of increased frequency of urine are discussed in **Table 3**.

## APPROACH TO DIAGNOSIS

A basic evaluation of a patient complaining of increased urinary frequency is required to determine the true nature of the problem. A primary assessment of *cognitive function* is vital to rule out falsely perceived increased frequency of urination as cognitive impairment can deter voluntary voiding by the patient. The level of cognitive function also influences further management as cognitively impaired elderly will not be able to co-operate with lifestyle modification. Additionally, drug therapies such as prescribing high-dose

**Table 1: Definition of lower urinary tract symptoms (International Continence Society).**

| *Symptom* | *Definition* |
|---|---|
| Voiding symptoms | • *Hesitancy*: Ready to pass urine → but difficulty in initiating micturition → delay in onset of voiding<br>• *Slow stream*: Perception of reduced urine flow (compared to others/previous performance)<br>• *Splitting/spraying*: Intermittent stream (urine flow that starts and stops on one or more occasions)<br>• *Straining to void*: A muscular effort to initiate/maintain/improve urine stream<br>• *Terminal dribble*: The prolonged final part of micturition when the flow has slowed to a trickle/dribble |
| Storage symptoms | • Increased urinary frequency during the day or night<br>• *Urgency*: A sudden compelling desire to pass urine that is difficult to defer<br>• *Incontinence*: Involuntary leakage of urine |
| Postmicturition symptoms | • Feeling of incomplete emptying after passing urine<br>• *Postmicturition dribble*: Involuntary loss of urine after micturition (usually after leaving the toilet) |

**Table 2: Prevalence of lower urinary tract symptoms (LUTS) in various age groups.**

| *Prevalence (in percentage)* | *Age group (in years)* |
|---|---|
| 22 | 50–59 |
| 45.3 | 70–80 |
| 70 | >80 |

antimuscarinic therapy may further adversely affect cognition. Maintaining *bladder diaries* by noting the date, time, and amount of voiding along with fluid intake charts by the patient or caregiver will aid in determining the pattern of voiding. Overall, a *focused history* addressing all the common urologic and systemic conditions (as listed in **Table 3**) and reviewing current medications is essential to arrive at a diagnosis. A *frequency-volume chart* (FVC), prescribed in patients with severe LUTS, is a self-recorded measurement of the volume and time of each void over a minimum of 3 days in order to calculate voiding frequency, total voided volume, and fraction of urine produced during the night. FVC can be used to rule out polyuria and nocturnal polyuria, which can be easily managed with lifestyle modifications and reduced fluid intake **(Table 4)**.

Initial evaluation should comprise a mandatory *physical examination* that includes a systemic examination by abdominal palpation and urogenital examination, a digital rectal examination (DRE) in men, and a urine dipstick. Abdominal palpation can detect large volumes of retained urine in the bladder, and urogenital examination can rule out risk factors of increased urinary frequency such as urogenital atrophy, prolapse, or phimosis. DRE can assess the presence of fecal loading (that can precipitate or worsen urinary symptoms) and evaluate the prostate to rule out benign prostatic hyperplasia (BPH) and prostate cancer (DRE findings of BPH vs. prostate cancer are given in **Table 5**). A *urine dipstick* will detect blood, glucose, white blood cells, and nitrites in the urine and hint at possible etiologies. **Box 1** lists the important points of the initial evaluation.

Tests such as urinalysis, renal function test, renal ultrasonography, and serum levels of prostate-specific antigen (PSA) are performed to supplement diagnosis. Urinalysis helps screen for urinary tract infection (UTI), diabetes mellitus, and hematuria through

**Table 3: Causes of increased urinary frequency.**

| *Causes of increased urinary frequency* | *Suggestive findings* | *Diagnostic approach in brief* |
|---|---|---|
| ***Male-specific causes*** | | |
| BPH or prostate cancer | The progressive onset of urinary hesitancy, incontinence, poor urine stream, a sensation of incomplete voiding | • Rectal examination<br>• Ultrasonography<br>• Cystometry |
| Prostatitis | Urgency, dysuria, nocturia, purulent urethral discharge with fever, chills, low back pain, myalgia, arthralgia, and perineal fullness | • Prostate tender to palpation<br>• Rectal examination<br>• Culture of secretions after prostatic massage |
| Phimosis | Inflammation, redness, dysuria | *Clinical evaluation*: Inability to retract the foreskin |
| ***Female-specific causes*** | | |
| Cystocele | Urinary incontinence<br>A sensation of vaginal fullness pain or urinary leakage during sexual intercourse | • Pelvic examination<br>• Voiding cystourethrography |
| Pregnancy | Third trimester, although highly unlikely in the geriatric population | Clinical evaluation |
| ***Sex nonspecific causes*** | | |
| Urinary tract infection | Dysuria, increased frequency, sometimes fever, and flank pain, particularly in women | • Urinalysis and culture<br>• STI testing |
| Overactive bladder (bladder detrusor overactivity) | Nocturia, urge incontinence, weak urinary stream, and sometimes urinary retention | Cystometry |
| Radiation cystitis | History of radiation therapy of the lower abdomen, prostate, or perineum for treatment of cancer | • Clinical evaluation<br>• Cystoscopy and biopsy |
| Medications, illicit drugs, dietary factors:<br>• Caffeine<br>• Alcohol<br>• Ketamine<br>• Diuretics<br>• Decongestants<br>• Calcium channel blockers (dependent edema → nocturia)<br>• Gabapentin/glitazones/ NSAIDs (edema → nocturia)<br>• Lithium (diabetes insipidus → polyuria)<br>• Cholinesterase inhibitors (increase bladder contractility) | Urinary frequency in an otherwise healthy patient | Empiric elimination of offending substance (to confirm that frequency resolves) |

*Continued*

*Continued*

| *Causes of increased urinary frequency* | *Suggestive findings* | *Diagnostic approach in brief* |
|---|---|---|
| Reactive arthritis | Asymmetric arthritis of knees, ankles, and metatarsophalangeal joints<br>Unilateral or bilateral conjunctivitis small, painless ulcers on the mouth, tongue, glans penis, palms, and soles 1–2 weeks after sexual contact | STI testing |
| Urethral stricture | Hesitancy, tenesmus, reduced caliber and force of the urine stream | Urethrography |
| Neurogenic bladder dysfunction | In spinal cord injury or lesion—lower-extremity weakness, decreased anal sphincter tone, absent anal wink reflex<br>Loss of sensation at a segmental level | The injury is usually clinically obvious on an MRI of the spine |
| Urinary tract calculi | Colicky flank or groin pain | • Urinalysis for hematuria<br>• Ultrasonography or CT of the kidneys, ureters, and bladder |
| Diabetes mellitus | Poor diabetic control → hyperglycemia → osmotic diuresis and polyuria | • Urinalysis may show glucose in the urine<br>• Impaired fasting/postprandial glucose levels or HbA1c levels |
| Congestive heart failure (CHF)/ lower extremity venous insufficiency | Increased nighttime urine production → nocturia | • Echocardiography<br>• Management of CHF, leg elevation and support stocking, late afternoon dosing of diuretic |
| Sleep apnea | May increase nighttime urine production by increased atrial natriuretic peptide (ANP) production | Diagnosis and treatment of sleep apnea (by continuous positive airway pressure machines) |

*Other causes*:
- *Decreased bladder capacity due to*:
  - Anxiety
  - Operative procedures
  - A thickened inelastic fibrotic wall due to:
    - Interstitial cystitis
    - Irradiation
    - Chronic infections such as tuberculosis and schistosomiasis
    - Inflammatory conditions that increase bladder sensitivity (pressure from intrinsic or extrinsic masses, calculi, or infections)
- Very low or high urinary pH rarely causes frequency
- Psychiatric disturbances
- Emotional stress

*Environmental factors*:
- Inaccessible toilets
- Unsafe toilets
- Caregivers unavailable for toileting assistance

(BPH: benign prostatic hyperplasia; CT: computed tomography; HbA1c: glycated hemoglobin; MRI: magnetic resonance imaging; NSAIDs: nonsteroidal anti-inflammatory drugs; STI: sexually transmitted infection)

**Table 4: American Urological Association (AUA) self-reported questionnaire for the severity of lower urinary tract symptoms (LUTS).**

| | *Not at all* | *Less than once in 5* | *Less than half the time* | *Almost half the time* | *More than half the time* | *Almost always* |
|---|---|---|---|---|---|---|
| **Incomplete emptying:** Over the last month, how often have you had a sensation of not emptying your bladder completely after you finish urinating? | 0 | 1 | 2 | 3 | 4 | 5 |
| **Frequency:** During the last month, how often have you had to urinate again <2 hours after you finished urinating? | 0 | 1 | 2 | 3 | 4 | 5 |
| **Intermittency:** During the last month, how often have you stopped and started again several times when you urinate? | 0 | 1 | 2 | 3 | 4 | 5 |
| **Urgency:** During the last month, how often have you found it difficult to postpone urination? | 0 | 1 | 2 | 3 | 4 | 5 |
| **Weak stream:** During the last month, how often have you had a weak urinary stream? | 0 | 1 | 2 | 3 | 4 | 5 |
| **Straining:** During the last month, how often have you had to push or strain to begin urination? | 0 | 1 | 2 | 3 | 4 | 5 |
| | None | 1 time | 2 times | 3 times | 4 times | 5 or more times |
| **Nocturia:** During the last month, how many times did you most typically get up to urinate from the time you went to bed until the time you got up in the morning? | 0 | 1 | 2 | 3 | 4 | 5 |
| **Total symptom score:**<br>• 1–7 is mild<br>• 8–19 is moderate<br>• 20–35 is severe | | | | | | |

**Table 5: Digital rectal examination (DRE) findings of benign prostate hyperplasia (BPH) versus prostate cancer.**

| *Prostate cancer* | *BPH* |
|---|---|
| Areas of induration/ frank nodules | Prostate symmetrically enlarged, nodularity present |
| Stony hard induration | Rubbery generalized enlargement |

**BOX 1: Initial evaluation.**

- Cognitive assessment
- Bladder diaries
- Focused history
- Frequency-volume chart (FVC)

*Physical examination*:

- Systemic evaluation (abdominal palpation and urogenital examination)
- Mandatory digital rectal examination (DRE) in men
- Urine dipstick

detection and quantification of white blood cells, nitrites, pH, glucose, and red blood cells. The presence of hematuria warrants further investigations such as diagnostic flexible cystoscopy and upper urologic tract imaging. Renal function tests are indicated in cases of suspected renal impairment from history and clinical examination or during consideration of surgical treatment. Elevated levels of serum creatinine, hematuria, or UTI mandate renal ultrasonography.

Further tests can be ordered on the basis of results from history and physical examinations. For example, *uroflowmetry* is a noninvasive test where the patient voids into a device that measures the volume of urine voided over time and is used to assess the maximum urinary flow rate (known as $Q_{max}$). Although the test is valid only if the patient voids >150 mL of urine, a $Q_{max}$ of <10 mL/s is highly suggestive of bladder outlet obstruction. An estimate of *postvoid residual (PVR) volume* of urine can be made either by a bladder ultrasound scan after urination or by in-out catheterization where retained urine in the bladder is removed and measured with the help of a catheter. Increased PVR can suggest an obstruction of the outflow tract or decreased contractility of detrusor muscles as in overflow incontinence. *Computer urodynamic pressure-flow studies* where an electronic transducer is passed into the bladder through the urethra can differentiate between low urine flow rate caused by impaired detrusor contraction and that caused by bladder outlet obstruction.

Refer to **Flowchart 1** for a holistic approach to the diagnosis of increased urinary frequency.

## THERAPY AND MANAGEMENT

Geriatric populations with multiple comorbidities and affections often are already on a multidrug regimen. Hence, to avoid the adverse effects of polypharmacy, initially, the symptoms should be managed with a trial of lifestyle modification and behavioral interventions. Weight loss, fluid selection, and alleviation of constipation may improve symptoms. However, *behavioral interventions* remain the mainstay of treatment. These primarily include *prompted voiding*, where individuals are *prompted* to use the washroom and rewarded socially upon successful toileting, and *habit retraining*, where the patient is made to void timely at fixed intervals according to a toileting schedule created on the basis of his toileting pattern identified from his bladder diaries. Additionally, *functional interventions* such as 30-minutes' walk daily and pelvic floor muscle strengthening by Kegel exercises have been shown to improve daytime and night urinary frequency. *Drug therapies* are reserved for refractory cases and include *anticholinergics* such as tolterodine, solifenacin, and oxybutynin; $\beta_3$ *agonists* such as mirabegron; and oral or intranasal

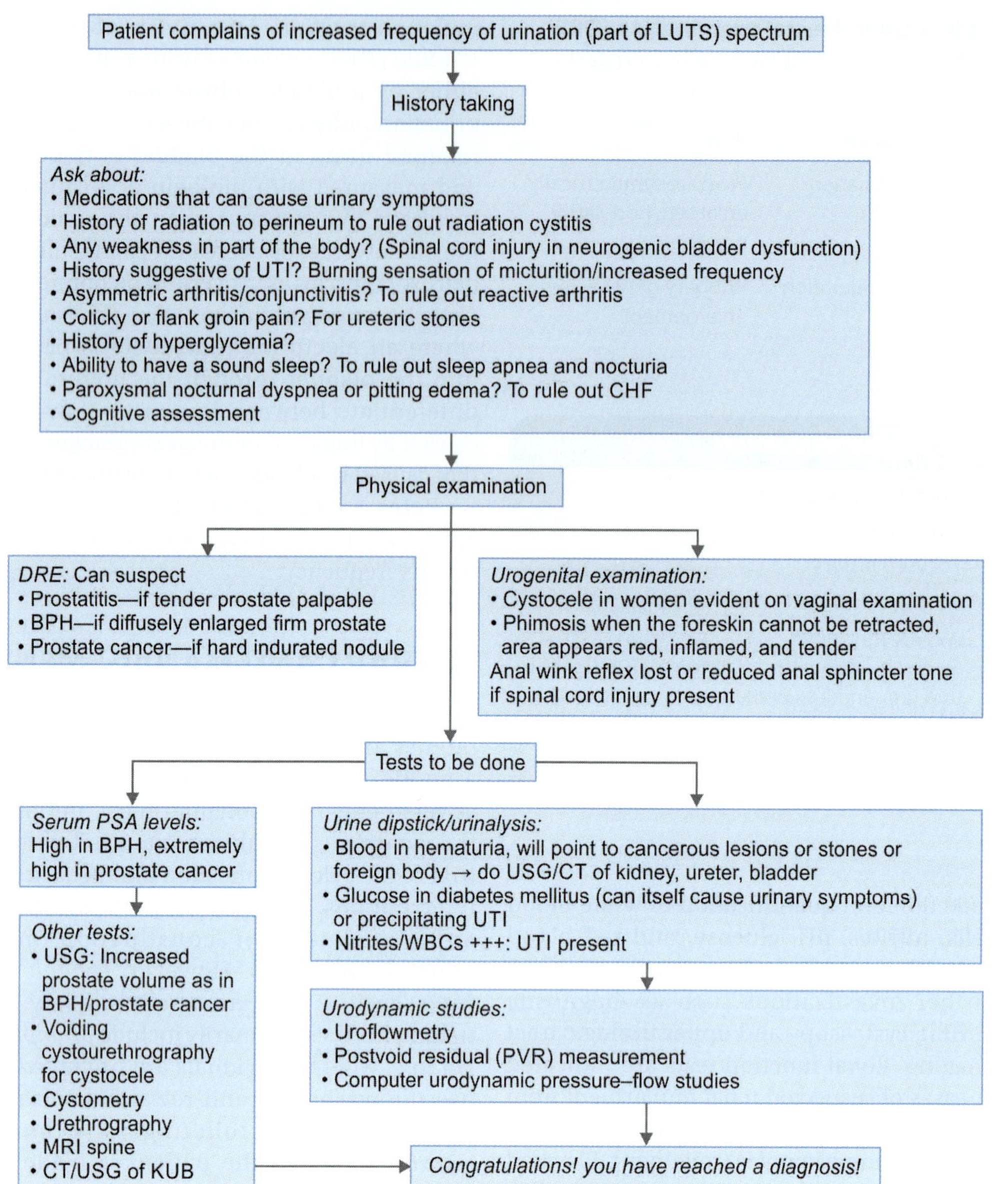


**FLOWCHART 1:** A holistic approach to diagnosis of increased urinary frequency.

(BPH: benign prostate hyperplasia; CHF: congestive heart failure; CT: computed tomography; DRE: digital rectal examination; KUB: kidneys, ureters, bladder; LUTS: lower urinary tract symptoms; MRI: magnetic resonance imaging; PSA: prostate-specific antigen; USG: ultrasound; UTI: urinary tract infection; WBCs: white blood cells)

synthetic *vasopressin*. Indications and further notes on drug therapies are provided in **Table 6**. Physically impaired individuals may use *appliances* such as handheld urinals, bedpans, and collection devices. *Surgical options* include transurethral resection of the prostate (*TURP*) in males for outflow tract obstruction, *tension-free vaginal tape* and *intravesical botulinum toxin* in females, and *intermittent catheterization*. Handrails, low-

**Table 6: Management and therapy for specific problems with adverse effects.**

| *Indication* | *Treatment* | *Further information* |
|---|---|---|
| For increased frequency/ urgency symptoms | Anticholinergics | • Side effects include urinary retention, dry mouth, constipation, postural hypotension<br>• The dose needs to be titrated slowly<br>• Minimum 6 weeks to see the effect<br>• Can precipitate confusion and cognitive impairment with long-term use; hence, risk–benefit ratio needs to be assessed every 3 years |
| Overactive bladder syndrome | $\beta_3$ agonists | No anticholinergic side effect as above but can cause hypertensive crisis |

level lighting, proper seating, and adapted clothing are some examples of *environmental changes* that can be incorporated to ease the afflictions of these patients. Furthermore, specific therapies can be instated based on etiology and diagnosis.

## CLINICAL PEARLS

- Increased urinary frequency is a common symptom in older adults that can have a profound negative impact on quality of life
- It is defined when an individual voids >8 times in 24 hours or more than once during the night
- There are a number of reversible and nonreversible causes of increased frequency of micturition that should be carefully evaluated
- Patient should be managed keeping comorbidities in mind

## FURTHER READINGS


1. Wrenn K. Dysuria, frequency, and urgency. In: Walker HK, Hall WD, Hurst JW (Eds). Clinical Methods: The History, Physical, and Laboratory Examinations, 3rd edition. Boston: Butterworths; 1990.
2. Maddukuri G. (2022). Urinary frequency—genitourinary disorders. MSD Manual Professional Edition. [online] Available from https://www.msdmanuals.com/en-in/professional/genitourinary-disorders/symptoms-of-genitourinary-disorders/urinary-frequency#:~:text=Urinary%20frequency%20usually%20results%20from,of%20the%20need%20to%20urinate. [Last accessed August, 2023].
3. Goldberg RP, Lobel RW, Sand PK. The urinary tract in pregnancy. In: Bent AEODR, Cundif CW, Swift SE (Eds). Ostergard's Urogynecology and Pelvic Floor Dysfunction. Philadelphia: Lippincott Williams & Wilkins; 2003.
4. Parsons JK, Bergstrom J, Silberstein J, Barrett-Connor E. Prevalence and characteristics of lower urinary tract symptoms in men aged > or = 80 years. Urology. 2008;72:318-21.
5. Araki I, Zakoji H, Komuro M, Furuya Y, Fukasawa M, Takihana Y, et al. Lower urinary tract symptoms in men and women without underlying disease causing micturition disorder: a cross-sectional study assessing the natural history of bladder function. J Urol. 2003;170:1901-4.
6. Barry MJ, Fowler FJ, O'leary MP, Bruskewitz RC, Holtgrewe HL, Mebust WK, et al. The American Urological Association symptom index for benign prostatic hyperplasia. J Urol. 2017;197:S189-97.
7. Sugaya K, Nishijima S, Owan T, Oda M, Miyazato M, Ogawa Y. Effects of walking exercise on nocturia in the elderly. Biomed Res. 2007;28:101-5.
8. Sooriakumaran P, Brown C, Mark E. Frequency volume charts should be used in men with lower urinary tract symptoms. Int J Surg. 2005;3(2):147-50.

# CHAPTER 43

# Retention of Urine

*Arshdeep Maman, Amanjot Kaur, Saumya Singh, Ashish Goel*

## DEFINITION

Retention of urine is defined as the inability to voluntarily void completely or incompletely. The normal adult bladder capacity is from 400 to 600 mL. In acute urine retention, the patient will present with pain in the lower abdomen, an inability to void urine despite the pain, and a palpable urinary bladder. On the other hand, patients with chronic urine retention will present with painless decreased urine output and palpable urinary bladder even after passing urine.

## MECHANISM OF MICTURITION

Knowledge of normal bladder functioning is necessary to understand how and why retention happens. Voiding is neurally mediated and is generally a reflex response to a full bladder so-called micturition reflex. Micturition reflex needs bladder distention, followed by transmission of sensory input from the bladder to the midsacral region of the neural structure, involuntary synchronal contraction of the bladder, and reflex inhibition of the internal urethral sphincter. There should be voluntary relaxation of the external urethral sphincter to complete the process **(Table 1)**.

**Table 1: Neural control of urine storage and voiding.**

| | ***Storage*** | ***Voiding*** |
|---|---|---|
| Brain | Pontine storage center | • Periaqueductal gray<br>• Pontine micturition center |
| T10–L2 | • Hypogastric nerve (sympathetic) (+)<br>• + Trigone<br>• – Detrusor | • Hypogastric nerve (sympathetic) (–)<br>• – Trigone<br>• + Detrusor |
| S2–S4 | • Pelvic nerve (parasympathetic) (–)<br>• Pudendal nerve (+) | • Pelvic nerve (parasympathetic) (+)<br>• Pudendal nerve (–) |
| Bladder | External urethral sphincter (+) | External urethral sphincter (–) |

*Note*:
(+) Sign indicating facilitation.
(–) Sign indicating inhibition of voiding of urine.

Visceral sensory afferents from the bladder travel primarily in the pelvic splanchnic nerves to synapse in the midsacral spinal cord (S2–S4), with projections to the micturition center in the brain. The neuromotor limb of this reflex consists of the following:

- Preganglionic parasympathetic fibers originating at S2–S4 travel in pelvic splanchnic nerves to peripheral cholinergic

receptors among the bladder wall and stimulate bladder contraction throughout the active session of micturition.
- Sympathetic neuromotor fibers originating from T10 to L2 travel via the superior and inferior hypogastric plexuses to the internal urethral sphincter. Their output maintains sphincter muscle tone throughout continence and the reflex is inhibited throughout the micturition.
- Somatic neuromotor fibers course within the pudendal nerves to the striated muscle of the external urethral sphincter muscle, which should be voluntarily relaxed throughout micturition.
- Barrington's nucleus [pontine micturition center (PMC)] is present in the brainstem, which works in coordination with other regions of the brain to stimulate urination. PMC acts through the activation of parasympathetic neurons leading to detrusor muscle contraction and inhibiting somatic nerves to relax the external urethral sphincter.

## ETIOLOGY OF CONDITION

The patient can present with urine retention due to various causes.

The most common cause of urine retention is benign prostatic hyperplasia (BPH) and there are many other surgical causes in literature, but for a physician, other causes such as neurogenic causes, infective causes, and drug-induced urine retention are more important. Commonly encountered medical and surgical causes for urine retention are given in **Table 2**.

### Infections and Inflammation-related Urine Retention

The most common infective cause leading to acute urine retention is acute prostatitis, caused by gram-negative organisms such as *Escherichia coli* leading to local inflammation and obstruction of the urine tract. Urethritis can also lead to local inflammation and urinary tract obstruction. In females, conditions such as vulvovaginitis and other local painful lesions can cause urine retention **(Table 2)**.

### Neurogenic Bladder

Neurogenic bladder is a condition involving the lower urinary tract due to the involvement of central or peripheral control disruption of micturition. Common causes include cerebrovascular accident (CVA), dementia, Parkinson's disease, multiple sclerosis, spinal cord tumors, trauma, transverse myelitis, intervertebral disk disease, cauda equine syndrome, and diseases such as Guillain-Barré syndrome (GBS) and diabetes **(Table 3)**.

Patients with a neurogenic bladder can come with symptoms of urine retention and/or incontinence according to the level of neural lesion. According to Lapides classification, patients can be categorized into different groups according to their bladder functioning:

- *Sensory neurogenic bladder*: Neurological process damaging sensory fibers from the bladder to the spinal cord. Diseases such as diabetes mellitus, tabes dorsalis, and pernicious anemia can present with this condition and the patient will have no bladder sensation and further leading to loss of motor function.
- *Motor paralytic neurogenic bladder*: Damage to parasympathetic motor innervations to detrusor muscle like in surgery, pelvic trauma, and herpes zoster. Bladder sensation will be normal and motor function is impaired.
- *Uninhibited neurogenic bladder*: Conditions such as stroke, brain trauma or tumor, Parkinson's disease, and demyelinating diseases can lead to this type. There will be normal bladder sensation and motor function, and the patient will have urge incontinence and urinary frequency and urgency.
- *Reflex neurogenic bladder*: Diseases involving the spinal cord such as cord trauma and transverse myelitis can lead to

**Table 2: Common medical and surgical causes of urine retention.**

| | *Medical causes* | *Surgical causes* |
|---|---|---|
| Males | • Balanitis<br>• Prostatic abscess<br>• Prostatitis | • Benign prostatic hyperplasia<br>• Meatal stenosis<br>• Paraphimosis<br>• Penile constricting bands<br>• Phimosis<br>• Prostatic cancer |
| Females | • Acute vulvovaginitis<br>• Vaginal lichen planus<br>• Vaginal lichen sclerosis<br>• Vaginal pemphigus | • Organ prolapse like cystocele, rectocele, uterine prolapse<br>• Pelvic mass (gynecologic malignancy, uterine fibroid, ovarian cyst)<br>• Retroverted gravid uterus<br>• Instrumental delivery<br>• Prolonged labor<br>• Cesarean section |
| Both genders | • Cystitis<br>• Herpes simplex virus<br>• Lyme disease<br>• Periurethral abscess<br>• Tuberculous cystitis<br>• Urethritis<br>• Varicella-zoster virus<br>• Schistosomiasis<br>• Echinococcosis<br>• Guillain–Barré syndrome<br>• Transverse myelitis<br>• Autonomic neuropathy<br>• Diabetes mellitus<br>• Pernicious anemia<br>• Poliomyelitis<br>• Cerebrovascular accident (CVA)/stroke<br>• Multiple sclerosis<br>• Normal pressure hydrocephalus (NPH)<br>• Parkinson's disease | • Aneurysmal dilatation<br>• Bladder neck calculi<br>• Urethral calculi<br>• Bladder neoplasm<br>• Fecal impaction<br>• Gastrointestinal or retroperitoneal malignancy/ mass<br>• Urethral strictures<br>• Foreign bodies<br>• Edema<br>• Spinal cord trauma<br>• Pelvic trauma<br>• Radical pelvic surgery<br>• Spina bifida occulta<br>• Spinal cord hematoma/abscess<br>• Spinal cord tumors |

this condition. The patient will have poorly coordinated bladder function, loss of bladder sensation, and urine incontinence.

- *Autonomous neurogenic bladder*: This condition will result from both motor and sensory nervous system control disruption of the bladder like in pelvic trauma and low myelomeningocele. There will be no ability to initiate bladder contraction and loss of bladder sensations.

## Drug-induced Urine Retention

Drugs having anticholinergic properties and alpha-adrenergic agonists are the culprit for many cases of urine retention. Drugs used for general anesthesia, opioid, and nonsteroidal anti-inflammatory drugs (NSAIDs) are also involved in cases with urine retention. Drugs causing urine retention are listed in **Table 4**.

**Table 3: Neurologic causes of urine retention (causes of neurogenic bladder).**

| | |
|---|---|
| Autonomic or peripheral nerve | • Autonomic neuropathy<br>• Diabetes mellitus<br>• Guillain–Barré syndrome (GBS)<br>• Pernicious anemia<br>• Poliomyelitis<br>• Radical pelvic surgery<br>• Spinal cord trauma<br>• Tabes dorsalis |
| Brain | • Cerebrovascular accident (CVA)/stroke<br>• Multiple sclerosis (MS)<br>• Normal pressure hydrocephalus (NPH)<br>• Parkinson's disease |
| Spinal cord | • Intervertebral disk disease<br>• Meningomyelocele<br>• MS<br>• Spina bifida occulta<br>• Spinal cord hematoma/ abscess<br>• Spinal cord trauma<br>• Spinal stenosis<br>• Transverse myelitis<br>• Tumors<br>• Cauda equina syndrome<br>• Spina vascular disease |

**Table 4: Drugs causing urine retention.**

| | |
|---|---|
| Antiarrhythmics | Disopyramide, procainamide, quinidine |
| Anticholinergics | Atropine, belladonna alkaloids, dicyclomine, glycopyrrolate, hyoscyamine, scopolamine |
| Antidepressants | Amitriptyline, amoxapine, imipramine, nortriptyline |
| Antihistamines | Brompheniramine, chlorpheniramine, cyproheptadine, hydroxyzine |
| Antihypertensives | Hydralazine, nifedipine |
| Antiparkinsonian agents | Amantadine, benztropine, bromocriptine, levodopa, trihexyphenidyl |
| Antipsychotics | Chlorpromazine, fluphenazine, haloperidol, prochlorperazine, thioridazine, thiothixene |
| Hormonal agents | Estrogen, progesterone, testosterone |
| Muscle relaxants | Baclofen, cyclobenzaprine, diazepine |
| Sympathomimetics (alpha-adrenergic agents) | Ephedrine, phenylephrine, pseudoephedrine |
| Sympathomimetics (beta-adrenergic agents) | Isoproterenol, metaproterenol, terbutaline |
| Miscellaneous | Amphetamines, carbamazepine, dopamine, nonsteroidal anti-inflammatory drugs (NSAIDs), opioid analgesics, vincristine |

## APPROACH TO DIAGNOSIS AND MANAGEMENT (FLOWCHART 1)

As in any other clinical condition, detailed history and clinical examination followed by relevant investigations will lead to a diagnosis.

History related to urinary symptoms, neurological history, drugs-related history, trauma, or any surgery in detail is required.

## CLINICAL PRESENTATION

Urine retention can present as an acute or chronic disease and according to the condition, the patient can have clinical signs and symptoms.

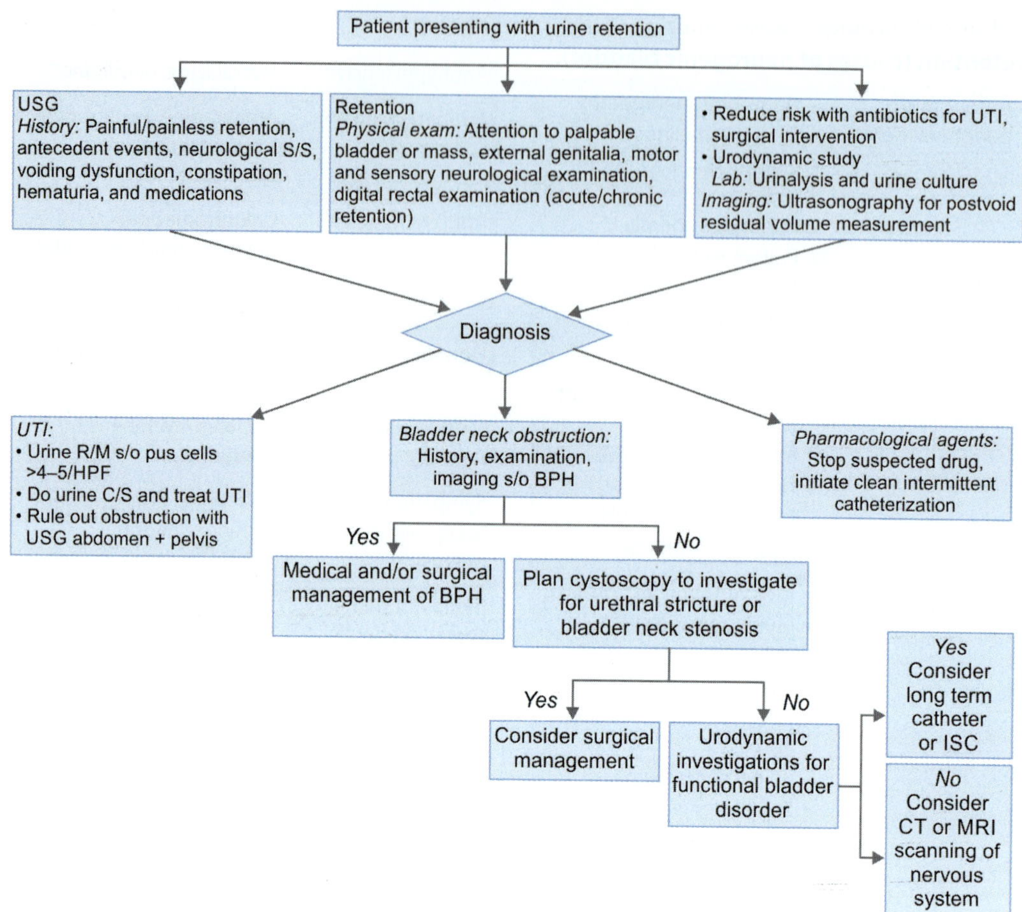


**FLOWCHART 1:** Approach to a patient with urine retention.

(BPH: benign prostatic hyperplasia; C/S: culture and sensitivity; CT: computed tomography; HPF: high power field; ISC: intermittent self-catheterization; MRI: magnetic resonance imaging; R/M: routine microscopy; s/o: suggestive of; S/S: signs and symptoms; USG: ultrasonography; UTI: urinary tract infection)

A patient with retention would be unable to pass urine despite the painful and urgent desire for micturition. There will be pain in the lower abdomen and discomfort. In addition, distension of the lower abdomen associated with a suprapubic swelling may be appreciable. This is caused by the distension of the bladder and may be painful and tender.

The symptoms of chronic urine retention may include frequency of urine and difficulty in initiating the stream of urine, which may be interrupted or be weak. The patient may complain of urgency and hesitancy. There may be a feeling of incomplete emptying associated with dribbling of urine. There may be mild constant discomfort in the lower abdomen and urinary tract. On examination, one may be able to identify a distended bladder.

A patient with an infective cause of urine retention can present with a history of fever, rectal or perineal pain, urethral or vaginal discharge, dysuria, hematuria, and genital rash.

Neurological diseases result in urine retention. A thorough history of newly diagnosed or preexisting disorders such as multiple sclerosis, Parkinson's disease, stroke, overflow incontinence, and diabetic neuropathy is important.

A detailed drug history of pharmacologic agents such as anticholinergics, antidepressants, antiarrhythmics, and antiparkinsonian drugs causing urine retention should be taken.

Postoperative urine retention is relatively common. Its frequency depends on the nature and location of surgery, the type of anesthesia used, the drugs given, and the patient's underlying physiology and medical conditions.

A detailed history taking of the previous history of urine retention, weight loss, constitutional signs, and symptoms may be seen in BPH and prostatic cancer.

In women, pelvic pressure, palpation of pelvic organs from the vagina, or a feeling of something coming out from the vagina may reveal prolapse of the bladder, rectum, or uterus. A history of dysmenorrhea, lower abdominal pain, difficulty conceiving, and bloating may suggest uterine fibroid, pelvic mass, or malignancy. A history of painless, gross hematuria with clots may reveal a bladder tumor on further investigation.

A history of abdominal pain or distension associated with rectal bleeding along with constitutional symptoms points toward gastrointestinal malignancy.

Apart from its impact on physical health, urine retention has many social and psychological implications. Patients with chronic urine retention tend to have decreased daily life activities and a lower quality of life. Moreover, lack of sleep due to symptoms causes daytime fatigue and emotional distress.

## PHYSICAL EXAMINATION

*Examination of the abdomen* is an important step toward revealing the etiology of the condition. Suprapubic tenderness and costovertebral angle tenderness/renal angle tenderness are pointers of cystitis, pyelonephritis, and urinary tract infections. Lower abdominal palpation may have palpable uterus, ovaries, or adnexa.

*Local examination of the genital area* is also important, such as urethral discharge, genital vesicles in urethritis, and sexually transmitted diseases. Edema of the penis without a retractable foreskin is seen in phimosis and paraphimosis.

A *rectal examination* and a per vaginal examination in women can delineate the exact etiology. A tender, boggy, warm prostate and penile discharge on digital rectal examination are suggestive of acute bacterial prostatitis. An enlarged, firm, nontender, nonnodular, or normal prostate examination is seen in BPH, whereas a normal or an enlarged prostate with or without palpable nodules is seen in prostatic cancer. A palpable rectal mass might reveal gastrointestinal (GI)/rectal malignancy, whereas impacted stools in the rectum also cause urine retention. In women, inflamed or erythematous vulva or vagina and vaginal discharge on per vaginal and per speculum examination are suggestive of vulvovaginitis, common causes being *Candida*, trichomonas, herpes simplex, or bacterial vaginosis.

*Neurological examination* for motor/sensory deficits relative to S1–S5 distribution is important.

Neurological examination to assess strength, sensation, muscle tone, and reflexes relative to lower thoracic, lumbar, and sacral spinal levels.

## LABORATORY INVESTIGATION

Laboratory investigation includes prostate-specific antigen, serum blood glucose, serum blood urea nitrogen, creatinine, electrolytes, and urine analysis.

*Imaging studies*: The most basic and first imaging is ultrasonography of kidneys, ureters, bladder, and prostate along with postvoid residual urine (PVRU) evaluation. If there is any diagnosis conflict or requirement to know the extent of the disease; other imaging studies are pelvic ultrasonography, computed tomography (CT) abdomen and pelvis, and magnetic resonance imaging (MRI) brain and/or spinal cord. Cystoscopy and retrograde cystourethrography are indicated for suspected bladder tumors and bladder or urethral stones or strictures. Ultrasonography is recommended for postvoid residual (PVR) urine evaluation.

## MANAGEMENT

### Acute Urine Retention Management

The initial management of acute urine retention involves prompt bladder decompression. This can be accomplished with urethral or suprapubic catheterization (SPC). Depending upon the condition, different sizes of catheters can be tried in the patient. The first line of catheterization therapy is with 16–18 Fr catheters. Usually, in obstructive urine retention, a normal adult-sized catheter does not work and in that case, the smaller urinary catheter can be tried and if after repeated attempts catheterization cannot be successfully done, SPC is required wherever urologists are available. In an emergency when both catheterization and SPC cannot be done, suprapubic aspiration with a needle is another temporary option to relieve symptoms.

Depending upon the cause of urine retention, the course of urinary catheterization is decided in patients with temporary urine retention like in drug-induced, a patient can be started upon voiding trials earlier. Patients with neurological causes of urine retention may need a longer duration of catheterization therapy.

Once bladder decompression is accomplished, alpha-blockers are started, followed by a voiding trial after 72 hours and elective urologic consultation throughout 2–3 weeks.

Benign prostatic hyperplasia is the most common cause in men and should be started on oral medications after successful urinary catheterization. Medication therapy includes alpha-1 adrenergic antagonists (alfuzosin 10 mg or tamsulosin 0.1 mg). Alpha-1 adrenergic antagonists work by relaxing the smooth muscle at the bladder neck and the capsule of the prostate. Medications such as 5 alpha-reductase inhibitors decrease the incidence of urine retention in BPH patients. Further, a urologist's opinion is required for BPH for procedures such as transurethral resection of the prostate (TURP), if indicated.

In the rest of the cases, treatment of underlying etiology is required to treat retention **(Flowchart 2)**.

### Chronic Urine Retention Management

The treatment of chronic urine retention should be based on its underlying cause. For patients with non-neurologic chronic urine retention, the American Urological Association has proposed a treatment algorithm that recommends classifying patients with chronic urine retention first by risk and then by symptoms. Patients with urine retention with underlying neurological diseases should be followed in conduction with a neurologist and urologist **(Flowchart 3)**.

### Neurogenic Bladder Management

Neurogenic bladder can present with acute or chronic retention of urine. The primary goal for management is the prevention of damage to the upper urinary tract and further damage to the urinary bladder and the secondary goal is to improve the quality of life of the patient and continence. Management will depend upon the patient's neurologic condition, underlying comorbidities, age, and history of medications.

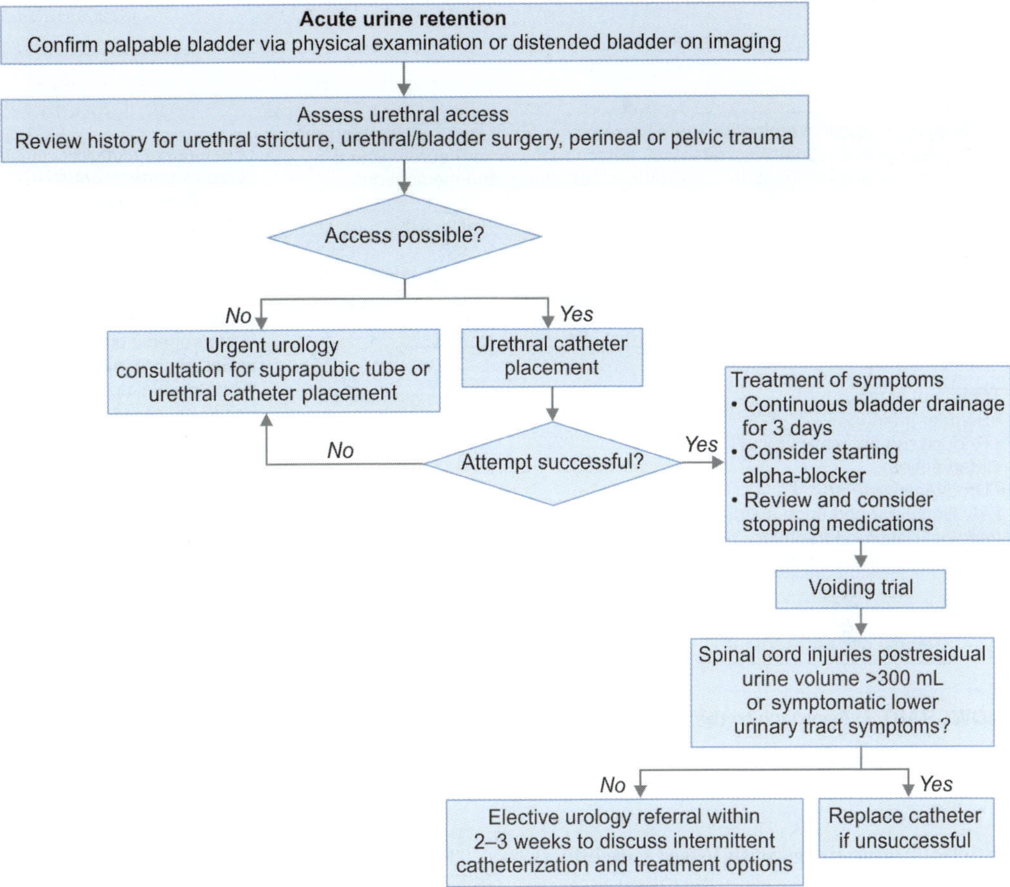


**FLOWCHART 2:** Approach to a patient with acute urine retention.

Treatment is divided into behavior therapy, medications, catheters, neuromodulation, and surgery.

## Behavior Therapy

Behavior therapy is helpful in patients with stroke, Parkinson's disease, spinal cord injury, multiple sclerosis, and transverse myelitis. It includes timed voiding, habit retraining, pelvic floor exercises, prompted voiding, and pelvic floor physiotherapy.

## Medications

Anticholinergic drugs (oxybutynin, tolterodine, darifenacin) are the first line of treatment with neurogenic bladder as they reduce detrusor overactivity leading to reduced intravesical pressure and improve storage. But on the other hand, these drugs can lead to an increase in residual volume in patients with CVA, Parkinson's, and multiple sclerosis. Hence, PVRU should be reviewed periodically in these patients. Alpha-blocker medications (tizanidine, clonidine) are used in selected neurogenic bladder conditions as these drugs decrease bladder outlet resistance, decrease the residual volume of urine, and improve continence and bladder capacity. Beta-3 agonists (mirabegron and vibegron) are newer agents designed to relax overactive detrusor muscle; these drugs are equally effective to

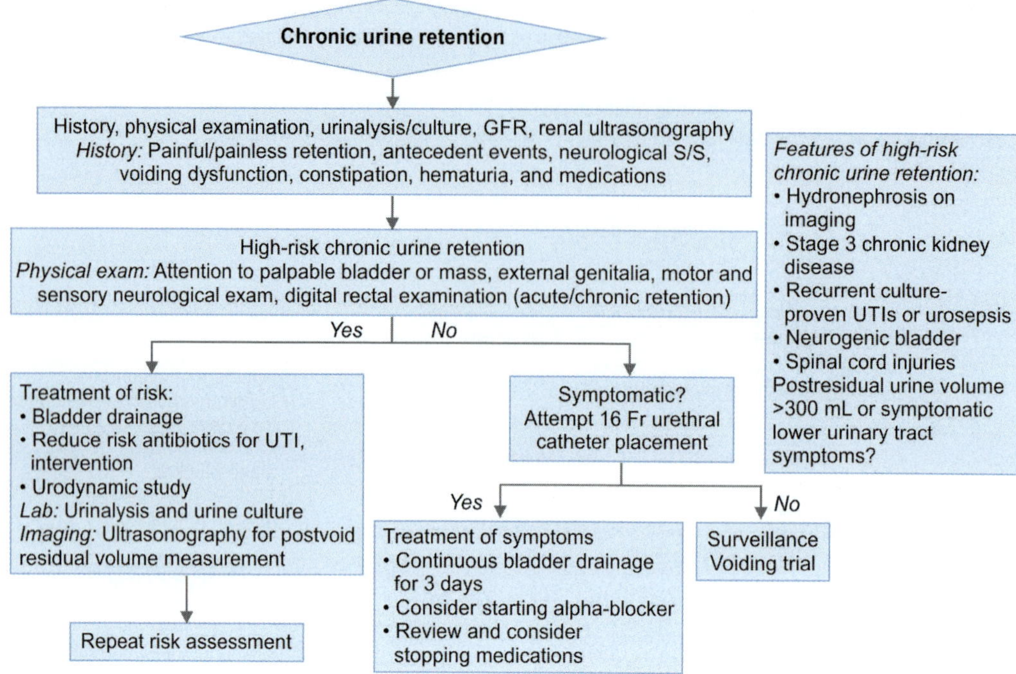


**FLOWCHART 3:** Approach to the patient with chronic urine retention.

(GFR: glomerular filtration rate; S/S: signs and symptoms; UTI: urinary tract infection)

anticholinergic drugs with lesser side effects. Desmopressin and onabotulinumtoxin A are other drugs used in the neurogenic bladder.

### *Clean Intermittent Self-catheterization*

Patients with urine retention, not able to drain bladders, and large postvoid volume (>200 mL) are advised for clean intermittent self-catheterization. This therapy cannot be advised in patients with abnormal urethral anatomy. Small bladders, autonomic dysreflexia, poor cognition, dementia, and Foley catheter insertion are preferred in these cases. Complications include urethral strictures, urinary tract infections, hematuria, and autonomic dysreflexia.

In patients requiring long-term Foley catheter therapy, suprapubic tubes are considered due to their lesser catheter-related side effects on the patient.

Patients who cannot be managed with the above therapies can undergo sacral neuromodulation and surgical therapies such as augmentation cystoplasty, sphincterotomy, and urinary diversion surgery.

## CONCLUSION

Urine retention is a common emergency presentation in elderly males. The most common etiology for urine retention in males is BPH. Females have less frequent visits to the emergency for urine retention. Thorough medical history related to urinary tract infection, inflammation, drug history, and neurological history is required, followed by relevant clinical examination and investigations. Ultrasonography is the initial investigation of choice to look for BPH and PVRU. Patients with acute urine retention require urgent bladder decompression with urinary catheterization or SPC. In cases where both urine catheterization and SPC cannot proceed, suprapubic needle aspiration is the procedure for relieving urine retention symptoms. Mostly, in neurological causes of urine retention, chronic urine retention is seen and, in these cases, clean intermittent self-urinary catheterization is advised as first-line therapy to avoid complications such as renal failure, upper urinary tract deterioration, and urosepsis. Medications such as anticholinergics, alpha-blockers, and beta-3 agonists can be used according to the case.

Interdepartmental coordination between medicine, surgery, urology, nephrology, and neurology is required for the management of a patient with urine retention.

## CLINICAL PEARLS

- Retention of urine is defined as the inability to voluntarily void completely or incompletely.
- The most common cause of retention of urine is benign prostate hyperplasia. Other causes include urinary tract infections, neurogenic bladder caused by cerebrovascular accidents, multiple sclerosis, trauma, etc., and drug induced with anticholinergics being the main culprit.
- A patient with acute retention will have inability to void urine with a painful and distended lower abdomen.
- Chronic urinary retention presents with increased frequency of micturition with an interrupted or weak stream, along with urgency, hesitancy and dribbling of urine.
- The most basic investigation is ultrasound pelvis with postvoid residual volume evaluation. CT, MRI, cystoscopy and retrograde cystourethrography may be indicated depending upon the case scenario.
- The initial management of acute urinary retention involves prompt bladder decompression with urethral or suprapubic catheterization. The management of chronic urinary retention is based on treating the underlying cause.

## FURTHER READINGS

1. Meigs JB, Barry MJ, Giovannucci E, Rimm EB, Stampfer MJ, Kawachi I. Incidence rates and risk factors for acute urinary retention: the health professionals followup study. J Urol. 1999;162(2):376-82.
2. Jacobsen SJ, Jacobson DJ, Girman CJ, Roberts RO, Rhodes T, Guess HA, et al. Natural history of prostatism: risk factors for acute urinary retention. J Urol. 1997;158(2):481-7.
3. Leslie SW, Rawla P, Dougherty JM. Female urinary retention. In: StatPearls [Internet]. Treasure Island, FL: StatPearls Publishing; 2023.
4. SerlinDC,HeidelbaughJJ,StoffelJT.Urinaryretention in adults: evaluation and initial management. Am Fam Physician.2018;98(8):496-503.
5. Lapides J. Neuromuscular, vesical and ureteral dysfunction. In: Campbell MF, Harrison JH (Eds). Urology. Philadelphia: Saunders; 1970. pp. 1343-79.
6. Stöhrer M, Blok B, Castro-Diaz D, Chartier-Kastler E, Del Popolo G, Kramer G, et al. EAU guidelines on neurogenic lower urinary tract dysfunction. Eur Urol. 2009;56(1):81-8.
7. Selius BA, Subedi R. Urinary retention in adults: diagnosis and initial management. Am Fam Physician. 2008;77(5):643-50.
8. Hallett J, Stewart GD, McNeill AS. The management of acute urinary retention: treating the curse of the aging male. Curr Bladder Dysfunct Rep. 2013;8.

# PART 7

# Hematology

# CHAPTER 44

# Pallor

*Shuvra Neel Baul*

## DEFINITION

Pallor comes from the Latin word "palleo," a faded appearance of skin and mucus membranes.

## PATHOGENESIS OF PALLOR

Its exact pathogenesis is varied and may result from alterations of cutaneous blood flow, anemia, or unknown mechanisms. Possible causes include decreased blood flow, which may be locoregional due to thrombosis or systemic in situations of shock, and most commonly normal blood flow with decreased oxygen-carrying capacity that is anemia. Anemia, the most common cause of pallor, can result from decreased production of hemoglobin from bone marrow due to nutritional deficiency essential for erythropoiesis, inherited causes of hemolytic anemia due to thalassemias, hematolymphoid malignancy such as acute leukemias, and lastly peripheral destruction of circulating red blood cells.

## WHAT ARE THE POSSIBILITIES?

Pallor is a clinical sign, the presence of pallor in a patient are due to:

- Anemia, which may be the result of:
  - Chronic blood loss
  - Nutritional deficiency (iron and vitamin B12)
  - Hereditary (thalassemia major)
  - Acute leukemias
  - Pregnancy
  - Chronic renal failure
- White skin
- Cold exposure
- Shock due to any etiology
- Hypopituitarism
- Blockage in the artery of a limb
- Aplastic anemia
- Long-standing chronic inflammation

*Pallor with palpable lymph nodes*: When pallor is present with associated lymph nodes' enlargement, the possible differential diagnosis is:

- Acute leukemias
- Non-Hodgkin's lymphoma
- Chronic lymphoproliferative disorder
- Tuberculosis
- Human immunodeficiency virus (HIV) infection
- Collagen vascular disease [e.g., systemic lupus erythematosus (SLE)]

*Pallor with hepatosplenomegaly*: When pallor is present with associated liver and spleen enlargement, the possible differential diagnosis is:

- Thalassemia major
- Acute leukemia

- Chronic myeloid leukemia
- Chronic lymphocytic leukemia
- Non-Hodgkin's lymphoma
- Autoimmune hemolytic anemia
- Myelofibrosis
- Hairy cell leukemia

# PATH TO DIAGNOSIS

## History

Majority of patients with anemia complain of fatigue, decreased stamina, and light-headedness. It depends on temporal onset of anemia; most individuals are asymptomatic at hemoglobin 7–8 g/dL. Loss of appetite is also a frequently associated complaint. Diet history is also helpful in patients with nutritional anemia. Other important aspects of information from patients are history of chronic blood loss from the gastrointestinal tract and bowel habits. Another important aspect is drug history such as intake of aspirin, clopidogrel, nonsteroidal anti-inflammatory drugs (NSAIDs), and also any chemotherapeutic agents. In ladies, one needs to take in detail menstrual history to rule out heavy menstrual bleeding (HMB).

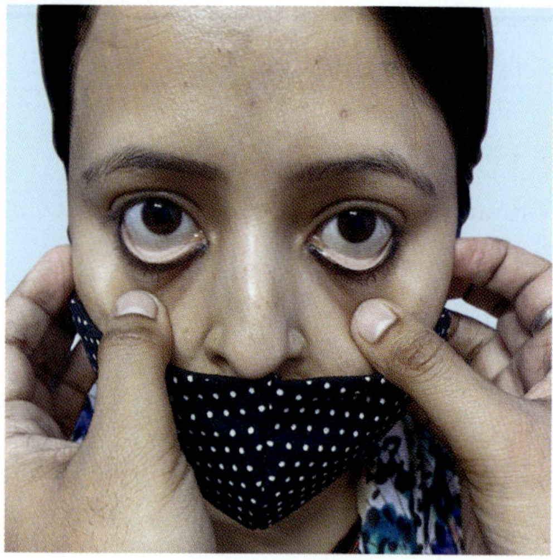

**FIG. 1:** Examination of pallor at palpebral conjunctiva.

## Clinical Examination

Pallor is most commonly examined in the lower palpebral conjunctiva by retracting the lower eyelids downward and asking the patient to look upward **(Fig. 1)**. The tip and dorsum of tongue are also examined for pallor; however, the color of food one eats may interfere with accurate interpretations. However, one should not forget the soft palate for pallor, which is the earliest site for pallor. Nail bed blanching and flushing is another method to examine pallor compared to physician's nail beds after pressing the base of nail. Palms, soles, and the overall skin surface are to be examined for pale appearance. Palmar creases become pale if hemoglobin is <8 g/dL **(Fig. 2)**.

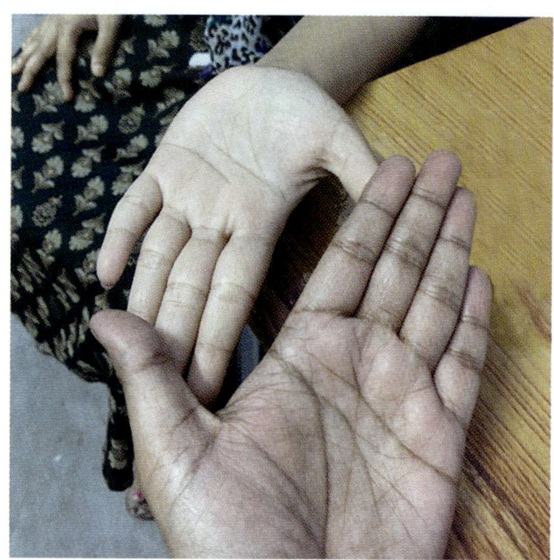

**FIG. 2:** Examination of palm with palmar crease demonstrating pallor.

One should meticulously examine the cardiovascular system for tachycardia, water hammer pulse, cervical venous, and location of apex beat for cardiomegaly. Auscultation over the pulmonary area for hemic murmur and mitral systolic murmur due to functional mitral regurgitation are evident when hemoglobin is below 6.5 g/dL.

## Investigations

The most important aspect for evaluation of pallor is complete blood count (CBC) followed by examination of peripheral smear of blood. In CBC besides hemoglobin estimation, one should check for blood indices such as red cell distribution width (RDW), mean corpuscular volume (MCV), mean corpuscular hemoglobin (MCH), and mean corpuscular hemoglobin concentration (MCHC). One should also check for reticulocyte count, which is an important key for classification of anemia. Based on MCV (<80 fL) classified as microcytic, if RDW is high one should ask for iron studies such as serum iron, serum total iron-binding capacity (TIBC), and serum ferritin. Based on peripheral smear evaluation for red blood cell (RBC) morphology and other formed elements of blood, needful investigations are to be planned. If MCV > 110 fL, one should ask for vitamin B12 and folic acid assay. If MCV <80 and RDW within normal limit, one should consider high-performance liquid chromatography (HPLC) to establish a thalassemia carrier state. If other formed elements of blood are low or circulating immature cells in peripheral smear, then one can plan for bone marrow studies. Ultrasonography of the whole abdomen, stool for occult blood, upper gastrointestinal endoscopy, and colonoscopy are important tools to rule out gastrointestinal malignancy in elderly people with iron deficiency anemia.

# THERAPY

The exact etiology of pallor has to be established first and foremost; therapy can only be effectively initiated based on etiology. However, blood transfusion should be avoided as far as possible by clinicians in patients with hemodynamically stable anemia. Thalassemia major patients need regular blood transfusion to maintain pretransfusion hemoglobin at 9 g/dL. Intravenous ferric carboxymaltose and iron isomaltoside are effective options in patients with iron deficiency anemia associated with oral iron therapy intolerance, inflammatory bowel disease, and celiac disease and in patients with heart failure.

# RED FLAG SIGNS

*Pallor with*:

- Shock
- Ongoing bleeding from trauma
- High fever
- Upper gastrointestinal hemorrhage
- Heart failure
- Unexplained weight loss

# CLINICAL PEARLS

Establish clinical pallor by astute examination.

One needs to establish the exact cause of pallor.

Therapeutic intervention can be effective after the exact cause is established.

Emergency situation in patients with pallor associated with red flags needs swift and effective therapeutic interventions.

# FURTHER READINGS

1. Ludwig S, Ku BC. Pallor. In: Shah SS, Ludwig S (Eds). Symptom-based Diagnosis in Pediatrics. New York: McGraw Hill; 2014 [chapter 10].
2. Drozd M, Jankowska EA, Banasiak W, Ponikowski P. Iron therapy in patients with heart failure and iron deficiency: review of iron preparations for practitioners. Am J Cardiovasc Drugs. 2017;17(3):183-201.
3. Jameson J, Fauci AS, Kasper DL, Hauser SL, Longo DL, Loscalzo J (Eds). Harrison's Principles of Internal Medicine, 20th edition. New York: McGraw Hill, 2018.
4. Greer JP. Wintrobe's Clinical Hematology, 14th edition. Alphen aan den Rijn: Wolters Kluwer Health Pharma Solutions (Europe) Ltd; 2018.

CHAPTER 45

# Bleeding Gums and Spots

*Shuvra Neel Baul*

## DEFINITION

Oozing of blood from gingival tissue, with occasional spots of blood on gums, is called bleeding gums **(Fig. 1)**.

## PATHOGENESIS

Most commonly, gum bleeding happens due to gingivitis, which is due to plaque deposits along the gingival sulcus. This plaque hardens over time to form tartar, which can lead to inflammation due to microbial infection and can cause gum bleeding. Fluctuation in estrogen and progesterone levels during pregnancy exerts an influence on subgingival microbiota and the gingival vasculature, and a spectrum of inflammatory responses in gingival tissues leads to gum bleeding in pregnancy. Mechanical trauma due to usage of hard bristles in a toothbrush and hard food particles can lead to gum bleeding. Gingiva, being a highly vascular tissue with an intact vascular system, is essential for the continued delivery of oxygen and nutrients to the tissues to maintain proper tissue function, this being the crucial reason for gum bleeding in patients with primary hemostatic defects such as low platelet number, platelet dysfunction due to drug effects, Von Willebrand disease, and lastly coagulation factor deficiency.

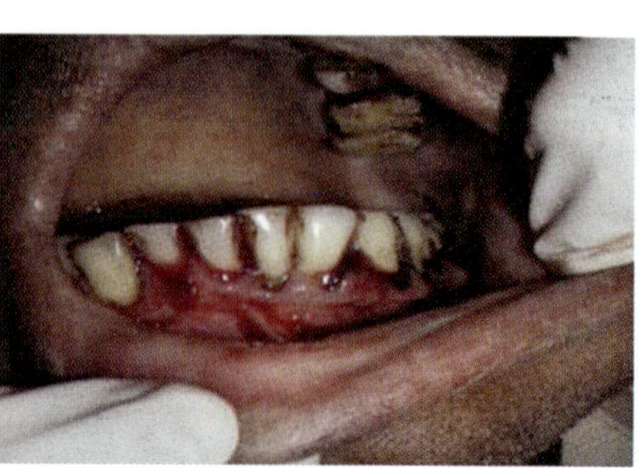

**FIG. 1:** Blood oozing from gums.

## WHAT ARE THE POSSIBILITIES OF BLEEDING GUMS AND SPOTS?

### Differential Diagnosis

The etiological causes of bleeding gums and spots are given in **Box 1**.

## PATH TO DIAGNOSIS

### History

Majority of patients with gum bleeding initially visit a dental surgeon as most causes are local gum and dental problems in which history of diabetes mellitus is important as poorly controlled diabetes mellitus are prone

**BOX 1: Possibilities of bleeding gums and spots.**

*Local*:
- Gingivitis
- Periodontitis
- Improper use of floss
- Vigorous brushing
- Poor oral hygiene
- Decayed tooth

*Systemic*:
- Drug-induced bleeding
- Diabetic mellitus
- Pregnancy
- Vitamin K deficiency
- Vitamin C deficiency (scurvy)
- Immune thrombocytopenia
- Leukemias
- Von Willebrand disease
- Hereditary platelet disorders
- Aplastic anemia
- Hemophilias

to poor oral hygiene, but if systemic causes are the reason for gum bleeding, detailed history is needed regarding any other bleeding manifestations such as epistaxis, vomiting of blood, frank blood in stool, or melaena. Another important aspect is drug history such as intake of aspirin, clopidogrel, nonsteroidal anti-inflammatory drugs (NSAIDs), and also any chemotherapeutic agents. In ladies, one needs to take in detail menstrual history to rule out heavy menstrual bleeding (HMB), and in pregnancy, gum swelling with bleeding is not uncommon. Family history of bleeding is also an important aspect. If one needs to rule out hemophilias, history of joint bleed with chronic joint arthropathy is also important.

## Clinical Examination

Oral cavity examination is of utmost importance to look for inflamed gingival tissues, caries tooth, and any wet purpura. Bleeding in the skin in the form of petechiae, purpura, perifollicular hemorrhage (common in scurvy), and bruises is important to rule out systemic causes of gum bleeding, especially in platelet-related bleeding. The clinician should meticulously examine the sites of pallor and any history of blood transfusion. Meticulous examination of lymph nodes, sternal tenderness, and palpation of liver and spleen is crucial for ruling out both acute and chronic leukemias. Examination for jaundice is essential to rule out chronic liver disease. In hemophilias, joint bleed and arthropathy are common, predominantly in large joints of leg, especially the ankle and knee.

## Investigations

The clinician should first ask for complete hemogram and check for hemoglobin and platelet count. Besides one should also check for circulating immature cells in peripheral smear of blood and to know the exact platelet count as sometimes platelet count is not accurately reflected every time in cell counters. The exact platelet count to predict gum bleeding or spots varies from patient to patient as drug-induced effects (such as aspirin, clopidogrel) cause platelet functional defect rather than quantitative deficiency. Uremia is also such a clinical situation of platelet dysfunction in renal failure patients. Size and granularity of platelet on peripheral smear of blood are important to know about hereditary platelet disorders. Prothrombin time (PT) is also an essential investigation of choice to rule out liver dysfunction or defects in factors I, II, V, VII, and X. International normalized ratio (INR) is required if the patient is on warfarin therapy to maintain it within the therapeutic range. Last but not the least, one should also do activated partial thromboplastin time (APTT) and mixing studies with normal plasma, and then needful factor assays to establish the exact deficiency of factors VIII, IX, and XI. Bleeding time and clotting time have nowadays largely been replaced with the above tests. Platelet aggregation studies with various agonists also help us to know about functional platelet disorders. However, the screening test may fail to detect all bleeding disorder; hence, other sophisticated tests may be required.

## THERAPY

Gum bleeding is best managed with proper dental consultation if the cause is local gingival factors; however, if it is due to systemic causes, the clinician needs to act prudently by dissolving tranexamic acid tablets in half glass of clean and plain water and ask the patient to swirl in mouth for 1 minute followed by spitting which is to be repeated every 2–3 hours till bleeding stops. However, if the cause is due to low platelet count, one needs to give platelet support, and if it is drug induced, one needs to stop the offending drug. Oral hygiene is another aspect of management because blood is a good source for infection. Eating fruits rich in vitamin C also helps in prevention of gum bleeding in scurvy.

## RED FLAG SIGNS

*Gum bleeding associated with*:

- Fever
- Other anatomical site bleeding
- Wet purpura
- Severe pallor
- Significant palpable lymphadenopathy
- Gum hypertrophy
- Sternal tenderness

## CLINICAL PEARLS

- Gum bleeding is a heralding sign for a serious underlying systemic illness.
- Dental- and gingival-related issues need to be properly managed for good oral hygiene.
- Gum bleeding needs meticulous history taking and clinical examination.

## FURTHER READINGS

1. Wu M, Chen SW, Jiang SY. Relationship between gingival inflammation and pregnancy. Mediators Inflamm. 2015;2015:623427.
2. Penmetsa GS, Baddam S, Manyam R, Dwarakanath CD. Comparison of the number of gingival blood vessels between type 2 diabetes mellitus and chronic periodontitis patients: an immunohistological study. J Indian Soc Periodontol. 2015;19(2):164-8.
3. Jameson J, Fauci AS, Kasper DL, Hauser SL, Longo DL, Loscalzo J (Eds). Harrison's Principles of Internal Medicine, 20th edition. New York: McGraw Hill; 2018.
4. Greer JP. Wintrobe's Clinical Hematology, 14th edition. Alphen aan den Rijn: Wolters Kluwer Health Pharma Solutions (Europe) Ltd; 2018.

CHAPTER 46

# Splenomegaly

*Debmalya Bhattacharyya*

## WHAT IS SPLENOMEGALY?

An increase in the size of the spleen, more than the normal range as a result of mechanical enlargement, is defined as splenomegaly. Signs and symptoms associated with splenomegaly may vary from being asymptomatic, mild lump, heavy lump, swelling, mechanical discomfort to serious pain, and heaviness in abdomen.

## WHAT CAUSES SPLENOMEGALY?

The anatomical structure as well as the physiological function of spleen gives a scope for its enlargement. As an important organ of the reticuloendothelial system, it gets enlarged due to various infective, inflammatory, congestive, or infiltrative pathologies.

## WHAT ARE THE POSSIBILITIES?

The current discussion is restricted to more common causes of splenomegaly, and the list of causes is not complete and takes into account possibilities to be considered in daily practice **(Box 1)**.

**BOX 1: Causes of splenomegaly.**

*Congestive*:
- Cirrhosis
- Heart failure
- Hepatic failure

*Malignancy*:
- Leukemia
- Lymphoma
- Myeloproliferative neoplasm
- Metastatic cancer

*Infective*:
- Malaria
- Kala-azar
- Histoplasmosis
- Tuberculosis
- Typhoid

*Others*:
- Hemoglobinopathy
- Autoimmune cytopenia
- Rheumatological disorders
- Storage disorders

*Systemic*: Cirrhosis of liver, heart failure, hemolytic anemia, hemoglobinopathy

*Infections*: Viral, bacterial, protozoal, fungal

*Local cause*: Thrombosis of portal vein, hepatic vein, or splenic vein

*Noninfectious immunological disorders*: Autoimmune cytopenia, systemic lupus erythematosus (SLE), rheumatoid arthritis

*Infiltration*: Metastasis, storage disorders

*Neoplasms*: Lymphoma, leukemia, myeloproliferative neoplasm

## WHAT IS THE PATH TO DIAGNOSIS?

### History

- Fever, alcohol intake, painful or painless lump in abdomen, associated jaundice
- Past history of anemia, blood transfusion, malaria, kala-azar

#### *Associated History*

- *Rigor*: Malaria, endocarditis, typhoid, abscess
- *Abdominal pain*: Infarction, infection, venous thrombosis, sequestration crisis
- *Jaundice*: Hepatitis, hemolytic anemia, decompensated cirrhosis of liver
- *Chest pain, palpitation, and shortness of breath*: Severe anemia, endocarditis
- *Gum bleeding and purpuric spots*: Hematological malignancy
- *Skin rash and joint pain/swelling*: Rheumatological disease
- Alcohol addiction history
- Travel to malaria/kala-azar-endemic areas

### Clinical Examination

Clinical examination is conducted to look for pallor, jaundice, cyanosis, clubbing, edema, lymphadenopathy, sternal tenderness, skin, and mucosa.

It is preferable to have a syndromic approach to splenomegaly, which facilitates narrowing down the differential diagnosis according to pattern of involvement.

#### *Systemic Examination*

*Respiratory system*: Evidence of consolidation, collapse, and effusion—miliary tuberculosis or malignancy

*Gastrointestinal system*: Hepatomegaly or lump (lymph node mass)

*Cardiovascular system*: New murmur, S3 gallop—infective endocarditis

### Investigations

- Complete blood count with peripheral blood smear, reticulocyte count, hemoglobin (Hb) electrophoresis
- Erythrocyte sedimentation rate (ESR) and C-reactive protein (CRP) level
- Total protein, alkaline phosphatase, alanine aminotransferase, aspartate aminotransferase
- Malarial parasite (MP) dual antigen, immunoglobulin M (IgM) for scrub typhus (after fifth day), Typhidot IgM, hepatitis profile, human immunodeficiency virus (HIV) serology
- Fasting blood glucose (FBG), postprandial blood glucose (PPBG), and glycated hemoglobin (HbA1c)
- Lactate dehydrogenase, creatine kinase, ferritin
- Antinuclear antibodies and rheumatoid factor
- Blood cultures
- Chest X-ray, abdominal ultrasonography, and tuberculin skin test
- Computed tomography (CT)/magnetic resonance imaging (MRI) scan if required for better visualization

It may be required to go for a fluorodeoxyglucose (FDG) positron emission tomography (PET) scan, which can reveal hidden inflammatory or malignant foci. Lymph node biopsy, liver biopsy, bone marrow aspiration, and biopsy from mass lesions may be performed if required.

## RED FLAG SIGNS

Seek immediate medical attention if any of these signs or symptoms accompanies splenomegaly:

- Severe pain in the abdomen, high fever
- Sever pallor—acute onset
- Difficulty breathing, cough or chest pain, palpitation
- Orthostatic hypotension and dizziness
- Icterus or ascites
- Bleeding in skin, gum, or elsewhere

## THERAPY

The treatment of the primary cause is the mainstay of therapy. Splenectomy is only indicated when there is huge splenomegaly causing mechanical discomfort and/or increased splenic sequestration. Often, a diagnosis of lymphoma is established only after histopathological examination of the removed spleen.

## CLINICAL PEARLS

Fever and splenomegaly may be associated with infection or hematologic malignancy. Splenic tenderness suggests the possibility of infarction, rupture, or abscess/infection. Ascites may be seen if there is severe liver disease and/or vascular obstruction.

The size of the spleen may be indicative of certain diagnoses but actually does not have reliable sensitivity or specificity. A massively enlarged spleen is often due to myeloproliferative neoplasms, lymphoma, transfusion-dependent thalassemia, or storage disorder.

Mild-to-moderate splenomegaly is seen mainly in chronic liver disease, acute leukemia, hemolytic anemia, or malaria. These are the most common diseases associated with splenomegaly, seen in the Indian subcontinent.

## FURTHER READINGS

1. Cesta MF. Normal structure, function, and histology of the spleen. Toxicol Pathol. 2006;34:455.
2. McIntyre OR, Ebaugh Jr FG. Palpable spleens in college freshmen. Ann Intern Med. 1967;66: 301.
3. Yang JC, Rickman LS, Bosser SK. The clinical diagnosis of splenomegaly. West J Med. 1991; 155:47.
4. O'Reilly RA. Splenomegaly at a United States County Hospital: diagnostic evaluation of 170 patients. Am J Med Sci. 1996;312:160.
5. Fremont RD, Rice TW. Splenosis: a review. South Med J. 2007;100:589.
6. Compérat E, Bardier-Dupas A, Camparo P, Capron F, Charlotte F. Splenic metastases: clinicopathologic presentation, differential diagnosis, and pathogenesis. Arch Pathol Lab Med. 2007;131:965.

# CHAPTER 47

# Lymphadenopathy

*Debmalya Bhattacharyya*

## WHAT IS LYMPHADENOPATHY?

Unusual enlargement of lymph node or lymph node groups is defined as lymphadenopathy. Nodes usually are <1 cm in their longest diameter, except in the inguinal region where these may be 1–1.5 cm in diameter. These are frequently palpable in the inguinal region in healthy individuals due to trauma and infection in the feet. Lymph nodes may also be palpable in the neck because of previous infections in oral cavity, scalp, or pharyngitis and tonsillitis.

## PATHOGENESIS OF LYMPHADENOPATHY

The pathogenesis of lymph node enlargement is multifactorial. There may be more than one pathogenesis causing the same lymphadenopathy. Primarily, lymph nodes are enlarged due to proliferation of cells in response to antigenic stimuli as in infections or as a result of malignant transformation. Large numbers of cells exogenous to the node (e.g., neutrophils or metastatic neoplastic cells) may enter the nodal structure and cause enlargement of the node. Suppuration secondary to tissue necrosis or caseation due to granulomatous infection is another reason. Vascular engorgement and edema due to acute inflammation may also play a role in the pathogenesis of lymphadenopathy. There are a few relatively rare pathological causes behind enlarged lymph node such as deposition of foreign material within histiocytic cells of the node (as occurs in lipid storage diseases).

## WHAT ARE THE CAUSES OF LYMPHADENOPATHY?

There are several reasons behind lymphadenopathy as follows **(Table 1)**:
- *Systemic infections*: Viral, bacterial, protozoal, fungal

**Table 1: Common causes of lymphadenopathy.**

| *Region* | *Most common cause* |
|---|---|
| Submandibular | Gum infection, head and neck cancer |
| Right supraclavicular | Lung, esophageal cancer, infection |
| Left supraclavicular | Gastrointestinal cancer, lymphoma |
| Axillary | Breast cancer, infection |
| Epitrochlear | Lymphoma, sarcoidosis, syphilis |
| Inguinal | Infections of foot, scrotum, sexually transmitted infection, plague, pelvic malignancy |

- *Localized infection*: Abscesses, empyema
- *Noninfectious immunological disorders*: Systemic autoimmune diseases, granulomatous diseases, vasculitis, autoinflammatory syndromes
- Neoplasms

# PATH TO DIAGNOSIS

## History Taking

- Duration, type, and pain of the lymph node
- Associated fever, weight loss, B symptoms
- Past history of tuberculosis (TB), lymphoma, other malignancies
- Associated lethargy, bone pain, any bleeding manifestations

## Clinical Examination

### *Physical Examination*

Lymph node groups should be examined with the following points in hindsight:

- *Location*: Localized lymphadenopathy suggests local causes and should prompt a search for pathology in the area of node drainage, with exceptions such as early stage lymphoma and TB. Generalized adenopathy usually suggests a systemic disease.
- *Size*: Abnormal nodes are generally >1 cm in diameter and are considered as pathogenic. But they vary with the region examined.
- *Consistency*: Hard nodes are found in cancer, whereas firm and rubbery nodes are seen in lymphomas and chronic diseases. Nodes in acute leukemia and inflammation are usually softer.
- *Fixation*: Normal lymph nodes are freely movable in the subcutaneous space, whereas pathological nodes can become fixed to adjacent tissues.
- *Tenderness*: Tenderness suggests recent and rapid enlargement, which typically occurs with inflammatory processes but can also result from hemorrhage into a node and in early cancers.

A complete physical examination should also be performed to look for signs of systemic disease.

**Differential Diagnosis Associated with Lymphadenopathy**

*Fever with lymphadenopathy*:

- Human immunodeficiency virus (HIV), infectious mononucleosis, cytomegalovirus infection
- Disseminated TB, brucellosis, secondary syphilis, toxoplasmosis, histoplasmosis coccidioidomycosis
- *Hematological disorders*: Leukemia, lymphoma
- Systemic lupus erythematosus (SLE), Sjögren's syndrome, rheumatoid arthritis, sarcoidosis

*Lymphadenopathy with purpura*: Dengue, leptospirosis, leukemia

*Lymphadenopathy with hepatosplenomegaly*: Lymphoma, leukemia, kala-azar, systemic vacuities, TB, brucellosis

*Lymphadenopathy with clubbing*: Lung carcinoma, infective endocarditis

*Lymphadenopathy with jaundice*: Lymphoma, carcinoma head of the pancreas, carcinoma, TB

### *Systemic Examination*

*Respiratory system*: Evidence of consolidation, collapse, and effusion—pneumonia, abscess, pulmonary TB, or malignancy

*Gastrointestinal system*: Hepatosplenomegaly or lump (lymph node mass)

*Cardiovascular system*: New murmur, S3 gallop—infective endocarditis

*Central nervous system (CNS)*: Neck rigidity, papilledema, cranial nerve palsy, weakness of limbs—TB meningitis

### Investigation

- Complete blood count with peripheral blood smear
- Erythrocyte sedimentation rate (ESR) and C-reactive protein (CRP) level
- Total protein, alkaline phosphatase, alanine aminotransferase, aspartate aminotransferase
- Hepatitis profile, HIV serology
- Lactate dehydrogenase
- Antinuclear antibodies and rheumatoid factor
- Chest X-ray, abdominal ultrasonography
- Computed tomography (CT)/magnetic resonance imaging (MRI) scan if required for better visualization
- Lymph node biopsy
- Bone marrow aspiration/biopsy and biopsy from any mass lesions if found
- If the diagnosis is still elusive, one may have to go for a fluorodeoxyglucose (FDG) positron emission tomography (PET) CT scan which can reveal hidden inflammatory or malignant foci from where directed biopsy can be done for histopathology or culture if indicated.

## RED FLAG SIGNS

- Severe headache, confusion, stiff neck, seizures
- Persistent vomiting, abdominal pain
- Difficulty breathing, cough or chest pain, palpitation
- Diminished urine output
- Icterus or ascites
- Bleeding in skin, gum, or elsewhere

## THERAPY

Treatment of the primary cause is the mainstay of therapy. Therapy targeting the lymph node only is seldom required unless it is hugely enlarged causing obstruction or pain or there is a discharging sinus or abscess formation. Proper treatment of the primary cause usually results in decrease in lymphadenopathy. In case of malignancy, a PET CT is often required after completion of treatment to find out lymphadenopathy and their metabolic activity.

## CLINICAL PEARLS

*Concern for malignancy*: In patients with lymphadenopathy, the probability of an underlying carcinoma, especially head, neck, and breast, rises rapidly with age. In children, retroperitoneal or mediastinal lymph nodes raise strong suspicion for malignancy.

*Latent TB*: In this era of antibiotics, often a diagnosis of TB is missed. Proper histopathological examination of the excised lymph node may be helpful.

## FURTHER READINGS

1. Ferrer R. Lymphadenopathy: differential diagnosis and evaluation. Am Fam Physician. 1998; 58:1313.
2. Pangalis GA, Vassilakopoulos TP, Boussiotis VA, Fessas P. Clinical approach to lymphadenopathy. Semin Oncol. 1993;20:570.
3. Lee Y, Terry R, Lukes RJ. Lymph node biopsy for diagnosis: a statistical study. J Surg Oncol. 1980;14:53.
4. Hurt C, Tammaro D. Diagnostic evaluation of mononucleosis-like illnesses. Am J Med. 2007; 120:911.e1.
5. Heinrich WA, Judd Jr ES. A critical analysis of biopsy of lymph nodes. Proc Staff Meet Mayo Clin. 1948;23:465.
6. Brindley P, Miller GV. Analysis of 600 lymph node biopsies. Texas State J Med. 1950;46:230.
7. Weiss LM, O'Malley D. Benign lymphadenopathies. Mod Pathol. 2013;26 Suppl. 1:S88.

# PART 8

# Neurology

# CHAPTER 48

# Headache

*Uddalak Chakraborty*

## INTRODUCTION

*"A detailed systematic history is the key to diagnosing and effectively managing patients with this common and disabling condition."*

The frequency of headache disorders in the general population is 48.9%, making them among the most prevalent nervous system illnesses. All ages, ethnicities, and socioeconomic statuses are affected by headaches, which afflict women more frequently than men. Certain headaches can be quite incapacitating and seriously affect a person's quality of life, costing the healthcare system a lot of money and indirectly harming the economy as a whole. Just a tiny percentage of headache diseases need a specialist's help. With a proper clinical diagnosis that does not call for further testing, the great majority can be successfully treated by a primary care physician or generalist.

## EPIDEMIOLOGY

Almost one in two persons report having headaches in a given year, which accounts for around 95% of the overall population. One in ten visits to a general practitioner (GP), one in three referrals to a neurologist, and one in five hospitalizations for acute medical conditions are due to headaches. The World Health Organization lists headache as one of the top 10 causes of disability, and among the top 5 in women, with an impact comparable to that of diabetes and arthritis, and worse than that of asthma. For instance, 25 million working days are missed annually in the United Kingdom due to migraines alone, with direct medical expenses such as medication, GP visits, and specialist visits amounting to approximately £2 billion annually.

## CLASSIFICATION

Primary headaches and secondary headaches are two different types of headaches. Primary headaches, such as migraine or tension-type headaches, are those with no known underlying disease. By far, the most typical forms of headaches are primary headaches. Headaches with a secondary cause are those caused by an organic pathology. In clinical practice, primary headaches predominate. A tiny percentage of individuals will get subsequent headaches, nevertheless. Knowing how to spot warning signs of organic pathology is crucial.

## HISTORY TAKING IN HEADACHE

- When did your headache begin?
- How many distinct kinds of headaches have you experienced?

- How often are your headaches? (To distinguish between chronic and episodic)
- How long does a bout of headache last? (Whether or not treated)
- Have you recently noticed a difference in the way your headaches behave?
- What are the pain's type, location, severity, and quality?
- What accompanying symptoms do you experience? (Such as dizziness and nausea)
- Are there any things that make it worse or better? (Early morning headaches that become worse with effort point to increased intracranial pressure)
- Are there any focal neurological symptoms present? (Aura-suggestive speech, sensory input, and visual cues)
- How do you deal with a headache? (Migraine sufferers often refrain from physical activities)
- Why does your headache worry you? (Many patients fear developing brain tumors)

## RED FLAGS IN HEADACHE

The warning signs (adapted from BASH, 2010).

- A pounding headache (intense, exploding, and hyperacute onset)
- A new headache in people who are 50 years or younger
- Continual morning headache and nauseous
- A patient with a history of malignancy has a new start of headaches
- A patient with a history of human immunodeficiency virus (HIV) infection has headaches for the first time
- A progressively developing headache over several weeks
- Headaches brought on by postural adjustments
- Symptoms of an aura that last more than an hour include motor weakness, differ from prior auras, and appear for the first time when taking an oral contraceptive.

## PRIMARY HEADACHE (TABLE 1)

Difference between the primary headaches are given in **Table 1**.

**Table 2** shows the difference between chronic migraine and chronic cluster headache.

## PATHOPHYSIOLOGY OF HEADACHE

The trigeminal, vagus, or glossopharyngeal cranial nerves, as well as the upper cervical roots, include nociceptive neurons that get depolarized to cause headaches. Direct electrical or mechanical stimulation of brain regions involved in pain processing may also result in headaches, according to data from operations involving intracerebral electrode implantation. In addition to direct mechanical, pharmacological, or inflammatory activation of pain-generating tissues, some less well-known activities that take place in primary headache disorders can also contribute to head pain. No matter what the initial trigger was, the transmission and processing of the unpleasant information were probably pretty comparable.

## WORKUP IN HEADACHE

*Infections*: Complete blood counts, CRP, ESR (nonspecific markers for infection).

A *metabolic panel* searches for metabolic reasons for headaches, while *endocrine tests* seek for abnormalities in the pituitary gland.

The preferred imaging technique for the brain is *magnetic resonance imaging (MRI)*.

**Table 1: Differentiating between the primary headaches.**

| *Migraine* | *Tension-type headache* | *Cluster headache* |
|---|---|---|
| *Episodic* | | |
| Unilateral (although often bilateral) | Bilateral | Unilateral (never bilateral) |
| Pulsating | Pressing, tightening, nonpulsating | |
| Moderate or severe | Mild or moderate *but not disabling* | Very severe |
| Aggravated by, or causing avoidance of, routine physical activity | No aggravation by, or avoidance of, routine physical activity | • Restlessness<br>• No aggravation by physical activity |
| • Nausea and/or vomiting<br>• Photophobia<br>• Phonophobia | No nausea, vomiting, photophobia, or phonophobia | *Ipsilateral to pain, there* may *be*:<br>• Conjunctival injection<br>• Lacrimation<br>• Nasal congestion<br>• Rhinorrhea<br>• Eyelid swelling/drooping |
| Attacks last hours to days (usually 4–72 hours) | Attacks last hours to days | Attacks last from 15 minutes to 3 hours |
| Frequency 1–2 attacks per month | | Frequency 1–3 attacks per day (up to 8) and usually occur daily for 2–3 months at a time |

**Table 2: Differentiating between chronic migraine versus chronic cluster headache.**

| *Chronic migraine* | *Chronic cluster* |
|---|---|
| *Chronic migraine or chronic tension-type headache*: At least 15 headache days per month for >3 months with the above clinical description, in the absence of medication overuse | *Chronic cluster headache*: Attacks occurring for >1 year without remission, or remission periods lasting <3 months |
| *Medication-overuse headache*: Ergotamine, triptans, or opioids taken on 10 or more days per month, or 15 days for simple analgesics, for >3 months. Chronic migraine is fulfilled 2 months after medication has been withdrawn without improvement | *No medication overuse headache*: Medication-overuse headache only reported in patients with a predisposition to migraine and/or tension-type headache; clinical syndrome of the headache exacerbated by the acute-relief medication overuse is of the migraine and/or tension-type headaches |

In order to improve the sensitivity and specificity of the structural abnormality detection, a contrast study is frequently advised. The differential diagnosis determines if vascular imaging is necessary. Depending on the underlying problem, more research could be necessary.

They might include *magnetic resonance spectroscopy (MRS)*, *biopsies*, and *positron emission tomography (PET) scan.*

If there is a possibility of a brain infection or idiopathic intracranial hypertension, a *lumbar puncture* may be necessary.

# TREATMENT OF HEADACHE

## Tension-type Headache

Most persons who get headaches of this sort are self-sufficient. Episodic tension-type headaches are self-limiting and seldom cause worry, but when they start to occur often and may no longer be responsive to medications, individuals consult specialists.

- Reassurance and treating the predisposing factors
- Over-the-counter analgesics (aspirin 600–900 mg, paracetamol 1,000 mg, and ibuprofen 400 mg) are sufficient without running the risk of consumption escalation.
- The goal of care for frequently occurring episodic or chronic tension-type headaches is long-term remission.
- The pillars of treatment for stress-related illnesses include modifying one's lifestyle to lower stress levels and engaging in relaxation or cognitive therapy to create coping mechanisms.
- The medicine of choice for treating depression is amitriptyline (10 mg at night, rising in increments to 50–150 mg when side effects permit); it should be discontinued if recovery has been sustained for 4–6 months. Sodium valproate (400–1,500 mg/day) can also be useful occasionally.

## Migraine

### *Elements of Good Management in Migraine*

- Accurate and prompt diagnosis
- Justification and necessary reassurance
- The doctor and the patient agreed upon high but practical goals.
- Identification of risk factors and advice on how to prevent them.
- Intervention (drug or nondrug, or both)
- Referral if these efforts are unsuccessful.

Several patients report success with straightforward oral analgesics, such as aspirin 900 mg, paracetamol 1,000 mg, or ibuprofen 400 mg, administered early and in soluble form before stomach stasis occurs.

The best option for treating nausea and vomiting is a prokinetic antiemetic (metoclopramide 10 mg or domperidone 20 mg), which increases the analgesic impact by encouraging stomach emptying.

Those who require triptans should not be denied medication. Patients may rationally attempt each triptan in turn since one triptan may help but not another.

### *Prophylactic Therapy*

- Beta-blockers without partial agonism [propranolol (long acting) 80–320 mg daily or atenolol (unlicensed indication) 50–200 mg]
- 0.6–2.5 g of sodium valproate daily (unlicensed indication)
- Daily 1.5 mg of Pizotifen
- 50–150 mg of amitriptyline at night (unlicensed indication)
- 1–2 mg of methysergide three times each day (hospital supervision recommended; restrict use to <6 months)

### *Cluster Headache*

*Acute*:

- Sumatriptan 6 mg subcutaneously
- Oxygen 100% at 7 L/min (requires special mask and regulator) helps some people.
- Analgesics have no place in treating cluster headache.

*Prophylaxis*:

- Verapamil (240–960 mg/day)
- Prednisolone (60–80 mg/day for 2–4 days, discontinued by dose reduction over 2–3 weeks)

- Lithium carbonate (600–1,600 mg/day), with higher doses and serum concentrations (0.8–1.4 mmol/L) over short periods in episodic cluster headache
- Ergotamine (2–4 mg/day per rectum, usually omitted every 7th day)
- Methysergide (1–2 mg three times daily)

## CONCLUSION

One of the most typical symptoms in the general population is a headache. The majority of headaches are migraines and tension-type headaches, which may be identified and treated in primary care settings or by general and emergency physicians practicing acute medicine with little knowledge and training.

## CLINICAL PEARLS

- Headache is one of the most basic and common symptom in the general population.
- Effort must be made to differentiate between the primary and secondary headaches.
- It is very important to go for proper investigations if one is dealing with a secondary headache.
- Treatment can be pin pointed if the headache type is diagnosed. Therapy should be individualized and tailored to each individual and his/her presenting complaint.
- To be vigilant of which headache should be evaluated immediately and which ones can be managed on an OPD basis.

## FURTHER READINGS

1. BASHH guidelines [Internet]. [cited 2024 Jan 2]. Available from: https://www.bashh.org/guidelines
2. Guidelines/ICHD [Internet]. 2023 [cited 2024 Jan 2]. Available from: https://ihs-headache.org/en/resources/guidelines/
3. Guidelines & Position statements [Internet]. 2023 [cited 2024 Jan 2]. Available from: https://americanheadachesociety.org/resources/guidelines/

# CHAPTER 49

# Convulsions

*Uddalak Chakraborty*

## INTRODUCTION

Although epilepsy is one of the most prevalent and severe neurologic disorders, our knowledge of its intricate pathophysiology and, consequently, the rationale for most of its therapy is still limited. In order to introduce neuroscientists to areas that could be subject to scientific inquiry, this chapter addresses the clinical features of seizures and epilepsy. Neuroscientists can design fundamental and translational research topics by understanding seizures and epilepsy, diagnostic techniques, numerous clinical syndromes, differential diagnosis, therapy, prognosis, and diverse clinical syndromes.

## SEIZURE

An abnormal, hypersynchronous firing of neurons in the brain results in a "seizure," which is a paroxysmal disruption of neurologic function. A seizure brought on by aberrant neuronal activity is referred to as an "epileptic seizure" in contrast to a nonepileptic occurrence, such as a psychogenic seizure. The medical term for repeated, unprovoked seizures is "epilepsy." Many factors can induce epilepsy, each of which reflects underlying brain dysfunction. As a seizure brought on by a temporary illness, such as a fever or low blood sugar, does not meet the criteria for epilepsy, it is not considered to be a chronic disorder.

Epilepsy is one of the most prevalent neurological disorders, with an incidence of about 50 new cases per 100,000 people annually. One-third of epilepsy patients develop refractory epilepsy, which affects around 1% of the population overall (i.e., seizures not controlled by two or more appropriately chosen antiepileptic medications or other therapies). Because the growing brain is more susceptible to seizures, around 75% of cases of epilepsy start in infancy.

## PATHOPHYSIOLOGY

The natural balance between excitation (E) and inhibition (I) in the brain might be thought of as being distorted during a seizure. A change in the way the brain functions, from genes and subcellular signaling cascades to extensive neural networks, can cause this E/I imbalance. Both hereditary and acquired variables can affect the E/I balance. For example, aberrant synaptic connection in cortical dysplasia, defective $\gamma$-aminobutyric acid (GABA) receptor subunits in Angelman syndrome, and improper ionic channel activity are examples of genetic diseases that can cause epilepsy [e.g., potassium channel mutations in benign familial neonatal epilepsy (BFNE)]. Similarly, acquired brain injuries can change how circuits work.

For a variety of physiological reasons, the growing brain is especially susceptible to seizures. Excitatory synaptic activity develops before inhibitory synaptic function, even in the normal growing brain, promoting increased excitation and seizure genesis. Moreover, early in development, GABA produces excitement rather than inhibition in the brain. These findings help to understand why the developing brain is particularly prone to seizures. Yet, compared to the adult brain, the growing brain is less damaged by seizures structurally.

## HISTORY AND EXAMINATION

Laboratory assessments are used as supplemental tests to the history and neurologic examination in the diagnosis of seizures and epilepsy. The clinical environment in which the seizure occurred, including premonitory indications, the specifics of the seizure itself such as phenomenology, responsiveness, focal characteristics, and the postictal state are all significant historical facts. If an epilepsy syndrome is present, it will define the kind and scope of the examination, the course of therapy, and the likelihood of recovery.

The neurological examination evaluates specific symptoms that might point to or locate brain disease. Increased tone on one side of the body, for instance, might be a sign of disease in the hemisphere across, such as cortical dysplasia. To ascertain whether the patient has an underlying disease, the general physical examination is crucial. For instance, aberrant skin markings might point to a neurocutaneous illness such as tuberous sclerosis or neurofibromatosis, where epilepsy is widespread.

## DIAGNOSTIC TESTS AND EVALUATION

- Routine blood investigations including a comprehensive metabolic and infection panel
- *Electroencephalogram (EEG)*: The electrical activity of the brain is captured by an EEG. It is capable of detecting aberrant electrical activity, such as diffuse bilateral spike waves or localized spikes or waves (which are consistent with focal epilepsy and generalized epilepsy). A typical EEG should ideally capture all three states of consciousness: Awake, sleepy, and drowsy. This is because the incidence of epileptiform abnormalities changes in each of these states. During an EEG, activation techniques such as hyperventilation and photic stimulation are used to boost the yield of epileptic activity. In a person who is predisposed to generalized epilepsy, photic stimulation may cause paroxysmal epileptiform activity or perhaps a generalized seizure. The diagnostic yield can be improved or an epileptic seizure can be distinguished from a nonepileptic event with continuous video-EEG monitoring for hours to days.
- *Magnetic resonance imaging (MRI)/ computed tomography (CT) imaging*: When evaluating a person with seizures, CT and MRI scans are crucial supplements to the clinical examination and EEG. For structural lesions of the central nervous system (CNS), neuroimaging methods are very sensitive. When a patient has focused seizures, unusual neurologic symptoms, or focal EEG discharges, MRI is more likely to reveal an anomaly. MRI is used over CT because it is more sensitive, particularly when looking for cortical malformations, dysgenesis, or hippocampal sclerosis. Asymmetries that are not immediately noticeable upon visual interpretation of the scan may be found using quantitative, computer-assisted volume analysis of the temporal lobes. In the acute context,

CT is useful for finding malignancies, calcification, and bleeding.

- *Newer imaging techniques*:
  - Functional MRI [blood-oxygen-level dependent (BOLD) technique]
  - Positron emission tomography (PET)
  - Single-photon emission computed tomography (SPECT)
  - Magnetoencephalography (MEG)
- Metabolic evaluation
- Genetic testing

## INTERNATIONAL LEAGUE AGAINST EPILEPSY CLASSIFICATION OF SEIZURES

This categorization now includes the following new seizure types:

- *Focal motor*: Epileptic spasms, hyperkinesia, and automatism
- *Focal nonmotor*: Emotional or behavioral arrest
- *Generalized*: Epileptic spasms, myoclonic-atonic, myoclonic-tonic-clonic, and absence with eyelid myoclonia

## EPILEPSY SYNDROMES ACCORDING TO AGE

- *Neonatal*: Familial benign neonatal epilepsy (BFNE)
- *Infancy*: West syndrome/Dravet syndrome
- *Childhood*: Generalized epilepsy with febrile seizures plus (GEFS+)/absence epilepsy in children/Lennox-Gastaut disease/Landau-Kleffner syndrome
- Teenage years and adulthood/myoclonic epilepsy in children

## SYNDROMES MIMICKING SEIZURES

- *Nonepileptic seizures (NES)*: NES are paroxysmal alterations in motor activity or behavior that mimic epileptic seizures but lack an EEG correlation. They are also known as psychogenic seizures or pseudoseizures. While not epileptic seizures, NES can be incapacitating and frequently indicate serious underlying psychopathology.
- *Breath-holding spells (BHS)*: Despite their name, they are automatic reflex reactions. BHS reach their peak in young children and are often outgrown by the time they reach school age. Cyanosis (also known as cyanotic infantile syncope) and pallid are two kinds of BHS (also called pallid infantile syncope or reflex anoxic seizures).

  The more prevalent variety of cyanotic BHS is brought on by rage or frustration. The child will cease breathing (in expiration), get cyanotic, and lose consciousness while wailing, which is characteristic of the condition. The youngster could then start acting stiff, limp, or even shaken, which raises the possibility of a seizure. Expiratory apnea, the Valsalva maneuver, hyperventilation, and intrinsic pulmonary mechanics are likely to interact in the complicated etiology of cyanotic BHS.
- *Syncope*: History typically helps to distinguish between syncope (fainting) and an epileptic seizure. Attacks may be preceded by warning (presyncopal) symptoms such as dizziness, nausea, pallor, and light-headedness. In contrast to a more sudden fall that is typical of a myoclonic or atonic seizure, these warning symptoms are followed by a loss of consciousness and gradual slouch to the ground. Due to cerebral hypoperfusion and hypoxia, there may be a short tonic or clonic seizure late in a syncopal episode; these are not epileptic seizures. When a more protracted postictal state follows an epileptic episode, consciousness returns quickly. The neuronal circuitry that is activated during the seizure that follows BHS or syncope results in generalized tonic-clonic (GTC) activity;

however, it is important to understand the processes behind this hypoxia-related seizure activity.

- *Parasomnias*: Sleep problems, known as insomnias, can occasionally resemble seizures. Between the ages of 18 months and 8 years, children might develop night terrors, a frequent parasomnia. The infant wakes up during early [nonrapid eye movement (REM)] sleep with uncontrollable screams, perspiration, and unrhythmic flailing of the extremities and then goes back to sleep with no recollection of the incident. Most commonly, nocturnal terrors run in families. Clinical history is used to make the diagnosis; video-EEG is seldom required. The primary differential diagnosis includes nocturnal epileptic seizures with frontal lobe origin and nightmares (which happen during REM sleep).

## DRUGS AND TREATMENT OF EPILEPSY

Up to 70% of newly diagnosed epilepsy sufferers can be effectively treated with a toolbox of more than 20 medications **Table 1**. Drugs used to treat epilepsy work by reducing brain electrical activity, either by preventing neuronal depolarization by blocking sodium or calcium channels, enhancing potassium channel function, inhibiting excitation mediated by the neurotransmitter glutamate, or promoting inhibition mediated by GABA. Depending on the cause, these drugs' effectiveness varies. The majority of patients with no known cause may be managed, especially if their neurological examination and developmental history are both normal.

In general, it is best to start taking medicine at a low dose to prevent negative effects. If necessary, dose increases might be carried out at regular intervals. With the lowest dose possible, seizures are to be controlled. When a first medicine fails, most doctors decide to add a second one before choosing whether or not to stop the first medication altogether. A 2-month study that is therapeutic and well tolerated is regarded as suitable. Combination treatment has the potential for severe toxicity due to medication interactions, although some combinations have proven particularly effective, such as lamotrigine + valproic acid for generalized seizures.

All seizure medicines have CNS adverse effects due to their mode of action. For instance, practically all antiepileptic drugs (AEDs) frequently cause drowsiness as a side effect. Lamotrigine requires a very gradual dosage titration but is generally well tolerated. If seizures have not returned in the past 2 years or more, some doctors think about quitting a drug. Other possibilities include nutritional therapy (ketogenic diet), resective epilepsy surgery (lesionectomy, hemispherotomy), and palliative epilepsy

**Table 1: Mechanisms of antiepileptic drugs.**

| ***Antiepileptic drugs*** | ***Mechanism*** |
|---|---|
| Phenytoin, carbamazepine, oxcarbazepine, lamotrigine, topiramate | Block repetitive activation of sodium channels |
| Lacosamide, rufinamide | Enhance slow inactivation of sodium channels |
| Phenobarbital, benzodiazepines, clobazam | Enhance activity of γ-aminobutyric acid ($GABA_A$) receptors |
| Lamotrigine, topiramate, zonisamide, valproate | Block N- and L-calcium channels |
| Gabapentin, lamotrigine | Modulate H-currents |
| Gabapentin, levetiracetam | Block unique binding sites |

surgery if medicine is unable to control seizures (stimulation therapy, callosotomy). Immunotherapy's function in treating refractory epilepsy is still being determined.

## CONCLUSION

For the purpose of enabling neuroscientists to evaluate the state of the field and develop pertinent research topics, this review provides an introduction to the ideas of clinical epilepsy. In a recent opinion piece, several clinical mysteries that require research attention were explored, and the following issues were judged appropriate for neuroscientific investigation: Epileptogenesis, neuroprotection, methods to better localize seizure onset and identify at-risk circuits with a goal of surgical intervention, how to predict (and thereby avert) seizure occurrence, optimization of medication for specific ages and epilepsy syndromes, the roles of genes versus acquired factors in seizure predisposition, and the development of epilepsy in an otherwise normal brain.

## CLINICAL PEARLS

- Convulsions are one of the commonest presentations to an Emergency. One must be adept as to how to approach this and treat any reversible causes.
- The semiology, localization and laterization of epilepsy.
- How to start and titrate AED's should be properly known.
- Newer therapies that include surgical therapies and other immunotherapies that can be used in refractory epilepsy.

## FURTHER READINGS

1. Specchio N, Wirrell EC, Scheffer IE, Nabbout R, Riney K, Samia P, et al. International League Against Epilepsy classification and definition of epilepsy syndromes with onset in childhood: Position paper by the ILAE Task Force on Nosology and Definitions. Epilepsia. 2022; 63(6):1398-442.
2. Guidelines [Internet]. [cited 2024 Jan 2]. Available from: https://www.aesnet.org/clinical-care/clinical-guidance/guidelines

CHAPTER 50

# Giddiness

*Uddalak Chakraborty*

## INTRODUCTION

Dizziness can relate to a bothersome disruption of spatial orientation or, more precisely, to vertigo, which is the incorrect impression of movement. Vertigo is a condition in which a person feels as though their body is rotating or swaying, their surroundings are moving, or both. Dizziness and vertigo are among the more frequent symptoms that people come with to doctors in general, not only neurologists, along with headache.

Experience has shown that before the right diagnosis is made and the right course of treatment is started, the affected individuals frequently undergo an odyssey of visits to doctors from different specialties, starting with their family physicians and moving through ear, nose, and throat (ENT) specialists, neurologists, ophthalmologists, internists, and orthopedists. To put it another way, these individuals frequently straddle many medical disciplines.

## HISTORY TAKING

- *Type of vertigo*: Postural vertigo feels like being on a boat, whereas rotatory vertigo feels like being on a merry-go-round (with vestibular neuritis and other illnesses) (e.g., in bilateral vestibulopathy). Many patients refer to lightheadedness without any feeling of movement as "dizziness" (e.g., in drug intoxication).
- *Duration of dizziness/vertigo*: Attacks may last for seconds or minutes (as in vestibular paroxysm) or hours (as in Ménière's disease or vestibular migraine). Persistent vertigo lasting days or weeks is seen in vestibular neuritis, among other conditions. Attacks of postural vertigo lasting minutes to hours can be produced, for example, by brainstem transient ischemic attacks.
- *Sensations of dizziness and vertigo* can occur at rest in some disorders (such as vestibular neuritis), while the patient is moving around (as in bilateral vestibulopathy), or they might be triggered simply by rotating the head to the right or left (as in vestibular paroxysm). Additional potential triggering variables consist of turning in bed [as in benign paroxysmal positioning vertigo (BPPV)], coughing, pushing, and loud tones of a certain frequency (Tullio's phenomena, found in perilymph fistula), as well as specific social or environmental circumstances (e.g., phobic postural vertigo).
- If present, *the concomitant symptoms*, which include Ménière's disease-specific bouts of acute tinnitus, hearing loss, and an ear pressure sensation, may come from

the inner ear. Symptoms of a central origin, such as diplopia, sensory abnormalities, dysphagia, dysarthria, and paralysis of the limbs and legs, often start in the brainstem. While a headache or a history of migraine may suggest the diagnosis of vestibular migraine, brainstem ischemia or posterior fossa hemorrhage can also result in the same symptoms.

## COMMON TYPES OF VERTIGO, PRESENTATION, AND TREATMENT

### Benign Paroxysmal Positioning Vertigo

The lifetime prevalence of this kind of vertigo is 2.4%, and it primarily affects elderly people. It is characterized by transient episodes of rotating vertigo and vertical placement nystagmus that beats toward the forehead and rotates toward the lower of the two ears. The afflicted ear must be positioned downward, either by reclination of the head or by lateral placement of the head or body. Rotational vertigo and nystagmus appear after one of these sorts of positional changes, with a delay of a few seconds, and then they follow a distinctive crescendo-decrescendo pattern, lasting a total of 30–60 seconds. The nystagmus is associated with a posterior vertical semicircular (PVS) excitation known as ampullofugal excitation.

The remaining symptomatic occurrences are typically brought on by head injury, vestibular neuritis, or Ménière's disease; >90% of cases are idiopathic. Moreover, BPPV occurs more frequently than usual during extended bed rest caused by other conditions or following surgery. Rare BPPV of the horizontal semicircular canal is brought on by head rotation in the supine posture. BPPV is referred to as "benign" since it often goes away on its own within a few weeks or months; however, it can occasionally continue for years. Around 30% of people continue to have symptoms if untreated.

Positioning techniques are used to cure BPPV. A quick change in head position can shift the otoconial agglomeration out of the semicircular canal, preventing it from causing positional vertigo. The Semont and Epley techniques are the preferred therapies. **Figures 1A to D** depict the Semont technique, while the Epley maneuver rotates the patient while they are lying flat with their heads hanging down. After a limited training period, the majority of patients can do these actions on their own. According to several controlled research and meta-analyses, both treatments are equally successful, and the cure rate is >95% within a short period of time. BPPV recurrence rates range from 15 to 30% annually.

#### *Vestibular Neuritis*

- Persistent rotating vertigo and a pathological tilt of the visual vertical axis in the direction of the labyrinth's afflicted side
- Spontaneous nystagmus that rotates horizontally in the direction of the unaffected side, giving the impression that the environment is moving ("oscillopsia").
- Alteration in gait and a propensity to fall to the afflicted side
- Nausea and diarrhea
- Both caloric testing and the Halmagyi–Curthoys head impulse test for the vestibulo-ocular reflex showed unilateral impairment of the horizontal semicircular canal **(Fig. 2)**.

#### *Ménière's Disease*

The membrane between the endolymphatic and perilymphatic compartments ruptures periodically in this disease, which is likely caused by labyrinthine endolymphatic hydrops. These ruptures trigger paroxysmal episodes, which can last anywhere from a few minutes to hours. The endolymphatic sac's decreased capacity for resorption as a result of perivascular fibrosis or endolymphatic duct obliteration is the cause in the end. Attacks happen when an endolymphatic tube

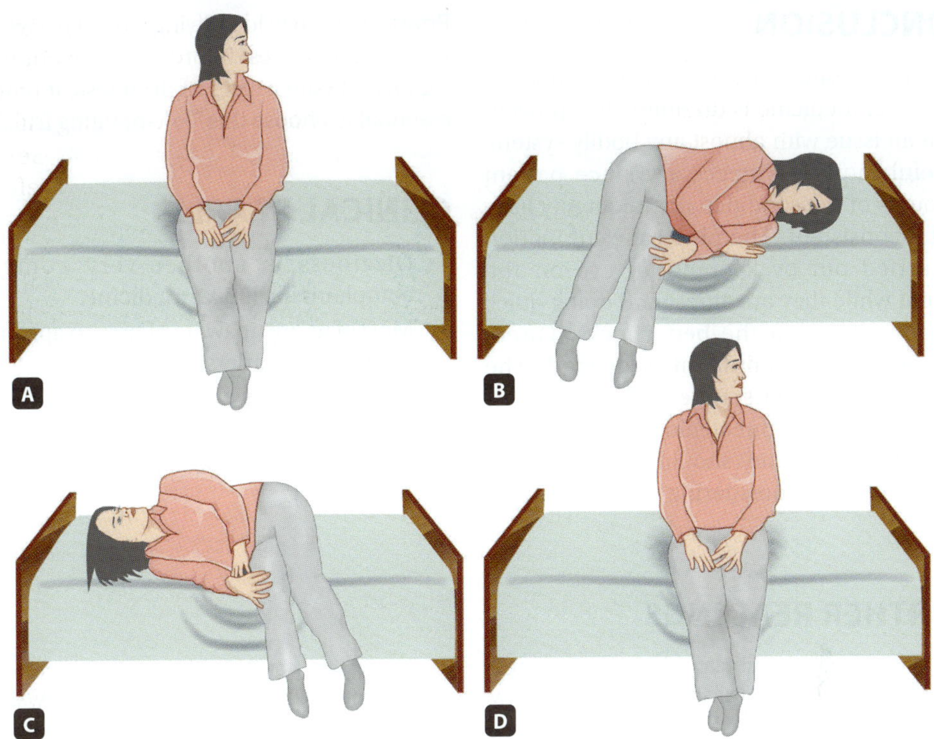


**FIGS. 1A TO D:** Semont technique.

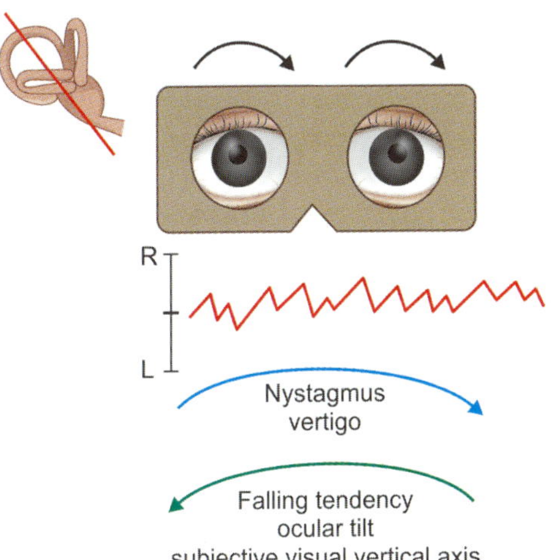


**FIG. 2:** Right vestibular neuritis symptoms and clinical findings.

rupture results in the vestibulocochlear nerve depolarizing due to calcium. Rotatory vertigo, tinnitus, hearing loss, and pressure in one ear are all hallmarks of a Ménière's episode. Around 0.5% of people will have this ailment throughout their lifetime. Attacks often start on one side, and the frequency might vary greatly. About 50% of instances of Ménière's disease result in bilateral involvement.

### *Vestibular Migraine*

Recurrent occurrences of rotatory vertigo that last anywhere from a few minutes to many hours are the hallmark of vestibular migraine. It is the most frequent reason for sudden bouts of vertigo. It has a 0.98% lifetime prevalence. The remaining individuals experience vertigo-only bouts; in >60% of patients, these attacks are accompanied by headache and/or photophobia or phonophobia. In certain instances, the diagnosis may only be made if the patient responds well to pharmacological prophylaxis and the drug used to treat the specific episodes. Similar to migraine with aura, the preventative therapy for vestibular migraine is giving patients beta-blockers, valproic acid, and topiramate.

## CONCLUSION

The most common symptom presentation in clinical medicine is dizziness. It can result from an issue with almost any bodily system. Careful inquiry is necessary since patient accounts of the condition are frequently hazy and inconsistent. The physical examination is carried out by keeping an eye on the patient while they are at rest and doing quick movements or at-the-bed checks. Often, no specialized equipment is needed. The characteristics that set these illnesses apart from benign to life-threatening conditions may be minor. Parsimony should be the guiding principle while considering diagnostic tests. Priority is given to identifying typical peripheral vestibular diseases. In order to rule out more significant core causes of dizziness, it may be essential to choose this "low-hanging fruit."

## CLINICAL PEARLS

- Dizziness is another very common complaint in clinical medicine.
- Most of us are unaware of how to approach vestibular disorders.
- Differentiating between central and peripheral vertigo.
- On when to take specialist opinion (ENT/ Neurology).

## FURTHER READINGS

1. International Vestibular Society [Internet]. [cited 2024 Jan 2]. Available from: https://www.intvest.org/
2. Medication for treating vestibular disorders [Internet]. 2022 [cited 2024 Jan 2]. Available from: https://vestibular.org/article/diagnosis-treatment/treatments/medication/

CHAPTER 51

# Abnormal Movements

*Srabani Ghosh*

## INTRODUCTION

Abnormal movements are a group of neurological motor disorders that cause either reduced and slow movements (bradykinesia or hypokinesia, such as seen in parkinsonian disorder) at one end of spectrum and increased movements (hyperkinesia) such as tremor, dystonia, chorea, athetosis, ballism, myoclonus, tics, and akathisia at the other end.

In most fields of neurology, the initial clinical approach is to determine where in the nervous system the disease process is located and then what is the cause. While dealing with an abnormal movement, the first step is to classify the disorder based on knowledge and recognition of the phenomenology. In spite of attempts at uniformity in definition, classification errors are common.

Abnormal movements may also occur with some systemic diseases.

## WHAT ARE THE TYPES OF ABNORMAL MOVEMENTS?

### Tremor

Tremor is a series of involuntary, relatively rhythmic, purposeless, oscillatory movements. It may be present at rest or action.

Rest tremor is present mainly during relaxation and is reduced when the part is used. It is seen mainly in Parkinson's disease.

Action tremor appears during some activity. It is divided into subtypes: Postural, kinetic, task-specific, and isometric.

Postural tremor becomes evident when the limbs are maintained in an antigravity position with outstretched arms. Common causes are enhanced physiologic tremor and essential tremor.

Kinetic tremor appears when making voluntary movement and may occur at the beginning, during, or end of the movement. The most common example is an intention tremor, which is found in cerebellar disease. The tremor appears when precision is required to touch a target, as in finger-nose-finger test. It progressively increases while approaching the target and is usually perpendicular to the line of travel.

Primary writing tremor is a type of task-specific tremor. It is a rare condition characterized by a 4–7-Hz tremor in the hand while assuming a writing posture or during writing. Men are affected more commonly than women.

Orthostatic tremor is a type of high-frequency (14–18 Hz) isometric tremor in the legs during standing. Affected subjects commonly complain of instability during standing. As soon as they sit or lean against a wall, the tremor stops.

## Dystonia

Dystonia is an abnormal involuntary movement characterized by co-contraction of agonist and antagonist muscles leading to deformed sustained posturing of body parts.

There is local pain due to excessive spasm and abnormal posturing. Initially, symptoms appear during specific activities such as writing, walking, and watching television; then it is called action dystonia.

Superficial sensory stimulus, such as touching skin of face, chin, or neck with finger, reduces muscle spasm in cranial and cervical dystonia. In cases of oromandibular dystonia, abnormal masseteric contraction leads to almost occlusion of mouth. Placing a piece of paper between teeth in some cases may relieve muscle spasm. The relief of muscle spasm by sensory stimulus is called sensory tricks. Prolonged spasm of the dystonic muscle may cause hypertrophy.

## Chorea/Athetosis

Chorea is a Greek word. It means dance. It is a type of hyperkinetic movement disorder. It consists of irregular unpredictable, brief, jerky movements that flow randomly from one body part to another. Athetosis means slow chorea, typically seen in cerebral palsy.

Most cases of Huntington disease (HD) occur in mid and late adult life; the onset of chorea is insidious and progression is slow. Initially, patients are often unaware of the involuntary movement, although there is incoordination and clumsiness, characterized by dropping of object from hands and bumping into things. In moderate-to-severe cases, there is involuntary jumping or jerking of the limbs or trunk. There is motor impersistence, manifested by inability to maintain protruded tongue (trombone tongue). Motor hypotonia may present with pendular reflexes. Dysarthria in HD is characterized by slurred, halting, and periodically interrupted speech. Disturbances in stance and gait may occur due to involuntary jerk. It may cause intermittent fall.

Causes of acute-onset chorea are Sydenham chorea, hyperthyroidism, cerebral infarct, systemic lupus erythematosus (SLE), antiphospholipid antibody (APLA) syndrome, and neuroleptic drug withdrawal. Chorea gravidarum may occur in women with a prior history of rheumatic chorea.

Chorea during pregnancy or history of previous fetal loss suggests possibility of SLE with APLA syndrome, even in the absence of other features of collagen vascular disease.

Hemichorea suggests a structural lesion in the contralateral basal ganglia.

## Ballism

There is abnormal high amplitude, continuous, rapid, nonpatterned, flinging movement of the proximal extremities such as chorea. Movement resembles normal throwing activity (ballism is a Greek word, meaning "to throw").

Chorea is more common and typically involves distal muscle group, lower in amplitude, less intense, more free flowing, and interrupted movement than ballism. Ballism is nearly exclusively unilateral, whereas chorea may be focal, hemichorea, or generalized. Ballism and chorea may coexist in the same patient or evolve into each other, particularly hemichorea or hemiballism.

The most common cause is stroke (either hemorrhagic or ischemic) involving subthalamic nucleus (STN).

Hyperglycemia patients may present with hemichorea-hemiballism. Characteristic imaging findings are putaminal computed tomography (CT) hyperintensity and T1-weighted magnetic resonance imaging (MRI) hyperintensity. Other causes of hemiballism are neoplasia (such as astrocytoma), infections (such as tuberculoma or abscess due to toxoplasmosis), surgery, autoimmune diseases (such as APLA syndrome, Sydenham's chorea, and multiple sclerosis).

## Myoclonus

Myoclonus is characterized by sudden, brief, jerky, shock-like, involuntary movement arising from the central nervous system (CNS) and involving extremities, face, and trunk. Occasionally, brief shock-like movements, clinically indistinguishable from CNS myoclonus, may occur from the peripheral nervous system disease.

Cortical myoclonus is the most common type of myoclonus. It is characterized by sudden-onset muscle jerk of cerebral cortical origin and distributed as focal myoclonus.

The subcortical myoclonus is usually generalized and associated with predominant involvement of axial, proximal, and flexor muscles causing neck flexion, shoulder elevation along with trunk, and knee extension.

Polyminimyoclonus is a small jerk in different areas of the body, commonly seen in spinal muscular atrophy and motor neuron disease.

## Akathisia

Akathisia means the inability to remain seated. There are two clinical components: One is sensory, characterized by inner restlessness and inability to remain still and another is motor, characterized by repetitive movement (such as tapping, body rocking, and leg swinging) to satisfy the inner urge to move.

The most common cause of akathisia is neuroleptic drug use that blocks dopamine receptor. It also occurs in Parkinson's disease, secondary to serotonin reuptake inhibitors, and in certain confusional states or dementia.

In mild cases, only subjective restlessness may be present, and it worsens with increase in dose of neuroleptics. Akathisia is a classic example of sensory movement disorder.

## Tics

Tics are very common and prevalent among children and adolescent. Affected subjects usually do not seek medical advice unless someone points them out or there is social, academic, or occupational interference.

Tics are sudden, abrupt, transitory, often repetitive, and coordinated brief and intermittent movements (motor tics) or sounds (phonic tics). They are voluntarily suppressible for variable periods, but this occurs at the expense of mounting inner tension which allows the tic to occur.

Motor and phonic tics may be simple or complex. Coprolalia (the utterance of obscenities) is an example of complex phonic tic.

In most cases, neurological examination is entirely normal.

## Parkinsonism

Parkinsonism is manifested by a combination of the six cardinal features: (1) Tremor at rest, (2) bradykinesia, (3) rigidity, (4) loss of postural reflexes, (5) flexed posture, and (6) freezing (motor block). The four major characteristics of parkinsonism are tremor, rigidity, akinesia, and postural disturbance (TRAP).

There is a clinical difference between idiopathic Parkinson disease (PD) and parkinsonism. PD usually starts unilaterally with prominent rest tremor and shows excellent response to levodopa. Parkinsonism indicates a person having bilateral symmetrical onset rigidity, bradykinesia, loss of postural reflex, mild tremor with or without additional clinical sign, and symptoms suggestive of involvement of other neurological systems.

# WHICH SYSTEMIC DISEASES CAUSE ABNORMAL MOVEMENT?

Some systemic diseases including autoimmune, endocrine, metabolic, hematologic, toxic and nutritional, infections, cerebrovascular, and paraneoplastic disorder may present with abnormal movements. So, careful systemic examination and relevant pathological test may identify the etiology.

## Thyroid Diseases

Enhanced physiological tremor may be the most common association of hyperthyroidism, occurring in as many as 97% patients. Beta blocker can effectively suppress the tremor.

Chorea may occur in hyperthyroid patients, which usually responds to dopamine-blocking agents.

Hypothyroid patients may present with truncal ataxia, which improves with L-thyroxine supplementation.

Antithyroid peroxidase (anti-TPO) and antithyroglobulin (anti-TG) antibodies may alter thyroid function in autoimmune thyroid disease and are responsible for Hashimoto's encephalopathy. It usually responds to steroid, so it is called steroid-responsive encephalopathy associated with autoimmune thyroiditis (SREAT). Brain MRI is usually normal or can show diffuse nonspecific white matter changes.

## Liver Disease

Asterixis and myoclonus can occur in hepatic encephalopathy, which is usually associated with a depressed level of consciousness and responds to ammonia-lowering agents.

Abnormal movements are more often observed in patients with acquired hepatocerebral degeneration (AHD), which is a chronic progressive disorder characterized by parkinsonism, ataxia, dystonia, and chorea. It is not associated with a depressed level of consciousness and does not respond to ammonia-lowering therapy. It occurs in advanced liver disease with portosystemic shunting. However, it is rarely found in cases with portosystemic shunting without any evidence of hepatocellular disease.

Parkinsonism in AHD is more symmetric, rapidly progressive, and associated with postural instability and action tremor, rather than rest tremor. Brain MRI shows T1 hyperintensity in pallidum with normal T2 and postcontrast images. The response to levodopa is variable. The patients often improve after liver transplantation.

## Renal Failure

Abnormal movements such as tremor, ataxia, asterixis, myoclonus, and restless leg syndrome (RLS) can occur in renal failure and uremic encephalopathy. A coarse action and postural tremor are often seen, which may respond to beta blocker partially. Multifocal myoclonus is effectively treated with benzodiazepine.

## Systemic Lupus Erythematosus

Chorea occurs in 2–4% of cases of SLE. It is the most common abnormal movement in SLE. Chorea may respond to low-dose dopamine-blocking agents. Intravenous immunoglobulin (IVIg) and plasmapheresis have also been used successfully to treat refractory chorea.

Dystonia, hemiballismus, tremor, parkinsonism, and stiff-person syndrome (SPS) may occur in SLE.

Stiff-person syndrome is characterized by stiffness and rigidity of the axial musculature with superimposed spasm. Muscle stiffness primarily affects the lower trunk and legs, but it can affect the arms, shoulders, and neck. Antiglutamic acid decarboxylase (anti-GAD) antibodies are frequently associated with SPS.

# OTHER SYSTEMIC DISEASES WITH ABNORMAL MOVEMENTS

Acute nonketotic hyperosmolar hyperglycemia may present with hemiballismus–hemichorea (HB-HC) syndrome, which improves with the correction of hyperglycemia.

Celiac disease is caused by autoimmunity against gluten, causing damage to the lining of the small intestine. It presents with gait ataxia caused by direct toxicity of antigliadin antibody to cerebellum, posterior column of the spinal cord, and peripheral nerves. MRI brain usually reveals cerebellar atrophy, both in the vermis and in the hemisphere. Sensory–motor axonal neuropathy is also common.

Parkinsonism is the most common movement disorder associated with Sjögren's syndrome.

Chronic vitamin E deficiency may present with spinocerebellar ataxia and peripheral neuropathy due to loss of myelinated nerve fibers in posterior column and CNS.

## WHAT INVESTIGATIONS SHOULD BE DONE?

When history and clinical features are typical of certain primary disorder, further investigation is unnecessary. Examples are physiological tremor, essential tremor, myoclonus, adult-onset focal dystonia, childhood tic disorder, and PD.

Wilson's disease must be excluded in chorea, dystonia, and early onset parkinsonism by slit-lamp examination, serum ceruloplasmin and copper estimation, liver function tests, 24-hour urinary copper estimation, and, if necessary, liver biopsy and genetic testing.

Chorea gravidarum may be a manifestation of the underlying SLE.

Hyperthyroidism, SLE, polycythemia vera, antiphospholipid syndrome, and neuroacanthocytosis should be excluded in chorea. Consider Sydenham chorea in a child and obtain antistreptolysin O (ASO) titer, antihyaluronidase, and electrocardiogram.

Search for vascular risk factor and hyperglycemia in case of hemiballism.

Antigliadin antibody should be tested in suspected cases of celiac disease.

Anti-GAD antibody for stiff person syndrome (SPS) and cerebellar ataxia.

Paraneoplastic movement disorder should be considered in patients with subacute-onset hyperkinetic movement disorder.

## CLINICAL PEARLS

Abnormal movement may occur in primary neurological disease or may be a manifestation of some systemic disease. History, thorough clinical examination, and relevant tests help us to reach a proper diagnosis and management.

## FURTHER READINGS

1. Jankovic J, Tolosa E. Parkinson's Disease and Movement Disorders, 6th edition. Philadelphia: Lippincott Williams & Wilkins; 2015.
2. Jankovic J, Lang AE. Diagnosis and assessment of Parkinson disease and other movement disorders. Bradly and Daroff's Neurology in Clinical Practice, 8th edition. Amsterdam: Elsevier; 2022. pp. 310-33.
3. Campbell WW, Barohn RJ. Abnormalities of movement. DeJong's The Neurologic Examination. Philadelphia: Lippincott Williams & Wilkins; 2019.

CHAPTER 52

# Facial Asymmetry

*Srabani Ghosh*

## INTRODUCTION

At rest, the face is generally symmetric, particularly in young individuals. An asymmetrical face is both normal and common. Often, it is the result of genetics, aging, or lifestyle habits. In some cases, an underlying medical condition may cause facial asymmetry. If asymmetry appeared suddenly or is causing discomfort or health problem, it may be a good idea to seek medical attention.

## WHAT ARE THE DISEASES CAUSING FACIAL ASYMMETRY?

- Note the tone of the muscles of facial expression and look for atrophy and fasciculations: Bulbar poliomyelitis and bulbar motor neuron disease (MND) may cause atrophy and fasciculation of facial muscle.
- In lower motor neuron (LMN) facial palsy, there is flaccid weakness of all the muscles of facial expression on the involved side, both upper and lower face. The affected side of the face is smooth, there is no wrinkle on forehead, the eye is open, the inferior lid sags, the nasolabial fold is flattened, and angle of the mouth droops.

The patient cannot raise the eyebrow, wrinkle forehead, frown, close the eye, laugh, whistle, or retract the angle of the mouth. A unilaterally widened palpebral fissure suggests loss of tone of orbicularis oculi muscle due to facial nerve lesion; this is sometimes confused with ptosis of the opposite eye.

Attempting to close the involved eye causes a reflex upturning of the eyeball (Bell's phenomenon). This is a normal response but only visible in the patient with orbicularis oculi weakness.

The patient talks and smiles with one side of the mouth, and the mouth is drawn on sound side.

The cheek is flaccid, and food accumulates in between the teeth and the paralyzed cheek.

Food, liquids, and saliva may spill from the corner of the mouth. The facial asymmetry may cause an apparent deviation of the tongue.

Leprosy may cause bilateral facial palsy with greater involvement of the upper face.

Causes of bilateral facial weakness and asymmetry are Guillain-Barré (GB) syndrome, diabetes, Lyme disease, human immunodeficiency virus (HIV) infection,

Melkersson–Rosenthal syndrome, and tubercular, fungal, and carcinomatous meningitis.

- In upper motor neuron (UMN) facial palsy, there is weakness of the lower face with relative sparing of upper face as the upper face has bilateral supranuclear innervation. Observe the depth and symmetry of a nasolabial fold. A flattened nasolabial fold with symmetric wrinkles suggests a UMN type of facial palsy. On the other hand, a flattened nasolabial fold with smoothening of the forehead wrinkles on the same side suggests an LMN type of facial nerve palsy.

  A lesion involving the corticobulbar fibers anywhere prior to synapse on the facial nerve nucleus will cause UMN facial palsy. The lesion may be in the cortex or internal capsule.

  Occasionally, a lesion in medulla may cause UMN facial palsy due to a lesion in the aberrant pyramidal tract. (The aberrant pyramidal tract is a normal descending fiber tract that leaves the pyramidal tract in the crus cerebri and travels in the medial lemniscus to the upper medulla and then ascends contralaterally in the dorsolateral medulla to reach the facial nucleus in the lower pons. Involvement of this tract explains the occurrence of ipsilateral UMN facial palsy in lateral medullary syndrome).

  Upper motor neuron facial palsy is of two types: (1) Volitional and (2) emotional.

  When facial asymmetry is more apparent during spontaneous expression, such as laughing, it is called emotional facial palsy (EFP). If weakness is more marked when the patient is asked to smile or show the teeth, it is called volitional facial palsy (VFP). VFP may result from a lesion involving the lower part of precentral gyrus (contralateral) that controls facial movements or the corticobulbar tract.

  In EFP, the weakness is more marked with spontaneous facial movements, and the patient can contract the lower facial muscles on command. The lesion is in thalamus, striatocapsular areas, or supplementary motor area of frontal lobe. The fibers that mediate the emotional response travel through pathway other than the corticobulbar tract.

- Infrequent blinking and an expressionless masked face may indicate Parkinson's disease. On examination, there will be rigidity, tremor, bradykinesia, and loss of postural reflex.
- Note the resting position of the face and whether there are any abnormal muscle contractions. Facial dystonia causes an abnormal fixed contraction of a part of the face, often imparting a curious facial expression.

  The procerus sign is seen in progressive supranuclear palsy (PSP) and corticobasal degeneration (CBD). There is contraction of forehead muscles, particularly procerus and corrugator supercilii, with knitting of the eyebrows, raised eyebrows, lid retraction, widening of palpebral fissures, and reduced eye blinking.

  Wilson's disease may present with facial dystonia (risus sardonicus).

  Spontaneous contraction of the face may be due to hemifacial spasm.

- In myasthenia gravis (MG), there is an expressionless face due to facial muscle weakness. When the patient attempts to smile, there is an upward contraction of the medial portion of lips, but the outer corner of mouth fails to move; it is called myasthenic snarl. There may be asymmetric weakness of facial muscle in MG.
- Some cases of muscular dystrophy can present with weakness and wasting of facial muscles. In facioscapulohumeral dystrophy (FSHD), there is wasting of facial muscle with severe weakness of orbicularis oculi and orbicularis oris. The patient is unable to close eyes during sleep. There is dryness and gritty sensation in the eyes.

The patient usually complains of difficulty in whistling, sucking, or blowing due to weakness of orbicularis oris. Sometimes, weakness is asymmetrical and appears unilateral.

They usually present with winging of scapulae and "Popeye sign" (wasting of arm muscles with sparing of forearm muscles).

Wasting and weakness of temporalis, masseter, facial, and sternocleidomastoid muscles give rise to "hatchet face" and "swan neck" appearance in myotonic dystrophy. There will be grip myotonia and wasting and weakness of forearm and leg muscles.

- In facial hemiatrophy (Wartenberg syndrome), there is either congenital failure of development or progressive atrophy of skin, subcutaneous fat, and muscles of one half of the face. Sometimes, there are trophic changes in connective tissue, cartilage, and bones. The disorder may be a form of localized scleroderma.

## THERAPY

Treatment of facial asymmetry depends on the treatment of underlying etiology and physiotherapy.

## CLINICAL PEARLS

Observing and analyzing the pattern of facial involvement has a significant impact on the anatomical localization and etiological diagnosis of neurological illness.

## FURTHER READING

1. Campbell WC, Barohn RJ. The optic nerve. DeJong's The Neurologic Examination, South Asian Edition. Lippincott, Williams & Wilkins; 2020. pp. 291-318.

CHAPTER 53

# Blurring of Vision

*Srabani Ghosh*

## INTRODUCTION

Blurring of vision can be due to neurological or non-neurological causes. Common causes of blurring of vision include uncorrected refractive error, corneal disease, cataract, glaucoma, diabetes, retinal disorder (such as age-related macular degeneration), and amblyopia. But our discussion will be restricted to neurological causes of blurring of vision.

## WHAT ARE THE CAUSES OF BLURRING OF VISION?

The localization and cause of visual loss can often be concluded from the pattern and temporal profile of visual loss.

### Pattern of Visual Loss

#### *Central Visual Loss*

A defect in the visual field surrounded by normal vision is called a scotoma (means darkness). Loss of central vision resulting in central scotoma (involves fixation point) is usually due to a lesion in the optic nerve or macula and is quickly noticed while peripheral visual field defects, such as homonymous hemianopia, can be asymptomatic. A cecocentral scotoma extends from the blind spot to the point of fixation. It is usually accompanied by loss of all central vision with preservation of a small amount of peripheral vision, and it strongly suggests optic nerve disease.

In general, scotomas caused by retinal disease are usually positive scotoma because they are perceived as a black or gray spot in the visual field. Positive scotomas are often due to exudate or hemorrhage involving the retina or opacity in the media. In contrast, optic nerve disease produces negative scotoma (areas of absent vision that are otherwise not perceivable, along with decreased color vision, contrast vision, and light brightness perception).

#### *Peripheral Visual Loss*

Visual field defect can be classified into one of the three groups: Prechiasmal, chiasmal, or retrochiasmal.

Prechiasmal lesion affects the visual field of one eye only, chiasmal lesion affects the visual fields of both eyes in a heteronymous bitemporal fashion, and retrochiasmal lesion causes homonymous visual field defects with varying degrees of congruity depending on their location.

## Temporal Profile of Visual Loss

Loss of vision can be *sudden onset or slowly progressive.*

### *Sudden-onset Visual Loss*

Sudden-onset visual loss can be transient, nonprogressive, and progressive. It may be monocular or binocular.

#### Transient Loss of Vision

*Transient monocular visual loss (TMVL)*: TMVL is caused by emboli from the carotid arteries, aorta, or heart to retinal circulation. It is called amaurosis fugax. These attacks are sudden in onset, last for several minutes, and are characterized by altitudinal visual field defect.

Retinal artery vasospasm may cause transient monocular loss of vision. It is called retinal migraine. It often responds to a calcium channel blocker.

Attacks of angle closure glaucoma may cause sudden-onset severe unilateral eye pain or headache, associated with blurring of vision. The patient complains of rainbow-colored halos around bright lights, and nausea and vomiting. Clinical examination reveals a fixed mid-dilated pupil and a hazy or cloudy cornea with marked conjunctival injection.

Transient monocular visual loss with increased body temperature is known as the Uhthoff phenomenon. This is due to a transient conduction block in the optic nerve and is found in multiple sclerosis (MS) patients with optic neuritis (ON). Vision returns to baseline when the body temperature returns to normal.

Monocular transient visual obscuration is brief episodes of visual loss in patients with optic disc edema with raised intracranial pressure. The visual loss lasts for only a few seconds. It usually occurs due to transient hypoperfusion of edematous optic nerve head, particularly during coughing and straining. Acute papilledema causes no impairment of visual acuity or color vision, except enlargement of the blind spot.

*Transient binocular visual loss*: Transient binocular visual obscuration can occur in patients with bilateral optic disc edema.

Simultaneous-onset complete or incomplete transient binocular visual loss may be due to transient dysfunction of the visual cortex. Cerebral hypoperfusion due to vasospasm, thromboembolism, systemic hypotension, hyperviscosity, or vascular compression may cause transient loss of binocular vision.

Visual migraine aura is probably the most common cause of transient binocular visual loss.

Although seizure disorder usually presents with visual hallucination (elementary or complex), transient loss of binocular vision may be associated with seizure disorder.

#### Loss of Vision without Progression

- *Sudden monocular visual loss without progression*: Anterior ischemic optic neuropathy (AION) is the most common cause of optic neuropathy in adults over 50 years after glaucoma. Predisposing factors are small crowded disc and vascular risk factors such as diabetes and hypertension. In AION, microangiopathy produces occlusion of the short posterior ciliary arteries and infarction of all or part of the disc. Visual loss is characteristically sudden in onset, painless, usually nonprogressive, and generally does not improve. Clinically, there is decreased acuity, impaired color perception, and altitudinal field defect. In the acute stage, fundus examination shows disc edema with hemorrhage. Later, there is optic atrophy.

  In patients older than 65 years with visual loss, giant cell arteritis (GCA) must be considered. The condition is associated with polymyalgia rheumatica, consisting of proximal muscle pain and stiffness, arthralgia, fever, malaise, scalp tenderness, and jaw claudication. The diagnosis is suggested by elevated erythrocyte sedimentation rate (ESR) and C-reactive protein (CRP), and confirmed by giant cell and endovascular inflammation on temporal artery biopsy. Vision loss is severe (decreased to hand movement perception or worse). In suspected cases, treatment with intravenous corticosteroid should not be delayed. The steroid helps to delay the progression of vision loss. Prognosis is poor, despite treatment.

Optic nerve ischemia almost never results from embolism. In contrast, central or branch retinal artery occlusions (BRAOs) are caused mostly by embolic or thrombotic events. Opacification of the retinal nerve layer with a cherry-red spot at the macula is the classic fundoscopic appearance of acute central retinal artery occlusion (CRAO). Retinal artery occlusion can cause altitudinal, quadrantic, or complete monocular vision loss.

- *Sudden binocular vision loss without progression*: Retrochiasmal stroke may cause sudden, permanent binocular homonymous visual field defect.

  Bilateral occipital lobe infarcts (involving posterior cerebral artery territory) can cause tubular visual field defect or complete loss of vision in both eyes (cortical/cerebral blindness). These may be due to sparing of the occipital pole (represents macular vision), which is supplied by the middle cerebral artery in some patients. Although acuity may be normal, the functional visual impairment is extreme because of constricted peripheral vision.

  Simultaneous or sequential bilateral ischemic optic neuropathy may cause bilateral vision loss.

### Sudden Vision Loss with Progression

Sudden-onset, painful monocular vision loss may occur due to inflammation and demyelination of the optic nerve (ON), caused by MS. Visual loss progresses rapidly over several hours or days (1–14 days). Pain on eye movement precedes the loss of vision in 90% of cases. The pain typically lasts for 3–5 days. If pain persists for >7 days, diagnosis of ON is less likely. Decreased acuity, impaired color vision, central or cecocentral scotoma, and an afferent pupillary defect (APD) are typical findings. Mild disc edema may be present in one-third of the affected cases. Prognosis for visual recovery is good in most of the patients.

Optic neuritis caused by neuromyelitis optica (NMO) and myelin oligodendrocyte glycoprotein antibody-associated disease (MOGAD) usually presents with simultaneous or sequential binocular loss vision with poor recovery even after treatment.

Progressive, painless vision loss may be a feature of Leber hereditary optic neuropathy (LHON). It is a maternally transmitted disease resulting from mitochondrial deoxyribonucleic acid (DNA) mutations. Vision loss may begin in one eye or simultaneously in both eyes. If vision loss starts in one eye, the other eye is usually affected within several weeks or months. There is severe loss of acuity, color vision, and loss of central vision.

### *Slowly Progressive Vision Loss*

Progressive vision loss usually occurs due to a compressive lesion over the optic nerve, such as pituitary tumor, aneurysm, craniopharyngioma, and meningioma.

Granulomatous diseases such as sarcoidosis and tuberculosis may cause chronic progressive vision loss.

Thyroid eye disease may cause optic nerve compression at the orbital apex.

Hereditary optic neuropathy such as LHON may cause painless, progressive loss of vision.

Glaucoma is a common cause of progressive bilateral, symmetrical visual field loss. The visual field defects are arcuate, and central vision is spared until late. Clinically, they have increased intraocular pressure and optic disc cupping.

Chronic papilledema from raised intracranial tension of any cause can produce optic neuropathy. Initially, there is a nasal field defect, later gradual constriction of the visual field occurs.

Toxic and metabolic optic neuropathies are bilateral and usually gradual onset progressive and painless. It develops over weeks to months, associated with dyschromatopsia, cecocentral scotoma, and development of optic atrophy later in the disease.

Medications that are toxic to the optic nerve are ethambutol, amiodarone, and linezolid.

Retinal toxicity is caused by vigabatrin, digitalis, chloroquine, hydroxychloroquine, and phenothiazines. There is painless progressive binocular vision loss.

Radiation therapy may cause damage to the retina and anterior visual pathway, particularly after direct radiation therapy to the eye or periocular region. There is a slowly progressive loss of vision. As there is radiation-induced capillary endothelial damage, radiation retinopathy is indistinguishable from diabetic retinopathy.

Paraneoplastic disorder may affect the retina and less commonly the optic nerve. Small cell lung cancer, gynecological, endocrine, and breast cancer are the cases of cancer-associated retinopathy (CAR).

*Functional or nonorganic vision loss*: A careful social and family history must be obtained when evaluating a patient with suspected nonorganic visual loss. Questions should be asked regarding abuse, peer pressure, and visually impaired friends and family members.

## CLINICAL PEARLS

Ophthalmic causes of visual loss are often not readily apparent to the neurologist, whereas neurological causes of visual loss often confuse the ophthalmologist. The neuro-ophthalmological examination by using ophthalmic tools and technique aims at neurological diagnosis. Many neurologists are not familiar with ophthalmic examination and ophthalmologists are often not experienced with neurological examination. So, the neuro-ophthalmological subspeciality helps to bridge between two disciplines. The approach to the blurring of vision should be systematic. Pattern of visual field loss and temporal profile help us with proper diagnosis and therapy.

## FURTHER READINGS

1. Thurtell MJ, Prasad S, Tomsak RL. Neuro-ophthalmology: afferent visual system. In: Bradly and Daroff's Neurology in Clinical Practice, Vol. 1. Amsterdam: Elsevier; 2002. pp. 164-90.
2. Campbell WW, Barohn RJ. The optic nerve. In: DeJong's The Neurologic Examination. Philadelphia, PA: Lippincott Williams & Wilkins; 2012. pp. 171-211.
3. Sadun AA, Currie JN, Lessell S. Transient visual obscuration with elevated optic discs. Ann Neurol. 1984;16:489-94.
4. Smetana GW, Shmerling RH. Does this patient have temporal arteritis? JAMA. 2002;287:92-101.
5. Newman NJ. Leber's hereditary optic neuropathy. New genetic considerations. Arch Neurol. 1993;50:540-8.

CHAPTER 54

# Slurring of Speech

Srabani Ghosh

## INTRODUCTION

*Phonation* is the production of vocal sounds without word formation; it is entirely a function of the larynx. Singing a note with mouth open is phonation.

*Speech* consists of words, which are articulated vocal sounds that symbolize and communicate ideas.

*Language is a mechanism for expressing thoughts and ideas as follows*: By speech (auditory symbol), by writing (graphic symbols), or by gestures and pantomime (motor symbol).

## WHAT IS SLURRING OF SPEECH (DYSARTHRIA)?

*Definition of dysarthria*: It is a motor speech disorder or disorder of speech articulation, without abnormalities of language.

## WHAT CAUSES DYSARTHRIA?

*Pathogenesis*: Dysarthria is neurogenic, related to dysfunction of the central nervous system (CNS), nerves, neuromuscular junction (NMJ), or muscle, with a contribution of sensory deficits in some cases. Abnormal neuromuscular (NM) activation of speech muscles, affecting speed, strength, timing, range, or accuracy of movements involving speech. So, there is abnormal articulation of sounds or phonemes.

Speech abnormalities secondary to the local structural problem of palate, tongue, or larynx do not qualify as dysarthria.

Complete loss of ability to articulate is called *anarthria*.

## WHAT ARE THE POSSIBILITIES?

### Types of Dysarthria

#### *Flaccid*

There is lower motor neuron (LMN) weakness of bulbar muscles, caused by polymyositis, myasthenia gravis (MG), bulbar motor neuron disease, and bulbar poliomyelitis. Speech pattern is breathy and nasal, with indistinctly pronounced consonants.

In pure dysarthria or anarthria, there is no abnormality of the cortical language mechanism. The patient is able to understand perfectly what is heard and, if literate, has no difficulty in reading and writing, although she may be unable to utter a single intelligible word.

In cases of bulbar palsy or LMN type of dysarthria, there is weakness or paralysis of articulatory muscles due to disease of the motor nuclei of the medulla and lower pons.

Tongue is atrophic and fasciculating (due to twelfth cranial nerve or nuclear involvement). Lips are lax and tremulous (seventh nerve/nuclear involvement). Saliva constantly collects in the mouth because of dysphagia and there is troublesome drooling (tenth cranial nerve/nuclear involvement).

Lesions of ninth and eleventh cranial nerves usually do not affect articulation.

As paralysis progresses lingual and labial consonants become difficult to be pronounced.

There may be nasal regurgitation of foods and liquids and nasal intonation of voice. Dysphonia may be present due to vocal cord paralysis.

Neuromuscular junction disorder, such as MG, causes progressive weakness of the voice with a decreased volume and at times the development of bulbar or nasal quality on prolonged speaking.

Differential diagnosis (D/D) in cases of bilateral acute-onset LMN dysarthria are diphtheria, poliomyelitis, Guillain-Barré syndrome, and Lyme disease.

Subacute-onset LMN dysarthria is caused by motor neuron disease and MG.

### *Spastic*

There are bilateral lesions of the motor cortex or corticobulbar tracts, such as bilateral strokes or multiple sclerosis (MS) and amyotrophic lateral sclerosis (ALS).

The patient may have had a clinically inevident vascular lesion at some time in the past, affecting the corticobulbar fibers on one side; however, since the bulbar muscles on each side are innervated by both motor cortices, there may be little or no impairment in speech or swallowing from the unilateral corticobulbar lesion. When another stroke occurs, involving the other corticobulbar tract, the patient immediately becomes dysphagic, dysphonic, and dysarthric. Although there is paresis of tongue and facial muscles, there will be no atrophy or fasciculation of paralyzed muscles. Tongue is weak and spastic. If tongue is protruded, it moves from side to side with difficulty. Patients often have the features of "pseudobulbar palsy," such as dysphagia, exaggerated jaw jerk and gag reflex, and also easy laughter and crying (emotional lability).

### *Ataxic*

Ataxic is associated with cerebellar disorder. "Scanning speech" is characterized by slow speech with excessively equal stress on every syllable. Ataxic speech is slow, slurred, irregular, labored, and jerky or explosive in type because of lack of coordination of the muscles of articulation. Causes are cerebellar stroke, tumors, MS, and cerebellar degeneration.

There will be gait ataxia, hypotonia, incoordination of limbs, intention tremor (tremor appears on reaching goal), and nystagmus with a fast component toward the side of the lesion.

### *Hypokinetic*

The voice is typically soft, breathy, and monotonous. Lack of movement or bradykinesia of the lips and tongue causes articulatory imprecision. This type of speech is found in Parkinson's disease. There may be pathologic repetition of syllables, words, or phrases (palilalia). Like parkinsonian gait, the speech may show festination, with a tendency to hurry toward the end of sentences or long words.

These patients usually have tremor, rigidity, bradykinesia, and loss of postural reflex on examination.

### *Hyperkinetic*

When chorea is present, the violent movements of the face, tongue, and respiratory muscles may make the speech jerky, irregular, and hesitant. There is marked variation in rate, loudness, and timing with distortion of vowel, harsh voice quality, and occasional sudden stoppage of speech. This speech pattern is seen in hyperkinetic movement disorder, such as Huntington's disease.

### *Mixed*

Mixed dysarthria involves a combination of the other five types of dysarthria. One common mixed dysarthria is spastic-flaccid dysarthria, seen in ALS. The ALS patient has the harsh, strain-strangle voice quality of spastic dysarthria, combined with the breathy and hypernasal quality of flaccid dysarthria.

Multiple sclerosis may feature a spastic–flaccid–ataxic or spastic–ataxic mixed dysarthria, in which slow rate or irregular breakdowns are added to the other characteristics seen in spastic and flaccid dysarthria.

Wilson's disease can cause hypokinetic, spastic, ataxic, and dystonic dysarthria.

## THERAPY

The management of dysarthria includes:

- Speech therapy techniques for strengthening muscles
- Training more precise articulation
- Slowing the rate of speech to increase intelligibility
- Teaching the patient to stress specific phonemes

*Devices*:

- Palatal lifts to reduce hypernasality
- Amplifiers to increase voice volume
- Communication boards to point to pictures
- Augmentative communication devices
- Computer techniques can be used when the patient is unable to communicate in speech.

*Surgical techniques*:

- Pharyngeal flap to reduce hypernasality
- Vocal fold Teflon injection or transposition surgery to increase loudness may help the patient to speak more intelligibly.

In Parkinson's disease, most patients have elements of dysarthria and dysphonia, and treatment can include speech therapy, drug treatment, deep brain stimulation, and even surgery.

## CLINICAL PEARLS

Analysis of pattern or type of dysarthria has immense value in anatomical localization and thus diagnosis of neurological diseases. So, it is very important to talk with the patient and listen attentively how her speech is deviated from normal.

## FURTHER READING

1. Krishner HS. Dysarthria and Apraxia of Speech, 8th edition. Neurology in clinical practice: Bradley and Daroff's; 2022. pp. 149-51.

CHAPTER 55

# Hemiplegia

*Amlan Kusum Datta*

## WHAT IS HEMIPLEGIA?

Hemiplegia is defined as weakness of one half of the body. Although hemiplegia is a motor phenomenon, sensory deficits are an integral feature that aid in clinical-anatomical localization. In certain circumstances, involvement of cranial nerves additionally helps in the localization of culprit lesion. A paucity of power must always be differentiated from a lack of volition, i.e., akinesia. Volition, or the motivation to initiate motor activity, originates from the prefrontal cortex, which projects to the motor strip in the frontal lobe to activate the corticospinal tract (CST).

## WHAT CAUSES HEMIPLEGIA?

Focal deficit, such as hemiplegia, is usually attributed to a discrete, well-defined structural lesion within the central nervous system (CNS); thereby, a crisp and clear understanding of the anatomy of the CST is paramount.

### Overview of the Corticospinal Tract (Fig. 1)

*Origin*: The pyramidal tract originates from layer V of the neocortex, specifically from the giant cells of Betz.

- Primary motor cortex (area 4)—30%
- Premotor and supplementary motor cortex (area 6)—30%
- Somatosensory cortex (areas 3, 1, 2), superior parietal lobule (area 5), and cingulate—40%

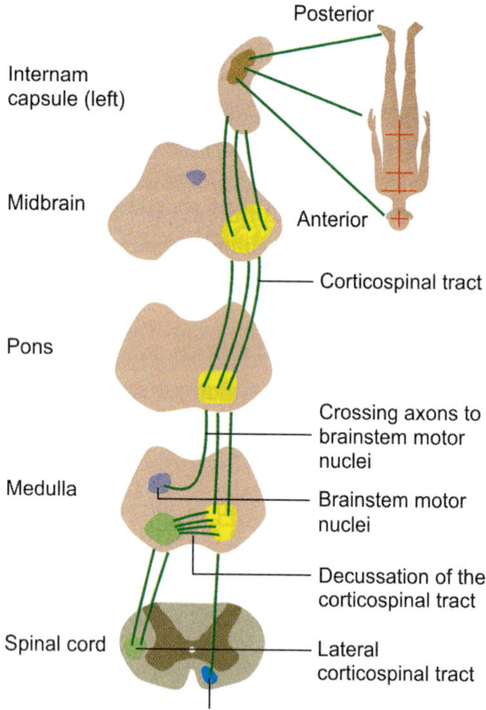


**FIG. 1:** Overview of corticospinal tract with somatotropic organization in cerebral cortex, brainstem and spinal cord. However, discrete lesions below the cerebral cortex are unlikely to produce topographically specific damage.

*Course and termination*: The fibers descend uncrossed and converge in the subcortical white matter of the corona radiata. The descent continues through the anterior two-thirds of the posterior limb of the internal capsule (PLIC), cerebral peduncle, ventral pons (basis pontis), and the pyramids of the upper medulla. It is here that decussation of most fibers occurs. The corticobulbar fibers converge on their respective contralateral cranial nerve nuclei in the brainstem. The lateral CST (75–80% of fibers) decussates at the lower medulla (upper extremity fibers decussate more rostrally than the lower extremity) and descends in the lateral funiculus of the spinal cord (lateral CST). The remaining 20–25% of fibers remain uncrossed, descend ipsilaterally, and decussate at the level of the local spinal synapse (ventral CST). Throughout its course, the somatotropic organization of the CST is maintained at all levels **(Fig. 1)**:

- *Cortex*: Face and arms are represented laterally and the legs medially. The cortical representation of the distal portion of the legs is situated on the central sulcus.
- *Subcortical*: Same as cortex
- *Midbrain*: CST fibers occupy the middle of the cerebral peduncle with the facial fibers situated medially.
- *Pons*: Hands—ventromedial; legs—dorsolateral
- *Medulla*: Hands—medial; legs—lateral
- *Spinal cord*: CST fibers of sacral segment lie most laterally, whereas those of the cervical lie medially [cervical, thoracic, lumbar, sacral *(CTLS)*: Medial to lateral].

  Possible sites of such lesions include the following:
- *Cortex*: It usually produces focal deficits such as weakness of the leg, face, and hand. Hemiplegia is unusual unless caused by a large lesion such as a cortical stroke due to occlusion of the ipsilateral internal carotid artery (ICA) or a large tumor.
- *Subcortical*: It is usually motor predominant or pure motor syndromes with involvement of the leg, arm, and face to equal degrees. Sensory signs are normally absent or subtle unless there is thalamic involvement, in which case deficits are sensory predominant with the presence of contralateral abnormal movements such as choreoathetosis or ballism with hemiplegia being unusual.
- *Cortical and subcortical*: Variable combinations of motor and sensory deficits with the presence of higher-order deficits (in the case of cortical lesion) such as aphasia (dominant hemisphere) and neglect (nondominant hemisphere). A lesion at internal capsule causes paralysis of the face, arm, and leg to equal extent along with ipsilateral hemianesthesia and hemianopia (*dense hemiplegia*).
- *Brainstem*: Brainstem lesions producing hemiplegia are always associated with cranial neuropathies, sensory signs and symptoms, and signs of brainstem dysfunction; hence, they are easy to localize.
  - Ipsilateral facial sensory deficit (mid-pons trigeminal lesion)
  - Ipsilateral hemiataxia (damage to cerebellar hemispheres, nuclei, or fibers)
  - Ipsilateral Horner's syndrome (damage to descending sympathetic tract above T1 level)
  - Crossed hemiparesis (ipsilateral cranial nerve dysfunction and contralateral motor weakness)
  - Crossed sensory deficit (lesions of the caudal medulla might cause ipsilateral loss of contralateral pain, temperature, ipsilateral position, and joint sense)
- *Spinal cord*: Noncompressive pathologies, such as demyelination or spinal infarction, can occasionally cause hemiplegia with sparing of the face and cranial nerves (except for high cervical lesions). Compressive pathologies, such as tumors or trauma, producing hemiplegia are usually intradural. Extradural lesions, such as spondylotic myelopathy, disc disease, and most extradural tumors, are expected to cause bilateral symmetric

deficits below the level of lesion. A spinal hemisection syndrome (Brown-Sequard syndrome) produces weakness ipsilateral to and below the lesion with affection of position sense on the same side, whereas loss of pain and temperature occurs contralateral to the lesion.

## WHAT ARE THE POSSIBILITIES?

*Differential diagnosis of hemiplegia is vast and needs meticulous exclusion by history, examination, and investigations* **(Table 1)**.

## PATH TO DIAGNOSIS

### History

- *Mode of onset*:
  - Abrupt/acute: Vascular (infarction or hemorrhage)
  - Subacute (over days to weeks): Demyelination, infection, tumors
  - Chronic (over months to years): Tumors (may be abrupt if there is hemorrhage within a tumor or if the tumor affects vasculature, producing infarction), amyotrophic lateral sclerosis (ALS)
- *Course of deficit*:
  - Monophasic with recovery: Transient ischemic attack (TIA) (over minutes to hours)
  - Monophasic without recovery: Stroke, acute demyelinating encephalomyelitis (ADEM)
  - Relapsing/remitting: Multiple sclerosis (MS)
  - Slowly progressive: Tumors
- *Progression*:
  - Over seconds to minutes: Migraine, epilepsy
  - Over minutes to hours: Stroke
  - Over days: Demyelination or infection, some cases of stuttering stroke (usually lacunar)
  - Over weeks: Mass lesion

**Table 1: Differential diagnosis of hemiplegia.**

| *Site of lesion* | *Etiology* | *Clinical clue(s)* |
|---|---|---|
| Cortex | Ischemic stroke | Cortical infarcts/hemorrhages are more likely to produce focal, discrete defects such as of leg, face, and hand rather than hemiplegia |
| | Seizure-related: Todd's palsy and ictal paralysis | Marching pattern of motor deficit with or without cortical signs; transient, lasting minutes to hours; abnormal EEG (slow waves or periodic lateralized epileptiform discharges) |
| | Alternating hemiplegia of childhood | Young child with bouts of recurrent hemiparesis particularly on awakening, without headache. Normal brain and vascular imaging |
| Subcortical | Stroke (infarction and hemorrhage) | Usually acute onset, however, might be steadily progressive or stuttering (lacunar infarctions more likely to be stuttering) |
| | Multiple sclerosis (MS) | Progression over days with prior history of neurological deficits or a relapsing-remitting course |
| Cortical, subcortical, and brainstem | Infarction and hemorrhage | • Acute onset; might be progressive or stuttering in some cases; cortical lesions can cause additional signs aphasia and neglect<br>• Usually associated with headache, fever, altered mental state, and/or seizures |

Continued

*Continued*

| *Site of lesion* | *Etiology* | *Clinical clue(s)* |
| --- | --- | --- |
| | Infection (abscess, encephalitis) | Combination of motor and sensory deficits not restricted to one vascular territory; associated with headache and seizures |
| | Mass lesion | Usually monophasic but may represent the first attack of MS |
| | *Autoimmune*:<br>• Acute demyelinating encephalomyelitis (ADEM)<br>• Sarcoidosis<br>*Migraine* | • Presence of aseptic meningitis, multiple mononeuropathies<br>• Young age + few or no vascular risk factors + marching pattern of deficit, with onset of hemiplegia before onset of headache; often familial |
| Spinal cord | *Noncompressive*: Demyelination (MS) | Brown–Sequard syndrome; peripheral enhancing cord lesions on MRI |
| | *Compressive*: Intradural tumors (meningioma, neurofibroma, lymphoma, metastasis) | Usually slowly progressive with late bladder involvement. Confirmation by MRI with gadolinium enhancement |
| Peripheral lesions | • Radiculopathy (multiple-level disc disease)<br>• Plexopathy (infection, inflammation, tumors)<br>• Mononeuritis multiplex (diabetes, leprosy, vasculitis, pressure palsies) | Pattern of weakness within the distribution of one nerve, plexus, or nerve root; widespread early LMN signs; confirmation by nerve conduction studies (NCS) and electromyography (EMG) |
| | Amyotrophic lateral sclerosis | Absence of sensory signs, slow progression, combination of UMN and LMN signs. Confirmation by EMG |
| Psychogenic hemiplegia | • Conversion disorder (patient is not conscious of the nonorganic nature of the deficit)<br>• Malingering (a conscious effort on part of the patient for secondary gains) | • Improvement in strength with entrainment<br>• Give-away weakness<br>• *Inconsistent examination patterns*: Inability to dorsiflex foot but able to walk on toes<br>• Hoover's sign (the patient lies supine with the examiner's one hand under the heel of apparently normal foot and another testing the power of apparently paralyzed leg. If the leg is truly paralyzed, the examiner feels a downward press on the opposite heel. Failure to do so constitutes the Hoover's sign)<br>• Paralysis in the absence of other signs of CST dysfunction such as changes in tone and reflexes |

(CST: corticospinal tract; EEG: electroencephalography; LMN: lower motor neuron; MRI: magnetic resonance imaging; UMN: upper motor neuron)

**Table 2: Differentiating migraine/stroke/seizure.**

| | *Migraine* | *Stroke/TIA* | *Seizures* |
|---|---|---|---|
| Warning | Often prodrome or aura | Usually none | Can begin with aura |
| Onset | Marching from one region to another | Acute onset, no march. Can be progressive or stuttering | Can march through an entire extremity and involve one or both sides (generalization) |
| Accompanying features | Usually but not always, headache. Nausea/ photophobia. Headache may accompany or follow motor deficit | No headache unless hemorrhage. Upper motor neuron facial weakness is very suggestive of stroke | Usually positive motor symptoms, rarely paretic. Postictal confusion |
| Distribution of deficit | Usually focal weakness; hemiplegia unlikely | Usually hemiplegia but arm/face or leg predominant depending on vascular territory involved | Usually focal tonic and/or clonic activity; paretic seizure rare and can be difficult to differentiate from strokes |
| Imaging of brain | Usually normal | Almost all strokes and 40% of TIA show restriction on diffusion-weighted imaging (DWI) of MRI | Can be associated with embolic strokes |

(MRI: magnetic resonance imaging; TIA: transient ischemic attack)

## Clinical Examination (Table 2)

- *Signs*:
  - Attitude:
    - Upper limbs: Preferential weakness of finger and wrist extensor, forearm supinator, elbow extensor, shoulder external rotator, and abductors (as a result, *hemiparetic upper limb is adducted and internally rotated at shoulder, flexed at elbow, pronated at forearm, with flexed wrist and fingers*)
    - Lower limbs: Preferential weakness of ankle/foot dorsiflexor, knee flexor, hip flexors, and internal rotators (*hemiparetic lower limb is extended, adducted, externally rotated at the hip, extended at the knee, with the foot plantar flexed and inverted)*
  - Atrophy: Minimal (disuse atrophy)
  - Tone: In acute lesion, muscle can be flaccid, followed subsequently by spasticity. In the case of slowly progressive lesions, spasticity may be present from onset.
  - Power: Characteristic distribution due to preferential innervation of certain muscle groups by CST.
  - Distal hand muscles receive more CST innervation than proximal muscle groups.
  - In contrast to lower motor neuron (LMN) lesion where specific muscles may be weak in a dermatomal or nerve distribution, upper motor neuron (UMN) weakness involves a group of muscles that participate in a joint movement.
  - *Deep tendon reflexes* are brisk; clonus may be present.
  - Absent or decreased superficial reflexes
  - Cranial nerves:
    - UMN facial on the same side of hemiplegia: Internal capsule
    - Crossed involvement, i.e., involvement of cranial nuclei contralateral to the side of hemiplegia: Brainstem

### Investigations

- *Computed tomography (CT) scan of the brain*:
  - May be normal up to 72 hours of infarction
  - Beneficial to rule out infection, tumors, or hemorrhage
- *Magnetic resonance imaging (MRI) (with or without gadolinium contrast)*:
  - Investigation of choice in cases of acute infarction, demyelination, tumors, and infection (abscess and encephalitis)
- *Cerebrospinal fluid (CSF)*: Done in cases of suspected vasculitis, infection, or demyelination
- *Electroencephalography (EEG)*: Useful in cases of Todd's palsy or postictal palsy [slow waves or periodic lateralized epileptiform discharges (PLEDs)] as well as encephalitis (PLEDs)
- *Nerve conduction studies (NCS)/ electromyography (EMG)*: Useful in peripheral lesions such as neuropathy, radiculopathy, plexopathy, or ALS

## THERAPY

- Treatment of cause
- Symptomatic:
  - Spasticity: Baclofen, tizanidine, tolperisone, gabapentin

## RED FLAG SIGNS

- *Headache at onset*: Hemorrhage, tumors, infection
- *Seizures at onset*: Hemorrhage, tumors, infection, embolic stroke
- *Slow progression (over weeks to months)*: Tumors

## CLINICAL PEARLS

Hemiplegia suggests involvement of the contralateral CST anywhere between the cerebral cortex and the caudal medulla or the ipsilateral CST at the rostral cervical cord.

In many cases, imaging and neurological examination might be normal, such as TIA, seizures, and migraine, where history is the only definitive way to reach a diagnosis.

Seizures commonly present with a positive phenomenon, such as clonic-tonic movements (rarely weakness), whereas strokes produce a negative phenomenon (weakness).

A marching pattern of progression of deficits is suggestive of migraine or seizure.

Stroke, mostly of abrupt onset, may on occasion be progressive or stuttering in course (lacunar or posterior circulation strokes).

## FURTHER READINGS

1. Jang SH. Somatotopic arrangement and location of the corticospinal tract in the brainstem of the human brain. Yonsei Med J. 2011;52(4):553-7.
2. Mehndiratta MM, Kumar M, Nayak R, Garg H, Pandey S. Hoover's sign: clinical relevance in neurology. J Postgrad Med. 2014;60(3):297-9.

CHAPTER 56

# Paraplegia

*Amlan Kusum Datta*

## WHAT IS PARAPLEGIA?

Paraplegia refers to complete loss of motor function in the lower extremities, in contrast to paraparesis which refers to partial weakness.

## WHAT CAUSES PARAPLEGIA?

*Possible sites of lesion include*:

- Cerebral cortex (parasagittal region)
- Brainstem (rare)
- Spinal cord
- Nerve roots and/or peripheral nerves
- Muscle

## WHAT ARE THE POSSIBILITIES?

- *Cerebral cortex:*
    - Superior sagittal sinus thrombosis
    - Thrombosis of unpaired anterior cerebral artery
    - *Demyelination*: Multiple sclerosis, acute demyelinating encephalomyelitis
    - *Space-occupying lesion*: Glioma, meningioma
    - *Penetrating injuries*: Gunshot injury
- *Spinal cord:*
    - Compressive myelopathies
    - *Extradural extramedullary*: Prolapsed intervertebral disk, Pott's spine, cervical spondylosis, trauma, metastasis, epidural abscess, leukemia, myeloma
    - *Intradural extramedullary*: Meningioma, neurofibroma, metastasis, arachnoiditis
    - *Intramedullary*: Glioma, hematomyelia, ependymoma, syringomyelia
    - Noncompressive myelopathies
    - *Infections*:
        - Bacterial: Tuberculosis, brucellosis, *Mycoplasma*, syphilis, Lyme disease
        - Viral: Human immunodeficiency virus (HIV), varicella zoster, human T-cell lymphotropic virus type 1 (HTLV-1), Epstein–Barr virus
    - *Demyelination*: Multiple sclerosis, neuromyelitis optica, postvaccine demyelination, Sjögren's syndrome, lupus
    - *Vascular*: Spinal artery thrombosis, embolism (Leriche syndrome), decompression sickness (caisson syndrome), postcardiac bypass surgery
    - *Nutritional*: Subacute combined degeneration, copper deficiency, vitamin E deficiency/excess, pellagra ("lathyrism")
    - *Traumatic*: Radiation, electric shock
    - *Degenerative*: Motor neuron disease
    - *Hereditary*: Hereditary spastic paraplegia, Friedreich's ataxia
    - Paraneoplastic

- *Toxins*: Nitric oxide (NO), bismuth, arsenic, lead, fluorosis

## PATH TO DIAGNOSIS

*Step 1: Upper motor neuron (UMN) versus lower motor neuron (LMN)*

- *UMN lesion*:
  - Increased (spastic) tone
  - History of flexor spasm
  - Hyperreflexia
  - Extensor plantar response
  - Differential pattern of weakness (greater weakness in lower limb flexors)
- *LMN lesion*:
  - History of cramps, twitching
  - Hypotonia
  - Hyporeflexia
  - Significant muscle wasting
  - Fasciculation
- *Clinical caveat*: An acute UMN lesion can mimic an LMN lesion as in spinal shock.

*Step 2: Localization of the lesion*

- *Pure UMN*
  - *Cerebral lesion*:
    - Headache
    - Seizure
  - *Spinal cord*:
    - Paralysis of all muscles below a certain level (corticospinal tract involvement)
    - Sensory loss below a circumferential level on the trunk (spinothalamic tract involvement)
    - Autonomic involvement (sphincter involvement)
    - Absence of superficial reflexes
    - Sensory perturbations:
      - ♦ Girdle-like sensation: Due to involvement of posterior column; common in compressive myelopathies and acute transverse myelitis
      - ♦ Local pain: Deep-seated and aching pain, which varies with change of posture and/or weight-bearing, as well as percussion over the spine. It arises from irritation of pain-sensitive spinal structures such as ligaments, periosteum, and dura.
      - ♦ Radicular pain: It commonly has a sharp and stabbing quality and is exacerbated by activities such as coughing or straining, which stretch the affected nerve root. It arises from any pathology which irritates the facet joints and nerve roots.
      - ♦ Central neurogenic pain/funicular pain: It is poorly localized, diffuse pain syndrome causing paresthesia (abnormal but not unpleasant sensation that is either provoked or spontaneous), dysesthesia (abnormal unpleasant sensation that is either provoked or unprovoked), allodynia (pain evoked by nonpainful stimuli), and hyperalgesia (augmented response to painful stimuli). The sensation may occur at the level, below the level, or rarely above the level of spinal cord injury. Central neurogenic pain possibly arises from local cellular changes in the dorsal horn and sensory roots due to segmental injury.

UMN + LMN

- *With sphincter/and sensory involvement*: Cauda equina or conus medullaris **(Table 1)**
- *Without sphincter/sensory involvement*: Anterior horn cell (amyotrophic lateral sclerosis)

*Pure LMN (no sensory or bladder involvement)*

- Anterior horn cell (poliomyelitis, postpolio syndrome, progressive muscular atrophy variant of motor neuron disease)

**Table 1: Comparison of clinical features between cauda equina and conus medullaris.**

| | *Cauda equina* | *Conus medullaris* |
|---|---|---|
| Pain | Severe, asymmetric | Uncommon |
| Sensory loss | Asymmetric, patchy | Symmetric saddle anesthesia |
| Motor deficit | Asymmetric, more marked with prominent wasting | Symmetric, less |
| Reflexes | Both knee and ankle jerks are lost or diminished, may be asymmetric | Only ankle jerk is lost |
| Plantar | Flexor | May be extensor |
| Sphincter involvement and erectile dysfunction | Less common, late feature | Common, early feature |

- Parapareitic variant of Guillain-Barré syndrome
- Myopathy
- Neuromuscular junction pathology (Eaton-Lambert syndrome)

*Step 3: If the lesion is in the cord, the following questions need to be answered:*

- *Longitudinal extent of the lesion?*
  - *Muscle power*: Weakness of all muscles below a certain level
  - *Sensory*: Sensory loss below a certain level/girdle-like sensation at the level of lesion
  - *Reflexes*: Deep tendon reflexes are lost at the level of the lesion and exaggerated below it.
  - *Local pain and deformity of the spine*: At the level of lesion
  - *Segmental LMN signs*: Loss of deep tendon jerks and wasting at the level of lesion
- *Which tracts are involved?*
  - *Complete spinal transection*:
    - Acute stage: Flaccid paralysis of limbs, loss of all sensations below the level of injury, and urinary retention
    - Chronic stage: Loss of all sensations below the level of lesion/spasticity and hyperreflexia below the level of lesion/detrusor hyperreflexia, detrusor sphincter dyssynergia
  - *Unilateral transverse lesion (Brown-Séquard syndrome)*:
    - Ipsilateral UMN pattern weakness below the lesion
    - Ipsilateral LMN pattern weakness at the level of lesion
    - Ipsilateral loss of vibration and joint sense below the level of lesion
    - Contralateral pain and temperature loss below the level of lesion
    - Segmental patch of ipsilateral pain and temperature loss with LMN weakness
    - Common etiologies: Multiple sclerosis, traumatic and penetrating injuries of the spinal cord, intradural cord compression
  - *Central cord lesion*:
    - Disproportionately more severe weakness of upper limbs than lower extremities (because of the placement of sacral fibers in the corticospinal tract laterally, they are involved to a lesser extent in central cord pathologies)
    - Bladder dysfunction, usually retention
    - Dissociated sensory loss: Loss of pain and temperature with preservation of vibration and joint sense
    - "Suspended sensory loss": A small lesion disrupts the crossing spinothalamic tracts bilaterally at the level of lesion, with sparing of

the ventrolateral spinothalamic tracts above and below it.
  - Sparing of sacral sensation (due to lateral predisposition of sacral fibers of spinothalamic cord in cord)
  - Common etiologies: Trauma (hyperextension injury, syringomyelia, neuromyelitis optica, intramedullary spinal cord tumor)
- *Anterior cord syndrome*:
  - Affection of both corticospinal and spinothalamic tracts with sparing of posterior columns
  - Paralysis below the lesion
  - Impairment of pain and temperature sensation below the lesion
  - Preserved proprioception and vibration
  - Autonomic dysfunction below the level of lesion
  - Common etiologies: Anterior spinal artery infarction, West Nile virus, poliomyelitis, multiple sclerosis
- *Anterior horn and pyramidal tract syndromes*:
  - Pure motor impairment with relative sparing of autonomic and sensory functions
  - LMN signs: Atrophy, fasciculations
  - UMN signs: Spasticity, hyperreflexia
  - Affection of different limbs to different degrees, with a progressive course
  - Spared bladder and bowel functions
  - Common etiologies: Amyotrophic lateral sclerosis, paraneoplastic subacute motor neuronopathy
- *Posterolateral cord syndrome*:
  - Affection of posterior and lateral white matter tracts
  - Spastic ataxic gait
  - Loss of vibration and proprioception with UMN weakness below the lesion
  - Extensor plantar reflex with loss of ankle jerks (due to involvement of large myelinated sensory fibers)
  - Common etiologies: Vitamin B12 deficiency, copper deficiency, HIV, tabes dorsalis (dorsal horn and column injury)
- *Dorsal horn (sensory neuronopathy)*:
  - Nonlength-dependent sensory loss below the level of lesion
  - Areflexia
  - Sensory ataxia
  - Pseudoathetosis
  - Common etiologies: Paraneoplastic, Sjögren's syndrome, pyridoxine excess, cisplatin toxicity

- *Is it compressive or noncompressive?* **(Table 2)**
- *Is it intramedullary or extramedullary?* **(Table 3)**
- *Is it extradural or intradural?* **(Table 4)**

Calculating the segment involved from the vertebral level is mentioned in **Table 5**.

**Table 2: Comparison between clinical features of compressive and noncompressive spinal pathologies.**

| | *Compressive* | *Noncompressive* |
|---|---|---|
| Local pain | Yes | No |
| Radicular pain | Yes | No |
| Funicular pain | No | Yes |
| Sensory level | Yes | May or may not be present |
| Vertebral deformity | Yes | No |
| Patterns of tract involvement | Sequential, nonselective | Selective, discrete tract involvement |

**Table 3: Comparison between clinical features of intramedullary and extramedullary pathologies.**

| | *Intramedullary* | *Extramedullary* |
|---|---|---|
| Onset | Symmetric | Asymmetric |
| Sphincter involvement | Early | Late |
| Local pain, radicular pain | No | Yes |
| Funicular pain | Yes | No |
| Upper motor neuron (UMN) signs | Late | Early |
| Lower motor neuron (LMN) signs | Early | Late |
| Progression | Descending | Ascending |

**Table 4: Comparison between clinical features of extramedullary extradural and extramedullary intradural.**

| | *Intradural* | *Extradural* |
|---|---|---|
| Root pain | Yes | No |
| Symmetry | Late | Early |
| Sphincter involvement | No/late | Yes/early |
| Vertebral deformity | No | Yes |

**Table 5: Calculating the segment involved from vertebral level.**

| *Spinal cord level* | *Corresponding vertebral body* |
|---|---|
| Upper cervical | Same as cord level |
| Lower cervical | One level higher |
| Upper thoracic | Two levels higher |
| Lower thoracic | Three levels higher |
| Lumbar | T10–T12 |
| Sacral | T12–L1 |

*Step 4: What is the etiology/what is the differential diagnosis?*

- *Mode of onset*:
  - *Acute*: Epidural hematoma, spinal cord trauma, hematomyelia, anterior spinal artery infarction, acute transverse myelitis, disk prolapse
  - *Subacute*: Spinal cord tumor, demyelination, epidural abscess, infections
  - *Chronic*: Tropical spastic paraplegia, HTLV-1-associated myelopathy, lathyrism, subacute combined degeneration, motor neuron disease
- *Course of illness*:
  - *Monophasic, with or without complete recovery*: Infection, abscess, trauma, hematomyelia
  - *Relapsing/remitting*: Demyelination
  - *Slowly progressive*: Nutritional, tumor, hereditary causes
- *Past history*:
  - *Vaccination*: Postinfective demyelination
  - *Vision loss*: Demyelination
  - *Koch's*: Pott's spine
- *Personal history*:
  - *Drug abuse*: Epidural abscess
  - *Vegetarian diet*: Subacute combined degeneration
  - *Sexual promiscuity*: HIV, syphilis
  - *Vascular risk factors*: Spinal artery infarction

*Investigations*

- *Blood*:
  - *Anemia, macrocytes*: Vitamin B12 deficiency

- *Basophilic stippling*: Lead poisoning
- *Anemia, raised erythrocyte sedimentation rate (ESR), hypercalcemia*: Myeloma
- *Antinuclear antibodies*: Lupus
- *Antiaquaporin 4 antibodies*: Neuromyelitis optica

- *Mantoux test*: Caries spine
- *Urine*:
  - *Bence Jones protein*: Myeloma
  - *Toxin/poisons*: Fluorosis, lead
- *Chest X-ray*: Koch's, sarcoidosis, lung tumor
- *Cerebrospinal fluid*:
  - *Oligoclonal band*: Multiple sclerosis
  - *Low glucose, pleocytosis with normal or increased protein*: Infections
- *Imaging*:
  - *Chest X-ray*: Lung neoplasm, Koch's
  - *Computed tomography (CT) scan of brain*: Parasagittal mass lesion, bleeding
  - *Magnetic resonance imaging (MRI)*: Investigation of choice for evaluation of spinal cord **(Fig. 1)**

*Therapy*

- *Demyelination*: Steroids, immunomodulators
- *Nutritional (e.g., vitamin B12, copper, vitamin E deficiencies)*: Replenishment of deficient nutrient
- *Infection/abscess*: Antibiotics with or without surgical decompression
- *Disk prolapse/spondylosis*: Surgical decompression

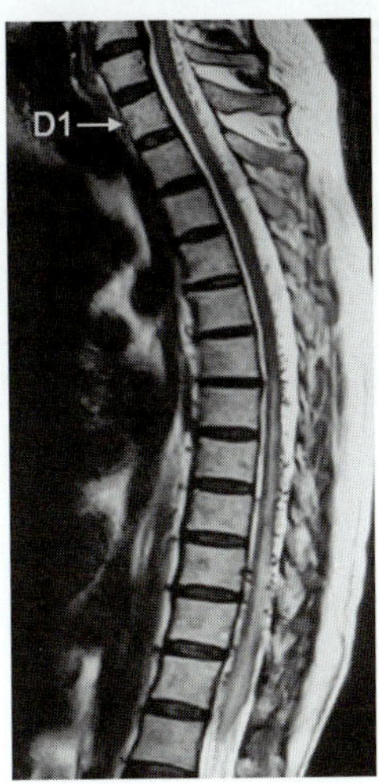


**FIG. 1:** T2-weighted sagittal magnetic resonance imaging (MRI) sequence showing T2 hyperintensity of dorsolumbar cord along with numerous flow voids along the epidural space, suggestive of a spinal arteriovenous malformation.

## CLINICAL PEARLS

- Careful neurological examination can help delineate exact pattern and distribution of sensory motor deficit, thereby helping to plan further diagnostic tests and imaging.
- Identification of type of bladder involvement can help in further localization:
  - Detrussor hyperreflexia, leading to urgency and frequency with or without loss of social inhibition localizes to paracentral lobule
  - Lack of coordination between overactive detrusor and external sphincter leading to urgency/frequency with interrupted flow, i.e., detrusor sphincter dyssynergia localizes to spinal cord above sacral level
  - Lack of detrusor contraction leading to distension of bladder and overflow incontinence, localizes lesion to level of T12 vertebrae and below as well as lesions of sacral nerve roots
- Sudden rise of blood pressure, with flushing of skin above lesion, headache, visual blurring signifying autonomic dysreflexia localizes to a cord lesion above T6.

## FURTHER READINGS

1. Kornegay JN. Paraparesis (paraplegia), tetraparesis (tetraplegia), urinary/fecal incontinence. Spinal cord diseases. Probl Vet Med. 1991;3(3):363-77.
2. Barcelos ACES, Scardino FB, Patriota GC, Rotta JM, Botelho RV. Paraparesis or incomplete paraplegia? How should we call it? Acta Neurochirurgica. 2009;151(4):369-72.

# CHAPTER 57

# Quadriplegia

*Amlan Kusum Datta*

## WHAT IS QUADRIPLEGIA?

Quadriplegia or tetraplegia is defined as weakness of all four limbs. The degree of involvement of all four limbs may be variable depending on the location and nature of lesion; however, in cases of predominant lower limb involvement in comparison to upper limbs, the term diplegia is preferred.

## WHAT CAUSES QUADRIPLEGIA?

Possible sites of lesion include:
- Cervical cord
- Brainstem
- Brain (bihemispheric lesion)

## WHAT ARE THE POSSIBILITIES?

- *Compressive lesions*:
    - *Trauma*: Vertebral body fractures/dislocation, hyperextension injury
    - *Spondylosis*: Cervical stenosis
    - Degenerative disk disease/herniation
    - *Infection*: Abscess, tuberculosis
    - *Inflammatory*: Rheumatoid arthritis, ankylosing spondylitis, sarcoid
    - *Hemorrhage*: Epidural hematoma
    - Congenital disorders
    - Arachnoid cysts
    - Paget's disease
    - Osteoporosis
    - Epidural metastasis
    - *Intradural extramedullary*: Neurofibroma, meningioma, leptomeningeal metastasis
    - *Intramedullary*: Glioma, ependymoma
- *Noncompressive lesions*:
    - *Demyelination*: Multiple sclerosis (MS), neuromyelitis optica spectrum disorder (NMOSD)
    - Hereditary (spastic paraplegia)
    - Viral myelitis [varicella-zoster, acquired immunodeficiency syndrome (AIDS)-related myelopathy, human T-lymphotropic virus type I]
    - Syringomyelia
    - Vitamin B12 deficiency
    - Infarction
    - Ischemia or hemorrhage from vascular malformation or cavernoma
    - Toxic myelopathies (radiation-induced)
    - Autoimmune disease (lupus, Sjögren's)
    - Paraneoplastic

## PATH TO DIAGNOSIS

- Determine upper motor neuron (UMN) or lower motor neuron (LMN)
  - *UMN lesion*:
    - History of flexor spasm
    - Spasticity
    - Hyperreflexia
    - Extensor plantar response
    - Differential weakness: Greater weakness of lower limb flexors and upper limb extensors
  - *LMN lesion*:
    - Hypotonia
    - Hyporeflexia
    - Presence of cramps, fasciculation
    - Marked muscle wasting
- Determine the level of lesion
  - *Foramen magnum and high cervical spine*:
    - Neck/occipital pain
    - Lhermitte's sign: Electric shock-like sensation radiating down the spine upon neck flexion; due to posterior column involvement
    - Lower cranial nerve palsies (IX–XII)
    - Diaphragmatic weakness (C3–C5 lesion)
    - Downbeat nystagmus
    - Facial numbness/paresthesia
    - Atrophy and LMN signs in upper extremities
    - Thoracic ("drop-down") sensory level
  - Lower cervical and upper thoracic spine:
    - Radicular pain
    - Segmental LMN signs:
      - ♦ C5–6: Paresthesia along the radial side of the upper limb, depressed biceps and/or brachioradialis jerks, brisk finger flexion jerks, weakness of elbow flexion
      - ♦ C7–T1: Sensory loss over the ulnar aspect of the upper limb, weakness of elbow extension, wasting of small muscles of the hand, and depressed triceps jerk
  - *Brainstem lesions*:
    - Cranial neuropathies
    - Internuclear ophthalmoplegia
    - Horner's syndrome
  - *Cerebral (bihemispheric lesion)*:
    - Pseudobulbar palsy (spastic dysarthria, emotional incontinence)
    - Frontal release reflexes
    - Causes: Recurrent stroke, leukodystrophies, hypoxic encephalopathy
- Etiology
  - *Mode of onset*:
    - Acute (over hours to days): Infarction, demyelination
    - *Subacute (over days to weeks)*: Infection (abscess)
    - Chronic (over months to years): Neoplastic, degenerative disk disease
  - *Disease course*:
    - Monophasic (with or without complete recovery): Vascular, acute disseminated encephalomyelitis (ADEM)
    - Relapsing or remitting: MS
    - Slowly progressive: Neoplastic, infection

### Clinical Examination

- *Inspection*: Segmental atrophy at the level of lesion, e.g., atrophy of upper extremities in high cervical cord lesions
- *Tone*: Hypertonia/spasticity (may be flaccid in the stage of spinal shock)
- *Power*: Weakness of muscles below the level of lesion
- *Sensory*:
  - Sensory loss below a certain level
  - Girdle-like sensation at the level of lesion

- *Reflexes*: Deep tendon reflexes are lost at the level of lesion and brisk below it, e.g., in a C6 lesion, absent brachioradialis jerk, and brisk finger flexion jerks (loss of all jerks below the level of lesion in the stage of spinal shock)
- Focal pain and spinal deformity (in an extramedullary extradural lesion)
- Cranial nerve examination (foramen magnum and high cervical cord lesions)
  - Downbeat nystagmus
  - Facial sensory loss in onion skin/ Balaclava pattern: Graded loss of pain, temperature over the lateral part of face with sparing of central areas (as fibers from the central part of the face are represented in the rostral part of the spinal sensory nucleus while those from the lateral part are represented more caudally)

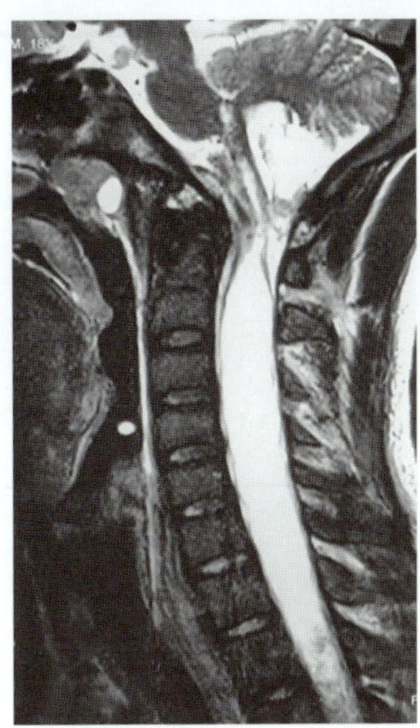

**FIG. 1:** Sagittal T2-weighted magnetic resonance imaging (MRI) sequence of the cervical cord and brainstem showing a syrinx extending from the cervicomedullary junction through the entirety of the cervical cord.

## Investigations

- Magnetic resonance imaging (MRI) of cord with or without gadolinium contrast injection: Investigation of choice **(Fig. 1)**
- Myelogram (if MRI is contraindicated)
- Spinal angiography/digital subtraction angiography: If spinal vascular malformation suspected
- *Cerebrospinal fluid (CSF) study*: Indicated in noncompressive myelopathies such as suspected infection or demyelination

# THERAPY

- *Compressive lesions (traumatic)*: Parenteral steroids in acute stage (<24 hours), surgical decompression
- *Demyelination/autoimmune*: Steroids, immunomodulatory drugs (interferons, mycophenolate, azathioprine)
- *Infection such as abscess*: Antibiotics, surgical decompression
- *Vascular malformation*: Embolization

# CLINICAL PEARLS

- Neurological examination should focus on the presence or absence of Horner's syndrome and/or INO, since it can aid localization at or rostral to brainstem
- Cranial nerve examination should be vital, particularly the lower ones.

# FURTHER READINGS

1. Martínez-Lage JF, Alarcón F, López-Guerrero AL, Felipe-Murcia M, Ruíz-Espejo Vilar A, Almagro MJ. Syringomyelia with quadriparesis in CSF shunt malfunction: a case illustration. Childs Nerv Syst. 2010;26(9):1229-31.
2. Vandertop WP. Syringomyelia. Neuropediatrics. 2014;45(1):3-9.

# CHAPTER 58

# Ataxia

*Swati Kumar*

## WHAT IS ATAXIA?

Ataxia is defined as impaired coordination of voluntary muscle movement; however, it is not a disease per se but a physical finding, and efforts should focus on determining its etiology. It can either be a patient's primary complaint or be a part of other presenting complaints.

## WHAT CAUSES ATAXIA?

*Balance* is the ability to maintain equilibrium, i.e., a dynamic state in which one's center of mass is regulated with respect to the lower extremities, gravity, and integrity of the support surface, despite external perturbations. The reflexes necessary to maintain balance and upright posture require input from cerebellar, vestibular, and somatosensory cues; the premotor cortex and corticospinal and reticulospinal tracts mediate output to axial and proximal limb muscles. Locomotion and bipedal walking are complex processes and are believed to be generated from locomotor centers in the midbrain, pontine tegmentum, and subthalamic nucleus and executed through the reticular formation and descending pathways in the ventromedial spinal cord as opposed to a "spinal pattern generator" in quadrupeds. Albeit walking and postural control is largely believed to be an unconscious and automatic process in which the center of mass is adjusted over the base of support throughout the gait cycle, cerebral control does provide a goal and purpose for locomotion with regard to avoidance of obstacles and adaptation to context and terrain **(Fig. 1)**.

Therefore, balance and posture are the end products of the integration and sound functioning of multiple neurological substrates at different levels, perturbation of any one of which can potentially cause ataxia **(Table 1)**.

## WHAT ARE THE POSSIBILITIES?

### Path to Diagnosis

The history and clinical examination form the basic framework for the diagnosis of ataxia and for narrowing down the etiological possibilities **(Table 2)**.

The evaluation starts with determining the type of ataxia and the chief neuro-anatomical substrates possibly affected as well as other associated features that also help in localization. Good history taking paves the path for a focused examination and allows the physical findings to be corroborative.

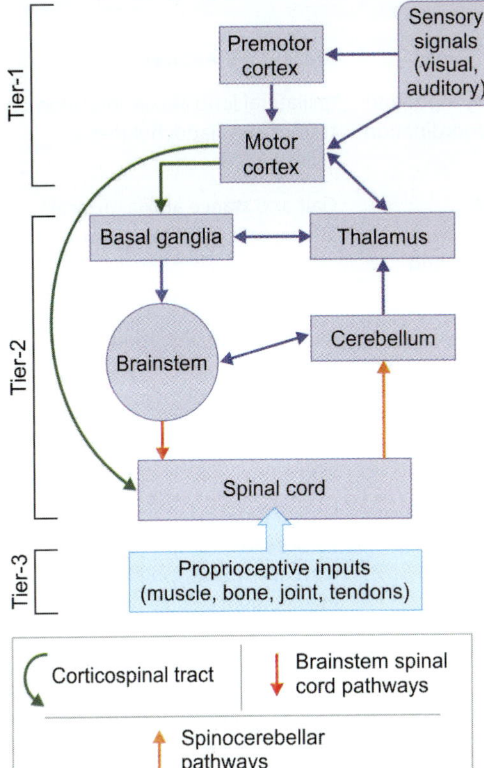


**FIG. 1:** Three tiers of gait control: Tier 1 consists of the premotor and motor cortices, which receive environmental cues via sensory modalities, plan and initiate gait, and generate environmental awareness during locomotion. Tier 2 comprises the basal ganglia, thalamus, brainstem locomotor centers, and cerebellum, which ultimately regulate and coordinate motor movements that participate in gait and locomotion via the spinal cord pattern generators. Tier 3 includes the musculoskeletal structures such as bones, joints, tendons, ligaments, and peripheral sensory pathways, which relay sensory proprioceptive cues to the higher gait centers via the spinal cord.

## History

- *Common symptoms of ataxia*:
  - Gait difficulty: One of the earliest manifestations of ataxia, which usually manifests as "walking as if one is drunk," with difficulty in running, turning, walking on heels, and walking up or down stairs.
  - Slurred speech: Ranges from occasional word pronunciation difficulty to persistent speech problems
  - Hand tremors: Often described as clumsiness or bad handwriting by patients or the tendency to spill on clothes while feeding oneself
  - Dizziness: Often associated with cerebellar ataxia
  - Double vision: Often precipitated by rapid head turns
- *Onset and progression*:
  - Acute: Stroke, demyelination, infection, toxins
  - Subacute: Immune-mediated causes, tumors
  - Chronic: Neurodegenerative and hereditary causes
  - Episodic: Episodic ataxia syndromes
- *Associated features*:
  - Cranial nerve deficits: Stroke, tumor, demyelination
  - Cognitive impairment, hallucinations: Korsakoff–Wernicke's encephalopathy, toxins
  - Sleep dysfunction, tremor, dysautonomia: Multiple system atrophy (MSA)
  - Symptoms increased in dark: Sensory ataxia
  - Drug history: Pyridoxine excess, anticonvulsants (phenytoin, carbamazepine, valproate), lithium, alcohol
  - Sexual history: Human immunodeficiency virus (HIV), syphilis
  - Weight loss, smoking: Paraneoplastic

## Neurological Examination of the Patient with Ataxia (Table 3)

- *Mental status examination*: Nonmotor functions of the cerebellum and its role in cognition are being increasingly appreciated. Salient functions of the cerebellum include executive functions, spatial orientation, motor memory, and language.
- *Cranial nerve examinations*: Special focus should be put on extraocular

**Table 1: Functional anatomy.**

| ***Neuroanatomy*** | ***Function*** | ***Presenting features*** |
|---|---|---|
| Cerebellar hemisphere | Integration of sensory input and motor planning for coordination of complex tasks | Ipsilateral limb ataxia, intention tremor, dysdiadochokinesia, scanning speech |
| Midline cerebellum | Motor execution, eye movements, balance, lower extremity coordination, and vestibular function | Gait and stance ataxia, truncal ataxia, titubation, nystagmus |
| Cerebral cortex (frontal lobe) | Planning and initiation of gait | Magnetic gait, initiation, and turning difficulty |
| Brainstem (vestibular nuclei, inferior olivary nuclei, pontine nuclei, cerebellar peduncles) | Relay signals in and out of cerebellum | Ataxia with associated cranial nerve deficits and long tract signs |
| Spinal cord (cuneate fasciculus, gracile fasciculus, and spinocerebellar tracts) | Conduction of sensory pathways | Sensory ataxia with nongraded sensory loss (proprioceptive) with or without sphincter involvement |
| Musculoskeletal (gluteal muscles) | Stabilization of weight-bearing hip | Waddling gait |
| Peripheral sensory system and visual system | Proprioceptive and visual cues | Sensory ataxia with Romberg's sign, graded sensory loss |
| Vestibular system (labyrinth of inner ear, vestibular nerve, and nuclei) | Balance and equilibrium | Ataxia with associated vertigo, tinnitus, nystagmus |

**Table 2: Etiological classification of ataxia.**

| ***Classification*** | ***Common etiologies*** |
|---|---|
| Time course | • *Acute (hours to days)*: Stroke, demyelination (multiple sclerosis), vestibular neuritis, infections (cerebellitis), acute poisonings<br>• *Subacute (over weeks)*: Posterior fossa mass lesions, meningeal infiltrates (metastasis, lymphoma, leukemia, sarcoidosis), human immunodeficiency virus, Creutzfeldt–Jacob disease, deficiencies such as vitamins B1 and B12, gluten and antiglutamic acid decarboxylase ataxias, paraneoplastic, hypothyroidism, alcohol<br>• *Chronic (months to years)*: Mass lesions such as meningiomas, craniovertebral junction abnormalities (Klippel–Feil syndrome), alcohol, sporadic ataxias, hereditary ataxias, neurodegenerative ataxias (multiple system atrophy, Friedrich's ataxia)<br>• *Episodic*: Inborn errors of metabolism, episodic ataxia syndromes |
| Distribution | • *Focal*: Posterior circulation strokes, primary or metastatic cerebellar neoplasms, abscess, congenital cysts (Dandy–Walker syndromes), multiple sclerosis, progressive multifocal leukoencephalopathy (PML)<br>• *Symmetric*: All other systemic, toxic, genetic, and neurodegenerative causes of ataxia such as intoxication (alcohol, phenytoin, lithium, barbiturates, toluene), postinfectious syndrome, paraneoplastic syndrome, immune-mediated ataxias, metabolic disorder, viral cerebellitis, tabes dorsalis, prion disease, hereditary ataxia |

**Table 3: Features of different types of ataxias.**

| | *Frontal ataxia* | *Cerebellar ataxia* | *Sensory ataxia* |
|---|---|---|---|
| Base of support | Wide-based | Wide-based | Narrow-based |
| Velocity | Very slow | Variable | Slow |
| Stride | Short, shuffling | Irregular, lurching | Regular with path deviation, high steppage |
| Romberg's test | ± | ± | Positive |
| Gait initiation | Hesitant | Normal | Normal |
| Falls | Early and frequent | Late | Frequent |
| Postural instability | ++++ | + | +++ |

**Table 4: Differences between central and peripheral nystagmus.**

| | *Peripheral nystagmus* | *Central nystagmus* |
|---|---|---|
| Direction | Unidirectional, fast phase beating away from the lesion | Bidirectional, changing with direction of gaze |
| Effects on visual fixation | Suppressed | Not suppressed |
| Vertigo | Yes, severe | Variable |
| Pattern of nystagmus | Mixed, horizontal–torsional | Pure vertical, pure horizontal |
| Tinnitus/deafness | Often present | Absent |
| Cranial nerve deficits (dysarthria, diplopia) | Absent | Present |

movements with respect to saccades, pursuit, opsoclonus, square-wave jerks, and saccadic oscillations. Papilledema may result from a posterior fossa mass lesion. Loss of ipsilateral corneal reflex and vestibular dysfunction might be a clue toward cerebellopontine angle tumor. Slowed saccades are a feature of spinocerebellar ataxia type 2 (SCA2), whereas perioral and tongue fasciculations are suggestive of SCA3.

- *Vestibular signs*: Associated hearing loss along with a unidirectional nystagmus is suggestive of vestibular dysfunction **(Table 4)**. The patient also tends to veer toward the affected side on walking.
- *Cerebellar signs*: Inability to tandem walk is the cardinal finding of cerebellar ataxia. The stance is broad with titubation. Other findings include scanning speech, hypometric saccades, impaired finger-nose-finger test with intention tremor, and nystagmus, which is bidirectional.
- *Extrapyramidal signs*: They are often indicative of a neurodegenerative process spreading beyond the brainstem and cerebellum. Etiologies include MSA and certain SCAs, namely SCA2, SCA3, and SCA17.
- *Motor strength*: Symmetric proximal muscle weakness suggests myopathy. Distal muscle weakness suggests a neuropathy. Gait dysfunction may also be due to muscle weakness rather than ataxia. For example, when the hip girdle is weak due to myopathy, the pelvis tends to shift toward the side, causing a waddling gait.

- *Proprioceptive sensory loss*: Impaired proprioceptive sensory cues to the brainstem and cerebellum result in sensory ataxia. The symptoms are markedly exacerbated in dark or with eyes closed (Romberg's sign) as opposed to cerebellar ataxia, where there is no significant difference with eyes closed or open. Absent vibration, absent or diminished deep tendon jerks, and proprioception at joints are clues to sensory ataxia.

### Salient Features of Gait of Prototypical Neurological Disorders

- *Spastic gait*:
  - Tendency to circumduct the hip joint and scuff the lateral border of the sole against the ground on the ipsilateral side
  - Tendency to walk on toes
  - In bilateral cases, tendency to cross legs ("scissoring") due to increased adductor tone
  - Causes: Cerebral (stroke, multiple sclerosis, cerebral palsy, motor neuron disease), myelopathy (demyelination, trauma, arteriovenous malformation)
- *Parkinsonism*:
  - Stooped posture, shuffling of feet
  - Tendency to accelerate (festination) and turn en block
  - Retropulsion, decreased arm swing
  - Freeing: Defined as a brief, episodic, cessation of forward progression of feet despite the intention to move forward. It is common in Parkinson's disease within the first 5 years of illness; other causes include progressive supranuclear palsy (PSP), corticobasal degeneration (CBD), and MSA.
  - A relatively erect posture with down-gaze restriction and falls occurring within the first year of illness are suggestive of PSP rather than idiopathic Parkinson's disease.
- *Frontal gait disorder*:
  - Short stride, shuffling along the floor
  - Difficulty with starts and turns
  - Freezing of gait
  - Signs of higher cerebral dysfunction such as pseudobulbar affect, dysphagia, dysarthria
  - Common causes: Subcortical small-vessel disease, normal pressure hydrocephalus
- *Cerebellar gait ataxia*:
  - Wide base of support
  - Lateral instability of trunk
  - Irregular foot placement
  - Inability to walk on a narrow base or in "tandem"
  - Difficulty maintaining balance during turns and while running is often an early feature
  - Truncal sway on narrow stance
  - Causes: Stroke, demyelination, tumors, degenerative, and hereditary diseases
- *Sensory ataxia*:
  - Narrow base, with tendency to look down while walking
  - Marked decompensation of standing balance upon eye closure

**Table 3** compares salient features of prototypical ataxias.

## Investigations

The investigations are planned according to the physical examination and history findings.

- *Laboratory testings*:
  - Drug level: Phenytoin, barbiturates, lithium, alcohol
  - Thyroid function
  - Vitamin B6, B12 levels
  - HIV, syphilis, Lyme, toxoplasmosis serology
  - Paraneoplastic panel (anti-Yo for ovarian cancer, anti-Hu for lung cancer, anti-Tr for Hodgkin's lymphoma, anti-Ri for breast cancer)
  - Antiglutamic acid decarboxylase, antigliadin antibodies
  - Low vitamin E and abnormal lipoprotein: Abetalipoproteinemia
  - High alpha-fetoprotein and low immunoglobulin: Ataxia telangiectasia

- High serum cholesterol and low albumin: Ataxia with oculomotor apraxia 1
- High alpha-fetoprotein: Ataxia with oculomotor apraxia 2
- High serum phytanic acid: Refsum's disease

- *Brian imaging*:
  - Plain computed tomography (CT): Can help to rule out posterior fossa bleed or mass lesion
  - Magnetic resonance imaging (MRI) brain: Ideal for ischemic stroke as well as demyelination. In some cases, MRI may be diagnostic such as hot cross bun sign (MSA-c), middle cerebellar peduncle sign (fragile X tremor ataxia syndrome), and molar tooth sign (Joubert's syndrome).
- *Genetic testing*:
  - CAG expansion: SCA1, SCA2, SCA3, SCA6, SCA7, SCA12, SCA17
  - CTG expansion: SCA8
  - Pentanucleotide repeat: SCA10 (ATTCT) and SCA31 (TGGAA)
  - Hexanucleotide repeat: SCA36 (GGCCTG)
  - POLG mutation: Mitochondrial recessive ataxia
  - APTX: Ataxia with oculomotor apraxia 1
  - SETX: Ataxia with oculomotor apraxia 2
- *Therapy*:
  - Stroke: Blood pressure (BP) control and mannitol for hemorrhagic stroke, intravenous thrombolysis for acute ischemic stroke
  - Demyelination: Steroids, immunomodulators
  - Paraneoplastic: Steroids, immunomodulators, tumor resection
  - Nutritional/metabolic: Thiamine replacement (Wernicke's encephalopathy), vitamin B12 replacement (sensory ataxia)
- *Fall prevention*:
  - High-resistance strength training to improve muscle mass, strength, and posture
  - Sensory balance training
  - Vestibular exercises
  - Environmental modification, such as installation of grab bars, removing slippery surfaces, and improving lighting at homes
  - Treatment of orthostatic hypotension (sitting cross-legged, midodrine, increasing salt intake)

## CLINICAL PEARLS

- Ataxia is a neurological sign, resulting in lack of coordination between muscles of the body
- It can involve a number of anatomical substrates and etiologies are myriad
- Careful physical and neurological examination can help narrow down the differentials and plan cost-effective, targeted investigations.
- Treatment involves a multidisciplinary approach.

## FURTHER READINGS

1. de Silva RN, Vallortigara J, Greenfield J, Hunt B, Giunti P, Hadjivassiliou M. Diagnosis and management of progressive ataxia in adults. Practical Neurology. 2019;19:196-207.
2. Zhang Q, Zhou X, Li Y, Yang X, Abbasi QH. Clinical Recognition of Sensory Ataxia and Cerebellar Ataxia. Front. Hum. Neurosci. 15:639871.

# CHAPTER 59

# Coma

*Joydeep Mukherjee*

## DEFINITION

Consciousness is a state of awareness of self and surroundings. Alteration in consciousness can be of several types. The physiological form of this alteration is sleep. But the pathological alteration of consciousness consists of various behavioral states ranging from lethargy to coma. A stuporous patient needs repeated strong stimuli to remain aroused. In contrast, a comatose patient is unresponsive to any form of stimuli for arousal. Lethargy has a place between alertness and stupor.

If the patient loses the proper content of mental function, she may have delirium, dementia, delusion, confusion, and inattention. But these patients do not have an abnormality in arousal.

## PATHOPHYSIOLOGY

Extensive brain dysfunction resulting from direct compression of brain tissue; obstructed supply of blood, oxygen, and glucose; and increased intracranial pressure lead to coma. The reticular activating system spreads from the upper pons to the diencephalon to the forebrain. It keeps the person aroused. The patient becomes unconscious if it becomes dysfunctional due to structural disintegration or metabolic suppression.

### Differential Diagnosis

- *Locked-in syndrome*: Bilateral ventral pontine lesion producing an alert, aware, and quadriplegic state with lower cranial nerve palsy
- *Persistent vegetative state*: No verbal or gestural interaction with the surroundings; no sustained, reproducible, purposeful, voluntary response to any stimulus with preserved sleep/wake cycles in patients with extensive gray matter or subcortical white matter involvement with preservation of brainstem
- *Minimally conscious state*: Limited but clear evidence of self or environmental awareness as an ability to follow simple commands or yes/no responses or intelligible verbalization or voluntary, purposeful, relevant behavior
- *Abulia*: Alert and aware patient neither speaks nor moves spontaneously with a bilateral medial frontal lesion.
- *Catatonia*: Usually psychiatric patient with severely reduced motor activity and mutism
- *Pseudocoma*: Patient acting as comatose

#### *Approach to the Patient*

As the patient's condition is serious, rapid clinical assessment followed by fast investigations and treatment can save the patient.

**General Approach**

Rapid initial examination to determine urgent medical or surgical care → airway to be protected → neck stabilized in trauma patients → assessment of Glasgow Coma Scale (GCS), vital signs, pupil size, and responsiveness, posturing or abnormal body movements → blood sugar, electrocardiogram (ECG), arterial blood gas → computed tomography brain

### *Glasgow Coma Scale*

*Best motor response (M)*

- Obeys—6
- Localizes—5
- Withdraws—4
- Abnormal flexion—3
- Extensor response—2
- Nil—1

*Verbal response (V)*

- Oriented—5
- Confused conversation—4
- Inappropriate words—3
- Incomprehensible sounds—2
- Nil—1

*Eye opening (E)*

- Spontaneous—4
- To speech—3
- To pain—2
- Nil—1

*Easy way to assess the GCS*

If a patient is in an eye-closed condition, we must call him by his name. If he opens his eye → E3 and obeys simple commands like showing tongue → M6.

We will give a painful stimulus to the sternum or forehead if he does not open his eyes. Now, if he opens his eye → E2; if not → E1.

After giving the painful stimulus, if either hand reaches up to the painful stimulus → M5; if he moves away → M4; if either upper limb flexed but does not reach up to the painful stimulus point → M3; if either upper limb gets extended → M2; if no movement → M1.

If he talks properly → V5; if he does not speak properly but starts coherent foul sentences after painful stimulus → V4; if the words have meaning but do not form a meaningful sentence → V3; if only sound is there but no word → V2; if no sound → V1.

If the patient came in an eye-opened state with normal talks and obeying instructions, he is E4, V5, M6 (GCS 15/15).

**Selective Approach**

- Progressive deterioration of consciousness—structural lesion or toxin
- Waxing and waning consciousness—metabolic causes
- Rapid, deep respiration—metabolic/pontine/neurogenic pulmonary edema
- Abnormality in pulse, blood pressure, and temperature will indicate a particular disease.
- Hyperthermia—infection, subarachnoid hemorrhage, hypothalamic lesions, heatstroke, thyrotoxic crisis, atropine, and other anticholinergic toxicity
- Shivering without sweating—brainstem origin, if unilateral—deep intracerebral hemorrhage
- Hypothermia—sepsis, hypothyroidism, hypopituitarism, severe cold exposure, barbiturate toxicity
- Abnormal heart, lung, abdominal examination, skin rashes, breath odor, urine color, lymphadenopathy, and signs of trauma will also indicate a specific disease.
- Vomiting—increased intracranial pressure, drug overdose, toxic-metabolic causes
- Cerebrospinal fluid (CSF) rhinorrhea, black eye, blood from ear—head trauma
- Small reactive pupil—toxic metabolic cause (except methyl alcohol poisoning causing dilated and unreactive pupil)
- Dilated nonreactive pupil or asymmetric ocular motility—structural cause (mostly require urgent neurosurgery intervention)

- Bilateral pinpoint pupil—pontine lesion, bilateral midposition fixed pupil—midbrain lesion
- Reflex eye movements are mostly retained in toxic metabolic causes.
- Papilledema/subhyaloid hemorrhage by ophthalmoscopic examination—raised intracranial pressure due to structural lesion. Papilledema is never in metabolic causes except for hypothyroidism and lead intoxication.
- Myoclonus—metabolic and anoxic
- Posturing—brainstem herniation/cerebral ischemia
- Motor restlessness, tremor, spasm—lithium/chlorpromazine
- Seizures indicate brain pathology, seizure semiology—focal onset in mostly structural causes, generalized onset in toxic-metabolic causes
- Neck rigidity may indicate meningitis or subarachnoid hemorrhage.
- Nystagmus in a coma—irritative lesion
- Roving eye movement—slow, conjugate, side-to-side movement—brainstem intact
- Cheyne-Stokes respiration—slowly oscillates between hypo- and hyperventilation—anywhere between forebrain and upper pons—good prognostic sign as brainstem intact if continuous—a sign of brainstem herniation if sudden appearance in a unilateral mass lesion—sudden change to other types of ventilation is ominous.
- Central neurogenic hyperventilation—40–70/min—central tegmental pontine lesion
- Kussmaul breathing—deep, regular respiration—metabolic acidosis
- Apneustic breathing—pause after full inspiration with a prolonged inspiratory gap—dorsolateral lower pons
- Cluster breathing—irregular frequency and amplitude with changing pauses between breath clusters—high medullary damage
- Ataxic breathing—irregular rate and rhythm—medullary lesion
- If partial pressure of oxygen ($PO_2$) <70–80 mm Hg or partial pressure of carbon dioxide ($PCO_2$) >40 mm Hg, hyperpnea is not due to a central nervous system (CNS) problem.
- Ocular bobbing—spontaneous conjugate rapid downward eye movement followed by slow upward movement to midline—acute pontine lesion—not pathognomonic
- Ocular dipping—spontaneous slow downward followed by fast upward eye movement—diffuse cerebral injury
- Doll's eye maneuver (oculocephalic reflex)—passive vertical or horizontal head movement leads to reflex conjugate eye movement to opposite direction maintaining position in space as a normal response. However, specific dysfunction leads to no eye movement in lateral head rotation (bilateral pontine gaze palsy, bilateral labyrinthine dysfunction, anesthesia, and drug intoxication) and vertical head movement (bilateral midbrain lesions). In addition, oculomotor nerve palsy leads to no movement in the ipsilateral eye.
- Caloric test—"COWS"—cold opposite, warm same—is the direction of fast phase following "cold caloric" test (10 mL ice-cold water instillation in one ear in 30° head forward tilt). There is slow conjugate eye movement to the stimulated ear followed by a fast return to the midline as a normal response. No response happens in the obstructed ear canal, dead labyrinth, vestibular nerve or nuclear dysfunction, or false negative. Patients have a normal slow phase but no fast phase in toxic-metabolic disorder, drugs, and structural lesions above the brainstem. If the patient has horizontal gaze palsy, he will only have downbeat nystagmus.
- Family stressors—more in malingering

*Misleading leads*:

- Hypoglycemia may unmask silent structural abnormalities.
- Sometimes, toxic-metabolic causes of coma have focal features such as hyponatremia, hypoglycemia, barbiturate or lead poisoning, and hepatic encephalopathy (HE).
- Sometimes, structural abnormalities mimic metabolic ones by becoming bilateral symmetrical and sudden onset like subarachnoid hemorrhage, bilateral subdural hemorrhage, meningitis, demyelinating diseases, and multifocal diseases like vasculitis.
- Sometimes, combined entity remains like hyponatremia in a multi-infarct state.

*Differentiate coma from pseudocoma*: History and clinical examination show various inconsistencies in pseudocoma patients. Passive eye opening is easy in coma patients but difficult in malingering patients. Moreover, coma patients have slow and gradual eye closing following the passive opening, which is difficult for malingering patients. Passive eye opening causes pupillary dilatation in a true coma and reverse in pseudocoma. Roving eye movement is a sign of a true coma. The coma is ruled out in cold caloric testing if the eyes have ipsilateral tonic deviation with present fast phases. Moreover, the vertiginous sensation of the "cold caloric" test awakens the malingering patient.

*Investigative approach*: Fast and holistic. We need to take a helping hand.

- The patient is brought by relatives/street people/police.
- Holistic history availability in doubt in emergency situations
- Capillary blood glucose (very low or high), arterial blood gas (severe acidosis, alkalosis, hypoxia, hypercapnia)
- ECG—cardiac ischemia or block
- Abnormality in sodium, potassium, calcium, magnesium, urine ketone
- Ammonia high in HE (HE may persist for 3 weeks after normalization of liver function)
- Lactate high in mitochondrial encephalopathy syndromes
- Creatine phosphokinase (CPK) high in neuroleptic malignant syndrome, rhabdomyolysis
- Thyroid function (very high or low), morning cortisol (Addisonian crisis), blood alcohol level, toxic screen
- Serum osmolality—osmolar gap, which is the difference between measured and calculated serum osmolality, indicates unmeasured osmotically active particles in patient's serum—may be alcohol or other substances.
- Electroencephalogram (EEG)—nonconvulsive status epilepticus, triphasic waves of metabolic encephalopathy, generalized slowing in toxic-metabolic causes, unilateral slowing in large hemispheric stroke or mass lesion
- CSF—bacterial, viral, fungal, other infective pathologies, myelin oligodendrocyte glycoprotein (MOG) antibody positive diseases, N-methyl-D-aspartate (NMDA)-voltage-gated potassium channel (VGKC) antibody-positive diseases
- Empirical use of supplemental oxygen, stabilization of airway, breathing, and circulation → intravenous 100-mg thiamine, intravenous 25-g dextrose.

## URGENT NEUROSURGICAL MANAGEMENT IN COMA

- Hydrocephalous—extraventricular drainage (EVD) of CSF
- Extradural or subdural hemorrhage—burr hole drainage of blood
- Thalamic/intraventricular hemorrhage—EVD
- Large hemispheric stroke—hemicraniectomy

- Uncal/subfalcine herniation—hemicraniectomy
- Large cerebellar hemorrhage or infarct causing brainstem compression—posterior fossa decompression

## URGENT NEUROINTERVENTION IN COMA

- Thrombolysis or mechanical thrombectomy in basilar artery thrombosis
- Thrombolysis in the artery of Percheron causing bilateral thalamic and rostral midbrain stroke
- Heparin therapy in basilar artery occlusion presenting the outside window period of thrombolysis

## PROGNOSIS IN COMA

Traumatic coma has a better prognosis than nontraumatic coma. Younger age, better motor response, good pupillary reactivity and eye movement, and lesser depth and duration of coma are the early predictors of a favorable outcome. Cerebrovascular accidents have the worst prognosis in the nontraumatic group, followed by hypoxia–ischemia from cardiac arrest. Hepatic and other metabolic encephalopathies have the best prognosis.

## BRAIN DEATH

The patient is deeply unconscious, i.e., having unarousable unresponsiveness. His pupillary, oculocephalic, corneal, and gag reflexes are absent. He does not have spontaneous respiration, even at a carbon dioxide pressure of at least 60 mm Hg. EEG is isoelectric, and there is no cerebral blood flow in cerebral contrast angiography or radionuclide angiography. All these features should be present without potentially reversible causes of marked CNS depression like hypothermia, barbiturate overdose, severe metabolic abnormalities, and continued use of sedatives and paralytic medicines.

## CLINICAL PEARLS

Coma is an emergency and needs urgent and fast holistic medical and surgical care in an intensive care unit.

Prognosis is poor.

Counseling of family members about the grave situation, diagnostic needs, treatment options, and probable outcome to be discussed with tender care.

## FURTHER READINGS

1. Berger JR and Price R. Stupor and coma. In: Jankovic J, Mazziotta JC, Pomeroy SL, Newman NJ (Eds). Bradley and Daroff's Neurology in Clinical Practice, 8th edition. Philadelphia: Elsevier; 2022. pp. 34-51.
2. Huff JS, Tadi P. Coma. StatPearls [Internet]. Treasure Island, FL: StatPearls Publishing; 2022.
3. Maiese K. Overview of coma and impaired consciousness—neurologic disorders. MSD Manual Professional Edition. [online] Available from https://www.msdmanuals.com/professional/neurologic-disorders/coma-and-impaired-consciousness/overview-of-coma-and-impaired-consciousness. [Last accessed August, 2023].

# PART 9

# Nephrology

CHAPTER 60

# Edema

*Koushik Bhattacharya*

## WHAT IS EDEMA?

Edema is the accumulation of excessive amount of fluid in the subcutaneous tissue or in the serous cavity due to an increase in interstitial volume of the extracellular fluid compartment. A weight gain of several kilograms commonly precedes overt manifestation of edema. Anasarca refers to gross, generalized edema. Ascites and hydrothorax are considered special forms of edema, characterized by excessive fluid in the peritoneal and pleural cavities, respectively. Edema is the result of an imbalance in the filtration system between the capillary and interstitial spaces. Edema is a frequently encountered problem in clinical practice and may indicate an underlying serious condition.

## WHAT CAUSES EDEMA?

About two-thirds of total body water is intracellular and one-third is extracellular. One-fourth of the extracellular fluid is in the intravascular compartment (plasma), and remainder is the interstitial fluid. There is constant exchange of fluid between intravascular and interstitial compartments of extracellular fluid. Edema represents the overt clinical manifestation of an excess of interstitial fluid. Development of edema depends on any of the following mechanisms: (1) Increase in intracapillary hydrostatic pressure, (2) reduction in plasma oncotic pressure, (3) inadequate lymphatic drainage, (4) increase in the oncotic pressure in the interstitial space, and (5) damage to the capillary endothelial barrier.

The kidneys have a central role in maintaining body fluid homeostasis: They control extracellular fluid volume by adjusting sodium and water excretion. Antidiuretic hormone, which is secreted in response to stimuli such as changes in blood volume, tonicity, and blood pressure, is the primary regulator of body water. The concept of effective arterial blood volume (EABV) is central to an understanding of the sodium retention that occurs to maintain plasma volume. In a volume-depleted state, EABV and extracellular fluid volume are reduced. Renal sodium retention is activated via the renin–angiotensin–aldosterone axis, and normal blood volume is restored. When kidney function is impaired, the partitioning of fluid in various compartments is disturbed. In the ensuing edematous states, the reduction in EABV activates volume/pressure sensors, including low-pressure baroreceptors in the venous circulation, high-pressure baroreceptors in the great vessels, intrarenal receptors, and intrahepatic receptors. In patients with primary sodium retention, the afferent stimuli are suppressed.

As extracellular volume increases, edema develops and EABV decreases. This change stimulates efferent pathways, causing sodium retention, activation of the sympathetic nervous system, stimulation of the renin-angiotensin-aldosterone axis, and secretion of arginine vasopressin.

Whether it is caused by decreased cardiac output or other conditions, edema persists because of compensatory mechanisms geared toward maintaining plasma volume.

# WHAT ARE THE POSSIBILITIES? CAUSES OF EDEMA

Etiology of edema always must be determined as the condition may indicate an underlying life-threatening disease such as congestive heart failure, or it may be caused by a benign condition.

## According to Generalized or Localized Edema

- *Generalized*:
  - Heart failure
  - *Edema of renal disease*: Nephrotic syndrome, chronic kidney disease (CKD)
  - Cirrhosis of liver
  - *Hypoalbuminemic states*: Protein-losing enteropathy, starvation, kwashiorkor (nutritional edema)
- *Localized*:
  - *Venous obstruction*: Pregnancy, superior vena cava (SVC) syndrome, inferior vena cava (IVC) syndrome, varicose veins in legs, prolonged recumbency, deep vein thrombosis, immobilized or paralyzed limbs
  - *Lymphatic obstruction (lymphedema)*: Filariasis, tuberculosis, carcinoma of the breast
  - *Allergic causes*: Allergic causes, angioneurotic edema
  - *Inflammatory*: Trauma, insect bite, snakebite

## Pitting or Nonpitting

- *Pitting edema*:
  - Congestive cardiac failure
  - Hepatic cirrhosis
  - Nephrotic syndrome
  - Pericardial effusion
  - Constrictive pericarditis
  - Hypoalbuminemia
- *Nonpitting edema*:
  - Myxedema
  - Lymphoedema
  - Angioneurotic edema
  - Scleroderma

# PATH TO DIAGNOSIS

A systematic approach is warranted to determine the underlying diagnosis. Detailed history and physical examination are required to ascertain the cause of edema.

## History Taking

### *Evolution of Edema*

- *Congestive cardiac failure*: Legs → face → ascites
- *Cirrhosis of liver*: Ascites → legs → face
- *Nephrotic syndrome*: Face (periorbital puffiness) → legs → ascites
- *Nutritional edema*: Pedal edema with facial puffiness → ascites

### *Distribution of Edema*

- Edema associated with heart failure is more extensive in the legs and accentuated in the evening. In patients who are bed bound, edema may be prominent in the presacral region.
- Edema resulting from hypoproteinemia, such as nephrotic syndrome, is generalized, but it is more prominent in the very soft tissue of the eyelids and face and tends to be more prominent in the morning.

- Edema secondary to venous or lymphatic obstruction is limited to one leg or to one or both arms.
- In patients with SVC obstruction, edema is limited to face, neck, and upper extremities.

### Other Relevant History

- *Edema of cardiac origin*: Dyspnea with exertion prominent in edema of cardiac origin; often associated with orthopnea or paroxysmal nocturnal dyspnea
- *Edema of CKD*: Edema often associated with uremic signs and symptoms, including decreased appetite, altered taste, altered sleep pattern, nausea, vomiting, and restless legs
- *Edema of nephrotic syndrome*: Associated with foamy urine
- *Edema of hepatic origin*: Dyspnea uncommon, except if associated with significant ascites. It is often associated with a history of yellowish discoloration of eye and urine and history of hematemesis and melena.
- History of intake of drugs that can cause edema such as nonsteroidal anti-inflammatory drugs (NSAIDs), vasodilators, steroids hormone, calcium channel blockers, cyclosporine, and thiazolidinediones
- A diet grossly deficient in calories and particularly in protein over a prolonged period may result in hypoproteinemia and edema.

## Clinical Examination

Clinical examination is done to ascertain whether the edema is unilateral or bilateral, generalized or local, pitting or nonpitting. Edema can be demonstrated at legs, that is, ankle, and sacral region. Careful observation should be made for puffy face, puffy lower eyelids, scrotal edema, and parietal edema of the abdominal wall. Edema can also be seen in the upper extremity (over wrist, lateral epicondyle at elbow), over sternum, vertebra, and forehead. Look for pallor, jaundice, cyanosis, clubbing, edema, pulses, blood pressure, jugular venous pressure, and respiratory rate.

### Systemic Examination

*Cardiovascular system*: Examine for displaced and dyskinetic apical impulse, murmur, S3 gallop, pericardial rub—pericarditis

*Respiratory system*: Evidence of pleural effusion

*Gastrointestinal system*: Look for ascites and hepatosplenomegaly

The following physical findings are frequently observed in major diseases associated with edema:

- *Edema of cardiac origin*: Elevated jugular venous pressure, S3 gallop, displaced cardiac apical impulse
- *Edema of hepatic origin*: Frequently associated with ascites, signs of chronic liver disease such as jaundice, palmar erythema, spider angiomata, male gynecomastia, asterixis, and other signs of encephalopathy may be present. Jugular venous pressure is normal or low; blood is lower than in renal or cardiac disease
- *Chronic renal failure (CRF)*: Elevated blood pressure, hypertensive retinopathy, pericardiac friction rub in advanced uremia

## Investigation

The following basic investigations will give a clue to diagnose the cause of edema:

- Complete blood count
- Liver function test
- *Renal parameters*: Urea, creatinine
- Total protein, serum albumin
- Free triiodothyronine (fT3), free thyroxine (fT4), thyroid stimulating hormone (TSH)
- Urine routine, spot albumin-to-creatinine ratio (ACR), and 24-hour urine protein
- Chest X-ray, echocardiography, ultrasonography (USG) W/A

Edema caused by major organ impairment is characterized by the following findings:

- *Cardiac origin*: Serum sodium often diminished, elevated natriuretic peptides, elevated urea nitrogen to creatinine ratio. Electrocardiogram (ECG) and echocardiography are often helpful.
- *Hepatic origin*: Altered liver function test including elevated liver enzymes and reduction in serum albumin. USG often shows coarse and contracted liver in cirrhosis.
- *CRF*: Normocytic anemia, elevation of serum creatinine and cystatin C, hypocalcemia, hyperphosphatemia, hyperkalemia, metabolic acidosis, albuminuria
- *Nephrotic syndrome*: Nephrotic range proteinuria (>3.5 g/day)

## THERAPY

Treatment of edema consists of reversing the underlying disorder, restricting dietary sodium to minimize fluid retention, and, usually, employing diuretic therapy. Not all patients with edema will require drug treatment; in some patients, sufficient sodium restriction and elevation of the lower extremities are effective. However, diuretics are required in most patients in addition to nonpharmacologic treatments, especially continued restriction of salt. The choice of diuretic, route of administration, and dosing regimen will vary based on the underlying disease, its severity, and the urgency of the problem. Knowledge of the pharmacokinetics and pharmacodynamics of the various agents is essential. Many medications have been implicated in pedal edema, especially vasodilators, estrogens, NSAIDs, and calcium channel blockers. Dihydropyridine drugs are more likely than other calcium channel blockers to cause pedal edema **(Figs. 1A and B)**. The edema appears to be dose-dependent and increases over time. Because medication-induced edema is caused by capillary hypertension, diuretics are not an effective treatment. However, angiotensin-converting enzyme inhibitors and angiotensin-receptor blockers seem to be effective.

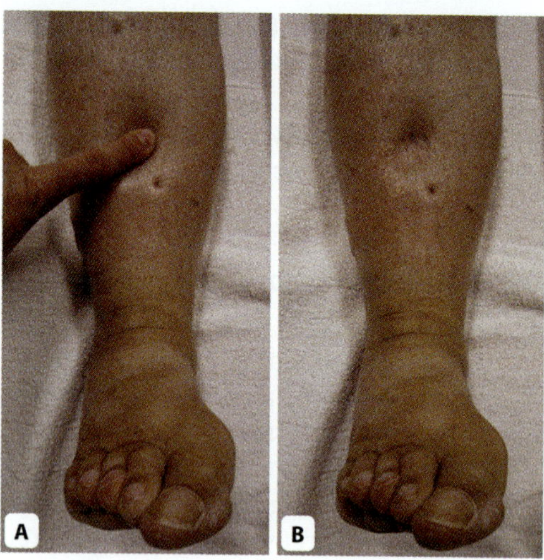


**FIGS. 1A AND B:** Pedal edema.

## CLINICAL PEARLS

Common etiologies of edema in the Indian subcontinent are congestive cardiac failure, CKD, proteinuric conditions, cirrhosis of liver, and hypoalbuminemic state such as malnutrition. The clinical association that may give clues are Evolution of edema, distribution of edema, associated clinical history, and physical examination findings. A systematic approach is helpful to pinpoint the cause of edema.

## FURTHER READINGS

1. Cho S, Atwood JE. Peripheral edema. Am J Med. 2002;113(7):580-6.
2. Miserocchi G, Negrini D, Passi A, De Luca G. Development of lung edema: interstitial fluid dynamics and molecular structure. News Physiol Sci. 2001;16:66-71.
3. Bhave G, Neilson EG. Body fluid dynamics: back to the future. J Am Soc Nephrol. 2011;22(12):2166-81.
4. Levick JR, Michel CC. Microvascular fluid exchange and the revised Starling principle. Cardiovasc Res. 2010;15:87(2):198-210.

# CHAPTER 61

# Dysuria

*Koushik Bhattacharya*

## WHAT IS DYSURIA?

Dysuria, or pain that occurs during voiding, is commonly perceived as burning, tingling, or stinging of the urethra and meatus. Dysuria is a symptom of several syndromes. These conditions are distinguished by the presence or absence of other symptoms. Dysuria is one of the most common symptoms that calls attention to the lower urinary tract.

## WHAT CAUSES DYSURIA?

Sensory nerves are located just beneath the urothelium. Chemical irritation and inflammatory conditions (e.g., acute bacterial infection) can alter the mucosal barrier and stimulate these nerves, causing pain. Chronic inflammation and other unknown factors can lead to altered nerve sensitivity and persistent pain. Inflammation from the adjacent abdominal structures, such as the colon, can also affect function and sensation in the bladder.

Inflammatory disorders of the bladder and urethra are the most common causes of dysuria. Among these, infections of the bladder, urethra, kidneys, and genital organs are the most prevalent, including uncomplicated cystitis, pyelonephritis, and urethritis. Distinguishing a complicated urinary tract infection (UTI) from cystitis is important because misdiagnosis increases the risk of treatment failure. In women, dysuria is also a common presentation of vaginitis. In men, prostatitis can present with dysuria. Sexually transmitted infections (STIs) can also cause dysuria.

Inflammatory, noninfectious conditions that can lead to dysuria include the presence of a foreign body (e.g., stent, bladder stone), noninfectious urethritis (e.g., reactive arthritis, formerly Reiter syndrome), and dermatologic conditions. Noninflammatory conditions can be divided into the following categories: Anatomic; endocrine; neoplastic; medication, food, or recreational drug-related; iatrogenic; and idiopathic. Any condition that causes hematuria with clots can cause dysuria, including renal neoplasms and nephrolithiasis. Interstitial cystitis (also known as bladder pain syndrome) refers to chronic bladder pain, often with voiding symptoms, lasting 6 weeks or more without an identifiable cause.

## WHAT ARE THE POSSIBILITIES?

- *Women*: Two major causes of dysuria are bacterial cystitis and lower genital tract infections.
    - *Bacterial cystitis*: It is usually caused by *Escherichia coli*, other gram-negative rods, and *Staphylococcus*

*saprophyticus*. Bacterial cystitis is acute in onset, and other lower urinary tract symptoms such as urinary frequency, urgency, suprapubic pain, and hematuria are usually present.
  - *Lower genital tract infections*: For example, vaginitis, urethritis, and ulcerative lesions. The onset of dysuria is more gradual than bacterial cystitis.
- *Men*: Prostatitis is the most common cause of dysuria and is usually caused by *E. coli* or other gram-negative rods. Acute bacterial prostatitis presents with fever and chills, and chronic bacterial prostatitis presents as a recurrent episode of bacterial cystitis.

*Causes of dysuria*:

- *Inflammatory*:
  - *Dermatologic*: Irritant or contact dermatitis, lichen sclerosis, lichen planus, psoriasis, Stevens–Johnson syndrome, Bechet syndrome
  - *Infectious*: Cystitis, urethritis, pyelonephritis, other STIs. In women, infections such as vulvovaginitis and cervicitis, and in men, prostatitis and epididymo-orchitis are the most common symptoms associated with dysuria.
  - *Noninfectious*: Foreign body (e.g., stent, stone), urethritis (e.g., reactive arthritis)
- *Noninflammatory*:
  - *Anatomic*: Urethral stricture or diverticulum. In men, benign prostatic hyperplasia
  - *Drug- or food-related*: Spermicides, topical deodorants, cyclophosphamide, opioids, ketamine, nifedipine, and others; bladder-irritating foods
  - *Endocrine*: In women, atrophic vaginitis, endometriosis
  - *Idiopathic*: Interstitial cystitis/bladder pain syndrome
  - *Neoplastic*: Bladder or renal cancer, lymphoma metastatic cancer. In women, vaginal or vulvar cancer, paraurethral leiomyoma. In men, prostate or penile cancer
  - *Trauma/iatrogenic*: Genitourinary instrumentation or surgery, pelvic irradiation, foreign body presence, horseback or bicycle riding

## PATH TO DIAGNOSIS

### History

Meticulous history taking is important to determine the etiology of dysuria. The medical history should characterize the timing, persistence, severity, duration, and exact location of the dysuria.

Pain occurring at the start of urination may indicate urethral pathology, whereas pain occurring at the end of urination is usually of bladder origin. Physicians should ask about other bladder symptoms, such as frequency, urgency, incontinence, hematuria, malodorous urine, and nocturia. The history should include the presence of flank pain, nausea, fever, and other systemic symptoms. A history of dysuria, UTIs, STIs, and recent sexual activity is crucial. Additionally, medication use, family history, and procedural history can help identify the cause of dysuria. In women, the history should also include the presence of vaginal discharge or irritation, most recent menstrual period, and type of contraception used.

Specific localization of the discomfort varies between men and women. Women with vaginitis often describe external dysuria as well as vaginal irritation or discharge. With cystitis, the dysuria is characteristically felt in the bladder or urethra. In addition to dysuria, men with prostatitis may have deep perineal pain and obstructive urinary symptoms, whereas those with epididymo-orchitis may have localized testicular pain. Lesions from herpes simplex virus of the vulvar or penile area may cause dysuria. Patients with interstitial cystitis may have suprapubic or abdominal pain related to bladder filling. These patients nearly always report urinary frequency and urgency, whereas dysuria is variable.

## Clinical Examination

The physical examination, especially when complicated UTI is a consideration, should include vital signs, evaluation for costovertebral angle pain, palpation for abdominal mass or tenderness, and inspection for dermatologic conditions and acute joint effusions. Often, the most relevant findings on physical examination are sex-specific, including inspecting for infectious or atrophic vaginitis and STIs in women, and prostatitis and STIs in men. The presence of costovertebral angle tenderness on examination modestly increases the likelihood of having a UTI, especially pyelonephritis.

## Investigations

Any complicating features or recurrent symptoms warrant a history, physical examination, urinalysis, and urine culture. Findings from the selected laboratory tests and directed imaging studies enable physicians to progress through a logical evaluation and determine the cause of dysuria.

### *Urinalysis*

Urinalysis is the most useful test in a patient with dysuria. Detection of leukocyte esterase, nitrites, and blood in urine dipstick and pyuria (presence of a significant number of pus cells) in urine microscopy is highly suggestive of UTI.

### *Cultures and Cytology*

Any patient with risk factors and clinical suspicion for a complicated UTI or whose symptoms do not respond to initial treatment should have a urine culture and sensitivity analysis.

### *Blood*

Patients with suspected pyelonephritis should have renal function assessed with serum creatinine measurement, and electrolyte levels should be measured if there is substantial nausea and vomiting. Blood cultures are usually not necessary but can be obtained in patients with high fever or risk of infectious complications.

### *Others*

- In women with vaginal symptoms, secretions should be evaluated with wet mount and potassium hydroxide microscopy or a vaginal pathogens deoxyribonucleic acid (DNA) probe.
- Urethritis should be suspected in younger, sexually active patients with dysuria and pyuria without bacteriuria; in men, urethral inflammation and discharge are typically present. In patients with suspected urethritis, a urethral, vaginal, endocervical, or urine nucleic acid amplification test for *Neisseria gonorrhoeae* and *Chlamydia trachomatis* is indicated.
- Genital ulcerations can be sampled for herpes simplex virus culture or polymerase chain reaction testing, as well as testing for other STIs.
- In men with suspected chronic prostatitis, urine culture after gentle prostatic massage can yield the causative bacterial agent. The prostate-specific antigen level is transiently elevated during acute prostatitis and should not be measured in patients with acute inflammatory symptoms.
- Urine cytology is helpful if bladder cancer is suspected, such as in older patients with hematuria and a negative culture result.

### *Imaging and Other Advanced Studies*

Imaging is not necessary in most patients with dysuria, although it may be indicated in patients with a complicated UTI, a suspected anatomic anomaly (e.g., abnormal voiding, positive family history of genitourinary anomalies), obstruction or abscess, relapsing infection, or hematuria.

- *Ultrasonography*: Preferred initial test for patients with obstruction, abscess, recurrent infection, or suspected kidney stones.
- Computed tomography urography is used to view the kidneys and adjacent structures and may be considered for further evaluation in patients with possible abscess, obstruction, or suspected anomalies when ultrasonography is not diagnostic.
- *Cystoscopy*: If urinalysis is unrevealing, cystoscopy can be performed to evaluate for bladder cancer, hematuria, and chronic bladder symptoms.
- Urodynamic studies can be performed for persistent voiding symptoms with otherwise unrevealing workup.
- Further investigation and urology referral should be considered in patients with recurrent UTI, urolithiasis, known urinary tract abnormality or cancer, history of urologic surgery, hematuria, persistent symptoms, or in men with an abnormal postvoid residual urine level.

## THERAPY

In the right clinical setting, symptoms alone can identify patients with a high likelihood of UTI who are candidates for empiric therapy. Women with an uncomplicated history who present with acute dysuria, urinary urgency or frequency, and no vaginal discharge can be treated for acute cystitis without other evaluation.

- *Interstitial cystitis/bladder pain syndrome*: Initiate conservative treatment (symptom diary to modify fluid intake, diet, and physical activity; bladder training)
- *Overactive bladder*: Fluid restriction, bladder training, pelvic floor muscle exercises, drug therapy as needed empirically
- *Potentially offending topical irritant*: Discontinue use of the offending agent
- *Suspected bladder irritants*: Dietary and medication modification
- *Urethral diverticulum or endometriosis (women)*: Urology or gynecology referral

## CLINICAL PEARLS

The most common cause of acute dysuria is infection, especially cystitis. Other infectious causes include urethritis, STIs, and vaginitis. Noninfectious inflammatory causes include a foreign body in the urinary tract and dermatologic conditions. Noninflammatory causes of dysuria include medication use, urethral anatomic abnormalities, local trauma, and interstitial cystitis/bladder pain syndrome. An initial targeted history includes features of a local cause (e.g., vaginal or urethral irritation), risk factors for a complicated UTI (e.g., male sex, pregnancy, presence of urologic obstruction, recent procedure), and symptoms of pyelonephritis. Women with dysuria who have no complicating features can be treated for cystitis without further diagnostic evaluation. Women with vulvovaginal symptoms should be evaluated for vaginitis. Any complicating features or recurrent symptoms warrant a history, physical examination, urinalysis, and urine culture. Findings from the selected laboratory tests and directed imaging studies enable physicians to progress through a systematic evaluation and determine the cause of dysuria.

## FURTHER READINGS

1. Michels TC, Sands JE. Dysuria: Evaluation and Differential Diagnosis in Adults. Am Fam Physician. 2015;92(9):778-86.
2. Geerlings SE. Clinical Presentations and Epidemiology of Urinary Tract Infections. Microbiol Spectr. 2016;4(5).
3. Wrenn K. Dysuria, Frequency, and Urgency. In: Walker HK, Hall WD, Hurst JW, editors. Clinical Methods: The History, Physical, and Laboratory Examinations. 3rd ed. Butterworths: Boston; 1990.

# CHAPTER 62

# Frequency of Urine

*Koushik Bhattacharya*

## WHAT IS NORMAL URINE FREQUENCY?

Abnormally frequent urination (e.g., once every hour or two) is termed urinary frequency. Urinary frequency should be differentiated from polyuria, which specifically relates to the passage of an abnormally large volume of urine in a relatively short period of time. Frequency of normal urination may vary considerably from individual to individual depending on age, personality traits, bladder capacity, or drinking habits. Because of this fact, a history of frequency is sometimes difficult to obtain. Changes in the pattern of frequency or a history of voiding more than once at night after retiring, however, are clues to urinary pathology. Frequency may be accompanied by a sensation of an urgent need to void (urinary urgency). Although the International Continence Society defines urinary frequency as the perception by the patient that he/she voids too often, epidemiological studies suggest that the normal micturition rate is approximately 8 micturitions per day and 1 or fewer episodes per night.

## WHAT CAUSES URINE FREQUENCY?

The urinary bladder is a hollow muscular organ that is lined by mucosa (urothelium) and is sensitive to both urine volume and its chemical composition. A healthy bladder is free of bacterial infection or tumors and stores urine without discomfort at low pressure with intermittent signals of filling. The normal functional bladder capacity in adults ranges from approximately 300 to 400 mL. Nerve fibers respond to increasing filling, and micturition is prompted at or near bladder volume capacity (approximately every 3–4 hours based on the volume of liquid consumed). Voiding typically occurs via initial relaxation of the pelvic floor muscles and the bladder neck followed by voluntary contraction of the detrusor muscle. Healthy voiding occurs promptly with strong continuous flow and complete emptying without pain or blood in the urine. When necessary, an individual should be able to defer voiding without leakage. Variations in any of these normal responses may be a sign of disease.

Anatomically, functional bladder capacity increases with age from childhood. Changes in the adult bladder and pelvic floor muscles with aging include decreased bladder sensation, decreased contractility during voiding, decreased muscle tone in pelvic floor muscles, and increased residual volume. Other physical changes include upregulation of purinergic receptors with increased prevalence of detrusor overactivity and increased acetylcholine release in the urothelium, both of which can produce lower urinary tract symptoms (LUTS).

Urinary frequency usually results from disorders of the lower genitourinary tract. Inflammation of the bladder, urethra, or both causes a sensation of the need to urinate. However, this sensation is not relieved by emptying the bladder, so once the bladder is emptied, patients continue trying to void but pass only small volumes of urine.

## WHAT ARE THE POSSIBILITIES?

Most common causes of urine frequency are urinary tract infections (UTIs), benign prostatic hyperplasia (BPH), drugs and substance related (caffeine, alcohol, diuretic), urine incontinence, neurogenic bladder, and overactive bladder (OAB).

Urinary frequency may occur because of either increased urine volume or decreased bladder capacity:

- Increased urine volume can result from diuretic use, diabetes mellitus with osmotic diuresis, diabetes insipidus, hypercalcemia, compulsive water drinking, or loss of renal concentrating ability. The latter occurs early in many types of renal parenchymal disease including infection. There is also a diuretic response after relief of urinary tract obstruction, during the recovery phase of acute renal failure, termination of supraventricular tachyarrhythmias, and with bedrest in the setting of edema.
- Decreased bladder capacity can result from anxiety, operative procedures, obstruction with resulting residual urine and decreased functional capacity, a thickened fibrotic wall (from interstitial cystitis, irradiation, chronic infections such as tuberculosis and schistosomiasis), or inflammatory conditions that increase bladder sensitivity (e.g., pressure from intrinsic or extrinsic masses, calculi, or infections). Spastic neurogenic bladders also cause a decreased bladder capacity, whereas hypotonic neurogenic bladders with chronic large residual volumes (>30 mL) mimic bladder outlet obstruction with a decreased functional capacity. Very low or high urinary pH can rarely cause frequency. Psychiatric disturbances are not infrequently reflected with symptoms of urinary frequency. Frequency is a common response to emotional stress.

Often, frequent urination is not a symptom of a problem but is the problem. In people with an overactive bladder syndrome, involuntary bladder contractions lead to frequent and often urgent urination.

## PATH TO DIAGNOSIS

Symptom of urinary frequency should be evaluated if it interferes with lifestyle or is accompanied by other symptoms such as fever, back or side pain, vomiting, chills, increased appetite or thirst, fatigue, bloody or cloudy urine, or a discharge from the genitourinary tract.

To diagnose the cause of frequent urination, meticulous history and physical examination are required.

### History

History should include:

- Acuity of onset of symptom
- Duration of symptoms
- Diet and addiction history (e.g., alcohol, caffeinated beverages)
- Medication history such as diuretics
- Associated with other LUTS such as irritative symptoms (e.g., irritation, urgency, dysuria) and obstructive symptoms (e.g., hesitancy, poor flow, sensation of incomplete voiding, nocturia)
- Diurnal variation of symptoms
- Pattern of daily fluid intake
- Any addiction history
- *Voiding diaries/bladder diaries*: Diaries that document intake and voiding behavior may be useful, particularly for

patient education and to document baseline symptoms and treatment efficacy
- Recent sexual contacts
- History of fever, flank or groin pain, hematuria
- History of back pain or lower limb weakness

*Past medical history* should ask about known causes, including prostate disease and previous pelvic radiation therapy or surgeries.

### Clinical Examination

Examination focuses on the genitourinary system.

Any urethral discharge or any lesions consistent with sexually transmitted infections are noted. Rectal examination in men should note the size and consistency of the prostate and rectal tone; pelvic examination in women should note the presence of any cystocele. Patients should be instructed to cough while the urethra is observed for signs of urinary leakage.

The costovertebral angle should be palpated for tenderness, and the abdominal examination should note the presence of any masses or suprapubic tenderness.

Neurologic examination should test for lower-extremity weakness and loss of sensation.

### Investigations

All patients require urinalysis and culture. Cystoscopy, cystometry, and urethrography can be done to diagnose cystitis, bladder outlet obstruction, and cystocele. Prostate-specific antigen level determination, ultrasonography, and prostate biopsy may be required, especially in older men, to differentiate BPH from prostate cancer.

- *Blood tests*: Routine blood test for fasting blood sugar (FBS), kidney function (urea, creatinine), electrolytes with serum calcium
- *Urinalysis*: The microscopic examination of urine with urine culture and sensitivity (C/S)
- *Cystoscopy*: Direct visualization inside the bladder and urethra using a thin, lighted instrument called a cystoscope.
- *Cystometry*: A test that measures the pressure inside the bladder to see how well the bladder is working; cystometry is done to determine if a muscle or nerve problem may be causing problems with how well the bladder holds or releases urine. There is a broader term called urodynamics that includes tests such as cystometry, uroflowmetry, urethral pressure, and others.
- *Ultrasonography*: This is done to look for kidney size, echotexture, prostatomegaly, urine bladder with postvoid residual (PVR) urine, presence of hydroureteronephrosis. PVR should be assessed in patients with obstructive symptoms, history of incontinence or prostatic surgery, neurologic diagnoses, and at clinician's discretion. Antimuscarinic drugs should be used with caution in patients with PVR—250–300 mL.

## THERAPY

Treatment for frequent urination will address the underlying problem that is causing it. For example, if diabetes is the cause, treatment will involve keeping blood sugar levels under control. Behavioral therapies (e.g., bladder training, bladder-control strategies, pelvic floor muscle training, fluid management) should be offered as first-line therapy to all patients with overactive bladder. Antimuscarinic agents may be used in combination with behavioral strategies. Limited evidence suggests that initiating behavioral and pharmacologic therapy simultaneously may improve outcomes, including frequency.

The treatment for overactive bladder should begin with behavioral therapies, such as:

- *Bladder retraining*: This involves increasing the intervals between using the bathroom over the course of about 12 weeks. This helps retrain bladder to hold urine longer and to urinate less frequently.

- *Diet modification*: Dietary advice to avoid any food that appears to irritate bladder or acts as a diuretic. These may include caffeine, alcohol, carbonated drinks, tomato-based products, chocolate, artificial sweeteners, and spicy foods. It is also important to eat high-fiber foods because constipation may worsen the symptoms of overactive bladder syndrome.
- *Monitoring fluid food intake*: Patients should drink enough to prevent constipation and overconcentration of urine. Avoid drinking just before bedtime, which can lead to nighttime urination.
- *Kegel exercises*: These exercises help strengthen the muscles around the bladder and urethra to improve bladder control and reduce urinary urgency and frequency. Exercising pelvic muscles for 5 minutes three times a day can make a difference in bladder control.

Treatment may also include anti-muscarinic drugs such as darifenacin, desmopressin acetate, imipramine, mirabegron, oxybutynin (Ditropan), oxybutynin skin patch, solifenacin, tolterodine extended-release. Darifenacin is specifically for people who wake up more than twice a night to urinate. Constipation and dry mouth are main side effects of this group of drugs. Clinicians must use caution in prescribing antimuscarinics in patients who are using other medications with anticholinergic properties. Medications with anticholinergic properties include tricyclic antidepressants, acetylcholinesterase inhibitors, and medications for Parkinsonism, other extrapyramidal diseases, and Alzheimer's disease. Certain antinausea medications and those with atropine-like properties may also potentiate adverse effects (AEs). Prescribers should be aware of precautions and contraindications for these medications. Clinicians should use caution in prescribing antimuscarinics in the frail OAB patient.

In refractory cases, especially those associated with overactive bladder, sacral neuromodulation and intradetrusor botulinum toxin A (Botox) may be offered.

## CLINICAL PEARLS

Urine frequency is one of the common LUTS challenged by clinicians. Varied causes, ranging from benign condition such as drug associated to serious condition such as complicated UTI, can be ascertained by proper history, physical examination, and directed investigations. Although the symptom of urine frequency will be ameliorated with specific treatment of the underlying condition, behavioral therapy and some antimuscarinic drugs have been shown to have some effect in clinical practice.

## FURTHER READINGS

1. Wang S, Mitu GM, Hirschberg R. Osmotic polyuria: an overlooked mechanism in diabetic nephropathy. Nephrol Dial Transplant. 2008; 23(7):2167-72.
2. Nocturia and nocturnal polyuria in men with lower urinary tract symptoms: oral desmopressin | Advice | NICE [Internet]. www.nice.org.uk. 2013 [cited 2024 Jan 22]. Available from: https://www.nice.org.uk/advice/esuom 10.
3. Cohen JF, Pauchard J-Y, Hjelm N, Cohen R, Chalumeau M. Efficacy and safety of rapid tests to guide antibiotic prescriptions for sore throat. Cochrane Database Syst Rev. 20204; 6(6):CD012431.
4. Fraser H, Gallacher D, Achana F, Court R, Taylor-Phillips S, Nduka C, et al. Rapid antigen detection and molecular tests for group A streptococcal infections for acute sore throat: systematic reviews and economic evaluation. Health Technol Assess. 2020;24(31):1-232.

CHAPTER 63

# Hematuria

*Rojina Choudhury*

## WHAT IS HEMATURIA? DEFINITION

Hematuria means presence of blood/blood cells in urine. It is defined as persistent presence of > 5 red blood cells (RBC)/high power field (HPF) in centrifuged urine sample. Minimum three sample should be taken at least 7 days apart. The word hematuria is derived from the Greek words haima (blood) and ouron (urine). Commercially available dipsticks are very sensitive and capable of detecting three to five RBCs/HPF.

A freshly voided midstream clean catch urine sample of 10–15 mL is needed for urine analysis.

Red urine without RBCs is seen in hemoglobinuria, myoglobinuria, drugs (rifampicin, chloroquine), and dyes (beets, blackberries, food coloring agents).

False-positive test is found in the presence of hydrogen peroxide ($H_2O_2$) and alkaline urine (urine pH > 8).

False-negative test is found in the presence of formalin, which is used as a preservative of urine sample and presence of high concentration of vitamin C in urine sample.

Hematuria can be gross (visible to the naked eye) or microscopic (not visible to the naked eye, detected by a microscope during urine analysis). It can be painful or painless and transient or persistent in nature. It can be isolated (only hematuria) or associated with proteinuria or other urinary problems.

Hematuria can be symptomatic or asymptomatic. It can be associated with the following local symptoms: Urinary frequency, urgency, hesitancy known as lower urinary tract symptoms (LUTS), flank pain, lower abdominal pain, back pain, flank fullness/mass, and passing stone or grits. Systemic symptoms can be the following: Fever, anorexia, cachexia, weight loss, joint pain, oral ulcers, rash, periorbital swelling, pedal swelling, hearing loss, hemoptysis, and recent throat or skin infection.

## WHAT CAUSES HEMATURIA? ETIOPATHOGENESIS

Hematuria occurs due to direct injury by trauma, tumor, or calculus on the mucosal surface of the urinary tract, that is, kidney, ureter, urinary bladder, and urethra. Apart from that prostate in men and cervix in women often contribute as a source of hematuria. Sometimes, hematuria occurs due to systemic illness causing injury to glomerulus. Glomerular injury results from either inflammatory or immunologic reaction.

## WHAT ARE THE POSSIBILITIES? ETIOLOGY

Causes of hematuria are grossly divided into two categories: (1) Upper urinary tract sources (glomerulus, tubular system, or interstitium) and (2) lower urinary tract source (pelvicalyceal system, ureter, bladder, or urethra).

Glomerular source of hematuria is characterized by the presence of cola- or brown-colored urine, proteinuria, RBCs cast, and deformed or dysmorphic RBCs, usually acanthocytes.

Tubular source of hematuria is characterized by the presence of tubular casts and sometimes leukocytes.

Gross hematuria that is bright red in color along with normal urinary RBCs (normal morphology) and minimal proteinuria is found in the lower urinary tract source of hematuria.

*Hematuria due to upper urinary tract causes*:

- *Hematuria due to renal disease*:
    - Poststreptococcal glomerulonephritis (PSGN)
    - Membranoproliferative glomerulonephritis (MPGN)
    - Membranous nephropathy
    - Rapidly proliferative glomerulonephritis (RPGN)
    - Focal segmental glomerulonephritis (FSGS)
    - Nephrotic syndrome
    - Immunoglobulin A (IgA) nephropathy
    - Alport syndrome
    - Thin glomerular basement membrane (GBM) disease
- *Hematuria due to multisystem disease*:
    - Systemic lupus erythematosus (SLE) nephritis
    - Henoch–Schönlein purpura (HSP) nephritis
    - Granulomatosis with polyangiitis
    - Goodpasture syndrome
    - Polyarteritis nodosa (PAN)
    - Hemolytic uremic syndrome (HUS) and thrombotic thrombocytopenic purpura (TTP)
    - Human immunodeficiency virus (HIV) nephropathy
    - Sickle cell nephropathy
- *Hematuria due to tubulointerstitial disease*:
    - Acute tubular necrosis
    - Pyelonephritis
    - Interstitial nephritis
- *Hematuria due to vascular disorder of the renal system*:
    - Arterial or venous thrombosis
    - Malformation (aneurysm, hemangioma)
- *Hematuria due to anatomic disorders*:
    - Polycystic kidney disease
    - Hydronephrosis
- *Hematuria due to neoplastic disorders*:
    - Wilms tumor
    - Rhabdomyosarcoma
    - Renal cell cancer
- Hematuria due to trauma

*Hematuria due to lower urinary tract causes*:

- Severe exercise
- Febrile illness
- Menstruation
- Nephrolithiasis
- *Infection*: Cystitis, urethritis, prostatitis
- Trauma or iatrogenic injury to the genitourinary tract (GU)
- Neoplastic disorders, that is, bladder cancer, prostate cancer, cancer of cervix
- Disseminated intravascular coagulation (DIC)
- Thrombocytopenia due to any cause
- Anticoagulation drug

The most common causes of gross hematuria are as follows:

- Urinary tract infection
- Trauma
- Obstruction due to urolithiasis or neoplastic conditions
- Postinfectious glomerulonephritis
- IgA nephropathy
- MPGN
- HSP
- SLE nephritis

- HUS
- Microscopic PAN
- Granulomatosis with polyangiitis

## APPROACH TO DIAGNOSIS

### History

Most of the cases of hematuria present to primary care physicians and need to take detailed history before referring to a specialist because isolated hematuria is often treated without any complication.

*Symptoms*:
- Recurrent episode of gross hematuria suggestive of (S/O) IgA nephropathy, Alport syndrome, or thin GBM disease
- Unexplained fever along with dysuria or LUTS S/O urinary tract infections (UTIs)
- Presence of family history S/O Alport syndrome, sickle cell disease
- History of (H/O) acute severe exercise S/O exercise-induced hematuria
- H/O hematuria associated with recent sore throat/skin infection/gastrointestinal infection S/O PSGN
- History of fever, joint pain, rash, oral ulcer, and constitutional symptoms S/O SLE nephritis or HSP
- Passing stone or grits during urination and colicky pain S/O urolithiasis
- H/O anticoagulant drug intake
- Hematuria along with epistaxis, altered mental status, headache, or heart failure S/O severe hypertension
- H/O fever, weight loss, and hematuria S/O renal cell carcinoma (RCC), Wilms tumor
- H/O hemoptysis and hematuria S/O Goodpasture syndrome

### Clinical Examination

- Presence of hypertension, anasarca, cola-colored urine, and oliguria S/O acute glomerulonephritis
- Fever with chill, rigor, and renal angle tenderness S/O pyelonephritis
- Presence of pallor, icterus S/O sickle cell anemia, and HUS
- Presence of recent diarrheal episode followed by pain in the abdomen and altered mentation along with acute kidney injury S/O TTP
- Presence of painless oral ulcer along with constitutional symptoms S/O SLE nephritis
- Presence of palpable purpura, pain in the abdomen, and fever in children S/O HSP
- Presence of lymphadenopathy along with constitutional symptoms S/O SLE/HIV
- Presence of sensory neural hearing impairment along with family history S/O Alport syndrome
- Presence of flank mass S/O hydronephrosis, renal cystic disease, and tumor
- Presence of suprapubic tenderness along with fever S/O cystitis
- Presence of bronchial asthma and hematuria S/O granulomatosis with polyangiitis
- Presence of sternal tenderness along with purpura in a febrile patient S/O acute leukemia

### Investigations

*Urine routine examination and microscopy* are the most important initial step. Turbid urine specimen with significant white blood cells (WBCs), positive nitrite, and leukocyte esterase test is S/O UTIs. Dysmorphic RBCs > 25%/HPF are highly specific for glomerulonephritis.

*Urine culture and sensitivity* (*C/S*) to know the causative organism.

*Complete hemogram with differential and platelet count and peripheral blood smear* are essential to exclude UTIs, HUS, and TTP. The presence of schistocytes is S/O HUS and TTP.

Raised serum urea and creatinine level indicate renal involvement.

*Liver function test (LFT)* with low serum protein and albumin is S/O nephrotic syndrome.

*Lipid profile* helps to diagnose nephrotic syndrome.

*Serology testing* is done to exclude HIV and hepatitis B virus infection.

*24-hour urine calcium or a spot urine calcium-creatinine ratio* is done to exclude hypercalciuria as a cause of hematuria.

*24-hour urinary protein* to differentiate nephrotic and nephritic range of proteinuria.

*Renal imaging*: Renal and bladder ultrasound is the initial imaging modality to exclude anatomic cause for hematuria. Computed tomography (CT) scan and magnetic resonance imaging (MRI) scan with or without renal vascular doppler are options other than ultrasonography (USG).

*High-performance liquid chromatography (HPLC)* is used to exclude sickle cell disease.

*Serum protein electrophoresis (SPEP) and urinary Bence–Jones protein* are used to exclude multiple myeloma and other light chain disease.

*Blood tests for antinuclear antibodies (ANAs) and double-stranded deoxyribonucleic acid (dsDNA)* are done to exclude SLE nephritis.

*Urine cytology* is done to detect malignant cell.

*C3 and C4 levels*: Low C3 along with positive ANA and anti-dsDNA is found in SLE nephropathy. Low C3 along with normal C4, high ASO titer, and anti-DNAse B is found in PSGN.

Blood for anti-GBM antibody tests are done to exclude Goodpasture's Syndrome (anti-GBM disease).

*Perinuclear anti-neutrophil cytoplasmic antibody (pANCA) and cytoplasmic anti-neutrophil cytoplasmic antibody (cANCA)* tests are done to exclude vasculitis.

*Renal scan* is used to know the anatomy and function of kidney in the presence of hydronephrosis.

*Micturating cystourethrogram (MCU)* is often useful to detect urethral stricture, presence of posterior urethral valve, and vesicoureteral reflux.

*Renal biopsy*: It is the gold standard investigation to diagnose glomerular pathology. Indications for renal biopsy in patients with hematuria are significant proteinuria, abnormal renal function, recurrent persistent hematuria, recurrent gross hematuria, and presence of abnormal complement, ANA, or dsDNA levels.

*Cystoscopy* is reserved because of cost and being a difficult procedure in children. It is done if a mass is detected in USG or there is presence of posterior urethral valve. In adults, negative imaging study of kidney, ureter, and bladder often needs cystoscopy as a next step of investigation. It plays a role in therapeutics also.

## THERAPY

Hematuria is a sign, so management depends on the underlying etiology. First, assure hemodynamic stability.

*Urinary tract infections* need a 7–14-day course of antibiotic therapy according to C/S report. Cystitis, urethritis, balanitis, and prostatitis are treated with antibiotics accordingly.

*Hypercalciuria*: Low-salt diet along with recommended daily amount (RDA) for calcium may be beneficial in children with hypercalciuria and hematuria.

*Nephrolithiasis*: Stone >5 mm in size often needs lithotripsy or nephrostomy.

*Ureteric stone*: It needs to be removed if it causes obstruction.

*Drug-induced hematuria*: Offending drug should be stopped immediately.

*Malignancy*: It needs proper staging, and management depends on the type and stage of malignancy.

*Henoch–Schönlein purpura nephropathy*: It is often self-limited, and symptomatic treatment is enough.

*Immunoglobulin A nephropathy*: IgA disease often has a benign course; angiotensin-converting enzyme (ACE) inhibitor or angiotensin receptor blocker (ARB) is needed for hypertension and proteinuria. Those who suffered from persistent proteinuria in spite of ACE inhibitor or ARB need corticosteroid or other immunosuppressant therapy.

*Poststreptococcal glomerulonephritis*: Treatment is mainly supportive and symptomatic with judicious restriction of salt and fluid to control hypertension and edema. Dialysis is needed sometimes. Antibiotics for streptococcal infection should be initiated.

*Systemic lupus erythematosus nephropathy*: Treatment and prognosis of SLE nephropathy depend on histologic classification and various combination therapies available. High-dose corticosteroid along with cyclophosphamide or mycophenolate mofetil is used for remission followed by maintenance therapy with low-dose steroid and mycophenolate mofetil or azathioprine. Other immunosuppressant options are cyclosporine, tacrolimus, rituximab, or belimumab. End-stage renal disease (ESRD) needs renal replacement therapy.

*HUS and TTP*: They are treated with plasma exchange and corticosteroid. Rituximab is added in refractory cases along with plasmapheresis.

*Anti-GBM disease*: It is treated with plasmapheresis along with corticosteroid and cyclophosphamide. Prognosis is often poor, especially for those who presented with advanced fibrosis in renal biopsy and serum Cr > 5–6 mg/dL.

*Vasculitis-associated glomerulonephritis*: It is treated with immunosuppressants along with supportive treatment. The dose and duration depend on the severity and type of vasculitis.

*Polycystic kidney disease*: It needs regular follow-up and control of hypertension. The goal is to reduce cardiovascular complication and progression of renal disease. Chronic flank or abdominal pain due to enlarged kidney needs pharmacotherapy with narcotic or nonnarcotic analgesic, with an occasional need for surgical decompression.

*Renal vein thrombosis*: Underlying causes need to be treated and anticoagulation therapy is recommended. Nephrectomy may be undertaken in a life-threatening condition. Vena cava filters are used for prevention of thrombi migration.

## RED FLAG SIGNS: POOR PROGNOSTIC INDICATORS

If hematuria is associated with the following signs and symptoms, then it carries poor prognosis.

- Gross hematuria along with proteinuria
- Hemodynamic instability
- Altered mental status
- Abdominal pain
- Anorexia, significant weight loss, and cachexia
- Rapid deterioration of renal function

## CLINICAL PEARLS

Asymptomatic patients with isolated hematuria should not need extensive evaluation, whereas symptomatic patients along with proteinuria often need thorough investigation. Asymptomatic hematuria with normal evaluation needs every 3–6 month follow-up till hematuria resolves.

## FURTHER READINGS

1. Loscalzo J. Harrison's Principles of Internal Medicine. 21st Edition (Vol. 1 & Vol. 2). McGraw-Hill Education; 2022.
2. Behrman R, Kliegman R, Schor N, Geme JWS, Stanton B, Nelson W. Nelson Textbook of Pediatrics. 21st Edition. Philadelphia: Elsevier Inc.; 2020.

# CHAPTER 64

# Pyuria

Rojina Choudhury

## DEFINITION

Pyuria means the presence of pus cells in urinalysis. Usually, it is defined as the presence of >5–10 pus cells or leukocytes per high-power field (HPF). Pyuria is usually associated with hematuria. Isolated pyuria is a very uncommon event. Females are most commonly affected than males.

Sterile pyuria is still not defined clearly, but its occurrence is common in day-to-day practice, and females are more affected than males. Approximately 9% of patients who presented with lower urinary tract symptoms (LUTS) are found to have sterile pyuria. In the simplest way, it is defined as the presence of white blood cells (WBC) in urinalysis without a positive urine culture report.

The ideal specimen for urinalysis is uncontaminated midstream clean catch morning urine sample. Suprapubic aspiration is the gold standard for urine sample collection. Avoid vaginal contamination during the collection of urine sample in females.

## WHAT CAUSES PYURIA?

### Pathogenesis

Pyuria most commonly occurs due to urinary tract infections (UTIs), but noninfective conditions also cause pyuria, particularly sterile pyuria. UTIs occur in any part of the urinary system, i.e., kidneys, ureters, bladder, urethra, and prostate in males. Risk factors compromising normal defense mechanisms are as follows: Prolonged indwelling catheter, frequent antibiotic use, female sex, pregnancy, sexual intercourse, vesicoureteral reflux, and susceptible uroepithelial cells. Pathogens (mostly gram-negative *Escherichia coli*) bacteria colonize the periurethral area and gradually ascend upward to penetrate bladder uroepithelial cells through fimbria and replicate there. After colonization in lower urinary tract bacteria ascend upward to involve upper urinary tract, i.e., kidney and result inflammatory cascades. As a result WBC number increases in urine. Apart from ascending infection through the urethra, there is also hematogenous route, lymphatic route, and direct spread from the surrounding organs for UTIs.

## WHAT ARE THE PROBABILITIES?

*Differential diagnosis (D/Ds) = etiology*: The causes of pyuria are as follows:

- *UTIs*: UTIs are the most common cause of pyuria. *E. coli* accounts for 80% of cases of UTIs. Other bacteria include *Klebsiella, Proteus, Pseudomonas, Streptococcus,*

*Staphylococcus*, and many others. Apart from bacteria fungi (*Candida, Histoplasma capsulatum*), viruses [rubella, mumps, and human immunodeficiency virus (HIV)] and protozoa (*Trichomonas vaginalis* and *Schistosoma haematobium*) also cause UTIs.

- *Infective cause of sterile pyuria*: Renal tuberculosis is one of the most common causes of sterile pyuria, particularly in a developing country. Other causes are Chlamydia, gonorrhea, mycoplasma, ureaplasma, fungal infections, parasitic infections (schistosomiasis), and viral infections (particularly adenovirus).
- *Noninfective causes of sterile pyuria*: They are renal or ureteric stone, catheterization, malignancy involving the urinary tract, malignant hypertension, allergic interstitial nephritis, systemic lupus erythematosus (SLE), sarcoidosis, post abdominal or pelvic surgery, drugs (aspirin, olsalazine, nitrofurantoin), and pregnancy.

## APPROACH TO DIAGNOSIS

### History Taking

Pyuria is not a disease. It is one of the most common laboratory findings, often detected as a part of routine investigations. Careful history-taking is essential for the proper management of pyuria.

- Pyuria along with history of LUTS usually suggestive of UTIs
- History of passing stone or grits along with hematuria suggestive of stone in the urinary system
- History of fever, anorexia, weight loss suggestive of underlying malignancy
- Pyuria along with recent history of drug allergy, contrast dye exposure suggestive of allergic interstitial nephritis
- Chronic recurrent sterile pyuria along with low-grade fever and weight loss suggestive of tuberculosis
- Ask about history of recent catheterization, instrumentations in the urinary tract, radiation to the pelvis, or any abdominal or pelvic surgery.

### Clinical Examination

- Check for blood pressure, pulse rate, presence of pallor, edema, and lymphadenopathy. Hypotension along with tachycardia suggestive of septic shock
- Presence of pallor, lymphadenopathy, abdominal or pelvic mass suggestive of underlying malignancy
- Presence of skin rashes, arthralgia, arthritis suggestive of autoimmune diseases.
- Suprapubic tenderness along with pyuria suggestive of cystitis
- Renal angle tenderness along with pyuria suggestive of acute pyelonephritis
- Per abdominal examination is to be done to look for organomegaly, pelvic mass, or retroperitoneal mass.

### Investigations

- Urine routine examination (RE)/ microscopic examination (ME)/culture and sensitivity (CS): Pyuria along with WBC casts are classically present in acute pyelonephritis. Pyuria along with muddy brown casts are found in acute tubular necrosis (ATN). Pyuria along with broad waxy casts are seen in chronic kidney disease (CKD). Dysmorphic red blood cells (RBCs) along with RBC cast are seen in glomerulonephritis or vasculitis.
- Dipstick leukocyte esterase test is rapid and specific test to detect pus cells.
- Urine albumin-to-creatinine ratio (ACR) or 24-hour urinary protein: To know the extent of proteinuria, i.e., microalbuminuria or macroalbuminuria, and nephritic or nephrotic range of proteinuria.
- Complete hemogram along with C-reactive protein (CRP) to know the extent and severity of infection.

- Liver function tests (LFTs) and kidney function tests are to be done accordingly.
- Urine cytology to detect malignant cells.
- Serum angiotensin-converting enzyme (ACE) is done as a screening test to exclude sarcoidosis.
- *Ultrasound of the whole abdomen (USG-W/A)*: To know kidney size, corticomedullary (CMD) differentiation, renal echogenicity, presence of stone, or any mass either in the renal system or in any part of the abdomen.
- *Noncontrast computed tomography (NCCT) of the pelvis*: Computed tomography (CT) scan is the investigation of choice for stones in the urinary tract.
- Cystoscopy and ureteroscopy have both therapeutic and diagnostic roles, particularly in renal stones.

## THERAPY

Treatment depends on the underlying causes:
- UTIs need 7–14-day course of antibiotic therapy according to CS reports.
- Withdrawal of offending drugs or contrast agents and adequate hydration is to be done for allergic interstitial nephritis.
- Ureteric stone is to be removed through ureteroscope. Bladder stone is to be removed by cystoscope.
- Renal tuberculosis is to be treated with antitubercular medication.
- Pelvic inflammatory disease is to be treated with combination of antifungal and antibiotics.
- Malignancy is to be treated with chemotherapy, radiotherapy or surgery, or combination.

## RED FLAG SIGNS: POOR PROGNOSTIC FACTORS

Severe pyuria in pregnancy, especially in untreated UTIs, carries the risk of premature birth and low birth weight baby. Sterile pyuria along with systemic symptoms, i.e., skin rashes, arthralgia, arthritis, and edema are of great concern to clinicians for serious underlying etiology.

## CLINICAL PEARLS

Almost all patients with symptomatic UTIs are found to have pyuria. Positive dipstick test for pyuria is not diagnostic of UTIs, but negative test excludes UTIs. Sterile pyuria is often a real challenge for clinicians, but systematic approach helps diagnose and treat the underlying condition. Isolated pyuria detected in routine tests without any symptoms often needs no treatment.

## FURTHER READINGS

1. Loscalzo J. Harrison's Principles of Internal Medicine, 21st Edition (Vol. 1 & Vol. 2). McGraw-Hill Education; 2022.
2. Behrman R, Kliegman R, Schor N, Geme JWS, Stanton B, Nelson W. Nelson Textbook of Pediatrics. 21st Edition. Philadelphia: Elsevier Inc.; 2020.

CHAPTER 65

# Retention of Urine

*Rojina Choudhury*

## DEFINITION

Retention of urine is defined as the inability to pass urine voluntarily, either completely or incompletely. It is also known as ischuria. It may be acute or chronic. It may be painless or painful retention of urine. Acute retention of urine is usually painful, and there is sudden inability to pass urine. Chronic retention of urine is usually painless, and there is an increased post-void residual urine (PVRU) volume following incomplete evacuation of the bladder chronically, usually >6 months.

The most vulnerable population is elderly people. Acute urinary retention most commonly occurs in men, and it is the most common urologic emergency that needs to be treated as early as possible. Women usually suffer from chronic retention of urine.

## WHAT CAUSES RETENTION OF URINE?

### Pathogenesis

Micturition occurs due to coordination between multiple pathways, that is, the central nervous system (CNS) (brain, brainstem, and spinal cord) and the peripheral nervous system, mediated by neurotransmitters.

Higher brain centers trigger downstream structures to suppress or stimulate urination according to social circumstances.

Pontine micturition center in the brainstem coordinates the detrusor muscle contraction along with sphincter relaxation to facilitate urination and vice versa, depending on afferent input from the spinal cord and efferent output from higher brain centers.

Bladder wall is composed of detrusor muscle, which is under autonomic control. Internal urethral sphincter is under autonomic control and absent in females, whereas external urethral sphincter is under somatic control. Bladder and urethra are supplied by three sets of nerve fibers. These are peripheral autonomic nervous system (pelvic nerve/parasympathetic nerve and hypogastric nerve/sympathetic nerve) and somatic nervous system (pudendal nerve). Sympathetic nerve relaxes the detrusor muscle and contracts the internal urethral sphincter for bladder filling, and parasympathetic nerve plays the opposite action to empty the bladder. Somatic nerve contracts and relaxes depending on social circumstances and voluntarily control the micturition reflex.

Loss of coordination between the higher brain, brainstem, and sacral spinal cord results in either retention or incontinence of urine.

## WHAT ARE THE POSSIBILITIES? ETIOLOGY

Retention of urine results from the following causes:

- *Obstructive causes*: Either there is mechanical obstruction or dynamic obstruction. Benign prostatic hyperplasia (BPH) is the most common cause of urinary retention in adult males, and meatal stenosis is the most important cause of urinary retention in children. Obstructive causes common in males are BPH, meatal stenosis, urethral stricture, penile constricting ring, prostate cancer, phimosis, and paraphimosis. Obstructive causes common in females are cystocele, rectocele, uterine prolapse, pelvic mass, and retroverted gravid uterus. Obstructive causes that occur in both genders are bladder stone, bladder neoplasm, fecal impaction, and retroperitoneal mass or neoplasm.
- *Infective and inflammatory causes*: In women, the most common causes are acute vulvovaginitis, vaginal pemphigus, and lichen planus. In men, the most common causes are balanitis, prostatitis, and prostate abscess. Other common causes occurring in both genders are cystitis, urethritis, and periurethral abscess.
- *Neurologic causes*: They mostly cause chronic urinary retention. The most important CNS causes are cerebrovascular accident, multiple sclerosis, normal-pressure hydrocephalus, and Parkinson's disease. The most important spinal cord lesions causing retention of urine are spinal cord trauma, transverse myelitis, spinal cord hematoma, abscess, spina bifida occulta, etc. The most important autonomic disorders causing retention of urine are autonomic neuropathy, Guillain–Barré syndrome (GBS), diabetes mellitus, poliomyelitis, and tabes dorsalis.
- *Pharmacologic causes*: Anticholinergics, such as atropine, glycopyrrolate, oxybutynin, and flavoxate; antipsychotics, such as haloperidol and fluphenazine; antidepressants, such as imipramine, amitriptyline, and nortriptyline; sympathomimetics, such as ephedrine, phenylephrine, isoproterenol, and terbutaline; anti-Parkinson's drugs, such as trihexyphenidyl, levodopa, and bromocriptine; muscle relaxants, such as diazepam and baclofen; and antihistaminic, such as diphenhydramine and hydroxyzine, often cause retention of urine. There are many other medications that cause retention of urine.
- *Traumatic causes*: Road traffic accident involving abdomen, spinal trauma, iatrogenic trauma during instrumentations to the urinary system, and prolonged labor are the other causes of urinary retention.

## APPROACH TO DIAGNOSIS

### History

History taking is often crucial and the most important step to search the etiology for retention of urine.

#### *Symptoms*

- Course of development that is acute or chronic and progression of the disease
- First episode or recurrent episode?
- Difficulty in starting of urination or difficulty in fully emptying the bladder?
- Ask about urinary flow and strained effort for urination.
- History of nocturia (waking up frequently for urination)
- History of fever suggestive of (S/O) infective, inflammatory, or neoplastic causes
- History of lower urinary tract symptoms (LUTS) S/O urethritis, cystitis

- Is there any previous history of BPH?
- Is there any important past medical history or neurological disorders?
- Detailed history of drug use
- Ask about sexual promiscuity.
- History of addiction to alcohol or substance abuse
- Is there a history of constipation?
- History of trauma or not
- History of recent catheterization, cystoscopy examination, or any lower abdominal operation

## Clinical Examination

- Check for temperature.
- Any local tenderness or not
- *Abdominal examination*: Tender, enlarged, globular mass is palpable, which is dull on percussion, S/O full bladder.
- Check for meatal stenosis, phimosis, and balanitis in male patients.
- Look for cystoceles, rectoceles, uterine prolapse, and signs of vulval infection in female patients.
- Per vaginal examination is performed to exclude pelvic mass.
- Look for gravid uterus.
- Digital rectal examination is done to exclude prostate enlargement.
- Neurological examination with lateralizing sign of plantar reflex suggestive of cerebrovascular accident.
- Presence of rigidity, tremor, and bradykinesia (classical triad) suggestive of Parkinson's disease.
- Neurological disease involving the brain, spinal cord, and optic nerve with relapsing and remitting course suggestive of multiple sclerosis.
- Areflexia with acute symmetric, flaccid, and ascending motor paralysis is a classical presentation for GBS.
- Detailed neurological examination is done to exclude the presence of neurogenic bladder.

## Investigation

- Complete blood count with differential counts
- Urine routine examination (RE)/microscopic examination (ME)/culture and sensitivity (CS) are done to exclude infective etiology.
- Blood for urea/creatinine
- Fasting blood sugar (FBS)/post-prandial blood sugar (PPBS)/glycated hemoglobin (HbA1c) are done to know glycemic status.
- Prostate-specific antigen (PSA) and free PSA are done to exclude prostate cancer.
- *Ultrasound of whole abdomen*: Measure PVRU volume and other structural abnormalities of the renal system.
- X-ray of kidneys-ureters-bladder (KUB) or computed tomography (CT) scan of the pelvis is done for calculi.
- CT scan of abdomen and pelvis is done to exclude intraabdominal mass.
- Magnetic resonance imaging (MRI) and CT scan of the brain are done to exclude space-occupying lesions (SOL) in the brain.
- MRI of the spine is done to exclude disc prolapse, spinal cord compression by tumor, metastasis, hematoma, and cauda equina syndrome.
- MRI of the brain, orbits, and spinal cord is done to exclude multiple sclerosis.
- Nerve conduction velocity (NCV) and cerebrospinal fluid (CSF) study (albumin cytological dissociation) are done to exclude GBS.
- Cystoscopy, urodynamic study, and cystourethrography are done to exclude bladder pathology, posterior urethral valve, and urethral stricture.

## THERAPY

The initial management step is urethral catheterization or suprapubic catheterization to empty the bladder in acute retention. The adult catheter size is usually 16–18 Fr as the initial step. The next management step is treating the underlying cause.

- Treat with adequate antibiotics according to culture sensitivity reports for cystitis, urethritis, and prostatitis.
- Clot retention is to be managed by bladder wash and cystoscopy-guided clot removal.
- BPH is treated by alpha-1-adrenergic blocker and 5-alpha reductase inhibitor. Transurethral resection of prostate (TURP) done if medical treatment fails.
- Urethroplasty for urethral stricture
- Endoscopic crusting of bladder stone is to be done for large bladder stone.
- Prostate cancer treatment is done by TURP, radiotherapy, chemotherapy, or combination, depending on the stage.
- Medications are to be stopped if they cause urinary retention.
- Cerebrovascular disease is treated with symptomatic treatment.
- GBS is treated with plasmapheresis or intravenous immunoglobulins and other supportive management.

## RED FLAG SIGNS/POOR PROGNOSTIC FACTORS

Urinary retention followed by RTAs to be managed very carefully with securing airway, breathing, and circulation. Contraindication for urethral catheterization is urethral trauma, blood at meatus, scrotal hematoma, or pelvic fracture. These are initially managed by suprapubic catheterization. Elderly patients with comorbidities are the most vulnerable. The presence of underlying chronic kidney disease (CKD), immunocompromised state, and malignancy carries a poor prognosis.

## CLINICAL PEARLS

Acute urinary retention in men with BPH is often prevented by long-standing treatment with 5-alpha-reductase inhibitors, that is, finasteride or dutasteride.

Suprapubic catheters or silver alloy-impregnated urethral catheters reduce the chances of urinary tract infections (UTIs) in patients who need catheterization for about 2 weeks.

Strict aseptic procedures must be followed during catheterization, and it must be done by properly trained health personnel.

Patient and their relative are to be informed regarding the complications of catheterization and how to care for the indwelled catheter.

## FURTHER READINGS

1. Loscalzo J. Harrison's Principles of Internal Medicine, 21st Edition (Vol. 1 & Vol. 2). McGraw-Hill Education; 2022.
2. Behrman R, Kliegman R, Schor N, Geme JWS, Stanton B, Nelson W. Nelson Textbook of Pediatrics. 21st Edition. Philadelphia: Elsevier Inc.; 2020.

# CHAPTER 66

# Oliguria

*Biva Bhakat*

## WHAT IS OLIGURIA?

Oliguria, diminished urine output, is an indirect measure of kidney function. It has importance in the early diagnosis of acute kidney injury (AKI), i.e., before the rise in serum creatinine level. It is defined as urine volume <0.5 mL/kg/h for 6 hours or 0.3 mL/kg/h for 24 hours. Oliguria associated with AKI has a poor prognosis. Urine output is also influenced by extracellular fluid volume depletion and renal blood circulation. In chronic kidney disease (CKD), oliguria is not common until the initiation of dialysis or end-stage renal disease. Oliguria can occur even in the absence of renal impairment. It may be due to the normal physiological response of increased salt and water reabsorption in response to dehydration.

## WHAT IS THE PATHOPHYSIOLOGY OF OLIGURIA?

Different underlying pathophysiological mechanisms can lead to oliguria. In cases of prerenal AKI, renal perfusion is decreased profoundly, resulting in diminished glomerular capillary filtration pressure. As a result, the glomerular filtration rate (GFR) may drop acutely. The tubules absorb sodium and water at an excess, resulting in low sodium, hyperosmolar urine. Any causes of extracellular fluid volume depletion may lead to impaired renal perfusion.

Acute tubular necrosis (ATN) is another important cause of oliguria. It could be due to ischemia or nephrotoxin-induced or both. The area of the tubules mostly affected is S3 segment of the proximal tubules and thick ascending limb of the loop of Henle (medullary). Renal autoregulation plays an important role in maintaining renal perfusion and GFR at a stable range. This autoregulation fails when systolic blood pressure falls below 50 mm Hg. Certain predisposing factors such as aging or CKD impair this autoregulation. So, the failure of dilatation of afferent arterioles and constriction of the efferent arteriole occur, resulting in a fall in GFR. Ischemia also causes an excess calcium content in afferent arterioles; this together with other vasoconstrictors such as adenosine, endothelin 1, and thromboxane A2 leads to intrarenal vasoconstrictions. The endothelial cells may also get involved because of decreased vasodilatory prostaglandins and nitric oxide synthetase. Involvement of endothelial cells of vasa recta leads to interstitial edema and exacerbates the hypoxic injury. All these factors lead to a reduction in GFR and oliguria.

In cases of postrenal AKI, there is obstruction at levels starting from the renal pelvis to the urethra. This causes an increased intratubular pressure, which further impairs glomerular filtration, thus causing oliguria.

## WHAT ARE THE DIFFERENTIAL DIAGNOSES?

- *Oliguria due to prerenal AKI*:
  - Intravascular volume depletion: Gastrointestinal losses (diarrhea, vomiting, nasogastric drainage), renal loss (use of diuretics, osmotic diuresis), dermal losses (burns), third spacing (pancreatitis, muscle injury)
  - Systemic arterial vasodilation: Sepsis, anaphylaxis, cirrhosis
  - Decreased cardiac output: Cardiogenic shock, congestive cardiac failure, cardiac tamponade
  - Renal vasoconstrictions: Early sepsis, hepatorenal syndrome, drugs such as nonsteroidal anti-inflammatory drugs (NSAIDs) and angiotensin-converting enzyme inhibitors (ACEI)
- *Oliguria due to intrinsic AKI*:
  - Tubular injury:
    - Ischemia: Hypovolemia, sepsis, hemorrhage, sepsis
    - Endogenous toxins: Hemoglobin, myoglobin, paraproteins
    - Radiocontrast agent
  - Interstitial injury:
    - Drugs: NSAIDs
    - Infections
    - Infiltrations: Lymphoma, leukemia
  - Glomerular injury:
    - Postinfectious glomerulonephritis
    - Membranoproliferative glomerulonephritis
    - Lupus nephritis
    - Infectious endocarditis
    - Immunoglobulin A (IgA) nephropathy
    - Cryoglobulinemia
  - Renal microvasculature:
    - Malignant hypertension
    - Toxemia of pregnancy
    - Thrombotic microangiopathy
    - Renal atherosclerosis
  - Renal vein: Thrombosis
  - Renal artery:
    - Occlusion or dissection
    - Large- and medium-vessel vasculitis
- *Causes of postrenal AKI*:
  - Retroperitoneal fibrosis
  - Ureteral trauma
  - Bladder neck obstruction
  - Neurogenic bladder
  - Nephrolithiasis
  - Tumors

## HOW TO APPROACH A PATIENT OF OLIGURIA?

While evaluating a patient with oliguria, one must focus on a detailed history and physical examination. Based upon the clinical evidence, one should proceed with investigations such as urinalysis, blood test, renal imaging, and even renal biopsy if indicated.

History should focus on the presence of excessive thirst, dizziness, diarrhea, vomiting, burns, drug history—diuretic, ACEI, angiotensin receptor blocker, NSAIDs, etc. (prerenal AKI), excessive exercise, crush injury, prolonged immobilization, use of contrast, colicky pain abdomen in flank, respiratory distress, and hemoptysis.

The clinical examination should focus on blood pressure (orthostatic hypotension), pulse rate (tachycardia, arrhythmia), signs of volume overload such as edema, raised jugular venous pressure (JVP), and S3. Skin should be examined for malar rash, livedo reticularis, palpable purpura, etc. Eye examination should focus on uveitis, keratitis, etc.

Urinalysis is a diagnostic tool that is inexpensive but very useful in differentiating causes of oliguria. Urine-specific gravity 1.015–1.020 suggests prerenal AKI, while

1.010 (isosthenuria) favors ATN. Urine should be examined for hematuria and proteinuria, casts, cells, and crystals. Proteinuria < 1 g suggests ATN but >1 g/day suggests glomerular proteinuria. Certain urine indices are very helpful, for example, fractional excretion of sodium (<1% indicates prerenal AKI, >2 indicates ATN), urine creatinine to plasma creatinine ratio, urine urea nitrogen to plasma urea nitrogen ratio.

Blood should be sent for blood urea nitrogen (BUN) and creatinine as their levels and timings of rise help in predicting the underlying etiology. BUN:creatinine >20:1 suggests prerenal AKI and 10:1 suggests intrinsic AKI. The timing of the rise in creatinine differs in different etiologies; for example, in ATN due to ischemia, creatinine starts to rise in 24–48 hours and peak occurs within 7–10 days; in contrast-induced nephropathy, the peak occurs in 5–7 days. Presence of anemia points to hemolysis, multiple myeloma, and thrombotic microangiopathy. Presence of hyperuricemia, hyperkalemia, and hyperphosphatemia in the presence of hypocalcemia points to rhabdomyolysis. Presence of eosinophilia favors the diagnosis of allergic interstitial nephritis, atheroembolism, and Churg–Strauss vasculitis.

Renal ultrasonography is very helpful in identifying the cause of AKI. It gives information regarding renal size, corticomedullary differentiation, cortical thickness, and pelvicalyceal system dilation.

Renal biopsy is indicated when prerenal and postrenal causes of AKI have been excluded and causes of intrinsic AKI need to be confirmed.

## WHAT IS THE TREATMENT FOR OLIGURIA?

While treating oliguria, the first consideration should be identifying the etiology. Specific therapy is available only in some cases of oliguria. Majority of cases need supportive therapy. Renal replacement therapy (RRT) is indicated in certain situations. When oliguria is due to prerenal AKI, supplementation of balanced crystalloid solution is helpful. Frequent monitoring of the patient's electrolytes and acid-base status is to be done to accurately identify the type of replacement fluid. If the patient develops hyperkalemia, urgent electrocardiogram (ECG) should be considered. If ECG changes are present, intravenous (IV) calcium gluconate 10 mL 10% should be given; another option is 10–20-unit IV insulin with 25% dextrose solution (25–50 g). $K^+$ binding resin, loop diuretics, and nebulizer with beta-2 agonist can be considered. Refractory cases should be considered for RRT. If oliguria is associated with metabolic acidosis, sodium bicarbonate should be supplemented if $HCO_3^-$ is <15. If hyperphosphatemia is present, dietary protein should be restricted, and phosphate-binding resin like calcium carbonate, calcium acetate, and sevelamer may be considered. Nephrotoxic drugs need to be avoided. NSAIDs need to be stopped. Doses of ACEI and ARB need to be modified or stopped. Ultrafiltration may be considered in volume-overloaded patients. RRT is indicated in the presence of refractory volume overload, persistent refractory hyperkalemia, severe metabolic acidosis, and uremic symptoms such as encephalopathy, pericarditis, and bleeding diathesis. It is also relatively indicated in the presence of persistent oliguria and progressive azotemia.

## RED FLAG SIGNS

- Pain abdomen and vomiting
- Chest pain
- Shortness of breath

## CLINICAL PEARLS

- Oliguria is defined by urine output <0.5 mL/kg/h for at least 6 consecutive hours.
- Proper history and clinical examination are necessary to accurately identify the underlying pathophysiology.

- Oliguria is associated with increased mortality.
- Life-threatening complications of oliguria should be searched for and treated on an urgent basis.

## FURTHER READINGS


1. Bhasin B, Velez JC. Evaluation of polyuria: the roles of solute loading and water diuresis. Am J Kidney Dis. 2016;67(3):507-11.
2. Bockenhauer D, Bichet DG. Pathophysiology, diagnosis and management of nephrogenic diabetes insipidus. Nat Rev Nephrol. 2015; 11(10):576-88.
3. Aleksandrov N, Audibert F, Bedard MJ, Mahone M, Goffinet F, Kadoch IJ. Gestational diabetes insipidus: a review of an under-diagnosed condition. J Obstet Gynaecol Can. 2010;32(3):225-31.
4. Balanescu S, Kopp P, Gaskill MB, Morgenthaler NG, Schindler C, Rutishauser J. Correlation of plasma copeptin and vasopressin concentrations in hypo-, iso-, and hyperosmolar states. J Clin Endocrinol Metab. 2011;96:1046-52.
5. Basile DP, Anderson MD, Sutton TA. Pathophysiology of acute kidney injury. Compr Physiol. 2012;2(2):1303-53.
6. Mehta RL, Kellum JA, Shah SV, Molitoris BA, Ronco C, Warnock DG, et al. Acute Kidney Injury Network: report of an initiative to improve outcomes in acute kidney injury. Crit Care.2007;11:R31.

CHAPTER 67

# Polyuria

*Biva Bhakat*

## WHAT IS POLYURIA?

Polyuria is defined as conventionally urine output of >50 mL/kg body weight in 24 hours. However, the physiological definition of polyuria is more appropriate, i.e., urine flow rate that is more than appropriate in a given setting. When vasopressin is acting normally, the urine volume depends on the rate of excretion of effective osmoles and medullary interstitium compartment osmolality. So, in this setting, even if the urine volume does not exceed the above-mentioned amount, polyuria is said to be present if the volume is higher for the rate of effective osmoles excretion.

## WHAT IS THE PATHOPHYSIOLOGY OF POLYURIA?

The urine output depends on the solute excretion rate and the concentrating ability of nephrons. Any disturbance of the balance leads to diuresis. Polyuria is mainly of two types: Water diuresis and osmotic diuresis. Urine osmolality <100 indicates water diuresis and >300 signifies osmotic diuresis. Sometimes, mixed osmotic and water diuresis occur as in arginine vasopressin (AVP) deficiency in the presence of solute diuresis. The urine osmolarity ranges between 100 and 300 mOsm/kg. Reduction in the basal AVP secretion by 10–20% causes a hypoosmolar urine. The plasma osmolarity is increased, which stimulates thirst mechanism, resulting in polydipsia. This stabilizes the plasma osmolarity at a slightly higher level, which approximates the osmotic threshold for thirst. If water intake is restricted, it leads to increased plasma osmolarity, hypernatremia, and associated complications. In the presence of diminished AVP secretion [central diabetes insipidus (DI)] or diminished renal response to AVP (nephrogenic DI), there is impaired activation of V2 subtype of AVP receptor. As a result, the osmotic water absorption via aquaporin 2 channel is hampered. AVP also contributes to medullary interstitium hyperosmolarity by stimulating the expression of Na–K–2Cl channel in the thick ascending limb of the loop of Henle. This mechanism, when affected, leads to further reduction of water reabsorption. Congenital or acquired causes of neurohypophysis destruction lead to central DI. The severity of polyuria depends on the degree of destruction. Nephrogenic DI is due to congenital (most common is mutation of AVP V2 receptor) or acquired (most common is lithium administration). Hypercalcemia, hypokalemia, lithium, and chronic urinary obstruction cause downregulation of AQP2 expression in renal collecting tubules, resulting in nephrogenic DI. In pregnancy, vasopressinase is released from the placenta that degrades the AVP. If hepatic dysfunction occurs [hemolysis, elevated liver enzymes, low platelets (HELLP) syndrome, acute fatty liver of pregnancy (AFLP)], the metabolism of vasopressinase is affected, further increasing the degradation of AVP, resulting in gestational DI. In patients with adrenal insufficiency, when treatment is given, i.e., glucocorticoid replacement, the blood pressure gets normalized, resulting in decreased secretion of AVP and unmasking the underlying DI. Primary polydipsia is characterized by excessive thirst and water intake. This leads to an expansion of body fluid and diminishes AVP secretion. As a result, the plasma osmolarity is set at a lower level approximating the osmotic threshold for AVP secretion. There is another terminology—dipsogenic DI, in which osmoregulatory control of thirst is abnormal. It is mostly idiopathic but can be associated with lesions in the hypothalamus.

## WHAT ARE THE DIFFERENTIAL DIAGNOSES?

- *Primary polydipsia*: Psychiatric problems like mania, obsessive compulsive disorder, schizophrenia, etc.
- *Defective tubular reabsorption of water*:
  - Central diabetes insipidus:
    - Congenital
    - Drug/toxin induced: Alcohol, snake venom
    - Granulomatous: Neurosarcoidosis, histiocytosis
    - Infectious: Tuberculosis, meningoencephalitis
    - Inflammatory: Lymphocytic infundibuloneurohypophysitis
    - Idiopathic
    - Post neurosurgery (present acutely)
    - Trauma
    - Infiltrative diseases affecting the pituitary stalk, hypothalamus
    - Tubercular meningitis
    - Multiple sclerosis
    - Neurosarcoidosis
    - Hypoxic injury
    - Tumor
  - Nephrogenic DI:
    - Hereditary
    - Drug induced: Lithium, cisplatin, demeclocycline
    - Hypercalcemia, hypokalemia
    - Infiltrating disease: Sarcoidosis, amyloidosis
    - Sickle cell anemia
    - Obstructive uropathy
- *Increased tubular solutes*: Diabetes mellitus, mannitol, diuretics, radiocontrast dye
- *Renal disorder*: Renal tubular acidosis, Barter's syndrome, Gitelman syndrome
- *Mixed water*: Solute diuresis—relief of prolonged urinary obstruction, infiltrative kidney disorder, etc.
- *Miscellaneous*: Treatment of adrenal insufficiency (unmask the underlying DI), gestational DI
- *Polyuria mimickers*: Urinary tract infections, overactive bladder, benign prostatic hypertrophy

## HOW TO APPROACH A PATIENT WITH POLYURIA?

When evaluating a patient with polyuria, a detailed history should be taken to identify the clinical setting in which polyuria is present **(Flowchart 1)**. The foremost important thing is to confirm the presence of true polyuria by quantitative measurement of 24-hour urine volume. History should include the presence of diabetes mellitus, pain in the abdomen or constipation (indicates hypercalcemia), weight loss (malignancy), headache, visual changes (indicates pituitary mass), and alteration in behavior (indicates psychiatric condition). Detailed drug history should be taken regarding the use of diuretics, mannitol, lithium, etc.

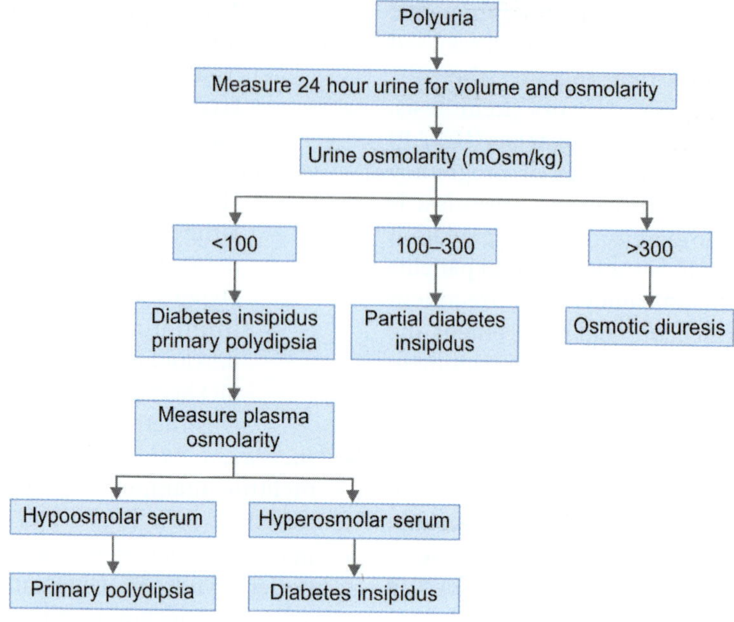


**FLOWCHART 1:** Approach to polyuria.

The approach to a patient with polyuria is cumbersome and time-consuming. It should include the measurement of urine osmolality, plasma sodium, and osmolarity.

Depending on the clinical context, serum calcium, intact parathyroid hormone (iPTH), computed tomography (CT) scan of the parathyroid gland, magnetic resonance imaging (MRI) of the posterior pituitary and pituitary stalk, and MRI of the brain should be considered.

Osmotic diuresis is to be diagnosed by measuring urine analysis for glucose and solute excretion rate. In patients with low urine osmolarity (<300 mOsm/kg $H_2O$) and hyperosmolar serum, the possibility of DI is to be considered. If plasma sodium and osmolality are low, the diagnosis of primary polydipsia is considered. But sometimes, patients with DI may present with normal serum osmolarity and sodium. A fluid deprivation test is helpful in these cases.

To differentiate between the two types of DI, the AVP stimulation test is helpful **(Flowchart 2)**. If urine osmolarity is increased by >50% within 1–2 hours of AVP administration, the diagnosis of central DI can be said accurately. An increase in urine osmolarity by <10% indicates nephrogenic DI. An increase by 10–50% is defined as indeterminate case (partial central and nephrogenic DI), and the fluid deprivation test is helpful here.

The relationship between plasma AVP and plasma osmolarity at the baseline and at the end of fluid deprivation test is measured. Baseline AVP > 3 pg/mL favors a diagnosis of nephrogenic DI over non-nephrogenic DI. Stimulated AVP > 1.8 pg/mL favors a diagnosis of primary polydipsia over partial central DI. AVP measurement is associated with some difficulties, so copeptin (C-terminal fragments of AVP prohormone) measurement is being preferred nowadays.

MRI brain posterior pituitary bright spot excludes the presence of central DI **(Flowchart 3)**. It has more importance in excluding rather than including. It is also helpful in the diagnosis of multiple sclerosis, tubercular meningitis, metastasis, etc.

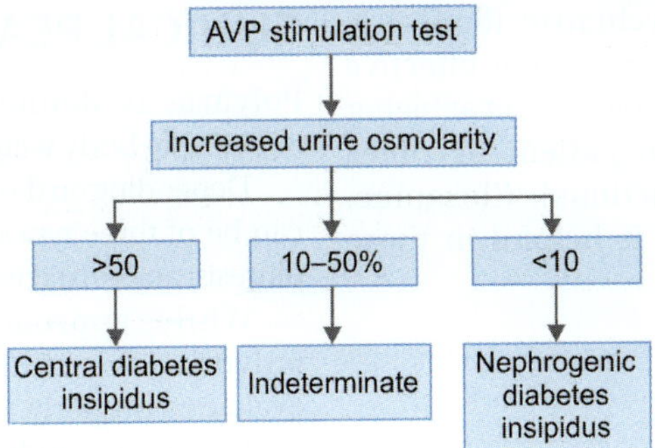


**FLOWCHART 2:** AVP stimulation test to differentiate between central and nephrogenic diabetes insipidus.

(AVP: arginine vasopressin)

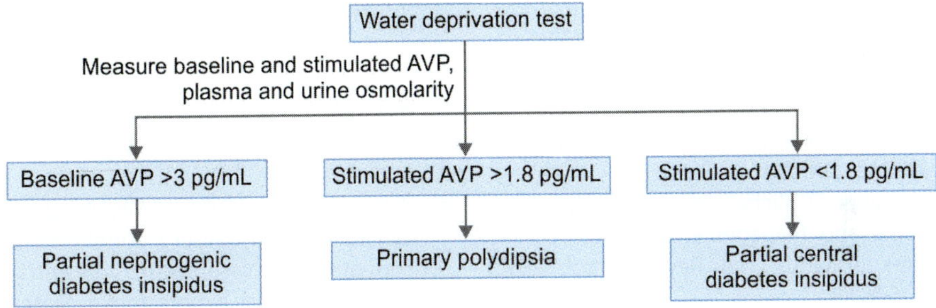


**FLOWCHART 3:** Water deprivation test the to differentiate between the types of indeterminate diabetes insipidus and some cases of primary polydipsia.

(AVP: arginine vasopressin)

## WHAT IS THE TREATMENT FOR POLYURIA?

Polyuria and associated polydipsia hamper the patient's daily activities. Therapy should focus on managing the underlying etiology as it differs markedly among different underlying causes. For the management of central DI, the mainstay of therapy is water substitution and antidiuresis. Desmopressin is the preferred drug. It is available in intranasal and parenteral forms. The parenteral form is more potent and its use is reserved for acute emergency settings. The dose of the intranasal formulation is 1–2 μg every 8–12 hours. Chlorpropamide, the sulfonylurea, has off-label indication for use in central DI. It reduces polyuria by 25–75%. This is contraindicated in the presence of hypopituitarism (may lead to hypoglycemia). Thiazide has a paradoxical effect on diuresis, so it can be used in central DI. The mainstay of therapy for nephrogenic DI is treating the underlying etiology such as stopping the drug lithium (if possible) and correcting the hypercalcemia. The administration of sodium should be restricted. The drug of choice is thiazide diuretic alone or can be used in combination with NSAIDS (prostaglandin synthesis inhibitor—indomethacin, ibuprofen) or amiloride. Interestingly some patient with NDI may respond to high dose of desmopressin. So desmopressin trial should be given in patients with NDI to identify any potential responsiveness. For patients with primary polydipsia behavioural modification and pharmacologic therapy (depending on the underlying psychiatric illness) is preferred. Fluid restriction is not effective (because the thirst threshold is reset at higher plasma osmolarity and patient becomes resistant to fluid restrictions). Clozapine, an antipsychotic drug, is helpful in these situations.

## RED FLAG SIGNS

- Absent or inappropriate thirst
- Drowsiness, convulsion, coma

## CLINICAL PEARLS

Polyuria is defined as urine output of >50 mL/kg body weight in 24 hours.

Depending on the urine osmolarity, polyuria can be of three types: Water diuresis, osmotic diuresis, and mixed water—osmotic diuresis.

While approaching a patient with polyuria, the clinical setting should be evaluated properly.

Desmopressin is the mainstay of therapy for central DI, but other causes of polyuria need treatment of the underlying etiology.

## FURTHER READINGS

1. Bhasin B, Velez JC. Evaluation of polyuria: the roles of solute loading and water diuresis. Am J Kidney Dis. 2016;67(3):507-11.
2. Bockenhauer D, Bichet DG. Pathophysiology, diagnosis and management of nephrogenic diabetes insipidus. Nat Rev Nephrol. 2015; 11(10):576-88.
3. Aleksandrov N, Audibert F, Bedard MJ, Mahone M, Goffinet F, Kadoch IJ. Gestational diabetes insipidus: a review of an underdiagnosed condition. J Obstet Gynaecol Can. 2010; 32(3):225-31.
4. Balanescu S, Kopp P, Gaskill MB, Morgenthaler NG, Schindler C, Rutishauser J. Correlation of plasma copeptin and vasopressin concentrations in hypo-, iso-, and hyperosmolar States. J Clin Endocrinol Metab. 2011;96:1046-52.

# PART 10

# Ophthalmology

CHAPTER 68

# Eye Pain

*Smiti Rani Srivastava*

## INTRODUCTION

*Pain in the eye*: It is one of the common causes for which patients consult doctors.

## WHAT CAUSES EYE PAIN?

Causes of eye pain can be divided according to the following etiologies:

- *Asthenopia*: The most common cause of strain and discomfort to the eye is uncontrolled refractory error. Other causes are phoria or tropia, convergence insufficiency, accommodative spasm, and pharmacologic (miotics).
- *Ocular*:
    - Typically mild-to-moderate: Dry eye syndrome, blepharitis, infectious conjunctivitis, episcleritis, inflamed pinguecula or pterygium, corneal or conjunctival foreign body, corneal disorder (e.g., superficial punctate keratopathy), superior limbic keratoconjunctivitis, ocular medication toxicity, contact lens-related problems, postoperative, ocular ischemic syndrome, etc.
    - Typically moderate-to-severe: Corneal disorder (e.g., abrasion, erosion, infiltrate/ulcer/keratitis, chemical injury, ultraviolet burn), trauma, anterior uveitis, scleritis, endophthalmitis, acute angle-closure glaucoma.
- *Periorbital*: Trauma, hordeolum, preseptal cellulitis, dacryocystitis, referred pain (e.g., dental, sinus), giant cell arteritis.
- *Orbital*: Sinusitis, trauma, orbital cellulitis, idiopathic orbital inflammatory syndrome, orbital tumor or mass optic neuritis, acute dacryoadenitis, migraine or cluster headache, diabetic cranial nerve palsy, postinfectious neuralgia (hepatic).

## MANAGEMENT

Every patient with complaints of headache, eye strain, and discomfort must get their visual acuity checked with either Snellen's chart or logmar chart. Visual acuity should be checked with the spectacle on if the patient was using one. Improvement of visual acuity with pinhole signifies the presence of refractory error. Near vision should also be checked. History of prolonged near work like reading and doing work on computer causes accommodative spasm. History of onset, type of pain, radiation, associated dimness of vision, redness of eye, discharge, trauma, or recent intraocular surgery are important. Pain due to infectious conjunctivitis, blepharitis, hordeolum, and dacryocystitis is generally not associated with visual disturbance. Any history of trauma or foreign body impaction is important. Patients should be examined under a slit lamp. Cornea and conjunctiva should be examined for any abrasion or foreign body impaction. Acute-onset pain in the eye with profuse discharge and redness is suggestive of infectious conjunctivitis (i.e., purulent discharge signifies bacterial cause, and watery discharge is associated with viral infection). A patient with a history of recent intraocular surgery with pain, eyelid swelling, redness, and pus in the anterior chamber of the eye suggests endophthalmitis and requires urgent referral to an eye hospital. Pain on movement of the eye and gradually deteriorated vision with headache must be suspected for optic neuritis. A patient with unilateral optic neuritis has a relative afferent pupillary defect in the ipsilateral eye. Color vision is also impaired. On ophthalmoscopy, the optic disc margin is often found blurred. Pain, swelling of eyelids, prolonged watering, and purulent discharge from the punctum on pressure over the lacrimal sac suggest acute dacryocystitis. Along with these symptoms if the patient has extraocular muscle movement restriction, proptosis, conjunctival chemosis, or orbital cellulitis must be thought of. Circumciliary congestion, irregular pupil margin, and posterior adhesion of the iris to the lens are signs of acute anterior uveitis. Herpes zoster ophthalmicus is a viral reactivation of varicella zoster virus that typically affects the dermatome of various branches of the trigeminal nerve. Hutchinson's sign (rash at the tip, side, and root of the nose) is a strong predictor of ocular inflammation and corneal denervation.

### Investigation

Computed tomography (CT) scan of orbit is recommended for patients with signs of orbital cellulitis. A patient with blunt trauma of the eye needs to be investigated with a CT scan orbit for bony fracture. A patient with clinically diagnosed optic neuritis must be investigated with magnetic resonance imaging (MRI) brain to look for retrobulbar optic nerve involvement and signs of multiple sclerosis (common cause of optic neuritis). B-scan ultrasound (USG B) scan should be done to look for posterior segment involvement in case of uveitis whose fundoscopy is not possible.

## MANAGEMENT

*Refractory error*: Prescription of appropriate glass or contact lenses.

*Infectious conjunctivitis*: Antibiotics drops, e.g., chloramphenicol (1%) or gentamicin (0.3%) or tobramycin (0.3%) or moxifloxacin (0.5%) eye drops 4–6 hourly in a day and maybe augmented with eye ointment at bedtime.

*Dry eye*: Lubricant drops (carboxymethyl cellulose 0.5%).

*Acute anterior uveitis*: Steroid eye drops (1% prednisolone 8 times daily), cycloplegic (1% atropine or 2% homatropine). If required oral steroids in tapering dose may be prescribed.

Traumatic corneal abrasion requires eye taping with antibiotics and lubricant eye drops. Traumatic rupture of the cornea or sclera needs urgent referral to an eye hospital.

*Acute dacryocystitis*: Oral antibiotics (amoxicillin + clavulanic acid 625 mg TDS), with antibiotics drops or ointments (moxifloxacin, azithromycin, chloramphenicol), hot compression.

*Orbital cellulitis*: Intravenous (IV) broad-spectrum antibiotics (ceftriaxone 1 g IV BD).

*Optic neuritis*: IV pulse methylprednisolone 1 g for consecutively 5 days followed by oral prednisolone 1 mg/kg/day.

*Herpes zoster ophthalmicus*: Oral acyclovir 800 mg 5 times daily for 7 days, topical 3% acyclovir eye ointment 5 times daily for 5 weeks with antibiotics eye drops for added bacterial infection.

## CLINICAL PEARLS

- Mild cases of eye pain are mostly due to refractive errors
- Moderate-to-severe cases of eye pain are due to infections, trauma, inflammatory diseases
- Schirmer's test value < 15 mm indicated dry eye
- Detailed evaluation under slit lamp biomicroscope is mandatory
- Foreign body must be excluded in cases of trauma
- Infective (bacterial) causes must be treated with antibiotics, topical and/or systemic
- Steroids must be avoided in viral etiologies, unless severe inflammation

## FURTHER READINGS

1. Salmon JF, Kanski JJ. Kanski's clinical ophthalmology: A systematic approach. 9th edition. Edinburgh: Elsevier; 2020.
2. Khurana AK, Khurana I, Khurana AK, Khurana B. Anatomy and physiology of eye. 2nd ed. New Delhi: CBS Publishers & Distributors Pvt Ltd; 2017.
3. 7 Oculofacial Plastic and Orbital Surgery [Internet]. [cited 2023 Dec 5]. Available from: https://www.aao.org/education/bcscsnip-petdetail.aspx?id=46febd1f-9f5d-4082-9e21-56ce9ebabf0d

CHAPTER 69

# Red Eye

*Smiti Rani Srivastava*

## WHAT IS RED EYE?

Red eye is one of the most common signs for which patients seek medical attention.

## WHAT CAUSES RED EYE?

Redness of eye is caused by: (1) Conjunctival congestion, (2) subconjunctival hemorrhage, (3) circumcorneal congestion, and (4) episcleritis and scleritis.

*Conjunctivitis*: It can be an infectious, allergic, autoimmune condition. Among the infectious causes, the causative agents might be bacterial (*Staphylococcus, Streptococcus, Haemophilus influenzae, Propionibacterium acnes*), viral (adenovirus, herpes simplex, etc.), or *Chlamydia trachomatis*. Allergic conjunctivitis is vernal keratoconjunctivitis and atopic keratoconjunctivitis. Among the autoimmune conditions, mucous membrane pemphigoid is significant. Hypersensitivity reaction like Stevens-Johnson syndrome presents with redness, scarring, and skin lesion.

*Subconjunctival hemorrhage*: It may occur due to hypertension, trivial trauma with fingernail scratch or blunt ocular trauma, Kaposi sarcoma, etc.

*Circumcorneal congestion*: Acute anterior uveitis (AAU) or acute angle-closure glaucoma presents with circumcorneal congestion with eye pain, watering, and dimness of vision.

*Episcleritis and scleritis*: It is often associated with pain and burning sensation; patients generally have arthritis or any systemic inflammatory condition.

## PATH TO DIAGNOSIS

All patients presenting with redness of eye must get their visual acuity checked. Infectious conjunctivitis and subconjunctival hemorrhage due to trivial causes are not generally associated with visual symptoms. Acute onset of redness, pain, and foreign body sensation, with discharge, signifies infectious causes (viral infection has watery or mucoid discharge, purulent discharge with matting of eyelids in the morning signifies bacterial infection). Viral conjunctivitis is often associated with keratitis. If keratitis is present, vision can be diminished along with photophobia. Chlamydial conjunctivitis is associated with conjunctival scarring and consequently cicatricial entropion. Chlamydial conjunctivitis patients may have other features of chlamydial infection such as urethritis, epididymitis (for male), and pelvic inflammatory disease (for female). Allergic conjunctivitis must have itching as the chief symptom with mucoid discharge. There may be a cobblestone appearance at the upper tarsal conjunctiva in vernal keratoconjunctivitis. Patients with acute-onset subconjunctival hemorrhage without any history of trauma must get their blood pressure (BP) checked. A sudden rise of BP may cause rupture of small conjunctival vessels and result in subconjunctival hemorrhage. Circumcorneal violaceous congestion signifies uveal tissue inflammation. Two significant causes are AAU and acute congestive angle-closure glaucoma. In AAU, the signs commonly associated are irregular pupillary margin, posterior synechiae formation, aqueous humor flare and cells, and keratic precipitate at the endothelium. These signs are generally examined under a slit lamp.

In acute congestive angle-closure glaucoma, the cornea is generally edematous, and intraocular pressure (IOP) may be as high as 50–80 mm Hg. Anterior chamber depth is shallow and the patient presents with severe pain. Scleritis or episcleritis patients generally have redness along the nasal or temporal quadrant of the eye associated with pain.

### Investigations

Most of the causes of red eye are clinically diagnosed. Chronic bacterial conjunctivitis not amenable by broad-spectrum antibiotics may seldom need conjunctival swab collection, bacterial culture, and drug sensitivity test. Allergic conjunctivitis patients often have an increased eosinophil level. A single mono-ocular acute attack of anterior uveitis does not need systemic investigation, but recurrent attack, both eye involvement, or granulomatous features (i.e., mutton fat keratic precipitate) may need to exclude systemic causes such as tuberculosis and sarcoidosis. Suspected patients should be tested with chest X-ray, sputum for acid-fast bacilli (AFB), and cartridge-based nucleic acid amplification test (CBNAAT) for tuberculosis. Angiotensin-converting enzyme (ACE) inhibitors are recommended for sarcoidosis. Patient with hazy media due to corneal edema, anterior chamber flare, cataract, or vitritis may need ultrasound (USG) B-scan to look for any posterior segment involvement.

## MANAGEMENT

### Infectious Conjunctivitis

Antibiotics drops, e.g., chloramphenicol (1%) or gentamicin (0.3%) or tobramycin (0.3%) or moxifloxacin (0.5%) eye drops 4–6 hourly in the day, are recommended and maybe augmented with eye ointment at bedtime. Patients with chlamydial conjunctivitis need oral azithromycin 1 g repeated after 1 week or doxycycline 100 mg twice daily for 10 days with topical erythromycin drops.

### Allergic Conjunctivitis

Mast cell stabilizers (e.g., sodium cromoglycate, lodoxamide, olopatadine), topical antihistamines (e.g., emedastine, epinastine), and combined antihistamine and vasoconstrictor (e.g., antazoline with xylometazoline) are recommended in mild cases. Topical steroids (e.g., fluorometholone 0.1%, prednisolone 0.5%, loteprednol etabonate 0.2 or 0.5%) are recommended in severe cases.

Patients with subconjunctival hemorrhage without any trauma do not need any medication; it resolves spontaneously.

Acute congested angle-closure glaucoma patients need to lower the IOP by oral acetazolamide 250 mg 3 times daily (with syrup potassium chloride) or intravenous (IV) mannitol 20% (1–2 g/kg) along with IOP lowering drops (e.g., timolol maleate, brimonidine, acetazolamide). Pilocarpine 2% drop should be repeated after 1 hour. Referral to an ophthalmologist is required once the IOP is controlled medically for further management.

Acute anterior uveitis needs topical steroids (e.g., prednisolone 0.5%, dexamethasone 0.1% 6–8 times daily with tapering dose) and cycloplegic (e.g., atropine 1%).

Scleritis and episcleritis patients need topical steroids along with lubricants (e.g., carboxymethyl cellulose 0.5%).

## CLINICAL PEARLS

- Acute cases and red eye are mostly due to foreign body, trauma, acute attack of glaucoma
- Chronic/acute-on-chronic causes are inflammatory and allergic mostly
- Slitlamp biomicroscope examination is mandatory in all cases
- Topical steroids must be avoided in cases of corneal damage, viral etiologies unless indicated
- Systemic illness and adnexal pathologies must be ruled out

## FURTHER READINGS

1. Salmon JF. Kanski's Clinical Ophthalmology, 9th edition. 2019.
2. Khurana AK, Khurana I. Anatomy and Physiology of Eye. 4th edition. CBS Publishers and Distributors Pvt. Ltd; 2024.

CHAPTER 70

# Watering of the Eye

*Smiti Rani Srivastava*

## INTRODUCTION

Watering of the eye is the overflow of tear from the conjunctival sac. It is the most common symptom of lacrimal disorder. It can be due to either increased tear production or decreased drainage. The term "epiphora" is reserved for overflow of tears from the eye due to drainage pathway obstruction.

## WHAT CAUSES WATERING FROM THE EYE?

*Watering due to excessive secretion of tear*: It is seen in corneal or conjunctival irritation or due to psychogenic stimuli such as tragedy. Among the irritants, few are foreign body impaction, conjunctivitis (infectious or allergic), corneal abrasion, keratitis, and rubbing of the cornea by misdirected eyelashes (trichiasis, entropion). Watering can occur due to reflex tear production due to dry eye disease.

*Watering due to drainage pathway dysfunction*: Obstruction of tear drainage pathway can occur at various levels such as punctum stenosis, malposition of punctum (seen in ectropion), both, and or common canaliculi block, nasolacrimal duct obstruction, functional nasolacrimal duct blockage, or lacrimal pump failure **(Flowchart 1)**.

## PATH TO DIAGNOSIS

Every patient coming with a chief complaint of excess lacrimation should be enquired about associated pain, redness, onset, foreign body sensation, discharge, etc. Every patient

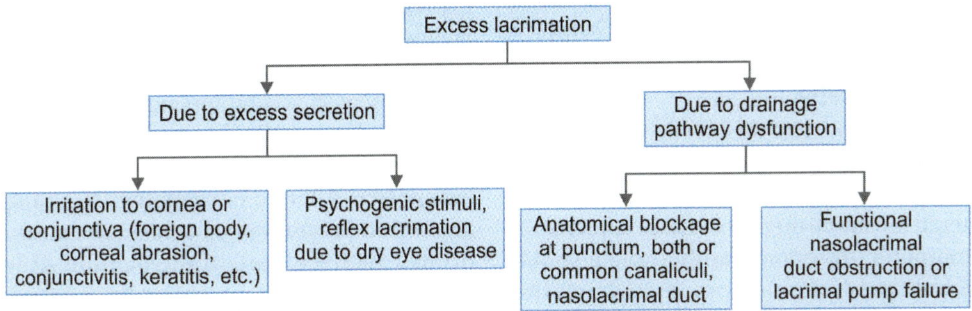


**FLOWCHART 1:** Causes of excess lacrimation.

should ideally be examined under a slit lamp to look for any corneal or conjunctival foreign body impaction. If no foreign body is detected, the upper eyelid must be everted to look for any impacted matter on the tarsal plate. In a patient having a history of any blunt trauma to the eye or a recent history of contact lens wear, corneal epithelial abrasion must be looked for. In case of doubt, the corneal epithelium can be stained with fluorescein sodium strips. Any defect in corneal epithelium takes up the stain and can be detected under cobalt blue filter light. In case of associated pain, redness, or purulent discharge, photophobia infectious conjunctivitis must be thought of. Allergic conjunctivitis is generally associated with mucoid discharge and itching. Virus conjunctivitis (most commonly by adenovirus) is often associated with superficial punctate keratitis. Intraocular pressure should be checked digitally and compared with the other eye if raised intraocular pressure is suspected.

If the patient has a chronic history of lacrimation with or without pain, dacryocystitis should be ruled out. There can be a history of chronic or recurrent lacrimal sac swelling, pain, or discharge. After the acute inflammation subsides, the site of tear drainage pathway obstruction is determined by doing a syringing test. Pressure should be applied over the lacrimal sac area to look for any regurgitation of pus (ROPLAS test).

The position of the eyelid margin and direction of the eyelashes must be checked to look for any irritation of the cornea by eyelashes or any symptom of dry eye.

## Investigations

All the patients should ideally be examined under a slit lamp. The pattern of conjunctiva congestion is noted. Intraocular pressure should ideally be measured by an applanation tonometer. Anterior chamber angle should be checked by gonioscopy if angle closure is suspected. Doubtful corneal abrasion is detected by fluorescein sodium stain. Diabetes mellitus status should be checked for patients with chronic or recurrent infectious conjunctivitis or dacryocystitis. Fluorescein dye disappearance test (FDDT) is done to screen for lacrimal drainage dysfunction. Lacrimal syringing test is done to determine the site of obstruction. Jones dye tests (tests 1 and 2) are performed for partial drainage pathway obstruction. Dacryocystography is helpful to determine the exact site, nature, and extent of obstruction. Radionucleotide dacryocystography (lacrimal scintillography) is a noninvasive technique for functional assessment of the lacrimal drainage system.

# THERAPY

A loose conjunctival foreign body can be removed by flushing with normal saline or manually by cotton pellets. An impacted corneal foreign body often needs removal under an operating microscope or a slit lamp. If bacterial conjunctivitis is suspected, in routine practice, broad-spectrum antibiotics are started, e.g., chloramphenicol (1%) or gentamicin (0.3%) or tobramycin (0.3%) or moxifloxacin (0.5%) eye drops 4–6 hourly in the day, which maybe augmented with eye ointment at bedtime. Irrigation of conjunctival sac with sterile lukewarm saline once or twice daily will help in removing obnoxious materials. In case of suspected adenovirus conjunctivitis, no topical antiviral drug is beneficial; topical antibiotics can be added to subside any superadded bacterial infection. In case of suspected gonococcal ophthalmia, neonatorum hourly saline water lavage is recommended till discharge is eliminated. 1% tetracycline or erythromycin eye ointment should be applied. A baby should be referred to a pediatric ophthalmologist for consideration of systemic intravenous (IV) antibiotics. Allergic conjunctivitis requires alleviation of symptoms by decongestant eye drops (naphazoline), antihistamine drugs (antazoline, azelastine, chlorpheniramine), or mast cell stabilizers (sodium cromoglycate, olopatadine, ketotifen, etc.). A short course of corticosteroid drops frequently gives relief in severe cases. Traumatic corneal abrasion is treated by topical antibiotics, lubricant drops (0.5% carboxy methyl cellulose), or ointment (2% hydroxymethyl propyl cellulose), cycloplegic eye drops. Eye taping is applied overnight to facilitate epithelial growth. Dry eye disease can be managed by topical lubricants or mild steroids. Acute dacryocystitis needs treatment with oral antibiotics along with topical antibiotic drops. Canaliculi or nasolacrimal duct blockage due to chronic dacryocystitis needs surgery such as dacryocystorhinostomy (DCR) or dacryocystectomy (DCT) according to the site of blockage. Trichiasis needs epilation as a temporary symptomatic relief **(Box 1)**.

**BOX 1: Computer vision syndrome.**

Computer vision syndrome, also referred to as digital eye strain is a common symptom in the current era due to prolonged exposure to digital screens. Headache, eye pain, and dry eye are few of the symptoms. Patients often present with burning sensation and hyperlacrimation. This excessive tearing is due to reflex lacrimation. Patients need to be advised for taking adequate interval between exposure to the screen and use of tear substitute drops or ointment

## RED FLAG SIGNS

Acute onset of pain, redness, and watering with corneal haziness may be a telltale sign of acute angle-closure glaucoma. The patient needs urgent lowering of intraocular pressure with oral carbonic anhydrase inhibition (acetazolamide), topical drops like beta-blocker (timolol maleate), carbonic anhydrase inhibitor (CAI) (acetazolamide, brinzolamide), and urgent referral to the hospital.

## CLINICAL PEARLS

- Epiphora is overflow of tears from eyes
- Hyperlacrimation is excessive tear production
- *Schirmer's test values*: ≤ 15 mm indicates dry eye
- Syringing helps in identifying the level of canalicular obstruction
- Pediatric eye inflammation demands urgent detailed examination, if necessary under general anesthesia

## FURTHER READINGS

1. Salmon JF, Kanski JJ. Kanski's clinical ophthalmology: A systematic approach. 9th edition. Edinburgh: Elsevier; 2020.
2. Khurana AK, Khurana I, Khurana AK, Khurana B. Anatomy and physiology of eye. 2nd ed. New Delhi: CBS Publishers & Distributors Pvt Ltd; 2017.
3. 7 Oculofacial Plastic and Orbital Surgery [Internet]. [cited 2023 Dec 5]. Available from: https://www.aao.org/education/bcscsnip-petdetail.aspx?id=46febd1f-9f5d-4082-9e21-56ce9ebabf0d

# CHAPTER 71

# Diplopia

*Sinjan Ghosh*

## INTRODUCTION

Diplopia or double vision is a clinical presentation that causes people to see two of the same images instead of one, which can be horizontal, vertical, or oblique.

## ETIOPATHOGENESIS

- *Causes of monocular diplopia*:
  - Uncorrected refractive error
  - Equipment failure (defective contact lens, ill-fitting bifocals in patients with dementia)
  - Corneal disease (e.g., astigmatism, dry eye, keratoconus)
  - After surgery for long-standing tropia (eccentric fixation)
  - Corrected long-standing tropia (eccentric fixation)
  - Foreign body in aqueous or vitreous media
  - Iris abnormalities (polycoria, trauma)
  - *Lens*: Multirefractile (combined cortical and nuclear) cataracts, subluxation
  - *Occipital cortex (bilateral monocular)*: Migraine, epilepsy, stroke, tumor, trauma (palinopsia, polyopia)
  - Psychogenic
  - Retinal disease (rare)

Generally, intraocular or ophthalmological causes are responsible for monocular diplopia. An exception: If a retinal distortion, such as an epiretinal membrane, displaces the fovea to an ectopic location, it can result in binocular diplopia due to impaired fusion of the two images.

- *Causes of binocular diplopia*:
  - Solely horizontal:
    - Abducens palsy (unilateral or bilateral)
    - Accommodative esotropia
    - Acute thalamic esotropia (following a thalamic stroke)
    - Chiari malformation
    - Cyclical oculomotor palsy (spastic phase)
    - Duane syndrome
    - Medial rectus entrapment (blowout fracture)
    - Nystagmus blockage syndrome (in congenital and latent nystagmus)
    - Posterior internuclear ophthalmoplegia (INO) of Lutz (pseudo-sixth)
    - Sagging eye syndrome
    - Spasm of the near reflex (near triad) (accompanied by miosis)
    - Stiff person syndrome (associated with abduction deficits, hypometric saccades)
    - Tonic convergence spasm (part of dorsal midbrain syndrome)

- Vertical ± horizontal
  - Common causes:
    - Superior oblique palsy
    - Thyroid-associated ophthalmopathy (muscle infiltration)
    - Myasthenia gravis (MG)
    - Skew deviation (brainstem, cerebellar, hydrocephalus)
  - Less common causes:
    - Orbital inflammation (myositis, idiopathic orbital inflammatory syndrome)
    - Orbital infiltration [lymphoma, metastases, amyloid, immunoglobulin G4 (IgG4)-related disease]
    - Primary orbital tumor
    - Entrapment of the inferior rectus (blowout fracture)
    - Brown syndrome (congenital, acquired)
    - Congenital extraocular muscle fibrosis or muscle absence
  - Other causes:
    - Chronic progressive external ophthalmoplegia (CPEO)
    - Miller Fisher syndrome
    - Botulism
    - Monocular supranuclear gaze palsy
    - Superior oblique myokymia
    - Dissociated vertical deviation (divergence)
    - Wernicke encephalopathy
    - Vertical one-and-a-half syndrome

*Physiological diplopia*: It occurs when a subject fixates on an object close to his eyes and then becomes aware of another object farther away in the direction of gaze. The nonfixed object is seen by noncorresponding parts of each retina and is perceived by the mind's (cyclopean) eye as double. Visual illusion can be induced by placing the index fingers of each hand horizontally in front of the eyes, at a distance of about 30 cm, with the fingertips touching, and one's gaze focused on a point in the distance. When the fingertips are then drawn apart, a finger can be perceived, with two ends, apparently floating in midair. This phenomenon is known as "floating finger" or "frankfurter illusion."

# DIFFERENTIAL DIAGNOSES

Differential diagnosis of diplopia is given in **Table 1**.

# PATH TO DIAGNOSIS

## History

A focused history is essential from a reliable informant that can provide a wealth of information for accurately narrowing down the cause of the diplopia, limiting the differential diagnoses, and directing the examination toward the underlying pathology.

*Monocular or binocular?*

*Horizontal, vertical, or oblique separation of the images?*
Diplopia that is horizontal in orientation suggests involvement of the medial or lateral rectus muscle. Diplopia that is vertical and torsional (with the lower image tilted) suggests an involvement of the superior oblique muscle (particularly if associated with a compensatory head tilt to the side opposite the weak muscle), while pure vertical diplopia is more likely to reflect brainstem or cerebellar pathology.

*Tilting of one image?*
Diplopia that is oblique/diagonal, reflecting dysfunction of both vertical and horizontal muscles, suggests dysfunction of the oculomotor nerve (involving some combination of the inferior rectus, superior rectus, and inferior oblique muscles).

*Effect of distance of target (worse at near or far)?*
Diplopia that is most pronounced at distance and on gaze to the left is supportive of dysfunction of the left lateral rectus

**Table 1: Differential diagnoses of diplopia.**

| | | | | |
|---|---|---|---|---|
| *Step 1*: High index of suspicion of stroke<br>• New-onset focal neurological deficit in favor of brainstem affection, hemiparesis, or cerebellar involvement<br>• Implement stroke protocol for prompt evaluation and treatment | | | | |
| *Step 2*: Diplopia with associated features | | | | |
| *Cavernous sinus pathology* | *Orbital apex syndrome* | *Trauma (head injury ± orbital trauma)* | *Infection* | *Increased ICP* |
| Ophthalmoplegia plus pain, chemosis, proptosis, periorbital swelling, facial numbness with ipsilateral absent corneal reflex and dilated nonreacting pupil (cranial nerves 3rd, 4th, 6th, V1, and V2 involvement)<br>D/D:<br>• Cavernous sinus thrombosis<br>• *Infection*: Bacterial or fungal (mucormycosis)<br>• *Inflammation*: Tolosa–Hunt syndrome<br>• Tumor infiltration<br>• *Caroticocavernous fistula*: Pulsatile proptosis | Optic nerve involvement plus cavernous sinus syndrome (Ophthalmoplegia with cranial nerves 3rd, 4th, 6th, V1, and V2 involvement)<br>D/D:<br>• Infection<br>• Inflammation<br>• Trauma<br>• Thyroid ophthalmopathy<br>• Neoplasms | Ophthalmoplegia with history and signs of trauma<br>D/D:<br>• Increased ICP (secondary to ICH)<br>• Retrobulbar hematoma<br>• Orbital wall fracture | Ophthalmoplegia plus fever, immunosuppression, facial or sinus infection<br>D/D:<br>• Orbital cellulitis<br>• Meningoencephalitis<br>• Abscess<br>• CVST | Ophthalmoplegia with headache, papilledema, cranial nerve 6th involvement: May be a false localizing sign<br>• SAH<br>• Idiopathic intracranial hypertension<br>• Intracranial SOL<br>• ICH |
| *Step 3*: Other systemic diseases—specific evaluation<br>• *Myasthenia gravis (ocular or generalized)*: Clinical signs with diurnal variation, serum autoantibodies, and electrophysiology (RNST or single fiber EMG)<br>• *Thyroid-associated ophthalmopathy*: MRI orbits, TSH receptor antibodies<br>• *Multiple sclerosis*: Internuclear ophthalmoplegia (INO) may be unilateral or bilateral. MRI brain and spinal cord for demyelinating plaques, CSF oligoclonal bands, and IgG index for supportive evidence | | | | |

(CSF: cerebrospinal fluid; CVST: cerebral venous sinus thrombosis; D/D: differential diagnosis; EMG: electromyography; ICH: intracerebral hemorrhage; ICP: intracranial pressure; IgG: immunoglobulin G; MRI: magnetic resonance imaging; RNST: repetitive nerve stimulation test; SAH: subarachnoid hemorrhage; SOL: space-occupying lesion; TSH: thyroid-stimulating hormone)

muscle/sixth cranial nerve. Difficulty with reading or other near tasks suggests dysfunction of convergence, reflecting possible involvement of third cranial nerve or medial rectus muscle or convergence insufficiency.

*Effect of fatigue? Worse in the morning or evening?*

In case of diurnal variation that is minimal or no diplopia at the beginning of the day and worsening of diplopia as the day progresses, can be due to fatiguability which is a key feature of neuromuscular junction disorder such as myasthenia gravis.

*Transient or persistent? If transient, consider giant cell arteritis.*

Diplopia is associated with headache, pain with (attempted) eye movement, ptosis, dysphagia, dyspnea, weakness, or, in patients older than 55 years of age, scalp tenderness, jaw/tongue claudication, fever, chills, unexplained weight loss, or body pain to suggest giant cell arteritis.

*Is there any history of head trauma, cancer, eye surgery, or botulinum toxin?*

*What other symptoms are present (i.e., headache, eye pain, dizziness, weakness)?*

## Clinical Examination

*Observation*: Head tilt or turn (review of old photographs for head tilt, pupil size, lids, and ocular alignment)?

- Ptosis (fatigue)?
- Pupil size? Anisocoria?
- Proptosis?

*Eye examination*: Visual acuity (monocular and binocularly)

### Fixation/Gaze-holding

The patient is instructed to keep looking at a distant target point in the primary viewing position.

Any instability of fixation should be noted. The following signs can be detected:

- Square-wave jerks, which are spontaneous, small-amplitude horizontal saccades away from fixation followed by a corrective saccade in the opposite direction. This implies an abnormality of the gaze fixation circuit.
- *Nystagmus*: The rhythmic involuntary oscillatory movements of the eyes which may be vertical, horizontal, or torsional. This implies a pathology affecting ocular coordination.

### Ductions

Ductions are performed by occluding one eye and asking the patient to follow a visual target through all cardinal gaze positions. Assessment should be made of any apparent restriction of eye movements; additionally, the pursuit movements (i.e., tracking) should be smooth and uninterrupted.

### Versions (Saccades, Pursuit, and Muscle Overaction)

Any abnormal resting head turns or tilt should be noted and then the version should be tested. This is about repeating the same procedure as done with duction but with both eyes open. Minor asymmetry and ocular misalignments are easily discerned with testing of versions.

### Saccades

The patient is asked to rapidly and alternately fixate on two different targets, a target held eccentrically and the examiner's nose in primary gaze. This should be performed in both vertical and horizontal planes. Any initiation delay, abnormal velocity of the saccades, and ocular dysmetria may imply brainstem or cerebellar dysfunction.

Diplopia/ocular misalignment that is unchanged with the direction of gaze is known as comitant and suggests congenital strabismus (or skew deviation if vertical). Ocular misalignment that changes with the direction of gaze is termed incomitant. It is frequently due to extraocular muscle dysfunction.

### Convergence

Adduction failure as observed during testing for saccades and pursuit evokes several possibilities including INO. Preserved convergence is noted in patients with INO, while it is impaired in nuclear or infranuclear nerve palsy.

### *Pupils*

*Miosis with ipsilateral ptosis*: Rule out Horner's syndrome

*Mydriasis with ipsilateral ptosis and impaired pupillary light reflex*: Third cranial nerve palsy

*Pupil sparing third cranial nerve palsy*: Diabetic third nerve palsy due to affection of vasa nervorum [Exception: In early stages of posterior communicating artery (PCOM) aneurysm, pupil sparing may be noted.]

### *Lids (Examine Palpebral Fissures, Levator Function, Fatigue)*

*Complete ptosis*: Third cranial nerve palsy

*Partial ptosis*: Horner's syndrome

*Bilateral ptosis with ophthalmoplegia*:

- In the elderly (around fifth decade): Rule out CPEO due to oculopharyngeal muscular dystrophy (OPMD). Enquire for family history
- *In young patients*: Consider CPEO due to mitochondrial myopathy. Positive family history may be supportive.
- *Lid edema with ophthalmoplegia*: Consider cavernous sinus pathology.

Signs that indicate a neuromuscular junction disorder (MG):

- *Fatigable ptosis*: Drooping of eyelids aggravating with the passing day
- *Peek sign*: Sustained tight eyelid closure induces fatigue of the orbicularis oculi muscles and a consequent mild widening of the palpebral fissures, exposing the sclera of the eye
- *Curtain sign*: In MG, extraocular involvement may be variable, leading to bilateral but unequal ptosis. Both lids receive equal innervation according to Hering's law. The neural firing innervating the levator palpebrae superioris (LPS) is an attempt to hold the lids open. The lid which is less affected by the disease process is open wider. Manually elevating the more ptotic lid sends a signal to the less ptotic lid and relaxation of LPS action on that side resulting in increased ptosis.
- *Cogan's lid twitch*: The patient is asked to maintain a downward gaze for 15 seconds and then gaze upward, finally returning to the primary gaze. A positive sign is manifested by the upper lid producing an overshoot or clear upward twitch when the patient has returned to the primary gaze.
- *Ice pack test for ptosis*: The ice pack test is a cheap, safe, and rapid bedside test to detect neuromuscular junction disorder. The palpebral fissure is measured pre- and post-testing for comparison. The test is considered positive if there is an improvement in ptosis by 2 mm after holding an ice pack for 3–5 minutes on the ptotic eyelid. In a study, the sensitivity of this test for the 5-minute application was 76.9% and the specificity was 98.3% with no reported false positives.

*Vestibulo-ocular reflexes (doll's eye reflex) and Bell's phenomenon*: If a conjugate defect is present, determine whether the eyes move reflexively by testing for the oculocephalic reflex (examiner moves the patient's head from side to side and notes the reflex movement of the eyes) and Bell's phenomenon which is the spontaneous upward deviation of the eyes, with lid closure.

*Cover–uncover test*: This test is useful to identify a tropia (manifest squint) and differentiate it from a phoria (latent squint). An opaque occluder is used to cover one eye for a few seconds and then removed. When the fixing eye is occluded, the examiner will observe the nonoccluded eye move to pick up fixation in the presence of tropia. A nasal deviation signifies exotropia and a temporal deviation signifies esotropia. In the absence of tropia, the nonoccluded eye remains stationary. To detect phoria, the examiner observes the eye behind the occluder. In the presence of phoria, the uncovered eye does not move but the eye behind the occluder deviates. It eventually returns to a straight position when the occluder is removed. The alternate cover test and alternate prism cover test can also be informative in specific cases.

*Other tests*:

- *Listen for bruits*: Orbital [caroticocavernous fistula or arteriovenous (AV) malformation], carotid (luminal stenosis)
- *Forced ductions test*: It is performed by grasping the anesthetized globe with forceps and pulling it through its range of motion. Any mechanical restriction during the excursion indicates a restrictive pathology (e.g., a mass abutting the muscle, inflammation, or post-traumatic impingement of muscle belly or tendon), while an unhindered passive movement confirms a nerve paresis.
- *Edrophonium (Tensilon) test*: For neuromuscular junction disorder
- Lights on–off test for the dragged-fovea diplopia syndrome

### Investigations

*Neuroimaging*: In post-traumatic cases, particularly with restricted ocular motility, computed tomography (CT) of the skull bones may be indicated. In nontraumatic cases, magnetic resonance imaging (MRI) (with dedicated skull base and orbital imaging) is preferable to CT. MRI of the orbits shows unilateral thickening and enhancement of the involved muscle and its myotendinous insertion signifies idiopathic orbital myositis. Similar orbital inflammation can be seen in IgG4-related diseases. Edema and hypertrophy of the extraocular muscles support a clinical suspicion of thyroid-associated ophthalmopathy. If other signs or symptoms of raised intracranial pressure are present, it is also important to visualize the brain parenchyma to exclude space-occupying lesions.

*Angiography*: MR angiography or CT angiography of the cerebral vessels might help in detecting an aneurysm (e.g., PCOM aneurysm). In general, neuroimaging has a low diagnostic yield in isolated fourth, pupil-sparing third, and sixth nerve palsies in older patients with vascular risk factors.

*Autoimmune markers*: Serum acetylcholine receptor (AchR) antibodies, anti-muscle-specific kinase (MuSK) antibodies, or anti-LRP4 antibodies are detected in MG.

Thyroid-stimulating hormone (TSH) receptor antibody correlates with disease severity and monitoring of treatment response in thyroid-associated ophthalmopathy.

*Neuroelectrophysiology*: Repetitive nerve stimulation test (RNST) and single-fiber electromyography (EMG) are sensitive tests for the detection of MG.

## SYMPTOMATIC THERAPY

The therapeutic aspects outlined below are symptomatic measures in cases with persistent diplopia. The definitive management targeting the primary etiology is beyond the scope of this chapter.

### Eye Patch

Covering one eye of patients with binocular diplopia is helpful in alleviating symptoms of diplopia. A long-term solution can be achieved using an eye patch or a translucent tape over spectacles. However, this has poor cosmetic implications. Patients should also be informed regarding the compromised depth perception due to disrupted binocular vision. Ensuring complete closure of the eyelid under the patch mitigates the chances of corneal injury.

### Prism Lenses

A prism lens can be applied to one or both lenses of spectacles to alter the disparity between images into a single vision. This is most effective for patients with comitant ocular misalignment. For patients with incomitant ocular misalignment, it will be beneficial for vision in the primary position only as the prism will not correct diplopia in all directions of gaze simultaneously. Once the appropriate prism strength is confirmed, a pair of spectacles for full-time wear can be used.

### Ocular Realignment Surgery

For patients with large-angle, incomitant ocular misalignment that has failed conservative management, surgery for repositioning the extraocular muscles to realign the eyes may be helpful. Surgical intervention for diplopia related to MG is rarely recommended because of the variable nature of the ocular misalignment.

## RED FLAG SIGNS

- Multiple cranial nerve involvement
- Headache
- Age > 60 years with headache
- Other neurological deficits may indicate a stroke
- Pain and proptosis

## CLINICAL PEARLS

The approach should be simple even if the manifestations seem to be apparently challenging during the initial presentation.

After completing the history and physical examination, clinicians need to ask the following questions:

*Where is the problem?* Probable anatomical localization of the lesion (supranuclear, internuclear, infranuclear, neuromuscular junction, extraocular muscle, or orbital dysfunction)

*What is the problem?* Pathophysiology suspected clinically and later confirmed on investigation

*Why is there a problem?* Syndromic diagnosis or etiology

While considering the etiopathogenesis of diplopia, the following acronym may be helpful:

- V—Vascular (stroke, aneurysms, cavernous sinus thrombosis)
- I—Infections (brainstem or orbital, e.g., tuberculosis, mucormycosis)
- T—Trauma (head injury and/or orbital fracture)
- A—Autoimmune (MG or Miller Fisher syndrome)
- M—Metabolic/endocrine (thyroid-associated ophthalmopathy, diabetes mellitus)
- I—Inflammation or infiltration (IgG4-related disease, Tolosa-Hunt syndrome, etc.)
- N—Neoplastic [primary—by direct tumor infiltration/metastasis involving brainstem or orbit and/or secondary—raised intracranial pressure due to central nervous system (CNS) tumor]
- S—Systemic causes

Judicious planning in terms of investigations and prompt initiation of management in case of ominous signs or impending threats to vision are essential.

## FURTHER READINGS


1. Rucker JC, Lavin PJM. Neuro-ophthalmology: ocular motor system. In: Jankovic J, Mazziotta JC, Pomeroy SL, Newman NJ (Eds). Bradley and Daroff's Neurology in Clinical Practice, 8th edition. Amsterdam: Elsevier.; 2021. pp. 208-11.
2. Sharp WL. The floating-finger illusion. Psychol Rev. 1928;35(2):171-3.
3. Gorelick PB, Rosenberg M, Pagano RJ. Enhanced ptosis in myasthenia gravis. Arch Neurol. 1981;38:531.
4. Cogan DG. Myasthenia gravis: a review of the disease and a description of lid twitch as a characteristic sign. Arch Ophthalmol. 1965;74:217-21.
5. Kearsey C, Fernando P, D'Costa D, Ferdinand P. The use of the ice pack test in myasthenia gravis. JRSM Short Rep. 2010;1(1):14.
6. Guyton DL. The "lights on-off test" in the diagnosis of the dragged-fovea diplopia syndrome. JAMA Ophthalmol. 2019;137(3):298-9.
7. Glisson CC. Approach to diplopia. Continuum (Minneap Minn). 2019;25(5):1362-75.

CHAPTER 72

# Dimness of Vision

*Sinjan Ghosh*

## WHAT IS DIMNESS OF VISION?

Dimness of vision may manifest as diminished color vision or gray areas and a lack of clarity of images. This encompasses both ocular and neurological causes such as optic neuritis, retinal detachment, diabetic retinopathy, macular degeneration, glaucoma, cataracts, or space-occupying lesions.

## WHAT CAUSES DIMNESS OF VISION?

### Etiologies of Ocular Pathology

- Central retinal artery occlusion
- Branch retinal artery occlusion
- Retinal vein occlusion
- Retinal detachment
- Central serous retinopathy
- Cystoid macular edema
- Diabetic retinopathy
- Hypertensive retinopathy
- Glaucoma
- Cataract
- Vitreous hemorrhage
- Acute idiopathic blind spot enlargement syndrome

### Etiologies of Optic Nerve Pathology

- Optic neuritis
- Nonarteritic anterior ischemic optic neuropathy (NAION)
- Arteritic anterior ischemic optic neuropathy (AAION)
- Posterior ischemic optic neuropathy (PION)
- Inflammatory conditions [e.g., neurosarcoidosis, vasculitis associated with systemic lupus erythematosus (SLE), and Sjögren's syndrome]
- *Infections*: Late syphilis (*Treponema pallidum*), varicella zoster, Lyme disease (*Borrelia burgdorferi*), human immunodeficiency virus (HIV), and opportunistic infections including toxoplasmosis, cytomegalovirus, *Cryptococcus*, mucormycosis, and aspergillosis
- Hereditary conditions such as Leber hereditary optic neuropathy (LHON)
- Neoplastic and paraneoplastic

## PATH TO DIAGNOSIS

### History

The evaluation of a patient with dimness of vision requires a meticulous history, which is imperative for narrowing down to a diagnosis.

Broadly, the distinction should be made between an ocular cause and a neurological cause.

*Primary presentation*: When patients complain of metamorphopsia or photopsia, it may indicate a retinal pathology. Metamorphopsia is an impression of distorted lines, which makes straight lines appear wavy and warped. This condition is usually associated with maculopathy. Positive phenomena such as photopsia or intermittent flashes of colored lights are associated with retinal involvement. Visual blurring with faded colors may suggest dysfunction of the optic nerve.

*Excluding field defects*: Occasionally, patients perceiving scintillating lights and having an undetected hemifield defect may misinterpret the hallucinations as originating in one eye. It is prudent to clarify whether the patient had ever covered one eye to discern if the visual difficulty had a monocular or binocular affection. Field defects are corroborated while performing the clinical examination.

*Temporal course and progression*: The progression and temporal course of the dimness of vision provide clues in terms of the potential etiology.

*Examples*:
- *Optic neuritis*: Quick evolution followed by gradual improvement
- *Ischemic optic neuropathy*: Sudden onset and static course
- *Compressive lesions*: Insidious onset and slowly progressive

*Associated features*: Orbital, neurologic, or associated systemic symptoms and signs may help in establishing or refuting a diagnosis.

*Examples*:
- *Painful dimness of vision*: Optic neuritis or giant cell arteritis
- *Painless dimness of vision*: Retinal diseases or NAION

Pertinent information regarding the patient's clinical profile, vascular risk factors such as hypertension or diabetes, malignancy, and autoimmune disorders are very useful.

## Clinical Examination

The role of a thorough examination cannot be overemphasized. When visual acuity is not correctable by pinhole, then retinopathy or optic neuropathy should be considered.

*Color vision*: Color vision impairment is detected using pseudoisochromatic color plates (Ishihara chart) or by testing for perceived color desaturation. Optic neuropathy can present with color vision affection.

*Red color desaturation*: The magnitude of red color desaturation is more prominent in asymmetric affection of integrity of the optic nerve. The prerequisite for this test is to ensure the best near-correction. The patient holds the test material at 30 cm from the eye in the presence of a bright light. After closing one eye, the patient is asked to focus on the dot in the middle of the screen. The patient should then confirm if he/she can spot four red circles in the corners. They must also identify the richness of the red color of these four circles or their faded color. Holding the circles slowly decreases the intensity of the red color, while pressing the same circle again increases the intensity of the red color. The goal is to equalize the tone of the perceived colors of all four circles. After completion, the middle white dot should be pressed **(Fig. 1)**.

*Amsler grid*: This is a series of horizontal and vertical lines in a grid pattern like a graph paper. The straight lines at places may be perceived as wavy or distorted by the patient and this is a test to detect metamorphopsia, which is a presentation of maculopathy **(Figs. 2A and B)**.

*Visual fields*: The confrontation method is a helpful bedside test to detect field defects. However, automated perimetry is comparatively more sensitive and an objective measure of patterns of field loss that aids in lesion localization.
- The affection of the central visual field is expected in maculopathy and optic neuropathy.

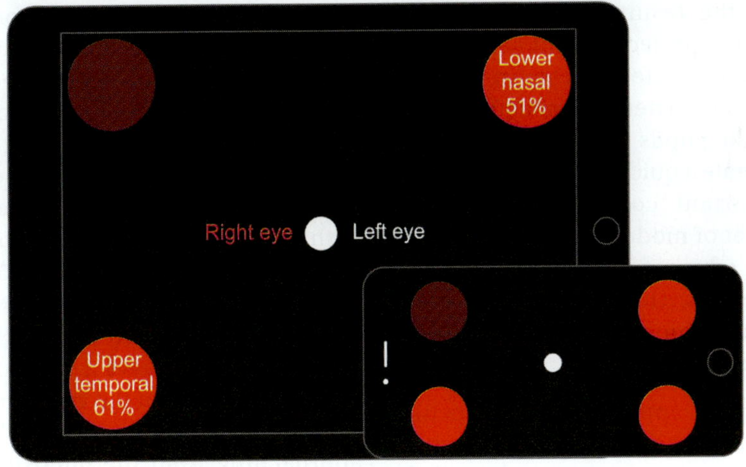


**FIG. 1:** Red desaturation.

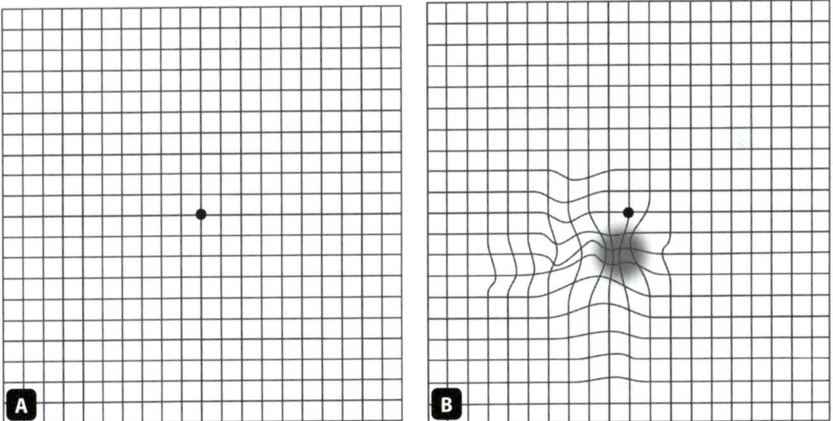


**FIGS. 2A AND B:** Wet macular degeneration—(A) A normal Amsler's grid. (B) How a patient perceives the straight lines as wavy and distorted in Metamorphopsia.

- In ischemic optic neuropathy, the field defect originates from the physiologic blind spot and respects the horizontal meridian.
- A homonymous visual field defect may be attributable to a retrochiasmal lesion, despite the patient's misperception that the change in vision is monocular.

*Swinging flashlight test*: The hallmark of unilateral optic neuropathy is the relative afferent pupillary defect (RAPD). The swinging flashlight test is usually performed by projecting light from a pen torch alternately directed toward each pupil.

*Unaffected eye*: When light is projected toward the unaffected eye, both pupils should constrict normally due to the direct and consensual reflexes in the ipsilateral and contralateral eyes, respectively.

*Affected eye*: When light is shone into the affected eye, the dilatation of both pupils indicates the presence of a RAPD. This is due to the dysfunctional afferent pathway, which involves the optic nerve on the affected side, because of which the stimulus required to give rise to a direct and consensual pupillary response is inadequate. The paradoxical pupillary dilatation in the affected eye is basically the result of the consensual response of the projected light being taken away from the unaffected eye. In cases of a subtler RAPD, when the affected eye is stimulated, the pupils may initially constrict but demonstrate a quicker redilatation.

An important consideration in this context is that of moderate or severe retinal dysfunction where a small RAPD may be observed as well. However, it is relatively more clinically pronounced with even mild asymmetric optic neuropathy.

*Fundoscopy*: The appearance of the ocular media, retina, and optic disc provides pivotal information regarding the likely causes of the dimness of vision. A detailed retinal examination following optimum pharmacologic pupillary dilation may reveal evidence of vitreous hemorrhage, features of hypertensive and diabetic retinopathy, retinal arterial or venous infarction, retinal detachment, or other macular pathology. The optic nerve head should be observed specifically for signs of swelling, pallor, or normal appearance.

- Optic disc swelling in a patient with dimness of vision indicates ischemia or inflammation of the optic nerve head.
- Normal optic disc is expected with retrobulbar processes, such as typical optic neuritis.
- Optic disc pallor due to optic atrophy may indicate chronic compression or prior optic nerve injury. Acute visual loss is unlikely in these cases unless the patient had an unrecognized previous subclinical injury.

*Photostress test*: In a patient presenting with a dimness of central vision, the two possibilities can be either a macular involvement or an optic nerve disease. Photo stress recovery test is a simple bedside test that can help in the preliminary distinction between the probable basis of visual affection. At the outset, a baseline visual acuity is recorded using Snellen's chart. The test involves exposing one eye at a time to the light from the ophthalmoscope or a pen torch for 10 seconds. This results in temporary bleaching of the retinal photoreceptors and measuring the time taken for acuity to return to within one line of prebleach acuity. Healthy subjects with normal macular function should be able to read the line in 50–60 seconds. Patients with maculopathy are expected to have longer recovery times lasting >1.5–3 minutes.

The practical relevance is noted while driving a car. Someone with macular degeneration will have a significant drop in visual acuity due to the bleaching effect on retinal pigments from the headlight of cars approaching from the opposite direction. The bleaching of the retina will have no effect on the recovery time in patients with optic neuropathy. Photostress recovery time increases with age.

## INVESTIGATIONS

The history and examination will guide an appropriate diagnostic workup that can confirm the correct diagnosis and eventually help in formulating a management plan.

- Orbital magnetic resonance imaging (MRI) sequences [including coronal T2-weighted images, fat-saturated postgadolinium images, and short tau inversion recovery (STIR) sequences] provide images of the prechiasmatic optic nerve. MRI in some cases may be helpful in differentiating between the different etiologies of optic neuropathy. Pathologic enhancement of the optic nerve reliably distinguishes optic nerve inflammation or demyelination from NAION. It is difficult to distinguish between inflammatory and demyelinating causes from MRI images, although the associated involvement of the meninges and meningeal enhancement makes an inflammatory condition more likely **(Table 1)**.
- Optical coherence tomography (OCT) provides high-resolution cross-sectional retinal images, which may distinguish retinal pathology from optic neuropathy.

**Table 1: Characteristic MRI features of optic neuropathies.**

| *Diagnosis* | *Optic nerve imaging* | *Brain and spinal cord imaging* |
|---|---|---|
| Multiple sclerosis | Unilateral, retrobulbar, and canalicular, short anterior segmental lesions, optic nerve enhancement | Periventricular ovoid lesions, subcortical and juxtacortical lesions |
| Neuromyelitis optica spectrum disorder | May be bilateral, often intracranial involving chiasm and optic tract, often longitudinally extensive, optic nerve enhancement | Longitudinally extensive transverse myelitis, posterior fossa and periaqueductal gray lesions, hypothalamic lesions |
| MOG-IgG | Frequently bilateral and retrobulbar, often longitudinally extensive, optic nerve and perineural sheath enhancement | Myelitis (thoracolumbar and conus predominance), lesions of deep gray nuclei |
| Seronegative (AON, RION, CRION) | Retrobulbar, optic nerve enhancement, occasional nerve swelling | Normal |
| Granulomatous (sarcoidosis, granulomatosis with polyangiitis) | Commonly unilateral, frequently combined optic nerve and sheath enhancement | • *Sarcoidosis*: Periventricular lesions, leptomeningeal lesions, pituitary and hypothalamic lesions<br>• *Granulomatosis with polyangiitis*: Pachymeningitis, nonspecific gray and white matter lesions due to vasculitis |
| Autoimmune (Sjögren's syndrome, systemic lupus erythematosus) | Retrobulbar, optic nerve enhancement | Systemic lupus erythematosus: Infarcts and dural thrombosis |
| GFAP-IgG | Normal | Linear radial perivascular enhancement, meningitis, myelitis, leptomeningeal and ependymal enhancement |
| Paraneoplastic (CRMP-5) | Bilateral, optic nerve enhancement | Cerebellar atrophy, mesial temporal lesions, cerebellar lesions, myelitis (may be longitudinally extensive) |
| Neuroretinitis | Normal, occasional high T2 signal or enhancement in proximal optic nerve | Normal |
| Syphilis | Optic nerve and perineural sheath enhancement | Leptomeningeal enhancement, encephalitis, myelitis, infarct |
| Lyme disease | Retrobulbar, optic nerve enhancement | Cranial nerve enhancement, periventricular and subcortical lesions |
| Tuberculosis | Retrobulbar, optic nerve and sheath enhancement | Leptomeningeal enhancement, ependymitis, tuberculoma |
| Viral infection | Retrobulbar, optic nerve enhancement | Variable depending on the pathogen |

(AON: autoimmune optic neuropathy; CRION: chronic relapsing inflammatory optic neuropathy; CRMP-5: collapsin response-mediator protein-5; GFAP-IgG: glial fibrillary acidic protein immunoglobulin G; MOG-IgG: myelin oligodendrocyte glycoprotein immunoglobulin G; MRI: magnetic resonance imaging; RION: relapsing isolated optic neuritis)

*Source*: Adapted from Bennett JL (2019).[4]

- Fluorescein angiography is used in some cases where there is suspicion of occult maculopathies, such as an ischemic lesion associated with diabetes.
- Visual evoked potentials (VEP's) are used in the diagnosis of optic neuritis. Prolonged P100 latency provides a reliable evidence in favour of optic nerve demyelination. A reduction in amplitude, in addition, signifies concurrent axonopathy.
- An electroretinogram may contribute to the diagnosis of acute retinal dysfunction, particularly when no overt lesions are evident and retinal dysfunction is suspected by history.
- Serologic and cerebrospinal fluid (CSF) tests can help diagnose an infectious, inflammatory, or neoplastic illness.
- Genetic testing can confirm a diagnosis of LHON.

## DIFFERENTIAL DIAGNOSES

*Central retinal artery occlusion*: Retinal whitening, cherry-red spot

*Branch retinal artery occlusion*: Segmental retinal whitening

*Retinal vein occlusion*: Retinal hemorrhages and engorged veins ("blood and thunder appearance")

*Retinal detachment*: Billowing, elevated retina

*Central serous retinopathy*: Macular subretinal fluid—confirmed by OCT

*Cystoid macular edema*: Subtle macular elevation—confirmed by OCT

*Acute idiopathic blind spot enlargement syndrome*: Photopsias, blind spot enlargement; subtle peripapillary retinal changes

- *Angle-closure glaucoma*:
  - Excruciating pain
  - Red eye with an enlarged, nonreactive pupil
- *Optic neuritis*:
  - Pain on eye movements
  - Normal-appearing optic nerve or mild swelling
  - Nadir at 7–10 days
  - Spontaneous recovery
- *Nonarteritic anterior ischemic optic neuropathy*:
  - Painless
  - Altitudinal visual field deficit
  - Optic disc edema may be sectoral
  - Increased age and vascular risk factors
  - Possibly nocturnal hypotension
- *Arteritic anterior ischemic optic neuropathy*:
  - Systemic symptoms (myalgias, jaw claudication, fevers, scalp tenderness, weight loss)
  - Optic disc edema, cotton wool spots (retinal ischemia)
  - Increased age
  - Elevated erythrocyte sedimentation rate (ESR) and C-reactive protein (CRP)
  - Giant cells and endovascular inflammation on temporal artery biopsy (preferably long segment biopsy or >1 cm)

*Posterior ischemic optic neuropathy* is rare and presents with acute, severe optic nerve dysfunction without nerve swelling. PION may be a consequence of severe blood loss or prolonged surgical procedures (e.g., spinal surgery). Giant cell arteritis is another important possibility. Nonarteritic PION is seldom seen.

### Inflammatory Conditions

Possibly associated with uveitis, systemic inflammatory symptoms

*Infections* such as "neuroretinitis" (optic neuropathy coexists with characteristic peripapillary or macular exudates) and macular star in cases like cat scratch disease are caused by *Bartonella henselae*. Lyme-associated optic neuritis is relatively rare but may be considered in a patient with a history of tick exposure, erythema migrans, arthralgias, or positive serologies (confirmed by Western blot).

*Hereditary conditions [LHON which is due to mitochondrial deoxyribonucleic acid (DNA) mutation]*:

- Painless sequential visual loss
- Predominantly, males are affected.
- Usually young men (second or third decade)
- Pseudoswelling of the optic disc
- Peripapillary telangiectasias

Genetic testing for LHON should be considered in any patient with unexplained sequential or simultaneous bilateral severe optic neuropathies.

*Neoplastic and paraneoplastic*: Primary malignant glioblastoma in adults occasionally originates in the optic nerve and may mimic optic neuritis early in its clinical course. Other neoplastic causes of optic neuropathy include disseminated lymphoma or leukemia, carcinomatous meningitis, and direct optic nerve metastasis (breast and lung tumors most likely).

Paraneoplastic optic neuropathy is more likely to cause bilateral visual loss. It may precede the manifestation of systemic malignancy and may present with coexisting retinitis, vitritis, limbic encephalitis, peripheral neuropathy, or ataxia. The antibody most commonly identified is directed toward collapsin response-mediator protein-5 (CRMP-5). Carcinoma-associated retinopathy (CAR) has antirecoverin antibodies, and melanoma-associated retinopathy (MAR) is usually associated with antibipolar cell antibodies.

## SYMPTOMATIC THERAPY

The treatment outlines mentioned below would cover only the symptomatic management of different causes of dimness of vision and not the disease-modifying therapies used in various conditions, such as multiple sclerosis (MS) and neuromyelitis optica (NMO), or specific management for the retinal causes.

- *Optic neuritis*: High-dose intravenous (IV) methylprednisolone (1,000 mg/day IV for 3 days) improves the speed of recovery. Lower dosages of oral prednisone (1 mg/kg) are contraindicated for acute optic neuritis treatment due to a higher risk of relapse. A complete response to high-dose corticosteroids is seen in only 36% of cases of NMO, which is lower than in MS-associated optic neuritis.
- *Steroid refractory optic neuritis*: Intravenous immunoglobulin (IVIg) (2 g/kg) failed to improve contrast sensitivity or visual function in patients with acute optic neuritis or MS with refractory vision loss. Plasma exchange improved visual outcomes in corticosteroid-refractory optic neuritis and neuromyelitis optica spectrum disorder (NMOSD) optic neuritis.
- *Inflammatory optic neuropathy*: Optic nerve involvement in neurosarcoidosis, SLE, and Sjögren's disease may be accompanied by anterior uveitis. There is also a clinical entity, known as chronic relapsing ischemic optic neuropathy (CRION). Unfortunately, the visual loss due to these conditions often is steroid-dependent, with recurrence of visual loss following the withdrawal of steroids.
- *Infectious optic neuropathy*: With a high index of suspicion for an infectious cause of optic neuritis, prompt initiation of antibiotics may lead to a better outcome. Corticosteroids may be initiated concurrently to salvage vision unless contraindicated. Appropriate therapy may be tailored in accordance to the clues from investigations. For optic neuritis associated with *Bartonella* infection, the role of antibiotic therapy remains unclear; however, significant vision loss, systemic infection, and immunocompromised status warrant antibiotics.
- *Giant cell arteritis and AAION*: In case of visual symptoms/loss or critical cranial ischemia, high-dose IV pulse

glucocorticoids (IV methylprednisolone 500–1,000 mg/day for adults or 30 mg/kg/day for children; maximum 1,000 mg/day or equivalent for 3–5 days) followed by high-dose daily oral glucocorticoids (prednisone 1 mg/kg/day up to 80 mg or equivalent) is used preferably with tocilizumab. In some instances, oral glucocorticoids with or without methotrexate may be administered. In case of remission, oral glucocorticoids should be tapered, while in case of persistent symptoms, addition or switchover to a nonglucocorticoid immunosuppressant like methotrexate or abatacept should be considered if the patient is already on tocilizumab. The lack of long-term follow-up data on tocilizumab and its cost may limit its use. According to the British Society for Rheumatology, oral glucocorticoids should be tapered according to the following protocol:

- Maintain the initial dose (40–60 mg) for at least 4 weeks, then
- Reduce by 10 mg, every 2 weeks, down to 20 mg, then
- Reduce by 2.5 mg, every 2–4 weeks, to 10 mg, then
- Reduce by 1 mg, every 4–8 weeks, provided there are no relapses.

Dose-reduction intervals can be prolonged, based on the patient's symptoms and history of relapses with previous dose reductions. A treatment duration of at least 1–2 years, often longer, may be expected in some cases.

- *Acute NAION*: In spite of limited data and no proven treatment options, some clinicians do offer a limited course of steroid treatment in patients with severe visual loss.

## RED FLAG SIGNS

- An unusual temporal course (progression beyond 2 weeks or lack of recovery within 1 month)
- An atypical scotoma (such as an altitudinal defect)
- Atypical fundus examination (including a nerve that is markedly swollen or atrophic, or retinal abnormalities such as hemorrhages, inflammation, or exudates)

## CLINICAL PEARLS

Papilledema or optic disc swelling secondary to raised intracranial pressure does not cause dimness of vision until late stages when optic atrophy sets in or in case of coexistent macular edema.

The dictums for fundoscopy findings and clinical possibilities are as follows:

- Doctor can see (optic disc swelling) and the patient can see (vision unaffected)—papilledema.
- Doctor can see (optic disc swelling) but the patient cannot see (vision affected)—anterior ischemic optic neuropathy.
- Doctor cannot see (optic disc changes) and the patient cannot see (vision affected)—retrobulbar optic neuritis.

Timely corticosteroid therapy is essential to salvage the vision in case of impending visual loss.

In cases of central serous retinopathy, clinicians should refrain from steroid therapy as it can worsen the condition. OCT is helpful in ruling out central serous retinopathy. It is usually a self-resolving condition due to subretinal fluid accumulation. In selective cases, minor laser surgery can curb the fluid leak.

## FURTHER READINGS

1. Prasad S, Galetta SL. Approach to the patient with acute monocular visual loss. Neurol Clin Pract. 2012;2(1):14-23.
2. O'Neill EC, Danesh-Meyer HV, Connell PP, Trounce IA, Coote MA, Mackey DA, et al. The optic nerve head in acquired optic neuropathies. Nat Rev Neurol. 2010;6:221-36.

3. Becker M, Masterson K, Delavelle J, Viallon M, Vargas MI, Becker CD. Imaging of the optic nerve. Eur J Radiol. 2010;74:299-313.
4. Bennett JL. Optic neuritis. Continuum (Minneap Minn). 2019;25(5):1236-64.
5. Mirza RG, Johnson MW, Jampol LM. Optical coherence tomography use in evaluation of the vitreoretinal interface: a review. Surv Ophthalmol. 2007;52:397-421.
6. Newman NJ. Hereditary optic neuropathies: from the mitochondria to the optic nerve. Am J Ophthalmol. 2005;140:517-23.
7. Kleiter I, Gahlen A, Borisow N, Fischer K, Wernecke KD, Wegner B, et al. Neuromyelitis optica: evaluation of 871 attacks and 1,153 treatment courses. Ann Neurol. 2016;79(2):206-16.
8. Noseworthy JH, O'Brien PC, Petterson TM, Weis J, Stevens L, Peterson WK, et al. A randomized trial of intravenous immunoglobulin in inflammatory demyelinating optic neuritis. Neurology. 2001;56(11):1514-22.
9. Roed HG, Langkilde A, Sellebjerg F, Lauritzen M, Bang P, Mørup A, et al. A double-blind, randomized trial of IV immunoglobulin treatment in acute optic neuritis. Neurology. 2005;64(5):804-10.
10. Deschamps R, Gueguen A, Parquet N, Saheb S, Driss F, Mesnil M, et al. Plasma exchange response in 34 patients with severe optic neuritis. J Neurol. 2016;263(5):883-7.
11. Kidd D, Burton B, Plant GT, Graham EM. Chronic relapsing inflammatory optic neuropathy (CRION). Brain. 2003;126:276-84.
12. Bhatti MT, Lee MS. Should patients with bartonella neuroretinitis receive treatment? J Neuroophthalmol. 2014;34(4):412-6.
13. Maz M, Chung S, Abril A, Langford CA, Gorelik M, Guyatt G, et al. 2021 American College of Rheumatology/Vasculitis Foundation Guideline for the Management of Giant Cell Arteritis and Takayasu Arteritis. Arthritis Rheumatol. 2021;73(8):1349-65.
14. Dasgupta B, Borg F, Hassan N, Alexander L, Barraclough K, Bourke B, et al. BSR and BHPR guidelines for the management of giant cell arteritis. Rheumatology (Oxford). 2010;49(8):1594-7.
15. Lee AG, Biousse V. Should steroids be offered to patients with nonarteritic anterior ischemic optic neuropathy? J Neuroophthalmol. 2010; 30(2):193-8.

CHAPTER 73

# Pupil and Its Abnormalities

*Agnibha Maiti, Siladitya Dewasi*

## INTRODUCTION

In the middle layer of the human eye, the layers from anterior to posterior are as follows:

- Iris
- *Ciliary body*:
  - Pars plana
  - Pars plicata
- Choroid

## WHAT IS PUPIL?

Iris is a muscular structure, and there is an aperture in the center of it called pupil **(Fig. 1)**.

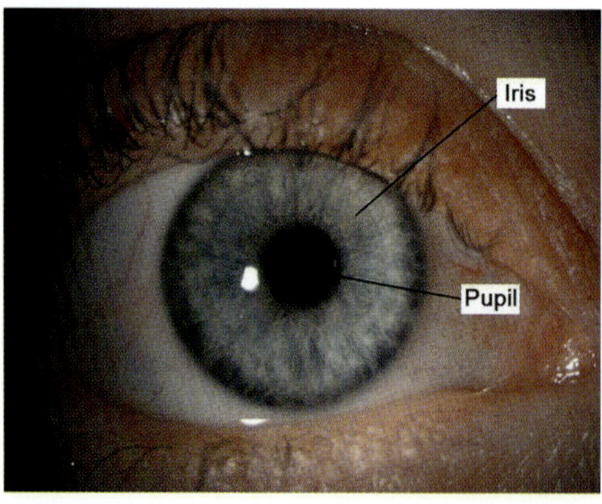


**FIG. 1:** Pupil.

According to the muscle of the iris, pupil will constrict and dilate **(Table 1)**.

## PUPILLARY REFLEXES

- *Near reflex*: Changes taking place in the eye while looking at a near object. It is a combination of miosis, accommodation, and convergence.
- *Ciliospinal reflex*: This reflex, which was first described by Budge, is present in

**Table 1: Muscle of iris.**

| | ***Sphincter pupillae*** | ***Dilator pupillae*** |
|---|---|---|
| Function | Constriction of pupil (miosis—**Box 1**) | Dilation of pupil (mydriasis—**Box 1**) |
| Nerve supply | Parasympathetic, short ciliary nerve | Sympathetic, long ciliary nerve |

**BOX 1: Causes of miosis and mydriasis.**

***Miosis***

Horner's syndrome, pontine hemorrhage, iridocyclitis, clonidine, organophosphate poisoning, opioids, parasympathomimetic, phenothiazines, pilocarpine, sleep, sedatives

***Mydriasis***

Belladonna poisoning, glaucoma (angle closure), internal ophthalmoplegia, oculomotor nerve palsy, sympathomimetics, tonic pupil

normal awake or sleeping humans as well as in comatose patients.

- *Ipsilateral dilation of pupil*: When there is pain in the neck/trunk due to any cause, the ipsilateral pupil will dilate. It is lost in Horner syndrome.
- *Psychosensory reflex*: Dilation of pupil in response to stress
- *Light reflex*: When exposed to light, the pupil will constrict (to control the excess amount of light getting into the eye).
    - Pupil will dilate in dark/dim light in order to let more light into the eyes.

## TYPES OF LIGHT REFLEXES

The types of light reflexes are direct and consensual.

- *Direct*: Constriction of the ipsilateral pupil when illuminated
- *Consensual*: Constriction of the contralateral pupil when not illuminated

*Light reflex pathway*: Light thrown in the ipsilateral eye → light falls in the retina → optic nerve → optic chiasma (temporal side) → ipsilateral optic tract → pupillomotor fibers leave the optic tract before they relay into lateral geniculate body (LGB) → then go to olivary pretectal nuclei (OPN) (center for light reflex) → interneurons/internuncial neuron—one half curves around periaqueductal gray and goes to ipsilateral Edinger-Westphal nucleus (EWN), the other half goes through the posterior commissure to contralateral EWN → third cranial nerve (CN) (both sides) → ciliary ganglion → short ciliary nerve → sphincter pupillae → both pupils constrict **(Fig. 2)**.

- *Afferent fibers*: Optic nerve second CN—sensory
- *Efferent fibers*: Oculomotor nerve third CN—motor
- Afferent and efferent pathway defect **(Box 2)**

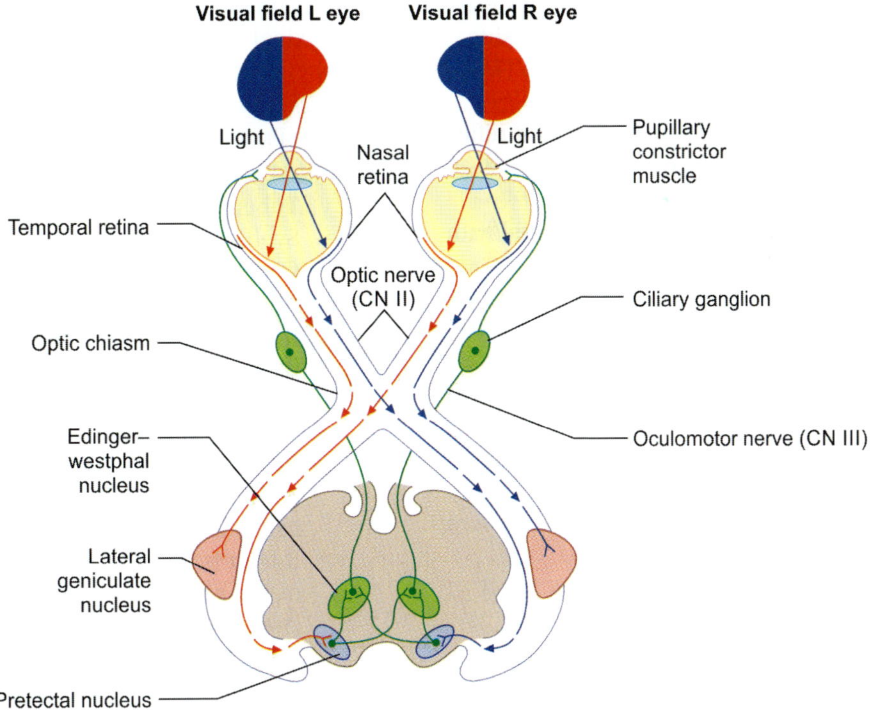


**FIG. 2:** Light reflex pathway.
(CN: cranial nerve; L: left; R: right)

**BOX 2: Afferent and efferent pathway defects.**

***Afferent pathway defects***
- Amaurotic pupil/AAPD/TAPD
- Marcus Gunn pupil/RAPD
- Wernicke's hemianopic pupil

***Efferent pathway defects***
- Argyll Robertson pupil (ARP)
- Tonic pupil or Adie's pupil
- Mydriasis

(AAPD: absolute afferent pathway defect; RAPD: relative afferent pathway defect; TAPD: total afferent pathway defect)

## Afferent Pathway Defect

1. *Amaurotic pupil/absolute afferent pathway defect (AAPD)/total afferent pathway defect (TAPD)*
    - *Cause*: End-stage optic atrophy/severe trauma
        - *Site*: Indicates lesion of optic nerve/retina on the affected side
        - Absence of direct light reflex (DLR) on the affected side
        - Absence of consensual light reflex (CLR) on the other eye
    - *Features*:
        - Ipsilateral anopia (blindness) with (–) DLR with (–) CLR
        - Near reflex is present due to normal eye (consensual).
        - Isocoria (same size of pupil)
2. *Marcus Gunn pupil/relative afferent pathway defect (RAPD)*
    - *Site*: Occurs due to partial optic nerve lesion
    - Incomplete optic nerve lesion/severe retinal diseases
    - *Causes*:
        - Optic neuritis
        - Retinal detachment
        - Central retinal artery/central retinal vein occlusion (CRAO/CRVO)
        - Anterior ischemic optic neuropathy (AION)
        - Primary open-angle glaucoma
    - It is the earliest sign of optic nerve disease, even in the presence of normal visual acuity on the affected side.
    - The presence of an RAPD is the hallmark of a unilateral afferent sensory abnormality or bilateral asymmetric visual loss.

    *Swinging flashlight test* ***(Figs. 3A to C)***:
    - This is a flashlight test for RAPD.
    - It leads to earlier fatigue of the partially lesioned optic nerve (right eye).
    - So, on drawing light from the normal side (left), for a brief moment as both pupils are in the dark, they start to dilate.
    - On reaching the right lesioned side, due to fatigue, the impulse for constriction is weaker than the impulse of already occurring dilation.
    - So, both pupils are seen to be dilated.
    - This phenomenon is known as "paradoxical dilation/pupillary escape phenomenon."
3. *Wernicke's hemianopic pupil*
    - *Site*: Proximal optic tract
    - *Causes*:
        - Tubercular meningitis
        - Syphilitic meningitis
        - Cerebral artery aneurysm
    - *Example*:
        - If light is thrown to the temporal half of the retina of the affected side (side of visual loss) and the nasal half of the retina of the opposite side eye, then ipsilateral (I/L) direct and contralateral (C/L) consensual light reflex will be absent.
        - If light is thrown to the nasal half of the retina of the affected side (where the vision is present) and the temporal half of the retina of the opposite side eye, then I/L direct and C/L consensual light reflex will be present.

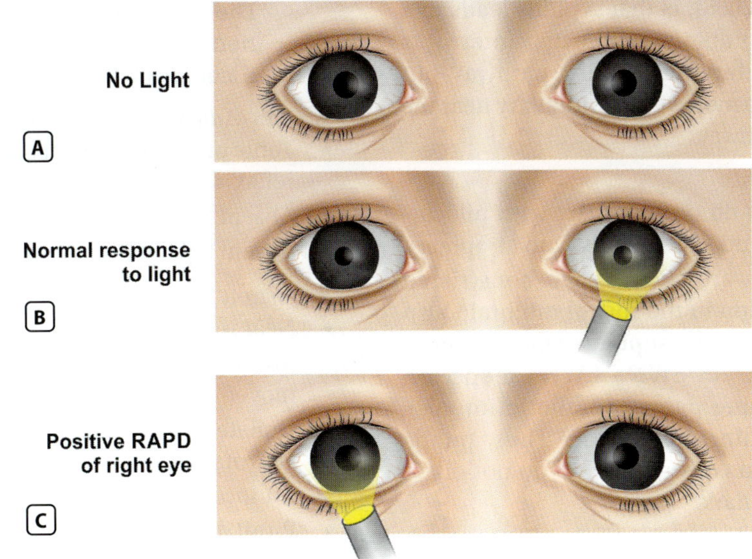


**FIGS. 3A TO C:** (A) On presentation, both pupils are contracted (isocoria); (B) Light on the left eye in a dark room; (C) Light on the right eye in a dark room [relative afferent pathway defect (RAPD) eye].

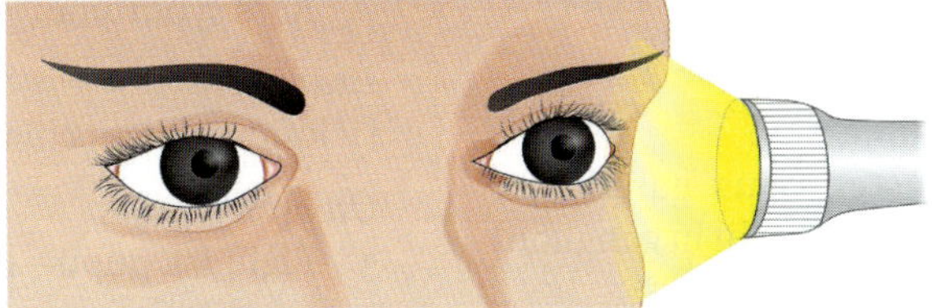

Pupils DO NOT constrict when exposed to bright light (light reflex)

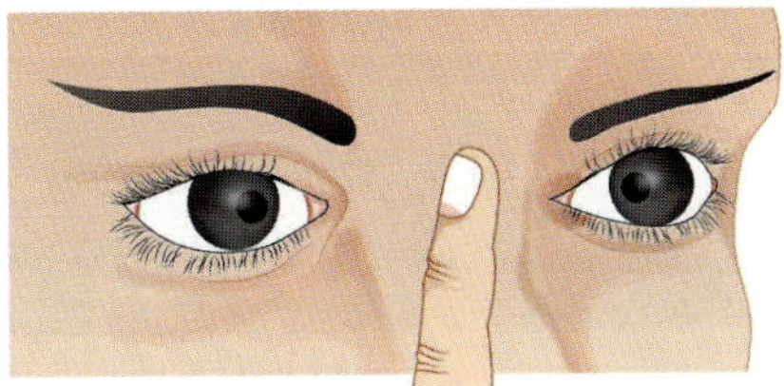

Pupils DO constrict on a near object (accommodation reflex)

**FIG. 4:** Argyll Robertson pupil.

## Efferent Pupillary Defect

1. *Argyll Robertson pupil (ARP)* ***(Fig. 4)***
   - *Site*: Rostral midbrain (aqueductal gray matter/Sylvius) or posterior commissure
   - *Causes*:
     - Neurosyphilis (tertiary syphilis) (tectum lesion)
     - Tabes dorsalis
     - Aortic regurgitation
     - Patient's history—unprotected intercourse way back + neurological symptoms ⇒ neurosyphilis
     - It is a bilateral presentation.
     - Pupils do not react to light.
     - Near reflex is present.

*Pathophysiology*: The current leading theory, proposed by Thompson and

Kardon (2006), is that syphilis leads to a "dorsal midbrain lesion that interrupts the pupillary light reflex pathway but spares the more ventral pupillary near the reflex pathway."

*Extra points*:
- Pupils do not constrict with pilocarpine and dilate poorly with atropine.
- Pupils are always seen constricted as lesion in the rostral midbrain also damages the supranuclear inhibitory fibers to EWN. EWN keeps on releasing parasympathetic impulse to sphincter pupillae. Thus, pupils remain constricted and do not dilate in the dark.
- No dilation lag is seen in ARP (Horner's syndrome).

2. *Tonic pupil/Adie's pupil* **(Fig. 5)**
   - *Site*: Parasympathetic pupillomotor damage (postganglionic), ciliary ganglion, short ciliary nerve
   - *Causes*:
     - Orbital trauma
     - Herpes zoster virus ganglionic (herpes virus dormant in ganglion)
     - Diabetes (pan peripheral autonomic neuropathy)
     - Alcoholism

*Holmes-Adie's pupil*:
- Tonic pupil + diminished deep tendon reflex
- Absent knee jerk
- Absent light reflex and slow near reflex

*Important points*:
- Near reflex is present.
- Absent light reflex or show "vermiform movement contraction"
- Unilateral involvement is observed in 80% of patients.
- *Anisocoria*: Affected pupil is larger.
- Pupil constricts with 0.125% pilocarpine (cholinergic supersensitivity).
- When Adie's pupil is accompanied by weakened or absent deep reflexes and segmental anhidrosis, it is known as Ross syndrome.

*Example*:
(If lesion in right ciliary ganglion)

*On presentation*:
- Right I/L pupil—dilated

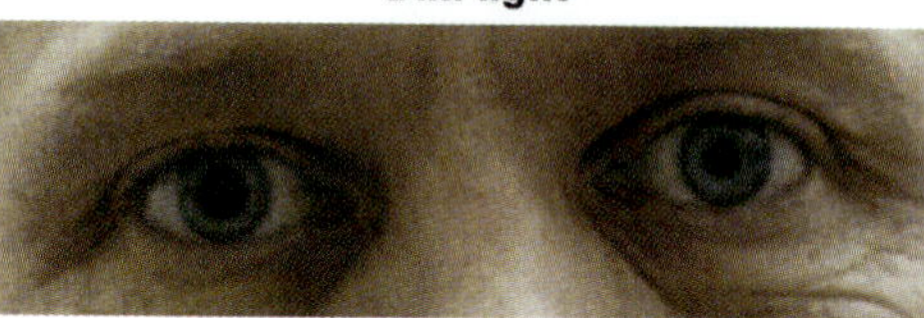


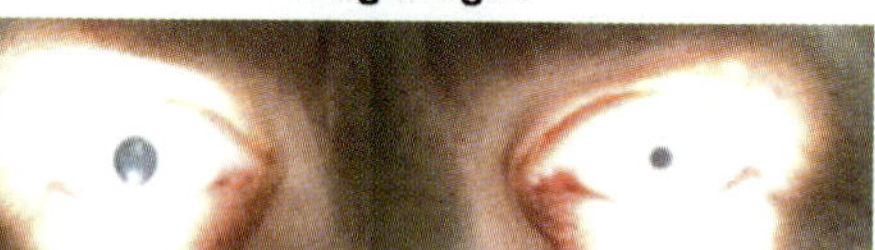


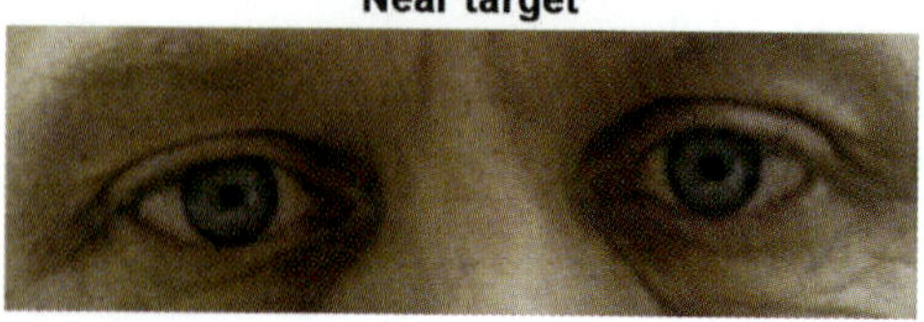


**FIG. 5:** Holmes–Adie's pupil.

- Left C/L pupil—constricted
- Anisocoria

*Light on left eye*:
- Right C/L pupil—does not constrict. Consensual absent
- Left I/L—constricts

*Light on right eye*:
- Right I/L pupil—does not constrict. DLR absent
- Left C/L—constricts. Consensual present

3. *Pharmacologic mydriasis*
   - *Due to the use of mydriatic agent*: Atropine
   - Affected eye never constricts, unaffected eye constricts normally (similarly to tonic pupil)
   - *Near reflex*: Absent (as atropine is cycloplegic)
   - Does not constrict even with 1% pilocarpine

## CLINICAL PEARLS

- *Pupillary light reflex*: The normal pupillary light reflex involves constriction of both pupils when light is shone into one eye. A brisk and equal response is expected.
- *Anisocoria*: Anisocoria, or unequal pupil size, can be physiological (normal in some individuals) or pathological. If anisocoria is greater in bright light, it may suggest a relative afferent pupillary defect (RAPD).
- *Horner's syndrome*: Horner's syndrome is characterized by miosis (constricted pupil), ptosis (drooping eyelid), and anhidrosis (lack of sweating) on the affected side. It results from disruption of sympathetic nerve pathway, often due to a lesion in the sympathetic pathway.
- *Adie's pupil*: Adie's pupil is a large, sluggish pupil that reacts slowly to light but constricts when the patient focuses on a near object. It is often caused by damage to the ciliary ganglion and is associated with absent or reduced deep tendon reflexes.
- *Argyll Robertson pupil*: Argyll Robertson pupils are small, irregular pupils that constrict when the patient focuses on a near object but do not react to light. This is classically seen in neurosyphilis.
- *Midbrain lesions*: Damage to the midbrain, such as with a pineal gland tumor, can cause Parinaud's syndrome, which includes impaired upward gaze, convergence-retraction nystagmus, and light-near dissociation.
- *Ocular trauma*: Trauma to the eye can result in a blown pupil, suggesting a severe injury to the globe or damage to the oculomotor nerve.
- *Medications and pupils*: Certain medications, such as opioids, can cause miosis, while anticholinergic drugs may induce mydriasis (dilated pupils).
- *Neurological causes*: Pupillary abnormalities can be indicative of neurological conditions, such as increased intracranial pressure (dilated pupils) or third nerve palsy (ptosis and mydriasis).
- *Pupil examination in coma*: Pupil examination is crucial in assessing brainstem function in comatose patients. Bilateral fixed and dilated pupils may suggest uncal herniation.
- *Photophobia*: Patients with abnormal sensitivity to light (photophobia) may have conditions affecting the pupils, such as iritis or anterior uveitis.
- *Pupillary assessment in ophthalmology*: Ophthalmologists use various tools, including a slit lamp, to assess the pupils and their responses in detail. Abnormalities may indicate specific eye conditions or neurological issues.

Always consider the broader clinical context when evaluating pupillary abnormalities, and if uncertain or concerned about the findings, consult with a neurologist or ophthalmologist for further evaluation and management.

# FURTHER READINGS

1. Wilhelm H. Disorders of the pupil. Handb Clin Neurol. 2011;102:427-66.
2. Tripathy K, Simakurthy S, Jan A. Ciliospinal reflex. StatPearls [Internet]. Treasure Island, FL: StatPearls Publishing; 2022.
3. Belliveau AP, Somani AN, Dossani RH. Pupillary light reflex. StatPearls [Internet]. Treasure Island, FL: StatPearls Publishing; 2022.
4. Simakurthy S, Tripathy K. Marcus Gunn pupil. StatPearls [Internet]. Treasure Island, FL: StatPearls Publishing; 2022.
5. Dichter SL, Shubert GS. Argyll Robertson Pupil. StatPearls [Internet]. Treasure Island, FL: StatPearls Publishing; 2022.
6. Adie WJ. Complete and incomplete forms of the benign disorder characterised by tonic pupils and absent tendon reflexes. Br J Ophthalmol. 1932;16(8):449-61.
7. Xu SY, Song MM, Li L, Li CX. Adie's pupil: a diagnostic challenge for the physician. Med Sci Monit. 2022;28:e934657.

CHAPTER 74

# Optic Fundus

*Agnibha Maiti, Siladitya Dewasi*

## INTRODUCTION

Human eye is anatomically divided by lens. The retrolenticular portion of the eye is very important not only for visual function but also due to various clinicopathological conditions. Optic fundus is one of the important structures among this.

Optic fundus **(Fig. 1)** is the portion of the retrolenticular eye that can be seen during an eye examination while looking through the pupil and probably the only place where the blood vessels can be visualized directly. So by doing fundoscopy, these vessels can be directly inspected. Optic fundus can be regarded as the mirror of the systemic circulation. Various clinical conditions can be detected through the optic fundus examination by fundoscopy or by direct ophthalmoscopy. So, any clinical examination would be incomplete without examination of the fundus. Not only for the ophthalmologist, optic fundus examination is very important for other clinicians also.

## PARTS OF OPTIC FUNDUS

Normally, the optic fundus includes the following:

- *Optic disc*: It is the area of the fundus where ganglion cells exit to form the optic nerve. It is located nasally and is around 1.5 mm in diameter, round or vertically oval in shape, and pale pink in color.

  Lamina cribrosa is a sieve-like structure present in the optic nerve head that surrounds and supports the retinal ganglion cell axon as they form the optic nerve head.
- *Physiological cup*: Normal optic disc has a central depression known as optic cup. Physiological cup is in the center of the optic nerve through which blood vessels pass. Normally, cup-disc ratio is around 0.3–0.5 of the optic disc. However, around

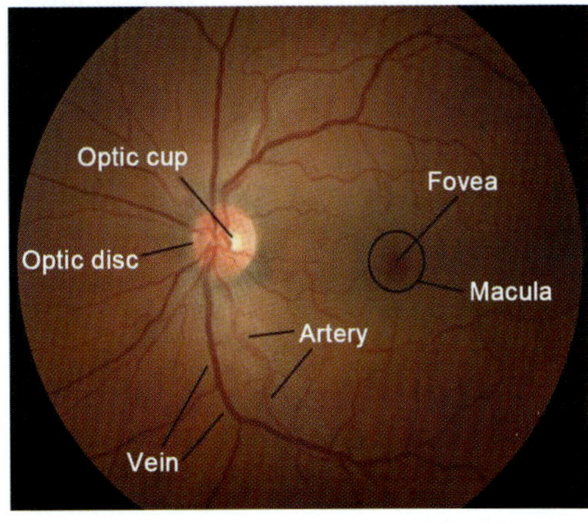


**FIG. 1:** Optic fundus.

15% of cases do not show cup. Generally, nasal border is steeper than temporal border.

This ratio is altered in certain pathological conditions like in glaucoma.

- *Optic papilla*: This is the slightly elevated portion in the periphery of the optic disc.
- *Macula lutea*: This is the oval-shaped pigmented area situated 2 disc diameter (DD) temporal to the optic disc around 3–5 mm in diameter at the center of the retina. The term *lutea* means yellow. The yellowish tinge is due to xanthophyll pigment. This is the most sensitive area of the retina and is rich in cone cells. The center of the macula has a depression known as *fovea*. Macula is responsible for visual acuity, color vision, and central vision.

  *Macula is subdivided into*:
- Umbo
- Foveola
- Fovea
- Parafoveolar region
- Perifoveolar region

  Foveola contains the highest cones with no rods and has the highest visual acuity.
- *Nerve fiber arrangements*:
  - *Papillomacular bundle (PMB)*: From macula through the PMB, nerve fibers directly reach the optic disc.
  - *Superior and inferior nerve fiber layers*: Some fibers are arranged superiorly and inferiorly of PMB to reach the optic disc.
- *Peripheral retina*: This portion is the area outside the macula. There is a high concentration of rods and it provides side vision and night vision.

## BLOOD SUPPLY OF FUNDUS

Two different vascular territories supply the fundus. These are:

1. Ciliary artery
2. Retinal artery

## EXAMINATION OF FUNDUS

Optic fundus can be examined via:

- Direct ophthalmoscopy
- *Indirect ophthalmoscopy*: Here, the fundus is visualized through a handheld condensing lens.
- Indirect slit-lamp biomicroscopy

*What to look for*: In optic fundus examination, we have to look for:

- Optic disc
- Retinal blood vessels
- Periphery of the fundus
- Macula

*Utility of fundus examination*:

- Used to identify any vitreoretinal damage
- Following any intervention to treat vitreoretinal pathology
- Monitor and screening of disease like in case of diabetic retinopathy (DR)

## PATHOLOGICAL FINDINGS IN THE OPTIC FUNDUS

*Some pathological findings in the optic fundus are as follows*:

- *Hemorrhage*: Retinal hemorrhage occurs when blood vessels of the retina rupture. Generally, a microaneurysm present in the retina may rupture and is generally seen most commonly in diabetic patients. Apart from that, it may be found in trauma, due to hypertension or due to a sudden change in air pressure. There are different variants of retinal hemorrhages, such as **(Fig. 2)**:
  - Dot blot hemorrhages
  - Flame hemorrhages
  - Boat hemorrhages

*Exudate*: Hard or soft exudates may be found in hypertension and diabetes. Hard exudates are nothing but leakage from precapillary arterioles. Soft exudates are retinal nerve fiber layer microinfarction. Soft exudates are

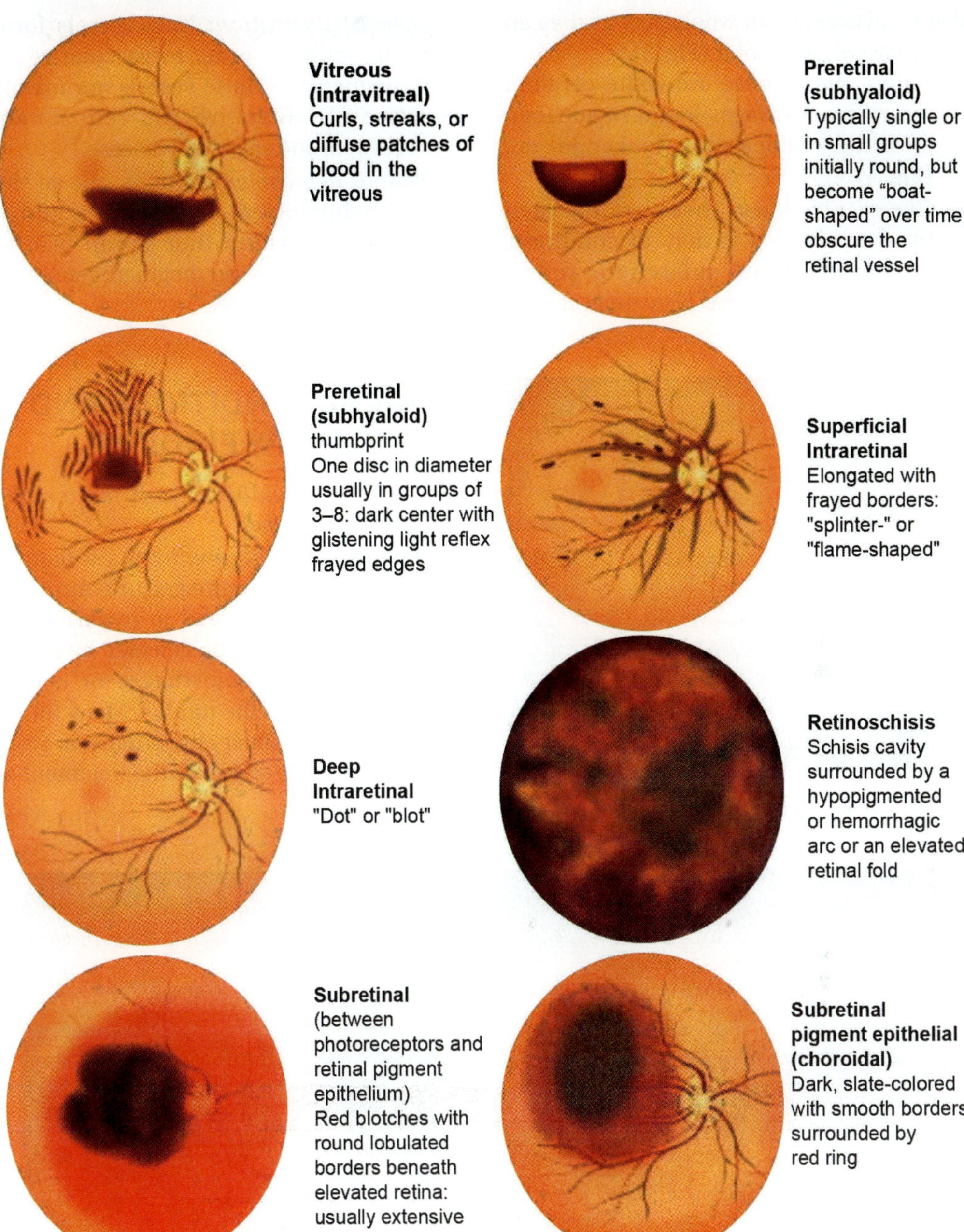


**FIG. 2:** Variants of retinal hemorrhages.

also known as cotton wool spots as they are fluffy gray-white in color **(Fig. 3)**.

- *Roth's spots*: These are white-centered retinal hemorrhages found in subacute bacterial endocarditis, leukemia, etc. **(Fig. 4)**.
- *Cherry red spots*: These are found in the macula in a variety of conditions including retinal infarction, retinal ischemia, and some lysosome-storage disorders **(Fig. 5)**.
- *Neovascularization*: New vessels form in the retina in order to vascularize an ischemic part. These vessels are mainly seen in proliferative DR, retinal vein occlusion, and sickle cell disease.
- *Retinal detachment*: This is one of the ophthalmological emergencies and if not treated within time it can lead to blindness. It may be rhegmatogenous or nonrhegmatogenous.

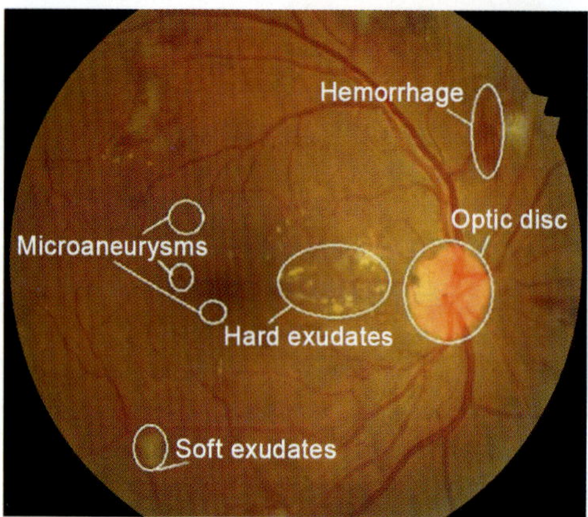


**FIG. 3:** Soft and hard exudate.

## CLINICAL CONDITIONS AND FUNDOSCOPY FINDINGS

*Some clinical conditions and fundoscopy findings are as follows*:

- *Hypertensive retinopathy*: As a feature of target organ damage, uncontrolled hypertension can lead to hypertensive retinopathy. It may be detected by seeing flame-shaped hemorrhages or cotton wool patches in the fundus. Many times, it is due to secondary hypertension. Strict blood pressure control is the treatment of choice.

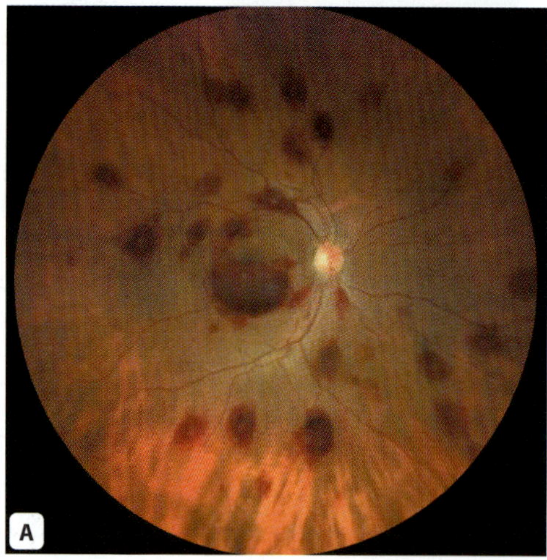

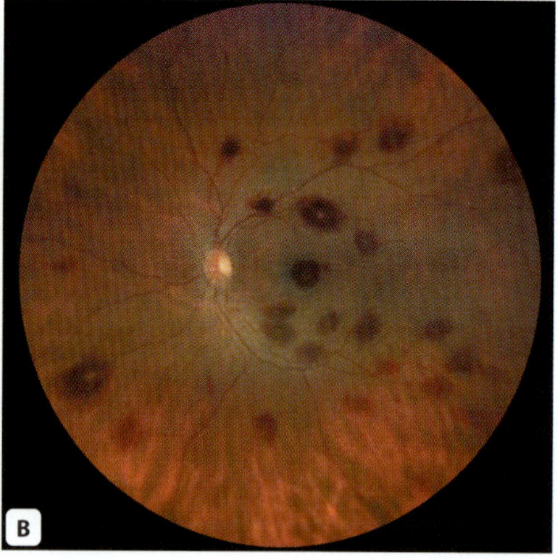


**FIGS. 4A AND B:** Multiple Roth's spot retinal hemorrhages in both eyes. (Left) Large premacular hemorrhage in right eye; (Right) Small premacular hemorrhage in left eye.

*Courtesy*: Andrew G Lee, MD.

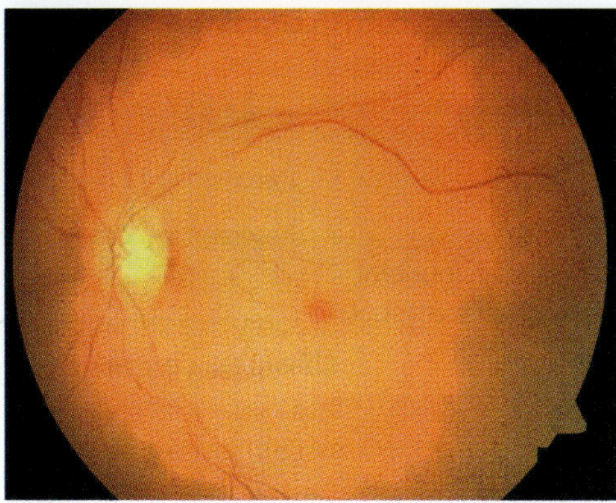

**FIG. 5:** Cherry red spots.

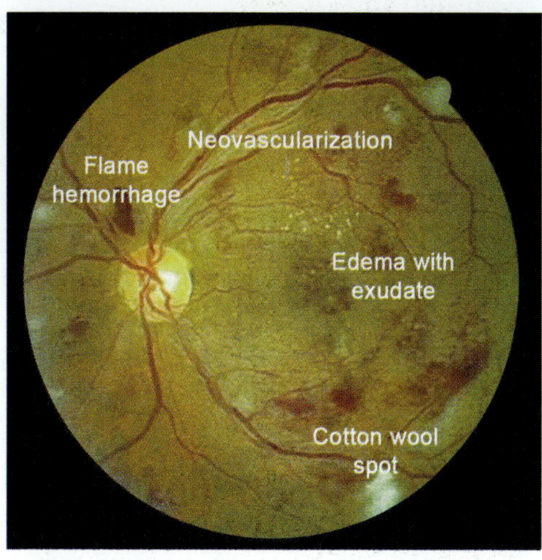


**FIG. 6:** Diabetic retinopathy.

**Table 1: Keith–Wagener–Barker classification.**

| Grade | Description |
|---|---|
| 1 | Slight narrowing, sclerosis, and tortuosity of the retinal arterioles; mild, asymptomatic hypertension |
| 2 | Definite narrowing, focal constriction, sclerosis, and arteriovenous (AV) nicking; blood pressure is higher and sustained; few, if any, symptoms referable to blood pressure |
| 3 | Retinopathy (cotton wool patches, arteriolosclerosis, hemorrhages); blood pressure is higher and more sustained; headaches, vertigo, and nervousness; mild impairment of cardiac, cerebral, and renal function |
| 4 | Neuroretinal edema, including papilledema; Siegrist streaks, Elschnig spots; blood pressure persistently elevated; headaches, asthenia, loss of weight, dyspnea, and visual disturbances; impairment of cardiac, cerebral, and renal function |

*Grading of hypertensive retinopathy*: The grading of hypertensive retinopathy is mentioned in **Table 1**.

- *DR*: It is one of the leading causes of blindness worldwide. As a part of microvascular damage, it can affect retinal vessels and cause microaneurysm. Routine checkup of all diabetic patients is mandatory for the screening of DR. DR **(Fig. 6)** is divided into proliferative and nonproliferative DR according to the presence of neovascularization. Strict glycemic control is the treatment of choice.

*Grading of DR*: The grading of DR is mentioned in **Table 2**.

- *Papilledema*: Meninges continues with the optic nerve sheath. So, any change in intracranial pressure (ICP) can directly affect the optic nerve. In case of raised ICP, it manifests as swollen disc termed papilledema **(Fig. 7)**.
- *Retinal vascular diseases*: These include central retinal artery, branch retinal artery, central retinal vein, branch retinal vein occlusion, and anterior ischemic optic neuropathy. These can lead to sudden and permanent vision loss and so require prompt diagnosis and treatment.
- *Infections*: Some infections, especially viral diseases like human immunodeficiency virus (HIV), cytomegalovirus, congenital rubella syndrome, and toxoplasma infection, can seriously affect the eye.
- *Connective tissue disorders*: Connective tissue disorders such as systemic lupus

**Table 2: Different grades of diabetic retinopathy (DR) in the Scottish Grading Protocol: Features and outcomes.**

| *Grade* | *Features* | *Outcomes* |
|---|---|---|
| R0 | No disease | Rescreen in 12 months |
| R1 | • Mild background DR<br>• Including microaneurysms, flame exudates, more than four blot hemorrhages in one or both hemifields and/or cotton wool spots | Rescreen in 12 months |
| R2 | • Moderate background DR<br>• More than four blot hemorrhages in one hemifield | Rescreen in 6 months |
| R3 | Severe nonproliferative or preproliferative DR: More than four blot hemorrhages in both hemifields, intraretinal microvascular anomalies (IRMA), venous beading | Refer |
| R4 | Proliferative retinopathy<br>NVD, NVE, vitreous hemorrhage, retinal detachment | Refer |
| M0 | No macular findings | 12-month rescreening |
| M1 | Hard exudates within 1–2 disc diameters of fovea | 6-month rescreening |
| M2 | Blot hemorrhage or hard exudates within 1 disc diameter of fovea | Refer |

(DR: diabetic retinopathy; NVD: neovascularization of the disc; NVE: neovascularization elsewhere)

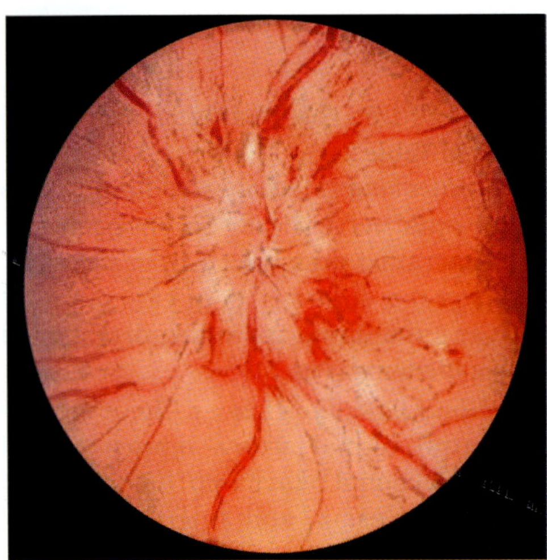

**FIG. 7:** Papilledema.

erythematosus, sarcoidosis, and Behçet's disease can involve the optic fundus along with other portions of the eyes.

- *Optic neuritis*: It is inflammation of your optic nerve. It can cause vision loss and pain when you move your eyes. Signs and symptoms of ON can be the first indication of multiple sclerosis (MS), or they can occur later in the course of MS. Apart from MS, neuromyelitis optica spectrum disorder (NMOSD) can also present with this; thus, it can be a potential clue to diagnose these demyelinating diseases.
- *Neoplasm*: Apart from these, there are certain malignancies that can evade the optic fundus. It may be a primary disease involving the optic fundus like choroidal melanoma or some metastatic deposits in the fundus.
- *Retinal detachment*: Primarily, retinal detachment is divided into rhegmatogenous or nonrhegmatogenous retinal detachment. Here, there is a separation of the sensory retina from the underlying pigment epithelium.
- *Roth's spot*: This is basically white-centered retinal hemorrhage. It can be a manifestation of most diabetes, subacute bacterial endocarditis, or sometimes life-threatening leukemia can present like this.

Apart from this, there are plenty of other conditions that can be diagnosed or sometimes manifestations of other disease conditions that can be identified by observing the optic fundus. Optic nerve is basically a direct extension of the human brain. Not only ophthalmological disease but also systemic conditions as well as some vascular disorders can reflect on the optic fundus. So, basically, by a simple observation of the fundus, a clinician can get a potential diagnostic clue to various disorders. So, it can be regarded as one of the important bedside examinations that can help the clinician to detect as well as to monitor certain disease conditions.

## CLINICAL PEARLS

- *Optic disc evaluation*: The optic disc is the region where the optic nerve enters the eye. It should have a distinct, sharp margin and a physiological cup (depression in the center).

  Cup-to-disc ratio (CDR) is an essential parameter. An increased CDR may indicate glaucoma.
- *Color and vessels*: A pale or atrophic optic disc may suggest optic atrophy, often seen in conditions like multiple sclerosis. Tortuous or abnormal vessels can indicate hypertension, diabetes, or increased intracranial pressure.
- *Optic disc edema*: Optic disc swelling or edema can be a sign of increased intracranial pressure, papilledema. Causes include intracranial mass, idiopathic intracranial hypertension, or severe hypertension.
- *Optic neuritis*: Optic neuritis, inflammation of the optic nerve, can cause disc swelling, pain with eye movement, and vision loss. It's commonly associated with multiple sclerosis.
- *Hypertensive retinopathy*: Hypertension can lead to changes in the optic fundus, like arteriolar narrowing, copper or silver wiring, and flame-shaped hemorrhages.
- *Diabetic retinopathy*: Diabetic patients are at risk for diabetic retinopathy, which can present with microaneurysms, dot-blot hemorrhages, and neovascularization.
- *Macular changes*: The macula, responsible for central vision, can be affected. Conditions like age-related macular degeneration (AMD) can cause drusen deposits and pigment changes.
- *Choroid*: Choroid provides blood supply to the retina. Disorders like choroiditis (inflammation) can present with fundus changes including exudates and hemorrhages.
- *Retinal detachment*: Retinal detachment can present with a characteristic 'shiny' appearance in the fundus, and patients often complain of floaters and flashes of light.
- *Optic fundus imaging*: Technologies like fundus photography and optical coherence tomography (OCT) are invaluable in documenting and monitoring fundus pathology.
- *Systemic disease indicators*: Optic fundus examination can provide insights into various systemic diseases such as hypertension, diabetes, and neurological disorders.
- Remember, accurate interpretation of the optic fundus requires a combination of clinical skills, experience, and sometimes, additional imaging studies. Always refer patients with fundus abnormalities to ophthalmologists for further evaluation and management.

## FURTHER READINGS

1. Brust AA. The eye-grounds in hypertension: a two-part slide [and cassette tape] series. Dallas: American Heart Association, undated.
2. Drews RC. Mirror fixation. Am J Ophthalmol. 1976;82:938-9.
3. Sapira JD. An internist looks at the fundus oculi. DM. 1984;30(14):1-64.
4. Schneiderman H. The Funduscopic Examination. In: Walker HK, Hall WD, Hurst JW (Eds). Clinical Methods: The History, Physical, and Laboratory Examinations. 3rd edition. Boston: Butterworths; 1990. Chapter 117.
5. Youssif AR, Ghalwash AZ, Ghoneim AR. Optic disc detection from normalized digital fundus images by means of a vessels' direction matched filter. IEEE Trans Med Imaging. 2008; 27(1):11-8.

# PART 11

# Otorhinolaryngology

CHAPTER 75

# Throat Pain

*Sudip Das*

## INTRODUCTION

Throat pain refers to any painful sensation localized to the pharynx or surrounding anatomy.

## CAUSES

- *Life-threatening conditions*:
  - Epiglottitis
  - Retropharyngeal abscess
  - Lateral pharyngeal abscess
  - Peritonsillar abscess
  - Infectious mononucleosis
  - Diphtheria
- *Common conditions*:
  - Pharyngitis
  - Tonsillitis
  - Stylalgia
- *Other conditions*:
  - Foreign body
  - Herpetic stomatitis

## APPROACH

### History

- *Age group*:
  - *2–7 years*: Epiglottitis, laryngeal diphtheria
  - *Below 3 years*: Laryngotracheobronchitis
- *Sore throat and respiratory distress*:
  - Epiglottitis
  - Retropharyngeal abscess
  - Parapharyngeal abscess
  - Peritonsillar abscess
  - Massive tonsillar hypertrophy
- *Hot potato voice*: Peritonsillar abscess
- *Fever*: Infective causes
- *Onset*:
  - *Abrupt*:
    - Pharyngitis
    - Epiglottitis
  - *Days/weeks*: Infectious mononucleosis
- *Immunocompromised*: *Candida albicans*

### Physical Examination

- *Stridor/drooling or respiratory distress*: Indicates airway obstruction:
  - Epiglottitis
  - Retropharyngeal abscess
- *Generalized inflammation of oral mucosa in a persistently febrile child*: Kawasaki disease
- *Specific asymmetry of tonsils*: Peritonsillar abscess

# MANAGEMENT

## Epiglottitis

Epiglottis is an acute inflammatory condition confined to supraglottic structures, i.e., epiglottis, aryepiglottic folds, and arytenoids. There is marked edema of these structures which may obstruct the airway.

### *Etiology*

Epiglottis is a serious condition and affects children of 2–7 years of age but can also affect adults. *Haemophilus influenzae* B is the most common organism responsible for this condition in children.

### *Clinical Features*

- Onset of symptoms is abrupt with rapid progression.
- Sore throat and dysphagia are the common presenting symptoms in adults.
- Dyspnea and stridor are the common presenting symptoms in children. They are rapidly progressive and may prove fatal unless relieved.
- Fever may go up to 40°C. It is due to septicemia. The patient's condition may rapidly deteriorate.

### *Examination*

- Depressing the tongue with a tongue depressor may show red and swollen epiglottis. Indirect laryngoscopy may show edema and congestion of the supraglottic structures. This examination is avoided in fear of precipitating complete obstruction.
- Lateral X-ray soft-tissue neck—Thumb sign **(Fig. 1)**

### *Treatment*

- Hospitalization
- Antibiotics
- Steroids
- Adequate hydration
- Humidification and oxygen

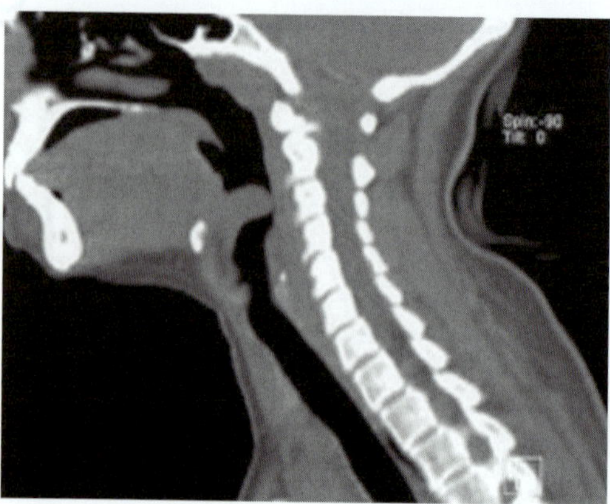

**FIG. 1:** X-ray soft tissue neck lateral view—thumb sign.

## RETROPHARYNGEAL ABSCESS

### *Acute*

#### Etiology

Retropharyngeal abscess is commonly seen in children below 3 years of age. It is the result of suppuration retropharyngeal lymph nodes secondary to infection in the adenoids, nasopharynx, posterior nasal sinuses, or nasal cavity.

In adults, it may result from penetrating injury of posterior pharyngeal wall or cervical esophagus.

#### Clinical Features

- Dysphagia and difficulty in breathing are prominent symptoms as the abscess obstructs the air and food passages.
- Stridor and croupy cough may be present.
- Torticollis
- Bulge in the posterior pharyngeal wall

X-ray soft-tissue neck—widening of prevertebral shadow and presence of gas **(Fig. 2)**

#### Treatment

- Incision and drainage
- Antibiotics
- Tracheostomy

### *Chronic*

#### Etiology

Chronic retropharyngeal abscess is tubercular in nature and is the result of (1) caries of cervical spine or (2) tubercular infection of retropharyngeal lymph nodes secondary to tuberculosis of deep cervical nodes.

#### Clinical Features

The patient may complain of discomfort in the throat. Dysphagia, though present, is not marked. The posterior pharyngeal wall shows a fluctuant swelling centrally or on one side of the midline.

#### Treatment

- Incision and drainage
- Full course of antitubercular therapy

## Lateral Pharyngeal Abscess

### *Etiology*

- Pharynx—acute and chronic infection of tonsils and adenoids, bursting of peritonsillar abscess
- Teeth—dental infection
- Ear—Bezold abscess
- Other spaces—infection of parotid, retropharyngeal, and submaxillary spaces
- External trauma—penetrating injuries of the neck, injection of local anesthetics for tonsillectomy, mandibular nerve block

### *Clinical Features*

- Prolapse of tonsil and tonsillar fossa
- Trismus
- External swelling behind the angle of jaw

### *Diagnosis*

Computed tomography (CT) scan

### *Treatment*

- Systemic antibiotics
- Drainage of abscess

## Peritonsillar Abscess

Peritonsillar abscess is a collection of pus in peritonsillar space **(Fig. 3)**.

### *Clinical Features*

*General*

- Fever
- Chills
- Rigor
- Malaise
- Body ache
- Headaches

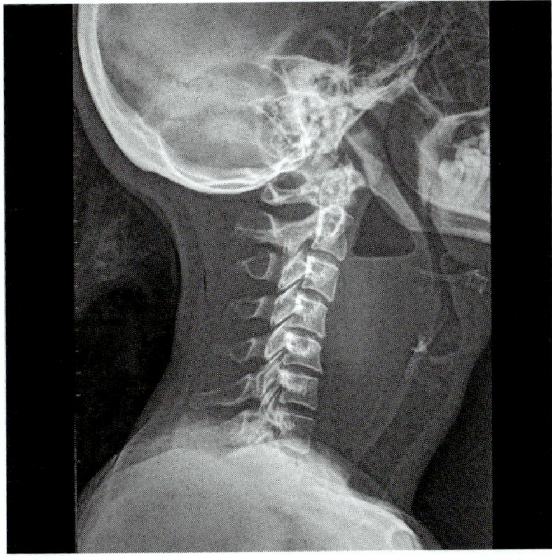

**FIG. 2:** Widening of prevertebral 'soft tissue' shadow.

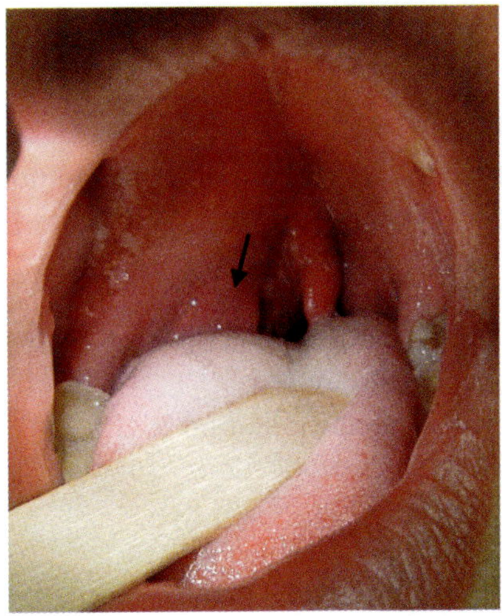

**FIG. 3:** Peritonsillar abscess.

*Local*:
- Severe pain in the throat
- Odynophagia
- Hot potato voice
- Foul breath
- Ipsilateral earache
- Trismus

### Examination

- The tonsil, pillars, and soft palate on the involved side are congested and swollen.
- Uvula is swollen, edematous, and pushed to the opposite side.
- Bulging of the soft palate and anterior pillar
- Cervical lymphadenopathy
- Torticollis

### Diagnosis

Computed tomography scan or magnetic resonance imaging (MRI) can be used for diagnosis.

### Treatment

- Intravenous (IV) fluids
- Antibiotics
- Analgesics
- Oral hygiene
- Incision and drainage

## Pharyngitis

Pharyngitis is an inflammatory condition of the pharynx **(Fig. 4)**.

### Etiology

- Persistent infection in the neighborhood
- Chronic irritants
- Environmental pollution
- Faulty voice production

### Symptoms

- Discomfort or pain in the throat
- Foreign body sensation in the throat
- Tiredness of voice
- Cough

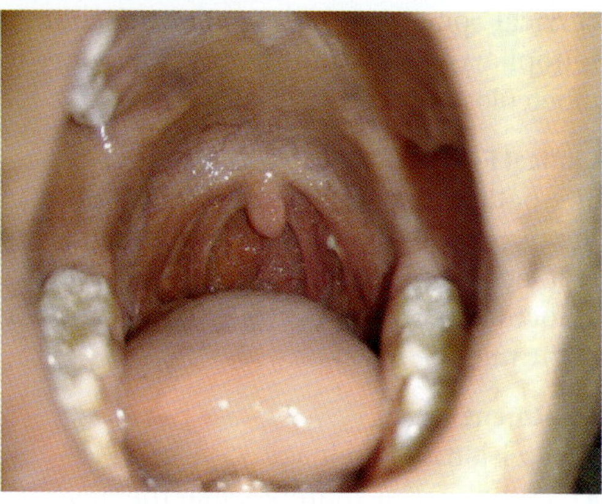

**FIG. 4:** Pharyngitis.

### Signs

- Congestion of posterior pharyngeal wall
- Lateral pharyngeal bands hypertrophied
- Pharyngeal wall appears thick and edematous with congested mucosa and dilated vessels.

### Diagnosis

Throat swab

### Treatment

- General measures
- Antibiotics
- Warm saline gargles

## Tonsillitis (Fig. 5)

Causative organism—Hemolytic streptococci, staphylococci, pneumococci, *H. influenzae*

### Symptoms

- Sore throat
- Difficulty in swallowing
- Fever
- Earache

### Signs

- Fetid breath and coated tongue
- Enlarged jugulodigastric nodes

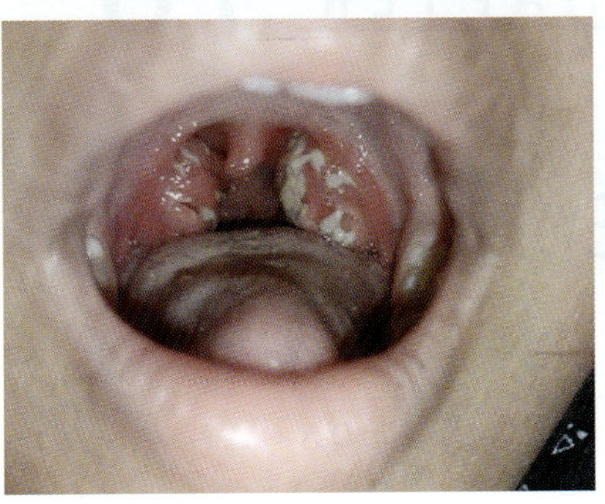

**FIG. 5:** Tonsillitis.

### *Treatment*

- Analgesics
- Antibiotics
- Gargle

## Stylalgia (Fig. 6)

### *Diagnosis*

Reverse Towne's view

### *Treatment*

- Styloid process excision
- Analgesics

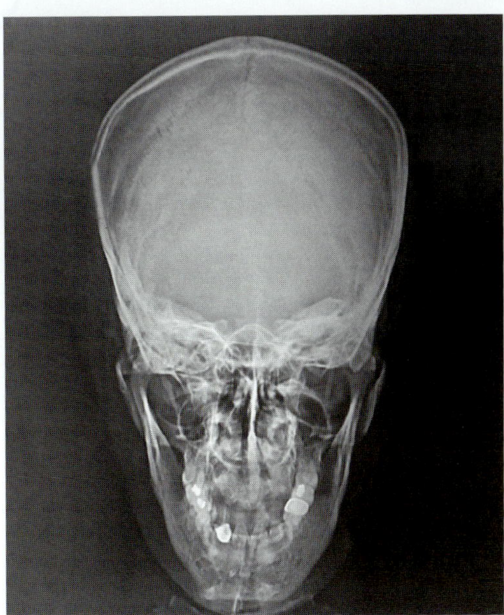

**FIG. 6:** Enlarge styloid process.

## CLINICAL PEARLS

Mild to moderate throat pain may be due to trivial cause but if it is severe and gradually increasing or persistent, it should be properly dealt with preferably by specialist.

## FURTHER READINGS

1. Watkinson J, Clarke R. Scott-Brown's Otorhinolaryngology and Head and Neck Surgery: Volume 2: Paediatrics, The Ear, and Skull Base Surgery (8th ed.). CRC Press; 2018. https://doi.org/10.1201/9780203731017.
2. Corbridge R, Steventon N. Oxford Handbook of ENT and Head and Neck Surgery, 3 edn, Oxford Medical Handbooks (Oxford, 2019; online edn, Oxford Academic, 1 Nov 2019), https://doi.org/10.1093/med/9780198725312.001.0001, accessed 19 Jan 2024.

# CHAPTER 76

# Epistaxis

*Sudip Das*

## INTRODUCTION

Epistaxis is defined as acute hemorrhage from the nostril, nasal cavity, or nasopharynx. It is a very common condition that can present as a life-threatening emergency. Epistaxis can be unilateral or bilateral. The site of bleeding varies with a number of factors including age, sex, anatomical and pathological abnormalities, occupation, climate, etc.

## HISTORICAL BACKGROUND

Nose bleed as a clinical entity was known since ancient times. Hippocrates is believed to be the first to stop nasal bleeding via packing.

Carl Michel (1871), James Little (1879), and Wilhelm Kiesselbach were the first to identify the nasal septum's anterior plexus as an important source of nasal bleeding.

Pliz was the first to surgically treat epistaxis with ligation of the common carotid artery (1869).

Seiffert ligated the internal maxillary artery via the maxillary sinus in 1928. Henry Goodyear performed the first anterior ethmoid artery ligation in the treatment of epistaxis.

## VASCULAR ANATOMY OF THE NASAL CAVITY

A rich vascular supply lies under this thin mucosal covering. Nasal erectile tissue results in a large number of venous sinuses, arteriovenous (AV) anastomoses, and venules. Multiple arterial vessels fed by the high-pressure carotid system course through the nose. The respiratory mucosa with its underlying vascular supply serves the regulate heat exchange and humidification during respiration.

The nasal cavity is basically supplied from two main sources **(Fig. 1)**:

1. *Branches of external carotid artery*:
    a. Sphenopalatine artery
    b. Greater palatine artery
    c. Superior labial branch
2. *Branches of internal carotid artery*:
    a. Anterior ethmoidal artery
    b. Posterior ethmoidal artery

These arteries intercommunicate in a rich plexus. These are two areas that are often implicated in nose bleeds—Kiesselbach's plexus (giving rise to anterior bleeds) and Woodruff's plexus (giving rise to posterior bleeds).

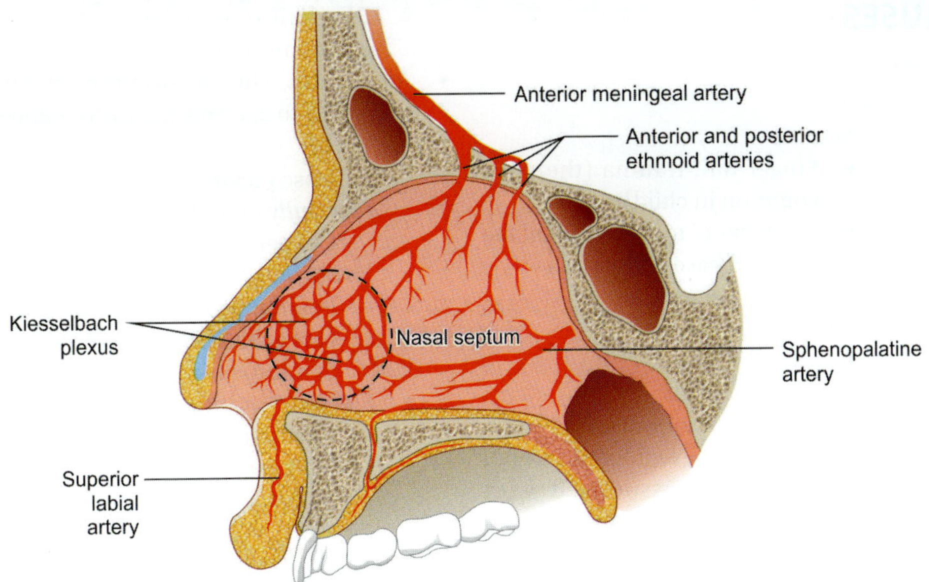


**FIG. 1:** Blood supply of nasal septum and nasal cavity.

The Kiesselbach's plexus is situated in the Little's area in the anteroinferior part of the septum. The plexus is contributed by four arteries of the nasal septum, namely:

1. Sphenopalatine artery
2. Greater palatine artery
3. Superior labial branch of the facial artery
4. Anterior ethmoidal artery

This plexus is the most common site of bleeding.

Woodruff's plexus is located over the area posterior to the middle turbinate and is made of anastomosis between branches of the internal maxillary artery, namely the posterior nasal, sphenopalatine, and ascending pharyngeal.

## CLASSIFICATION

1. *According to the site of bleeding*:
   - *Anterior epistaxis*: Bleeding from a vessel anterior to the plane of pyriform aperture (this includes bleeding from anterior septum, vestibular skin or mucocutaneous junction).
   - *Posterior epistaxis*: Bleeding from a vessel posterior to the plane of pyriform aperture (this includes bleeding from septum or lateral wall)
2. *According to the age*:
   - *Child*: Below 16 years of age
   - *Adult*: Above 16 years of age
3. *According to the cause*:
   - *Primary*: Idiopathic/Spontaneous
   - *Secondary*: Trauma, surgery or overdose of anticoagulant.

## SITES

- *Little's area*: The most common site for epistaxis in children and young adults
- *Above the level of middle turbinate*: Anterior and posterior ethmoidal arteries
- *Below the level of middle turbinate*: Branch of sphenopalatine artery
- *Post part of nasal cavity*: Woodruff's plexus (the most common site in elderly)
- *Just behind the columella*: Retrocolumellar vein

## CAUSES

- *Local*
  - *Nose*
    - Trauma
      - Finger nail trauma (the most common in child)
      - Fractures of middle third of the face and base of the skull
      - Violent sneezes
    - Infections
      - Viral rhinitis
      - Acute sinusitis
      - Granulomatous diseases
    - Foreign body: Neglected foreign body (usually associated with unilateral foul-smelling discharge)
    - Neoplasms of nose and paranasal sinuses (PNS)
      - *Benign*: Hemangioma, papilloma
      - *Malignant*: Carcinoma (commonly), sarcoma (rare)
    - Atmospheric changes
      - High altitude
      - Sudden decompression
    - Deviated nasal septum with spur
  - *Nasopharynx*
    - Juvenile angiofibroma
    - Malignant tumor
- *General*
  - *Cardiovascular system (CVS) diseases*
    - Hypertension
    - Arteriosclerosis
  - *Disorders of blood and blood vessels*
    - Aplastic anemia
    - Leukemia
    - Hemophilia (commonly in young males)
  - *Liver diseases*: Cirrhosis
  - *Kidney diseases*: Chronic nephritis
  - *Drugs*
    - Salicylates
    - Analgesics
    - Anticoagulant therapy
  - Vicarious menstruation
  - Acute general infection
  - *Bleeding dyscrasias*: Male consanguineous marriages
- *Idiopathic*: The most common causes according to age and sex are as follows—
  - *In kids*
    - Nose picking
  - *Especially in male babies*
    - Congenital bleeding disorders
  - *Young adult male*
    - Possibility of juvenile nasopharyngeal angiofibroma (JNA) to be kept in mind.
  - *Elderly*
    - Hypertension
    - Malignancy
    - Anticoagulant

## EVALUATION OF EPISTAXIS

In acute active epistaxis, priority is given to controlling the bleeding before doing the investigations to find out the cause. Hypovolemia and blood loss should be promptly dealt with. Vital signs should be regularly monitored and concentration is given on the following:

- Volume status
- Blood pressure
- Adequacy of airway
- Oral and nasal examination

Detailed medical and treatment history is taken as the patient is being managed and the bleeding is controlled.

### Anterior Rhinoscopy

Anterior rhinoscopy is the mainstay of evaluation. With a good light source using a head mirror or head light, the nasal cavity is inspected using a nasal speculum. Special attention should be paid to the plexus areas as these are areas that often bleed. In case of active bleeding, a suction cannula may be used to determine the site of bleeding. Sometimes, a cotton applicator may be used to find the bleeding point.

## Posterior Rhinoscopy

Posterior rhinoscopy is often difficult but is helpful in recurrent mild epistaxis or blood-stained nasal discharge following neoplasia, rhinosporidiosis in the nasopharynx, or fungal sinusitis.

It is almost replaced by nasal endoscopy.

## Nasal Endoscopy (Fig. 2)

Nasal endoscopy is a very useful tool in identifying and treating the bleeding point, especially in difficult cases where the bleeding vessel is located far posteriorly.

## Radiological Evaluation

- X-ray PNS helps in ruling out infective, traumatic, and neoplastic conditions (almost obsolete).

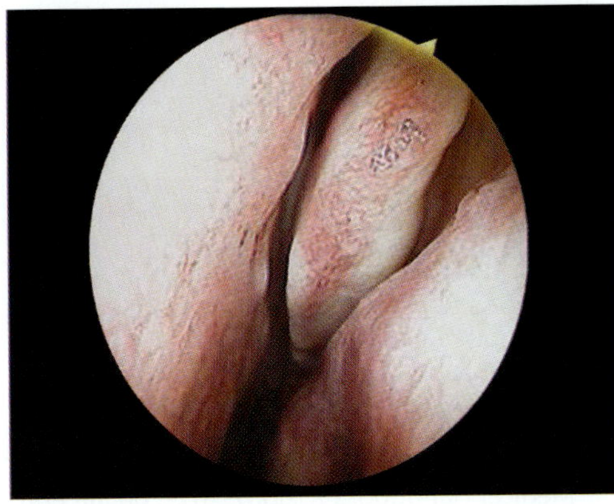

**FIG. 2:** Nasal endoscopy.

- Computed tomography (CT) scan (1 mm cuts; plain and contrast) is more useful in such cases.
- Digital subtraction angiography is more useful in the identification of bleeding vessels in profuse recurrent epistaxis. Embolization of the bleeder may be done selectively (done by interventional radiology—in limited sophisticated centers only).

## Hematological Investigations

Complete blood picture includes the following:

- *Clotting and bleeding profiles*: Bleeding time (BT), clotting time (CT), prothrombin time (PT) international normalized ratio (INR), activated partial thromboplastin time (APTT)
- Blood grouping and cross-matching
- Blood counts including total platelet count

# MANAGEMENT

The management of epistaxis is shown in **Flowchart 1**.

# CLINICAL PEARLS

Epistaxis is one of the most common ENT emergency. Initial management is to stop the bleeding; for final management cause has to be ascertained by ENT specialist.

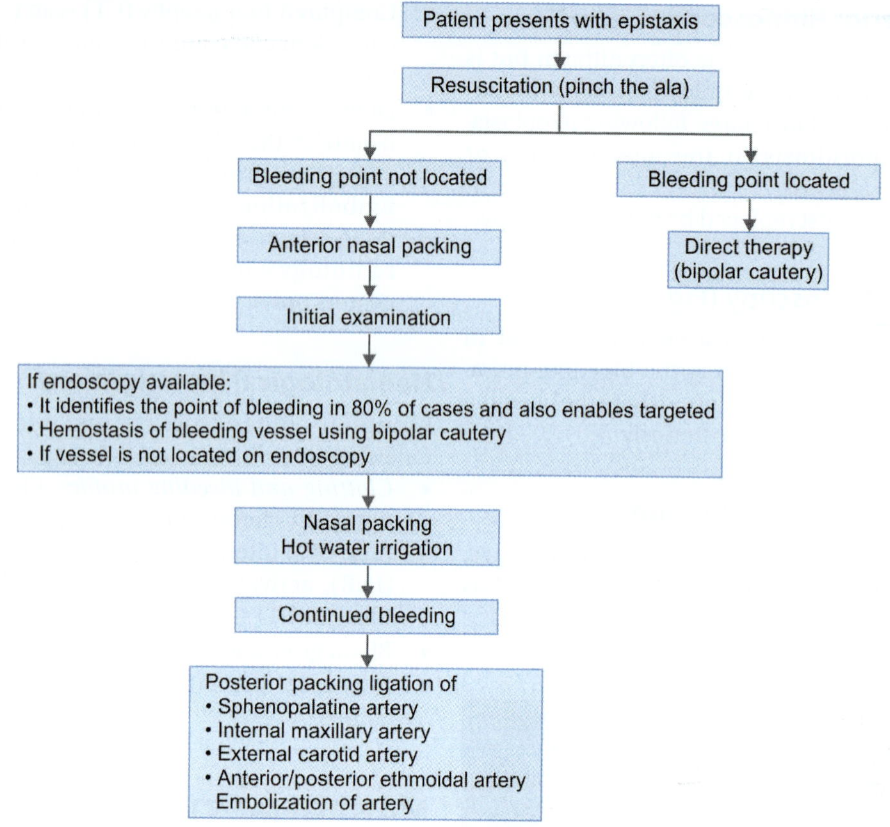


**FLOWCHART 1:** Management of epistaxis.

# FURTHER READINGS

1. Watkinson JC, Clarke RW. Scott-Brown's Otorhinolaryngology and Head and Neck Surgery, Eighth Edition. CRC Press; 2018.
2. Corbridge R, Steventon N. Oxford Handbook of ENT and Head and Neck Surgery, 3 edn, Oxford Medical Handbooks (Oxford, 2019; online edn, Oxford Academic, 1 Nov 2019).

CHAPTER 77

# Otalgia

*Sudip Das, Gautam Raghu*

## INTRODUCTION

Otalgia refers to pain in the ear and is one of the most common causes of visit to a physician. Although causes are multiple, they can be broadly divided into intrinsic and extrinsic causes depending on the etiology. The various causes have been summarized as follows:

- *Intrinsic causes of otalgia*:
  - Otitis externa
  - Acute otitis media
  - Perichondritis
  - Chronic suppurative otitis media (less common; pain may indicate complication)
- *Extrinsic causes of otalgia (referred pain)*:
  - Tongue ulcers/dental ulcers/aphthous ulcers
  - Dental caries/dental infections/unerupted wisdom teeth
  - Malocclusion of teeth
  - Tonsils (acute tonsillitis/tonsillar malignancy)
  - Arthritis of temporomandibular joint
  - Throat ulcers/laryngeal tumors
  - Cervical spondylosis (less common)

## TREATMENT

The treatment for some of the causes have been given in the following text.

### Otitis Externa

Otitis externa can be due to bacterial, viral, or fungal etiology.

#### *Bacterial*

*Furunculosis*: Painful reddish inflammation in the external auditory canal **(Fig. 1)**.

*Treatment*: Oral antibiotic (amoxycillin, cloxacillin), analgesics, and topical antibiotics.

It may require aural packing.

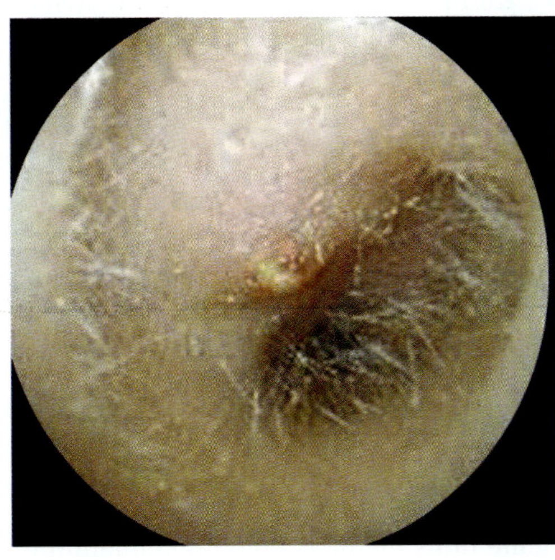

**FIG. 1:** Furunculosis in the external auditory canal.

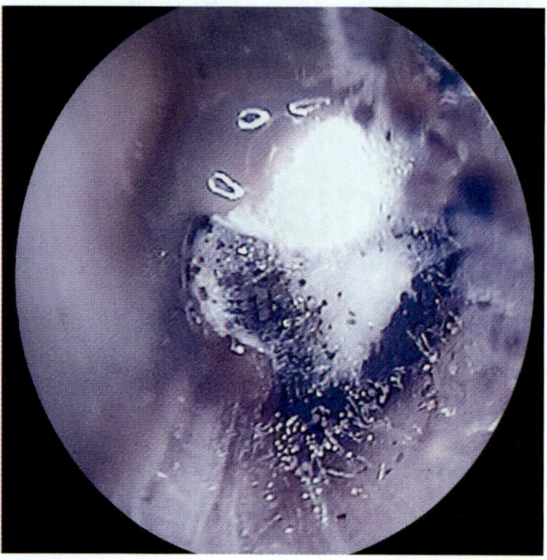

**FIG. 2:** Otomycosis with wet tissue paper discharge and black spots representing fungal mycelium.

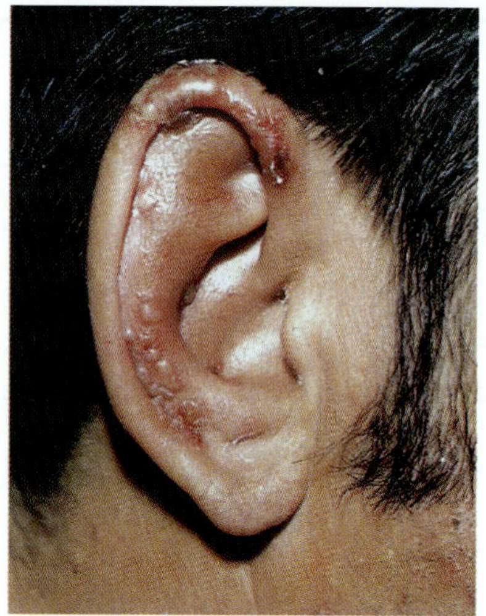

**FIG. 3:** Herpes zoster oticus with vesicles in the right pinna.

### *Fungal*

*Otomycosis*: Wet tissue paper-like whitish discharge from the ears. Increased incidence is seen during moist conditions **(Fig. 2)**.

*Treatment*: Topical antifungal and antibiotic ear drops. Aural mopping will be required after completion of treatment.

### *Viral*

- *Herpes zoster oticus* **(Fig. 3)**: Vesicular eruption on pinna and external auditory canal.
- Herpes Zoster Oticus associated with lower motor neuron facial palsy is also called *Ramsay Hunt syndrome.*

*Treatment*: Oral acyclovir 800 mg × 5 times/day for 7–10 days.

If a patient develops facial palsy, a course of oral steroids with facial muscle exercises and measures for eye protection may be required.

## Acute Otitis Media

Acute otitis media is cute inflammation of middle ear by pyogenic organisms **(Fig. 4)**.

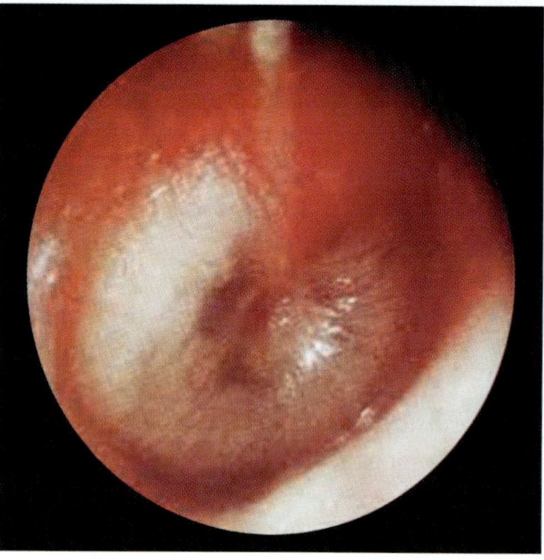

**FIG. 4:** Acute otitis media showing congested inflamed tympanic membrane.

It mainly occurs in children.

It is so common that before school-going age, almost 90% children have suffered from it.

It is usually preceded by upper respiratory tract infection (URTI).

It may be associated with ear discharge and impaired hearing.

*Treatment*: Oral antibiotic (third-generation cephalosporins/amoxycillin) and analgesics along with antibiotic ear drops and antihistaminics in case of ear discharge.

## Perichondritis

Perichondritis is infection of the cartilage and perichondrium of the pinna **(Fig. 5)**.

It is common after trauma, ear piercing, and in poorly controlled diabetics.

Oral antibiotics with good cartilage penetration, analgesics, and warm compress help in treatment. Control of blood sugar levels is important. If there is development of abscess, incision and drainage may be required in addition to above treatment. The patient also has to be counseled about the possibility of pinna deformity in severe cases.

## Chronic Suppurative Otitis Media

Chronic suppurative otitis media is long-standing infection of a part or whole of the middle ear cleft.

It is usually painless.

If otalgia is present, urgently refer to an ENT specialist to rule out complications of chronic suppurative otitis media (CSOM) **(Fig. 6)**.

## Tongue Ulcers/Dental Ulcers/ Aphthous Ulcer

Pain is referred via 5th cranial nerve.

Treatment includes oral antibiotic, topical analgesic gel, and oral hygiene. It may need consultation with the dental surgeon for dental ulcers.

Long-standing ulcers not responding to treatment may require further investigation to rule out malignancy.

## Dental Caries/Dental Infections/ Unerupted Wisdom Teeth

Pain is referred via 5th cranial nerve.

*Treatment*: Oral antibiotics and analgesics, oral hygiene, mouthwash, and referral to a dental specialist for further treatment.

## Tonsils (Acute Tonsillitis/Tonsillar Malignancy)

Pain is referred via 9th cranial nerve.

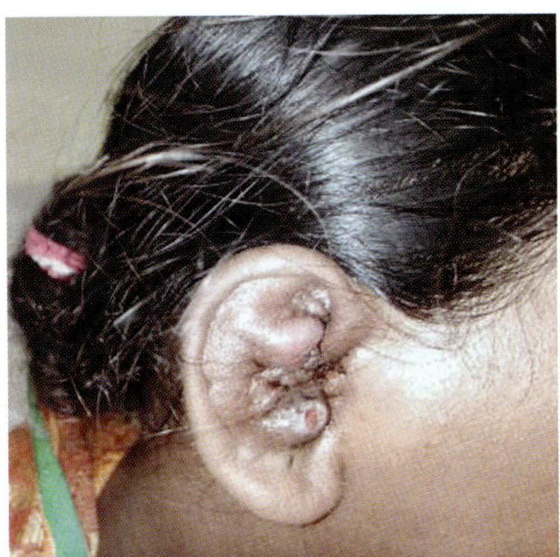

**FIG. 5:** Perichondritis of the right pinna.

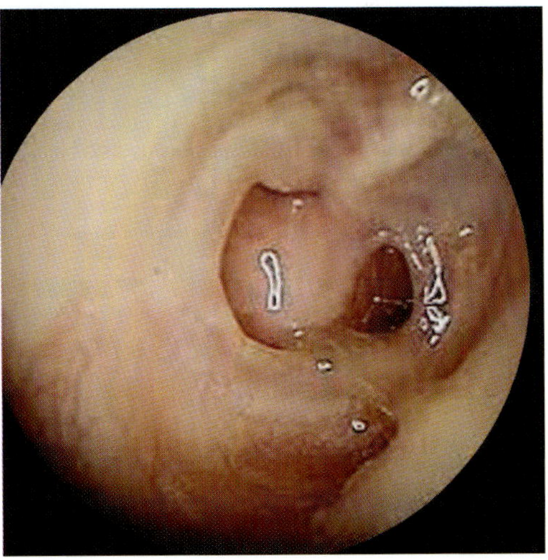

**FIG. 6:** Chronic suppurative otitis media showing large perforation in the tympanic membrane with mucoid discharge.

*Treatment*: For acute tonsillitis, treatment mainly includes oral antibiotics with analgesics.

Recurrent attacks of tonsillitis may require tonsillectomy.

Suspected tonsillar malignancies (indurated/unilateral tonsillar enlargement) require biopsy to determine the nature of malignancy followed by treatment as per biopsy report.

### Arthritis of Temporomandibular Joint/Malocclusion of Teeth/Bruxism

Pain is referred via 5th nerve.

Pain usually occurs during chewing, usually in the elderly.

*It is frequently overlooked.*

*Treatment*: Soft diet, hot compress for 3 weeks along with analgesics, muscle relaxants in case of muscle spasms.

Persistent symptoms need consultation with a dental surgeon for management of malocclusion.

### Throat Ulcers/Laryngeal Tumors

Pain is referred via 10th cranial nerve.

Treatment of suspected laryngeal tumors involves laryngoscopy followed by biopsy for suspicious lesions and radiotherapy or surgery depending on biopsy report and stage of tumor.

### Cervical Spondylosis or Injuries to Cervical Spine

It is less common.

Pain is referred via C2/C3 nerve fibers.

Treatment may require analgesics, cervical collar/immobilization, muscle relaxants, and physiotherapy.

Cervical spine injuries require immediate consultation with the neurosurgeon and orthopedic surgeon for further management.

## CLINICAL PEARLS

- Other than local pathology, otalgia may be caused due to pain referred via cranial nerves V, IX, X or C2, C3 nerve fibres.
- In all cases of otalgia, rule out other causes of referred pain such as tonsillitis, cervical spondylosis, etc.
- Arthritis of the TM joint is often overlooked as a cause of otalgia.
- CSOM presenting with pain should alert the clinician to the possibility of developing complications.

## FURTHER READING

1. Scott-Brown's Otorhinolaryngology and Head and Neck Surgery, Eighth Edition. CRC Press; 2018.

CHAPTER 78

# Ear Discharge

*Dipankar Datta*

## WHAT IS OTORRHEA?

### Definition

Otorrhea is the drainage that comes out of the ear. Sometimes, people refer to otorrhea as "runny ears" or "watery ears."

Most commonly, otorrhea is the result of a ruptured tympanic membrane from a middle ear infection (otitis media). When there is a hole in the tympanic membrane, the fluid in the middle ear drains out in the ear canal. But other conditions can cause otorrhea too, including external otitis (swimmer's ear), retained unknown foreign body, or less commonly, head injury.[1]

## WHAT CAUSES DISCHARGING EAR?

### Pathogenesis

Discharging ear is most common in children, but it affects adults too. A discharging ear is also the presentation of middle ear infection after grommet (ventilation tube) insertion. It occurs in up to 17% of cases.

There are five different types of ear discharge:

1. Purulent (contains pus)
2. Serous (contains serum)
3. Sanguineous (contains blood)
4. Mucoid (contains mucous)
5. Clear (thin and watery)

In the case of external otitis, in the preinflammatory stage, the ear is exposed to heat, humidity, maceration, the absence of cerumen, and an alkaline pH. Loss of acidity has been shown to be proportionate to the degree of infection. This can cause edema of the stratum corneum and occlusion of the apopilosebaceous units. In the inflammatory stage, bacterial overgrowth ensues, with progressive edema and intensified pain and otorrhea.

In the case of otomycosis, patients with diabetes and immunocompromised state are particularly susceptible. Patients with a mastoid bowl after a canal wall-down mastoidectomy are susceptible to otomycosis.

In the case of malignant otitis externa, the disease disseminates through the Haversian canals and vascularized spaces of the skull base. This progresses to cellulitis, chondritis, osteitis, osteomyelitis, and cranial neuropathy. The most frequently isolated causative organism is *Pseudomonas aeruginosa.*

Acute otitis media is thought to be caused by a combination of Eustachian tube anatomy, Eustachian tube malfunction, immune status, and infective organisms.

The pathogenesis of chronic suppurative otitis media is poorly understood. It seems probable that recurrent bacterial ingress into the middle ear in early childhood triggers inflammation, which in some (genetically) predisposed individuals leads to nonresolving mucosal inflammation, resulting in tissue dysfunction and damage. Mucosal dysfunction can disrupt gaseous exchange and lower middle ear pressure, and if combined with lysis and weakening of the fibrous layer of the tympanic membrane from chronic inflammation, it can lead to tympanic membrane retraction and perforation, although this may also occur secondary to acute otitis media, trauma, or nonhealing after grommet extrusion.

Cholesteatoma can be defined as "the presence of squamous epithelium in the middle ear cleft," as a result of active proliferation and medial growth of the epithelium. Cholesteatoma is more likely to occur within a retraction pocket. The clinical behavior of cholesteatoma can vary over time. It may grow insidiously at first and can attain a significant size without causing any symptoms other than hearing loss. Bone erosion is responsible for the invasive nature of cholesteatoma. The anatomic patterns of the growth of cholesteatoma are determined by the mucosal partitions of the middle ear and attic.

# WHAT ARE THE POSSIBILITIES?

## Differential Diagnosis

The common causes of otorrhea include:

- Ruptured tympanic membrane
- Middle ear infections (acute and chronic suppurative otitis media)
- External ear infections (external otitis), such as swimmer's ear or fungal yeast infections of the ear canal (otomycosis)
- Retained unknown foreign body

Less common causes of otorrhea include:

- An abnormal skin growth behind the tympanic membrane (cholesteatoma)
- Fracture of the skull base at the middle cranial fossa level [cerebrospinal fluid (CSF) otorrhea]
- Cancer of the ear canal
- Malignant external otitis (a severe necrotizing infection of the external auditory canal)

# PATH TO DIAGNOSIS

## History

The history of the patient with discharging ear should include the following:

- Duration of symptoms
- Presence of earache
- Presence of fever
- History of trauma to the upper body, especially above the shoulders
- History of swimming
- Habit of using earbuds
- Itching in the ear
- Upper respiratory symptoms compatible with viral infection
- Redness (erythema) of the skin around the ear
- History of recent air flight travel
- History of recent diving
- Hearing loss
- Tinnitus
- Vertigo
- Cranial nerve dysfunction
- If the patient looks toxic, the presence or absence of mental status changes as well as other systemic signs

## Clinical Examination

The physical examination should include:

- Checking vitals and ruling out fever
- Inspection of the external auditory canal to check for drainage, infection, and nature of the drainage
- Inspection of the tympanic membrane
- Inspection of the skin around the ear for any redness and inflammation
- Palpation of the mastoid bone
- Palpation around the ear, jaw, and neck
- Insufflation of air in the canal to document adequate movement of the tympanic membrane

- A neurological examination is appropriate in toxic patients and in those patients complaining of headache or with a history of trauma.

### Investigations

In the majority of cases, a physical examination is all that is necessary to diagnose a case of discharging ear. But some investigations are often recommended to confirm the diagnosis, including:

- *Audiometry*: To measure the range and sensitivity of hearing
- *Computed tomography (CT) scan*: To assess the extent of the disease and spread beyond the ear (if any)
- *Magnetic resonance imaging (MRI)*: Recommended in case of head trauma and suspected CSF otorrhea
- Test of cranial nerves
- *Culture*: Microbiological assessment of drainage

## THERAPY

Otorrhea treatment focuses on the cause of ear drainage. For example, if otorrhea is the result of a bacterial infection of the external or middle ear, the treatment is either by topical or systemic antibiotics. Occasionally, it needs local dressing also.

If there is perforation in the tympanic membrane, it may heal within 6 weeks with conservative medical management. But few patients need surgical reconstruction of the tympanic membrane (tympanoplasty).

In the case of chronically discharging ear and cholesteatoma, surgical exploration is mandatory. There are different types of mastoidectomies depending upon the extent of disease removal.

In the case of CSF otorrhea and/or head injury, collaboration with a neurosurgeon is recommended.

## RED FLAG SIGNS

### Poor Prognostic Indicators

- Severe pain and/or cellulitis
- Suspected intracranial sepsis
- Sudden onset or rapidly progressive hearing loss
- Facial palsy
- Vertigo and dizziness
- Suspicion of acute mastoiditis
- Bleeding from ear
- Evidence of congenital or traumatic deformity of the ear

## CLINICAL PEARLS

Discharging ear can be caused by many different things as mentioned earlier. Most of the time, it is the result of ear infection and ruptured tympanic membrane. It usually goes away in a few days with treatment. But in some instances, discharging ear means a serious health issue. So, it is best to consult an ENT doctor at the first sign of trouble.

## FURTHER READINGS

1. Senturia BH, Marcus MD, Lucente FE. Disease of the external ear. 2nd edition. New York: Grune & Stratton; 1980.
2. Sade J, Fuchs C. Secretory Otitis Media in adults: II. The role of mastoid pneumatization as a prognostic factor. Ann Otol Rhinol Laryngol. 1997;106:37-40.
3. Sundstrom J, Jacobson K, Munck-Wikland E, Ringertz S. *Pseudomonas aeruginosa* in otitis externa: A particular variety of the bacteria? Arch Otolaryngol Head Neck Surg. 1996;122(8):833-6.
4. Bojrab DI, Bruderly T, Abdulrazzak Y. Otitis Externa. Otolaryngol Clin North Am. 1996;29(5):761-82.

5. Lindeman P, Holmquist J. Mastoid volume and Eustachian tube function in ears with cholesteatoma. Otol Neurotol. 1987;8(1):5-7.
6. Sanna M, Russo A, Donato G. Colour atlas of otoscopy: from diagnosis to surgery. New York: Theime; 2002.
7. Wormald PJ, Browning GG, Robinson K. Is otoscopy reliable? A structured teaching method to improve otoscopic accuracy in trainees. Clin Otolaryngol. 1995;20:63-7
8. Doyle PJ, Anderson DW, Sipke P. The tuning fork: An essential instrument in otologic practice. *J* Otolaryngol. 1984;13:83-6.
9. Carhart R, Jerger J. Preferred methods of clinical determination of pure tone thresholds. J Speech Hear Disord. 1959;24: 330-45.
10. Watkinson JC, Clarke RW. Scott-Brown's Otorhinolaryngology Head & Neck Surgery, 8th edition. London: CRC Press; 2019.

CHAPTER 79

# Deafness

*Dipankar Datta*

## WHAT IS DEAFNESS?

Disabling hearing loss refers to hearing loss >40 dB in the better ear in adults (15 years or older) and >30 dB in the better hearing ear in children (0–14 years).

Deafness is a very common worldwide problem affecting all age groups and leading to marked disability and handicap. The World Health Organization (WHO) lists deafness in the 20 leading causes of burden of disease and as the most common cause of disability globally.

In 2012, the WHO estimated that there are 360 million people worldwide with a disabling hearing loss, which is 5.3% of the world's population. Of these, 91% are adults and 9% are children. The prevalence of disabling hearing loss is greatest in South Asia, Asia Pacific, and sub-Saharan Africa.

## WHAT CAUSES DEAFNESS?

The ear is divided anatomically into three parts: External, middle, and inner. Any abnormality in the normal anatomy and physiology of hearing can result in deafness. The human ear has a huge dynamic range and is able to hear frequencies of 2–20 kHz and intensities up to 120 dB.

The pinna reflects sound from various directions into the external auditory canal. The acoustic signal then travels down the canal, where it undergoes a resonance boost between 2.5 and 3.5 kHz in adults. Any abnormality in the pinna or external auditory canal, namely microtia, wax, and exostosis, can result in deafness.

The middle ear acts as an efficient transformer to conduct acoustic energy from the low-impedance, high-velocity tympanic membrane to the high-impedance, low-velocity fluid-filled cochlea. The impedance difference is mainly matched by the ratio of the surface area of the tympanic membrane to the stapes footplate. A much smaller part is played by the lever action of the ossicles. Aside from the air conduction, the cochlea can also be directly stimulated by the vibration of the bony skull. Any abnormality in the tympanic membrane, middle ear, or ossicles can result in deafness, namely perforation or retraction in the tympanic membrane, secretory otitis media, suppurative otitis media, ossicular fixation, or discontinuity.

Once sound is delivered into the cochlea through the stapes–oval window interface, a cochlear traveling wave is generated that traverses the basilar membrane. High-frequency sounds are best represented at the basal end and low frequencies at the apex. The movement of the basilar membrane creates relative motion between the tectorial membrane and the stereocilia of the inner hair cells. This allows ion channels to open and depolarize the cell, resulting in synaptic release of glutamate and firing of afferent nerve fibers. Afferent nerve fibers on outer hair cells form a feedback loop with efferent fibers, which results in a change in the shape of the outer hair cells and active modification of basilar membrane motion. This results in signal amplification at low-intensity levels, improving hearing sensitivity, and also improves spectral resolution. The outer hair cells are responsible for otoacoustic emissions (OAE) and the cochlear microphonic (CM) potential. Information on timing, frequency, and intensity of sound is encoded by the rate, number, location, and timing of auditory nerves firing. For sound localization, encoding of interaural time differences and interaural level differences in the auditory pathway is important. Any abnormality in the cochlea, auditory nerve, or higher auditory pathway can lead to deafness, namely presbyacusis, noise-induced hearing loss, infective sensorineural hearing loss, cerebellopontine angle tumors, etc.

## WHAT ARE THE POSSIBILITIES?

- *Conductive hearing loss*:
    - *External ear*:
        - Cerumen
        - Foreign body in the canal
        - External otitis
        - Exostoses and osteoma
        - Cysts and tumors of the canal
    - *Middle ear*:
        - Tympanic membrane perforation due to chronic or acute suppurative otitis media
        - Traumatic tympanic membrane perforation due to blunt trauma, water accidents, barotrauma, explosions, penetrating injuries, or temporal bone fractures
        - Glue ear or otitis media with effusion
        - Cholesteatoma
        - Myringosclerosis or tympanosclerosis
        - Otosclerosis
        - Osteogenesis imperfecta
        - Ossicular chain discontinuity
        - Glomus tumors
- *Sensorineural hearing loss*:
    - *Degenerative*: Age-related hearing loss
    - *Genetic*:
        - Syndromic
        - Nonsyndromic
    - *Ototoxic drugs*:
        - Aminoglycosides
        - Loop diuretic
        - Antimalarials
        - Antitumors such as platins
        - Industrial chemicals
    - *Infectious*:
        - Meningococcal meningitis
        - Encephalitis
        - Herpes virus
        - Cytomegalovirus
        - Measles
        - Rubella
        - Syphilis
        - Lyme disease
    - *Traumatic*:
        - Barotrauma
        - Perilymph fistula
        - Intense noise exposure
        - Temporal bone fracture
        - Blast injury
        - Ear surgery
    - *Neoplastic*: Cerebellopontine angle tumors
    - *Autoimmune*:
        - Rheumatoid arthritis
        - Lupus erythematosus
        - Sarcoidosis
    - *Neurologic*:
        - Multiple sclerosis
        - Migraine
    - *Miscellaneous*:
        - Idiopathic

- Ménière's disease
- Microvascular disease
- *Mixed hearing loss*: Concomitant conductive and sensorineural deafness

# PATH TO DIAGNOSIS

## History

A thorough history and careful physical examination are essential to the diagnosis and treatment of deafness.

Pertinent questions to ask patients are as follows:

- What is the duration of your hearing loss?
- Was your hearing loss sudden, or has your hearing slowly been getting worse?
- Does your hearing loss involve one or both ears?
- Any associated history of ear discharge, earache, ringing in the ear, fullness in the ear, or dizziness?
- Is there a history of early hearing loss in your family?
- What is your job and what is the noise level at your workplace?
- Do you have a history of ear infection, ear injury, or straining to hear?
- Do you have any history of diabetes, ischemic heart disease, or stroke?
- What medicines are you taking currently?
- Have you received any intravenous antibiotics, diuretics, salicylates, or chemotherapy?

## Clinical Examination

The physical examination begins with inspection and palpation of the auricle and periauricular tissue. An otoscope should be used to examine the external auditory canal and tympanic membrane. A pneumatic bulb is required to assess the ventilation status of the middle ear.

The next most important assessment is hearing by the tuning fork test and the whisper test. The most commonly used forks are the 256 Hz and 512 Hz forks, as these give more reliable responses than the 1,024 Hz fork. Weber's test is performed by softly striking a 512-Hz tuning fork. If the deafness is conductive, the sound will be heard best in the affected ear. If the loss is sensorineural, the sound will be heard best in the normal ear. The sound remains midline in patients with normal hearing.

The Rinne test compares air conduction with bone conduction. In the presence of normal hearing or sensorineural deafness, air conduction is better than bone conduction. In conductive deafness, bone conduction is better than air conduction.

Free-field speech testing is used as a screening tool to determine whether pure-tone audiometry is required. A number-letter combination is chosen, as this has a reasonable mix of consonants that allows a relatively broad range of frequencies to be tested. When standing behind at an arm's length, if the subject cannot repeat >50% of the words spoken in a whispered voice, they will have a hearing impairment of at least 25 dB hearing loss in that ear.

## Investigations

- *Pure tone audiometry*: Pure tones are used to measure hearing levels as they are easily characterized in terms of frequency and sound level.
- *Speech audiometry*: To understand the impact of hearing loss on communication, speech audiometry is done. Speech discrimination score gives a measure of speech discrimination and the cochlear reserve in a mixed hearing loss.
- *Tympanometry*: It is used to assess middle ear function. Parameters of the middle ear, such as compliance, pressure, and ear canal volume, are measured.
- *OAE*: Low-level sounds that reflect the active mechanism of the outer hair cells in the cochlea can be recorded in the canal. OAEs are typically absent or abnormal in cochlear hearing losses.

A key application of OAE is the diagnosis of auditory neuropathy and newborn hearing screening program.

- *Auditory evoked potentials (AEP)*: This gives important diagnostic information about the integrity of the peripheral and central auditory systems.
- *CM*: It indicates outer hair cell function. It is often measured in children as part of the auditory neuropathy test battery.
- *Electrocochleography (ECOG)*: It is a technique for assessing cochlear and auditory nerve function. A high summating potential (SP): Auditory nerve action potential (AP) ratio is associated with Ménière's disease.
- *Brainstem evoked response audiometry (BERA)*: It generates waves from different loci of the nerve tract, starting from the distal portion of the auditory nerve up to the lateral lemniscus and inferior colliculus. The great advantage of BERA is that a robust response can be measured even during sleep or general anesthesia. This test is very useful to rule out retrocochlear loss and in the diagnosis of auditory neuropathy.
- *Magnetic resonance imaging (MRI)*: It is done to rule out cerebellopontine angle, posterior fossa, and brainstem lesions, particularly in a case of asymmetric unilateral hearing loss.

# THERAPY

Treatment of deafness is, just like any other clinical condition, targeted toward the diagnosis and etiology, supplemented with symptomatic support.

Conductive deafness is managed either medically or surgically, depending upon the clinical condition. Most of the deafness arising out of pathologies in the external ear is managed conservatively, namely simple removal of wax or medical management of external otitis. If there is foreign body or any space-occupying lesion (SOL), it needs intervention and removal. Deafness arising out of pathologies in the middle ear is predominantly managed by micro-ear surgeries, except in secretory otitis media, where medical management is the first-line treatment.

Sensorineural deafness is tricky to manage. The main aim is to identify any treatable cause and the provision for supportive treatment and rehabilitation. The duration and speed of onset of symptoms, laterality, and other accompanying onto-logical symptoms should be assessed. Guidance should be given to patients to optimize their acoustic environment. Management includes the provision of hearing aids/auditory implants, auditory rehabilitation, and psychological support.

Sudden sensorineural hearing loss (SSNHL) is a treatable medical emergency and is extremely rewarding to treat, particularly if diagnosed and managed early. SSNHL is defined as hearing loss of rapid onset of ≥30 dB over greater than three consecutive frequencies developing over ≤72 hours with a subjective sensation of hearing impairment. The majority of cases are idiopathic, with a cause identified in only 5–10% of cases. The possible causes of "idiopathic" cases include labyrinthine viral infection, vascular insult, intracochlear membrane rupture, and autoimmune inner ear disease. Steroids are the mainstay of treatment of SSNHL. There is minimal benefit if started after 4–6 weeks. Antivirals, neurovitamins, and hyperbaric oxygen therapy have some role to play in the treatment of SSNHL.

# RED FLAG SIGNS

## Poor Prognostic Indicators

- Family history of permanent sensorineural hearing loss during childhood
- In utero infection (toxoplasmosis, rubella, herpes, cytomegalovirus)
- Illness requiring admission to the neonatal intensive care unit for at least 48 hours

- Syndromic babies
- Parental or caregiver concern about hearing, speech, language, or developmental delay
- Head injury
- Postnatal infection associated with sensorineural hearing loss (meningitis)
- Neonatal hyperbilirubinemia requiring exchange transfusion
- Neurodegenerative disorders
- Sudden onset
- Unilateral loss
- Associated facial palsy or altered sensations
- Associated otorrhea and/or otalgia

## CLINICAL PEARLS

- Universal neonatal hearing screening and "*catch them young*" policy are to be adapted so that prelingual deaf babies can be spared from being handicapped and brought back to the mainstream.
- Early presentation for sudden sensorineural hearing loss
- Noise pollution is to be avoided at any cost.
- Suppurative otitis media, particularly with complications, should be surgically treated as an emergency to avoid potential fatalities.

## FURTHER READINGS

1. World Health Organization. Deafness and Hearing Loss. Fact sheet 300. Updated February 2017. Available from: http://www.who.int/mediacentre/factsheets/fs300/en/
2. World Health Organization. The global burden of disease. 2004 update. Available from http://www.who.int/healthinfo/global_burden_disease/GBD_report_2004update_full.pdf
3. World Health Organization. WHO global estimates on prevalence of hearing loss: Mortality and burden of diseases and prevention of blindness and deafness. 2012. Available from www.who.int/pbd/deafness/WHO_GE_HL.pdf
4. Maria PLS, Oghalai JS. Anatomy and Physiology of the Auditory System. Sataloff's Comprehensive Textbook of Otolaryngology Head & Neck Surgery. Jaypee Brothers Medical Publishers. 2016.
5. Pacala JT, Yueh B. Hearing deficits in the older patients: "I didn't notice anything". (Review) JAMA. 2012;307(11):1185-94.
6. Wormald PJ, Browning GG. Otoscopy: a structural approach. London: Hodder Arnold; 1996.
7. Swan IRC, Browning GG. The whispered voice as a screening test for hearing loss. J R Coll Gen Pract. 1985;35:197.
8. Doyle PJ, Anderson DW, Sipke P. The tuning fork: An essential instrument in otologic practice. J Otolaryngol. 1984;13:83-6.
9. Browning GG. Clinical assessment of hearing: free-field voice testing and tuning forks. Open access guide to audiology and hearing airs for otolaryngologists. Available from: https://www.scribd.com/document/352826251/Clinical-assessment-of-hearing-with-free-field-voice-testing-and-tuning-forks-pdf
10. Stachler RJ, Chandrasekhar SS, Archer SM, Rosenfeld RM, Schwartz SR, Barrs DM. Clinical practice guideline: sudden hearing loss. Otolaryngol Head Neck Surg. 2012;146 (3 Suppl):S1-35.

# CHAPTER 80

# Tinnitus

*Dipankar Datta*

## WHAT IS TINNITUS?

The word tinnitus originates from the Latin word *tinnire* (to ring), and Dennis McFadden's classical description of the term is worth appropriate at the outset, which states that tinnitus is "the conscious expression of a sound that originates in an involuntary manner in the head of its owner, or may appear to him to do so."

The definition by McFadden, as described above, includes hallucinations of mental illness and excludes tinnitus that is perceived outside the body. Other attempts at a definition have included the sensation of hearing a sound in the absence of an external stimulus or a sound sensation in the absence of an external or internal acoustical source or electric stimulation.

A completely unambiguous definition has yet to be published.

Tinnitus can be divided into subjective or objective tinnitus. In subjective tinnitus, only the patient is aware of the sound sensation. In objective tinnitus, the sound can be perceived by others.

## WHAT CAUSES TINNITUS? (PATHOGENESIS)

The pathophysiology of subjective tinnitus is one of the most controversial aspects of medical science. Subjective tinnitus, often described as hallucination of sound, implies a subject's feeling or perception of sound in the absence of any physical sound. In objective tinnitus, there is a physical sound (usually of vascular origin) generated by biological activities in the subject's body.

Tinnitus can be divided into nonpulsatile and pulsatile tinnitus. Pulsatile tinnitus is considered to be either synchronous or nonsynchronous, depending on whether the sound is in synchrony with the patient's arterial pulse.

The most prevalent presentation of tinnitus in the general population is that of subjective nonpulsatile tinnitus. Although the link between high-frequency hearing loss and tinnitus might be considered evidence for a cochlear origin of tinnitus, most modern research emphasizes the importance of central auditory pathways in both the development and the maintenance of distressing tinnitus. That deafness or lesions in the peripheral auditory systems do not have any definitive relationship with tinnitus is borne out by the fact that tinnitus is not present in many deaf patients, irrespective of the type and severity of the deafness, and that tinnitus is not absent in many patients who have perfectly normal hearing. These observations have been drawn together in a concept that makes a distinction between the location, within either the peripheral or the central auditory system, at which an initial tinnitus signal is generated, and the subsequent central auditory mechanism by which this signal is misconstrued as a sound with the potential to become a clinical problem.

The point at which the initial signal generation occurs has been dubbed the *ignition site* and the ensuing central mechanisms have been entitled *promotion*.

Pathological events that create an ignition site do not inevitably generate tinnitus—the central promotion must also be there.

The following are some of the pathophysiological mechanisms that have been suggested as giving rise to tinnitus, but this list is far from exhaustive, and many other hypotheses have been proposed.

### Peripheral Mechanisms

- Discordant damage of cochlear hair cells
- Calcium channel dysfunction
- Accentuation of glutamate receptors

### Central Mechanisms

- Increased spontaneous firing
- Increased central neural synchrony
- Reorganization of the cortical auditory map

## WHAT ARE THE POSSIBILITIES? (DIFFERENTIAL DIAGNOSIS)

- *Nonpulsatile tinnitus*:
  - Subjective
  - Objective:
    - Spontaneous otoacoustic emission
    - Patulous Eustachian tube
- *Pulsatile synchronous tinnitus*:
  - Atherosclerotic carotid artery disease
  - Arteriovenous (AV) fistula
  - AV malformation
  - Intracranial aneurysm
  - Fibromuscular dysplasia of the carotid artery
  - Dissection of the carotid artery
  - Vascular anomaly of the ear
  - Vascular compression of the 8th nerve
  - Jugular bulb abnormality
  - Dural venous sinus stenosis
  - Glomus tumor
  - Cholesterol granuloma of the middle ear
  - Paget's disease and otosclerosis
  - Cavernous hemangioma
  - Increased cardiac output due to anemia, thyrotoxicosis, and pregnancy
  - Cochlear trauma
  - Benign intracranial hypertension
  - Superior semicircular canal dehiscence syndrome
- *Pulsatile nonsynchronous tinnitus*:
  - Middle ear myoclonus
  - Palatal myoclonus
- *Allied conditions*:
  - Musical hallucination
  - Acoustic shock
  - Low-frequency noise complaint
  - Exploding head syndrome
  - Typewriter tinnitus
  - Temporomandibular joint disorder

## PATH TO DIAGNOSIS

### History

History taking should include leading questions such as the presence or absence of hearing loss, hyperacusis, and ear blockage; whether there is any concomitant vertigo/instability and whether these are related to tinnitus; and lastly whether there are any associated cardiovascular/cerebrovascular/metabolic disorders. Tubotympanic dysfunction and diseases of the middle ear, such as otosclerosis, are treatable conditions that should be elicited during tinnitus history taking. A history of systemic diseases is very important because cardiovascular disorders, especially fluctuating hypertension; metabolic disorders such as hyperlipidemia, diabetes, thyroid disorders; and neuropsychiatric disorders are quite often associated with tinnitus. During history taking, it is also important to document the mental and psychological status of the patient and annoyance level as well.

### Clinical Examination

A number of medical disorders, in addition to otologic disorders, are known to cause or aggravate subjective tinnitus. These disorders are different kinds of metabolic disorders, neurological disorders, cardiovascular disorders, dental disorders, and psychological disorders. Hence, a general medical workup and requisite history taking with special reference to these disorders are very relevant. A drug history is important, as some drugs such as aspirin, quinine, some antibiotics, and some antidepressants are known to cause tinnitus with or without deafness. Depression is a comorbid condition, and many tinnitus patients suffer from mental depression. Treating the depression often relieves the tinnitus.

A routine ear, nose, and throat (ENT) examination with special emphasis on the ear, which should include auscultation of the neck, the ears, and adjacent areas of the head, is sometimes very informative. Auscultation helps to rule out any objective tinnitus also.

### Investigations

Investigations for tinnitus start with the basic audiological assessment consisting of pure tone audiometry, impedance audiometry, speech audiometry, brainstem evoked response audiometry (BERA), and tests for central auditory speech processing (particularly necessary if the pure tone audiometry test is normal). Vestibulometric evaluation is also a very important part in the diagnostic workup of tinnitus. Radiologic imaging, namely computed tomography (CT), magnetic resonance imaging (MRI), positron emission tomography (PET), and angiography, is appropriate when there are signs and/or symptoms that raise suspicions of a specific abnormality, such as unilateral tinnitus, pulsatile tinnitus, asymmetric hearing loss, vertigo, or cranial neuropathy.

## THERAPY

To date, a whole host of medicinal, device, and psychological treatments for tinnitus have been proposed. The evidence base to support these treatments is poor, mainly due to a paucity of well-designed randomized controlled trials (RCTs). For conditions such as tinnitus, where many treatments may work via a placebo effect and there being a general natural improvement in symptoms with time, it is difficult to consider any method other than double-blinded RCT as fit for the purpose.

Explanation and reassurance are key initial steps in the management of any patient with tinnitus.

As there is an association between tinnitus and hearing loss, it would make sense to provide hearing aids which would, in part, ameliorate a patient's symptoms. Currently, hearing aid is considered to be the primary intervention for a patient with tinnitus, even if patients feel that amplification is not yet required for the hearing loss.

Sound therapy can be used as part of tinnitus retraining therapy (TRT) or as a standalone treatment. According to a publication, it is possible to use sound to completely or partially suppress or mask tinnitus in 95% of tinnitus patients in a clinical setting.

Ultrasound has also been used to treat tinnitus.

Tinnitus retraining therapy combines directive counseling and sound therapy to counteract the pathological positive feedback process and promote habituation to the tinnitus.

Cognitive behavioral therapy (CBT) results in no significant difference in tinnitus loudness, but it results in a significant improvement in both depression and quality of life scores.

Modern psychological treatment modalities, namely mindfulness meditation and acceptance and commitment therapy (ACT).

Complementary and alternative modalities, namely acupuncture, homeopathy, ginkgo biloba, meditation, tai chi, and yoga.

Electromagnetic stimulation of the ear has been shown to suppress tinnitus in select few patients.

Systemic pharmacotherapy includes psychoactive drugs, antiepileptic and antispasmodic drugs, betahistine, local anesthetic agents, melatonin, hyperbaric oxygen, glutamate antagonists such as caroverine, botulinum toxin, and intratympanic drug treatments.

A large number of vitamins, minerals, and other dietary supplements have been given to tinnitus patients in an effort to alleviate the condition.

Surgery has a definite role in the management of tinnitus associated with certain conditions, such as otosclerosis. Destructive surgical procedures, including 8th nerve neurectomy or selective cochlear neurectomy, have been tried, but results are not validated. Surgery can play an important role in the management of pulsatile tinnitus.

## RED FLAG SIGNS (POOR PROGNOSTIC INDICATORS)

- Sudden tinnitus
- Pulsatile tinnitus
- Tinnitus associated with asymmetric hearing loss
- Tinnitus associated with significant neurological features
- Tinnitus associated with severe vertigo
- Tinnitus with psychological distress
- Tinnitus developed after head injury

## CLINICAL PEARLS

All patients with tinnitus should undergo a basic audiological assessment, and when it is associated with hearing loss, it is recommended to correct this hearing loss, surgically if appropriate, or via the use of hearing aids.

Tinnitus with red flag signs should be urgently investigated and treated.

Although there is currently no established drug treatment for subjective idiopathic tinnitus, drugs may have a role in the management of comorbid conditions such as anxiety and depression.

Negativity should be avoided at any cost, and patients should be offered helpful management strategies, particularly hearing therapy and mental health services.

## FURTHER READINGS

1. McFadden D. Tinnitus: Facts, Theories and Treatments. Washington, DC: National Academy Press; 1982.
2. Holgers KM, Hakansson BE. Sound stimulation via bone conduction for tinnitus relief: a pilot study. Int J Audiol. 2002;41:293-300.
3. Baguley DM. Mechanisms of tinnitus. Br Med Bull. 2002;63:195-212.
4. Eggermont JJ, Roberts LE. The neuroscience of tinnitus. Trends Neurosci. 2004;27:676-82.
5. Salvi RJ, Lockwood AH, Burkard R. Neural plasticity and tinnitus. In: Tyler RS (Ed). Tinnitus Handbook. San Diego: Singular; 2000. pp. 123-48.
6. Baguley DM. What progress have we made with tinnitus? The Tonndorf Lecture 2005. Acta Otolaryngol Suppl. 2006;126:4-8.
7. Duckert LG, Rees TS. Placebo effect in tinnitus management. Otolaryngol Head Neck Surg. 1984;92:697-9.
8. Vernon JA, Meikle MB. Masking devices and alprazolam treatment for tinnitus. Otolaryngol Clin North Am. 2003;36:307-20.
9. Jastreboff PJ, Hazell JWP. A neurophysiological approach to tinnitus: clinical implications. Br J Audiol. 1993;27:7-17.
10. Martinez-Devesa P, Perera R, Theodoulou M, Waddell A. Cognitive behavioural therapy for tinnitus. Cochrane Database Syst Rev. 2010;(9):CD005233.
11. Kreuzer PM, Goetz M, Holl M, Schecklmann M, Landgrebe M, Staudinger S, et al. Mindfulness and body-psychotherapy based group

treatment of chronic tinnitus: a randomized controlled pilot study. BMC Complement Altern Med. 2012;12:235.
12. Westin VZ, Schulin M, Hesser H, Karlsson M, Noe RZ, Olofsson U, et al. Acceptance and commitment therapy versus tinnitus retraining therapy in the treatment of tinnitus: a randomised controlled trial. Behav Res Ther. 2011;49:737-47.
13. Sismanis A, Butts FM, Hughes GB. Objective tinnitus in benign intracranial hypertension: an update. Laryngoscope. 1990;100:33-6.

# PART 12

# Psychiatry

# CHAPTER 81

# Anxiety Disorders

*Ranjan Bhattacharyya*

## HOW WILL YOU DEFINE ANXIETY DISORDERS?

Anxiety is defined as a subjective feeling of uneasiness, dreadfulness, or foreboding, which has an uncomfortable feeling of intense fear and apprehension presenting with physiological, cognitive, and behavioral symptoms. Anxiety disorders usually develop before the age of 30 years, are more common in women, and present as a heterogeneous group of illnesses.

*Prevalence of anxiety disorders*: The high prevalence and functional impairment associated with anxiety disorders have led to high economic cost and social burden.

## WHAT ARE THE NEUROBIOLOGICAL UNDERPINNINGS OF ANXIETY DISORDERS?

The molecular and neuropsychiatric abnormalities that lead to anxiety symptoms have been extensively researched, in both animal and human models.

- *Gamma-aminobutyric acid (GABA) system*: GABA is an inhibitory neurotransmitter. The potential involvement of this system is justified by the following neuroimaging and radioreceptor binding findings. For example:
  - In generalized anxiety disorder (GAD), decreased numbers of GABA-benzodiazepine (BZD) receptors are found in temporal lobe.
  - In post-traumatic stress disorder (PTSD), cortical BZD receptors have been found to be reduced.
  - In panic disorders, decreased GABA-A binding is noted.
- *Serotonergic system*: Abnormal regulation of serotonin release, or reuptake, or abnormal responsiveness to 5-HT signals has been found in anxiety disorders.
- *Amygdala (the center for emotions)*: It plays a role in detecting, coordinating, and maintaining fearful emotions. It integrates information from various sensory inputs, scans, and perceives a threat, and a rapid response is being coordinated.
- *Noradrenergic system*: Locus coeruleus in brainstem serves as alarm center and releases norepinephrine, which leads to overwhelming adrenergic symptoms (noradrenergic theory of anxiety disorders). The drugs yohimbine (alpha-2 adrenergic antagonist), isoproterenol, caffeine, and carbon dioxide inhalation can induce anxiety symptoms.

## HOW DO YOU CLASSIFY ANXIETY DISORDERS?

Anxiety disorders can be classified as per the Diagnostic and Statistical Manual (DSM) and International Classification of Diseases (ICD) classificatory systems:

- Panic disorder without agoraphobia
- Panic disorder with agoraphobia
- Agoraphobia without a history of panic disorder
- Specific phobia
- Social phobia
- Acute stress disorder
- PTSD
- Anxiety disorder not otherwise specified (NOS)
- Obsessive-compulsive disorder (OCD)

The last disorder OCD has now been separated from the anxiety group of disorders as per the latest DSM-V classification and has been given due weightage to be classified as obsessive-compulsive related disorder (OCRD).

## WHAT ARE THE ETIOLOGICAL FACTORS ATTRIBUTED FOR ANXIETY DISORDERS?

The following factors are attributed for causation of anxiety disorders as mentioned below:

- *Genetic factor (heritability 30–67%)*: The following genes have been implicated for anxiety disorders: *5HT1A, 5HTT, CCK-B, MAO-A, NPSR1, COMT, RGS2/7, ADORA2A, CHR1, FKBP5.*
- *Environmental factors (eco-anxiety)*: Cognitive, affective, physiological, psychological, behavioral, life stressor, and social factors are attributed for development of anxiety. Genetic and epigenetic factors come into play for development of anxiety disorders. Anxiety symptoms are the body's natural response to stress.

*Generalized anxiety disorders*: These disorders develop when excessive worries come in our day-to-day life, which is difficult to control. It is diagnosed when an individual experiences overwhelming anxiety and worry for at least 6 months. Three or more of the following symptoms should be present during this period, such as feeling restless or tensed, easily getting fatigued, irritability, difficulty in concentrating, and disturbances in sleep.

*Panic disorder*: It includes recurrent, unprovoked panic attacks (a period of sudden, intense fear which reaches peak in a very short period of time) and apprehension of having an attack. Each attack is a distinct episode of intense discomfort or fear associated with physical symptoms which usually peak in 10 minutes and does not last after 30 minutes. There should be unexpected panic attacks followed by a 1-month period of having persistent concerns of future attacks.

*Agoraphobia*: It is a fear of open or crowded places.

*Specific phobia*: Disproportionate and overwhelming on a specific object stimulus or situation, when there is no real danger. For example, blood, injection/needle, natural environment such as thunderstorm.

*Simple phobia*: Excessive fear of animals (dogs, cockroaches, snakes, or rodents), environmental type (fear of height, or acrophobia/altophobia, deep water), germs, and situational phobia (flying in aeroplane, dentist chair syndrome). Phobic disorders have a high community prevalence. 1 in every 10 individuals suffer from phobic anxiety disorders.

*Social anxiety disorder/social phobia*: It is characterized by disproportionate fear about social interaction, mixing with other people, and gatherings for irrational and excessive fear about humiliation. The common features include blushing, sweating, palpitation, and diarrhea.

*Acute stress disorder*: It is an acute reaction to trauma which has short- and long-term consequences. There is a history suggestive of peritraumatic dissociation.

*Post-traumatic stress disorder*: It happens following life-threatening events with features such as flashbacks, severe anxiety, and nightmares (e.g., Vietnam War, Gulf War, and tsunami).

*Anxiety NOS*: This does not fulfill the other groups of anxiety disorder and meeting the criteria of anxiety disorder.

*Obsessive–compulsive related disorder*: It is an exclusive diagnosis of DSM-V and has been given new weightage to mention in a separate chapter.

*Separation anxiety disorder*: It is classified under childhood behavioral disorders. It is characterized by fear of being separated and isolated from near and dear ones and home. This can be explained by attachment theory.

*Selective mutism*: It is another childhood behavioral disorder where there is a consistent fear of failure in school or class performances but unable to speak at home with parents and other family members.

*Substance-induced anxiety disorder*: Intense panic and other anxiety symptoms during the use of psychoactive substances/during withdrawal from drugs.

*Anxiety disorders due to GMC (general medical conditions)*: The following medical conditions can present with symptoms of anxiety: (1) Left atrial myxoma, (2) floppy mitral valve syndrome, (3) cardiac illnesses, (4) diabetes mellitus, (5) hypoglycemia, (6) hyperthyroidism, (7) Graves' disease, (8) thyrotoxicosis, (9) autoimmune thyroiditis, (10) Hashimoto's thyroiditis, (11) hypoparathyroidism, (12) tetany, (13) respiratory disorders such as chronic obstructive pulmonary disease (COPD) and bronchial asthma, (14) chronic pain syndrome, (15) irritable bowel syndrome, etc.

## Clinical Features

Anxiety is a normal behavioral response of all animals. Humans also have anxiety symptoms from the hunter-gatherer stage till date. The territory Anxiety was unique for not being killed by animals in higher place of hierarchy in ecosystem. The features of anxiety disorders can have a wide range of symptoms as follows:

- *Physical symptoms of anxiety*: Headache, light-headedness, breathing difficulties, profuse sweating, nausea, vomiting, diarrhea, restlessness, increased fatigability, irritability.
- *Behavioral symptoms of anxiety*: Pathological doubt, intense worry but can lead normal life (worried well), need to ask for reassurance, avoidance reaction to phobic situations and stimuli, compulsive behaviors such as washing hands and checking door locks. The details of symptoms are summarized in **Box 1**.

**BOX 1: Behavioral symptoms of anxiety.**

*Physiological*:
- Chest tightness
- Chills and hot flashes
- Choking sensation
- Dry mouth
- Hyperventilation
- Muscle tension
- Palpitation
- Paresthesia
- Sleep disturbances
- Sweating
- Tachycardia
- Urinary frequency
- Vertigo

*Cognitive*:
- Amnesia
- Apprehension
- Distractibility
- Derealization
- Depersonalization
- Carefulness
- Flashbacks
- Inclusive thoughts
- Irritability
- Racing thoughts
- Recurrent thoughts
- Recurrent images
- Recurrent dreams

*Behavioral*:
- Avoidance
- Hypervigilance
- Hyperkinesia
- Pressured speech
- Repetitive behaviors
- Ritualistic behaviors
- Stiffness
- Startle response

*Anxiety symptoms during COVID-19 pandemic*: A survey done on 288,830 participants from 19 countries shows that one in every three adults has experienced anxiety symptoms during the COVID-19 pandemic.

### Risk Factors for Anxiety Disorders

- Childhood physical and sexual abuse and trauma
- Stress due to chronic medical illness [cancer, coronary artery disease (CAD), type 2 diabetes mellitus (T2DM), hypertension, chronic kidney disease (CKD)]
- Significant life events (death of near and dear ones, break-in relationship, failure in examinations, loss of job, divorce)
- Comorbid mental illnesses such as depression and substance abuse
- Type A personality disorder
- Family history of anxiety disorder
- Societal factors such as unemployment and poverty

## WHAT ARE THE DIFFERENT TREATMENT OPTIONS IN THE MANAGEMENT OF ANXIETY DISORDERS?

The current treatments fall short to meet health burden attributed to anxiety disorders. This is summarized in **Table 1**.

### Pharmacological Treatments

- *Selective serotonin reuptake inhibitors (SSRIs)*: They are the first line of treatment. The medicine starts its action after 3–4 weeks, and at least a period of 6–8 weeks is required to get the optimum response.

**Table 1: Pharmacological management of anxiety disorders.**

| | *Dose (mg/day)* | *Adverse effects (FDA pregnancy category)* |
|---|---|---|
| ***SSRI*** | | |
| Escitalopram | 10–20 | GI symptoms, somnolence (C) |
| Fluoxetine | 20–60 | GI symptoms, sexual dysfunction (C) |
| Fluvoxamine | 100–300 | GI symptoms, sexual dysfunction (C) |
| Paroxetine CR | 12.5–37.5 | Anticholinergic effects, sedation (D) |
| Sertraline | 50–200 | GI symptoms, sexual dysfunction (C) |
| ***SNRI*** | | |
| Duloxetine | 60–120 | GI symptoms, hypertension (C) |
| Venlafaxine | 75–225 | GI symptoms, hypertension (C) |
| ***Benzodiazepines (GABA-A-receptor agonist)*** | | |
| Clonazepam | 1–4 | Cognitive impairment, dependence (D) |
| Alprazolam | 1–4 | Cognitive impairment, dependence (D) |
| Chlordiazepoxide | 15–30 | Cognitive impairment, dependence (C) |
| ***TCA (tricyclic antidepressants)*** | | |
| Clomipramine | 25–250 | Dry mouth, constipation, urinary retention (C) |
| ***MAO inhibitors*** | | |
| Phenelzine | 45–90 | Dry mouth, constipation, urinary retention |

(CR: controlled release; FDA: Food and Drug Administration; GABA: gamma-aminobutyric acid; GI: gastrointestinal; MAO: monoamine oxidase; SNRI: serotonin and norepinephrine reuptake inhibitor; SSRI: selective serotonin reuptake inhibitor)

Selective serotonin reuptake inhibitors block the reuptake of serotonin (5-HT) in presynaptic neurons; thus, more serotonin remains available in synaptic clefts and generates its potential action by improving mood and anxiety symptoms through greater postsynaptic neuronal activity.

- *Tricyclic antidepressants (TCAs)*: They act by inhibiting biogenic amines, mostly norepinephrine as well as serotonin. They also have anticholinergic and antimuscarinic activities. They have potential anticholinergic adverse effects such as dry mouth, constipation, urinary retention, oversedation, and orthostatic hypotension.
  - *Tertiary amine*: Amitriptyline, imipramine, trimipramine
  - *Secondary amine*: Desipramine, nortriptyline
- *Monoamine oxidase (MAO) inhibitors*: The substrate of MAO-A enzyme is serotonin, melatonin, and norepinephrine. By irreversible inactivation and further deactivation, this group of drug increases the stores of monoamines (serotonin, dopamine, norepinephrine) within the neurons resulting in diffusion of excess neurotransmitters in synaptic clefts. The adverse effects of MAO inhibitors include cheese reaction, especially with red wine, orthostatic hypotension, peripheral edema, weight gain, and insomnia.
- *Benzodiazepines (BZDs)*: They should be used judiciously, optimally for a brief period, due to their anxiolytic properties and capability of rapid symptom relief. All benzodiazepine groups of drugs have potential for causing dependence and may be abused as a psychoactive drug. Short-acting BZDs (triamcinolone) can cause rapid symptom relief but have high withdrawal symptoms causing rebound anxiety. Long-acting BZDs are less potent and take more time for symptom relief, but they have less chance of dependence. They can produce day-time drowsiness and hangover (chlordiazepoxide).
- *Buspirone*: It is a nonbenzodiazepine anxiolytic and acts by partial agonism of 5-HT1A-receptor, which reduces the firings of serotonergic neurons. Their potential adverse effects are mild in nature and include nausea, headache, gastrointestinal (GI) upset, etc.
- *Newer drugs*:
  - *Vortioxetine*: It has multiple receptor targeted action. It acts by 5-HT1A agonism, 5-HT1B partial agonism, and 5-HT1D,3,7 antagonism. It has less sexual adverse effects, less weight gain, and favorable drug–drug interaction profile. The $t_{1/2}$ of this molecule is 66 hours. Initially being an activating drug can increase anxiety symptoms.
  - *Vilazodone*: This is also known as SPARI (serotonin 1A partial agonist reuptake inhibitor). It is an SSRI with buspirone-like activity. Theoretically, it has a faster onset of action (onset of action in 7 days). It is a molecule which is suitable for women in the child-bearing age group.
  - *Agomelatine*: It is a melatonin agonist, restores circadian rhythm, and has antidepressant and anxiolytic actions.

## Other Lifestyle Measures

- Work–life balance
- Healthy balanced nutritious diet
- Connectedness with family, friends, colleagues, and mental health experts
- Regular brisk walking and exercises (20–30 min/day at least 5 days a week, which releases the feel-good substance endorphin)
- Relaxation exercises, deep breathing exercises, Jacobson's progressive muscular relaxation (JPMR)
- Mindfulness training, yoga and meditation, stress management
- Sleep hygiene (avoid mobile phone and television with stimulus control at least 2 hours before sleep)

- Avoid unhealthy practices and addictions (smoking, alcoholism, and other psychoactive substances)
- Practicing and enjoying hobbies such as listening music, painting, cooking, gardening, and reading books

### Nonpharmacological Treatments

- Psychoeducation to family members
- Supportive psychotherapy and reassurance
- Cognitive behavioral therapy (8–16 weeks)

## CLINICAL PEARLS

Anxiety disorders present with feelings of intense worry, fear, apprehension, withdrawal from social life, irrational fear, and avoidance reaction to a harmless object, place, or situation which is very common and interfere with the day-to-day activities. Avoiding alcohol and caffeine intake, quitting smoking, relaxation exercises, and stress management may be helpful but should be treated with combined pharmacotherapy and behavioral therapy.

## FURTHER READINGS

1. Garcia R. Neurobiology of fear and specific phobias. Learn Mem. 2017;24(9):462-71.
2. Ströhle A, Gensichen J, Domschke K. The diagnosis and treatment of anxiety disorders. Dtsch Arztebl Int. 2018;115(37):611-20.
3. Domschke K, Maron E. Genetic factors in anxiety disorders. Mod Trends Pharmacopsychiatry. 2013;29:24-46.
4. Showraki M, Showraki T, Brown K. Generalized anxiety disorder: revisited. Psychiatr Q. 2020; 91(3):905-14.
5. Roy-Byrne PP, Craske MG, Stein MB. Panic disorder. Lancet. 2006;368(9540):1023-32.
6. Crocq MA. The history of generalized anxiety disorder as a diagnostic category. Dialogues Clin Neurosci. 2017;19(2):107-16.
7. Deng J, Zhou F, Hou W, Silver Z, Wong CY, Chang O, et al. The prevalence of depression, anxiety, and sleep disturbances in COVID-19 patients: a meta-analysis. Ann NY Acad Sci. 2021;1486(1):90-111.
8. Murrough JW, Yaqubi S, Sayed S, Charney DS. Emerging drugs for the treatment of anxiety. Expert Opin Emerg Drugs. 2015;20(3):393-406.

# CHAPTER 82

# Phobia

*Ranjan Bhattacharyya*

## WHAT IS PHOBIA? WHAT IS THE PREVALENCE OF PHOBIA IN THE COMMUNITY?

Phobia is an anxiety disorder characterized by persistent and excessive fear of any object or situation. If fear becomes familiar, is out of proportion to the imminent danger, lasts >6 months' duration, and makes a significant impact on the day-to-day working, social, and personal life, then treatment is required. The person avoids the triggering object, place, and situation and is unable to enjoy his or her life when it causes intense and overwhelming fear. This subject knows that this fear is out of proportion to the imminent danger. The consequences of phobia may be severe and disabling, and such fears can interfere with their personal, family, work, and school activities.

The word "phobos" came after the name of Greek God "Phobos," the god of fear. The duration criterion is >6 months. The particular situation or stimulus is usually being avoided. The characteristics of phobia are fainting attacks, which may occur in blood injection or needle injury phobia. Agoraphobia is characterized by fear of open spaces. In the Epidemiologic Catchment Area (ECA) program (1981–1991), phobia has been found to be the most common psychiatric disorder (prevalence 4.0–11%) in the country, surpassing major depressive disorder and substance abuse. Around 75% of individuals can present with multiple phobias. The disease starts commonly during adolescence. The specific phobias are very common in women, and the overall prevalence lies between 1 and 12.5%. The earliest phobias to appear are animal phobia, and a slightly later age of onset is seen in social phobia and agoraphobia. The ICD-10 (International Classification of Diseases, 10th revision) describes the difference between phobic anxiety disorders (e.g., agoraphobia) and other anxiety disorders such as generalized anxiety disorder (GAD). The ICD-11 classification has combined both groups together as anxiety or fear-related disorders.

## BRIEFLY DESCRIBE ETIOLOGY, TYPES, AND SYMPTOMS OF PHOBIA

The etiology of phobia can be explained in various theories. In social and specific phobias, there could be a conflict regarding castration anxiety and sexual arousal. When the primary defense repression is not entirely successful, the auxiliary defense mechanisms such as displacement, symbolization, and avoidance come into play. Thereby a neutral, harmless object or stimulus turned out to become anxiety that satisfies ego. The most common types of specific phobias are fear of spiders, fear of snakes, and fear of heights. Specific phobia is a strong, inappropriate fear of any object or stimulus that is associated with avoidance reaction. Five common types of specific phobias have been recognized. They are given in **Table 1**.

## Symptoms of Phobia

The symptoms of phobias resemble a panic attack. The physical symptoms have a wide range of ideas, thoughts, and emotions. These include palpitations, hot flushes or chills, shortness of breath, numbness, chest pain, nausea or dizziness, choking sensation, tingling, numbness, paresthesia, tinnitus, etc. The other symptoms of phobia include fear of fainting, fear of dying, feeling out of touch of reality and self (derealization and depersonalization), and fear of fainting.

Specific phobias are more common in women. Animal and blood-injection-injury phobias generally begin in childhood, whereas situational phobia (claustrophobia, driving a car) usually appears in late adolescence and early adulthood.

Social anxiety disorder (SAD) is one of the most common types of anxiety disorders. The concerned person gets tensed in certain situations such as starting conversations, talking with strangers, making a speech in front of public, and going to shopping. Social phobia is characterized by a triad of (1) excessive self-consciousness, (2) fear of public humiliation in common social situations, and (3) fear of negative appraisal by others. Before confirming a diagnosis to be a case of SAD, one has to rule out normal shyness, other anxiety disorders, panic disorder, obsessive-compulsive disorder (OCD), avoidant personality disorder, etc. The different names of specific phobias are summarized in **Table 2**.

**Table 1: Types of specific phobia [Diagnostic and Statistical Manual of Mental Disorders, 5th edition (DSM-5)].**

| *Type of phobia* | *Definition* |
|---|---|
| Animal | Dogs, spiders, insects |
| Natural environment | Heights, storms, water |
| Blood-injection injury | Needles, surgery, invasive procedures |
| Situational | Elevator, crowded bus, airplanes |
| Other | Loud sound, vomiting, certain characters |

**Table 2: Nomenclature-specific phobias.**

| *Phobia* | *Definition* |
|---|---|
| Claustrophobia | Fear of being entangled in closed spaces |
| Agoraphobia | Fear in open, public, crowded places |
| Aerophobia | Fear of flying |
| Arachnophobia | Fear of spiders |
| Acrophobia/ Altophobia | Fear of heights |
| Escalaphobia | Fear of riding in escalator |
| Emetophobia | Fear of vomiting |
| Erythrophobia | Fear of blushing |
| Aquaphobia | Fear of water |
| Hypochondria | Fear of becoming ill |
| Zoophobia | Fear of animals |
| Glossophobia | Fear of speaking in front of public |
| Aviophobia | Fear of flying high |
| Cynophobia | Fear of dogs |
| Ophidiophobia | Fear of snakes |
| Nyctophobia | Fear of darkness |
| Xenophobia | Fear about strangers |
| Homophobia | Fear about homosexuality |
| Taphophobia | Fear of being buried alive |
| Trypanophobia | Fear of injections |
| Spectrophobia | Fear of ghosts |
| Brontophobia | Fear of thunder |
| Herpetophobia | Fear of lizards |
| Katsaridaphobia | Fear of cockroaches |
| Gelotophobia | Fear of laughing |

## WHAT IS THE NEUROBIOLOGY OF SPECIFIC PHOBIA?

In phobic anxiety disorder, there is aberrant and altered self-referential processing. In different researches, the altered activations have been noticed in medial prefrontal cortex (mPFC), which is responsible for self-representation; insula involved in interoceptive processing, amygdala (fear response), posterior cingulated and temporal lobes, etc. Alterations in both dopaminergic and serotonergic systems have been found in phobia. Neuropeptides such as oxytocin also play crucial roles in social anxiety. There is decreased inhibitory signaling in lateral temporal lobe, left medial inferior temporal lobe, bilateral orbitofrontal cortex (OFC). Low baseline GABA (gamma-aminobutyric acid) concentration and high excitatory glutamatergic signaling are associated with symptoms of phobia. Neuropeptide cholecystokinin (CCK) has also been attributed for development of symptoms of phobia, which could not be substantiated. The genes attributed to phobic anxiety disorders are: (1) *COMT*, (2) *CCK*, (3) *CCK-B receptor*, (4) *adenosine 2A receptor*, (5) MAO-A (monoamine oxidase-A), (6) *5-HT2A receptor*, (7) *SLC6A4*, and (8) *AVPR1B* or vasopressin 1B receptor gene, and CRF1 polymorphisms have been found to be linked with symptoms of phobic anxiety disorder.

## WHAT ARE THE DIFFERENT DRUGS USED IN PHOBIC ANXIETY DISORDER?

The current therapeutic approach is a combination of behavioral and pharmacotherapy approaches. Exposure therapy is based on changing the catastrophic response by gradual and repeated exposure. In cognitive behavioral therapy, the negative maladaptive thoughts/schema are being challenged by alternative thoughts. In pharmacotherapy, beta blockers are very helpful, which block the stimulating effects of adrenaline (tachycardia, hypertension, trembling, etc.). Benzodiazepines bring immediate relief but have to be used judiciously or else they can cause dependence. The different options in pharmacotherapy are summarized in **Table 3**.

**Table 3: List of drugs used in phobic anxiety disorder.**

| *Class of drugs* | *Example* |
|---|---|
| SSRIs | Escitalopram, paroxetine, sertraline, fluoxetine, fluvoxamine |
| SNRIs | Venlafaxine, duloxetine, milnacipran |
| NaSSA | Mirtazapine |
| TCAs | Amitriptyline, nortriptyline, imipramine, clomipramine |
| Calcium modulator, GABA agonist | Pregabalin, gabapentin |
| MAO inhibitors | Phenelzine, moclobemide |
| Azapirone | Buspirone |
| Melatonin agonist | Agomelatine |
| Beta blockers | Propranolol, pindolol |
| Antipsychotics (low dose) | Olanzapine, quetiapine, risperidone, ziprasidone |
| Antihistaminics | Phenelzine |

(GABA: gamma-aminobutyric acid; MAO: monoamine oxidase; NaSSA: noradrenergic and specific serotonergic antidepressant; SNRIs: serotonin and norepinephrine reuptake inhibitors; SSRIs: selective serotonin reuptake inhibitors; TCA: tricyclic antidepressants)

## WHAT ARE THE DIFFERENT NONPHARMACOLOGICAL TREATMENTS OF PHOBIC ANXIETY DISORDER?

The treatment aimed in specific phobias are exposure and response prevention, systematic desensitization, and flooding techniques. Among the pharmacological management, selective serotonin reuptake inhibitors (SSRIs), benzodiazepines, and beta blockers are first-line therapies. Phobias can be best managed by combined psychotherapy and pharmacotherapy. The aim of the therapy is to improve the quality of life, and the treatment of specific phobia should be directed one at a time. Lifestyle modification, mindfulness training and relaxation techniques (deep breathing exercises, Jacobson's progressive muscular relaxation techniques), and yoga therapy are often very helpful. Mindfulness meditation, relaxation techniques, physical activities, and exercises often help to curb down intense anxiety and fear related to phobic anxiety disorder. Challenging automatic negative thoughts (ANT), negative schema, maladaptive thoughts with alternate thoughts, addressing cognitive errors, attributes and biases such as catastrophization, behavioral techniques such as systematic desensitization (hierarchy construction), and flooding are very helpful in the management of phobic anxiety disorder. In the systematic desensitization (SD) technique, a strategy called "climbing up the fear ladder" may be formulated (make a list, build up your own fear ladder, work up on this fear ladder, and practice). Debriefing and eye movement desensitization and reprocessing (EMDR) have been found useful in the management of some types of specific phobias apart from their proven efficacy in post-traumatic stress disorder (PTSD).

## CLINICAL PEARLS

Phobia can be defined as excessive and irrational fear of any object or situation that leads to conscious avoidance. The presence or anticipation of phobic entity is very stressful. It is out of proportion to the demand of the situation, cannot be explained, and beyond voluntary control. It may occur after previous traumatic experiences and following biological and psychological response to a stimulus. It may present with intense anxiety features such as palpitation, respiratory distress, choking sensation, and sense of impending doom with vasovagal response such as fainting. The treatment approach should be a comprehensive management plan that includes pharmacotherapy and nonpharmacological therapy (cognitive behavioral therapy, exposure therapy, and response). In the pharmacological management, SSRIs, benzodiazepines, and beta blockers are very useful.

## FURTHER READINGS

1. Raeder F, Merz CJ, Margraf J, Zlomuzica A. The association between fear extinction, the ability to accomplish exposure and exposure therapy outcome in specific phobia. Sci Rep. 2020;10(1):4288.
2. Thng CEW, Lim-Ashworth NSJ, Poh BZQ, Lim CG. Recent developments in the intervention of specific phobia among adults: a rapid review. F1000Res. 2020;9:F1000 Faculty Rev-195.
3. Frumento S, Menicucci D, Hitchcott PK, Zaccaro A, Gemignani A. Systematic review of studies on subliminal exposure to phobic stimuli: integrating therapeutic models for specific phobias. Front Neurosci. 2021;15:654170.
4. Eaton WW, Bienvenu OJ, Miloyan B. Specific phobias. Lancet Psychiatry. 2018;5(8):678-86.
5. Abado E, Aue T, Okon-Singer H. Cognitive biases in blood-injection-injury phobia: a review. Front Psychiatry. 2021;12:678891.
6. Meule A, Voderholzer U. Life satisfaction in persons with mental disorders. Qual Life Res. 2020;29(11):3043-52.
7. Fumero A, Marrero RJ, Rivero F, Alvarez-Pérez Y, Bethencourt JM, González M, et al. Neuronal correlates of small animal phobia in human subjects through fMRI: the role of the number and proximity of stimuli. Life (Basel). 2021;11(4):275.

8. Reddy YCJ, Sudhir PM, Manjula M, Arumugham SS, Narayanaswamy JC. Clinical practice guidelines for cognitive-behavioral therapies in anxiety disorders and obsessive-compulsive and related disorders. Indian J Psychiatry. 2020;62(Suppl. 2):S230-50.
9. Benau EM, Wiatrowski R, Timko CA. Difficulties in emotion regulation, alexithymia, and social phobia are associated with disordered eating in male and female undergraduate athletes. Front Psychol. 2020;11:1646.
10. Chavanne AV, Robinson OJ. The overlapping neurobiology of induced and pathological anxiety: a meta-analysis of functional neural activation. Am J Psychiatry. 2021;178(2):156-64.

CHAPTER 83

# Obsessive-compulsive Disorder

*Ranjan Bhattacharyya*

## WHAT IS OBSESSIVE-COMPULSIVE DISORDER AND WHAT ARE THE DIFFERENT TYPES OF OBSESSIVE-COMPULSIVE DISORDER?

"Obsessive-compulsive disorder" (OCD) is a chronic, common, and uncontrollable disorder that is characterized by recurrent intrusive unpleasant thoughts, impulses, urges, and/or mental images that cause anxiety. Compulsions are repeated thoughts and/or behaviors to neutralize the obsessive thoughts. The common obsessions and compulsions are mentioned in **Box 1**.

**BOX 1: Common types of obsessions and compulsions in clinical practice.**

*Obsession*

- Fear of germs and contamination
- Pathological doubts
- Forbidden or taboo thoughts involving sex, religion, or herm
- Aggressive impulsive or thoughts directed to self or others
- Symmetrical or orderliness
- Ruminations
- Fear of making a mistake
- Need for repetitive reassurances
- Sexual thoughts

*Compulsion*

- Repetitive cleaning, bathing, and handwashing
- Repetitive checking, hoarding
- Praying
- Compulsive counting
- Arranging things in particular way
- Bothersome disturbing repetitive compulsive acts
- Eating food in a particular mannerism
- Compulsive touching
- Blinking eyes, jerking head, grunting, sniffling nose, clearing throat, shrugging shoulders

## WHAT IS THE PREVALENCE AND WHAT ARE THE RISK FACTORS FOR THE DEVELOPMENT OF OBSESSIVE-COMPULSIVE DISORDER?

In the 14th and 15th centuries, this disease was believed to be caused by devil and bad omens and used to be treated by exorcism. In the 17th century, it was thought that people were cleansing their guilt. In the successive centuries, it was considered with a medical model, and in the 20th century, the behavioral therapy model was advocated in the management of OCD.

## Prevalence and Risk Factors

Obsessive-compulsive disorder commonly occurs during late adolescence, earlier in boys than in girls. It is a fairly common disorder that affects approximately 1% of population and happens in all races, ethnicities, cultural backgrounds, and genders. It can affect 2.3% people globally at some point in their life. It is unusual to begin after the age of 35 years, and 50% of patients developed their symptoms before the age of 20 years. It is highly comorbid in other psychiatric illnesses such as depression, anxiety, tic disorder, eating disorder, body image disorder as well as a particular illness known as PANDAS (Pediatric Autoimmune Neuropsychiatric Disorder Associated with group A β-hemolytic Streptococcal infections). It is usually characterized by rapid onset and progression of OCD in children and adolescence and can be explained by an autoimmune process. In a child, symptoms start abruptly and peak to full intensity within 24–72 hours, which may disappear and come back again at a later date. This illness is also called pediatric acute-onset neuropsychiatric syndrome (PANS).

## WHAT ARE THE DIFFERENT GENETIC FACTORS INVOLVED IN OBSESSIVE-COMPULSIVE DISORDER? WHAT IS THE ETIOLOGY OF OBSESSIVE-COMPULSIVE DISORDER?

Obsessive-compulsive disorder is more common in first-degree relatives who have been diagnosed with OCD as found in twin and adoption studies. The genetic factors can account for 45–65% of variability in children having OCD symptoms. The specific genetic loci attributed in OCD are summarized in **Table 1**.

**Table 1: Genetic loci attributed in obsessive-compulsive disorder (OCD).**

| *Gene* | *Result* |
|---|---|
| Mutation in human serotonin transporter gene (*hSERT*) | In unrelated families with OCD |
| L allele in Caucasian, homozygous S allele | Increased risk of OCD |
| LS genotypes | Inversely related with OCD |
| Genome-wide association study (GWAS) found SNP (single nucleotide polymorphisms) near BTBD-3, BLGAP-1 | Increased risk of OCD |
| Polymerization of SLC1A1 | Increased risk of OCD |

*Autoimmune-related etiologies*:
- GABHS (group A beta-hemolytic strepto-cocci)
- Lyme disease
- H1N1 flu virus

*Behavioral causes*:
- Avoidance reaction is response to fear of any objects or situations.
- Following insurmountable pressure such as significant loss or traumatic events.
- Defense mechanisms involved in OCD are isolation of affect, undoing, and reaction formation.

*Cognitive causes*:
- Recurrent intrusive thoughts are unwelcome and gradually become more intense.
- Alternate cognitive schema leads to maladaptive functioning due to mental rigidity and inflexibility.
- Cognitive errors in OCD are mismatch signaling leading to catastrophization and dysfunctional cortico-striato-thalamo-cortical (CSTC) circuit.

## EXPLAIN THE NEUROBIOLOGICAL BASIS OF OBSESSIVE-COMPULSIVE DISORDER

The imaging studies have revealed involvement of frontal cortex and subcortical structure of brain in patients with OCD. The cascades of events triggered in the brain in a patient suffering from OCD are summarized in **Figure 1**.

*Environmental factors*: Restrictive upbringing and childhood are associated with OCD. Certain environmental stress can trigger individuals who have a high genetic load or propensity to have OCD as mentioned in **Box 2**.

## HOW TO DIAGNOSE A CASE OF OBSESSIVE-COMPULSIVE DISORDER?

Diagnosis is made by certain criteria as laid out in DSM-5 (Diagnostic and Statistical Manual, fifth edition by the American Psychiatric Association) and ICD-11 (International Classification Diseases, 11th edition); however, the severity of OCD can be assessed by Yale–Brown Obsessive-Compulsive Scale (Y-BOCS). This scale has 13 predefined symptoms, and after factor analysis, 4 symptom clusters usually being found CSTC loops: (1) Symmetric factor, (2) cleaning factor, (3) forbidden thought factors, and (4) hoarding factors.

## WHAT ARE THE NEUROIMAGING FINDINGS IN OBSESSIVE-COMPULSIVE DISORDER?

The functional neuroimaging such as positron emission tomography (PET) scan, single-photon emission computed tomography (SPECT), and functional magnetic resonance imaging (fMRI) studies have found significant abnormalities in different regions of the brain as mentioned below in **Table 2**.

This involves CSTC loop, which is also involved in ADHD (attention deficit hyperactivity disorder). Similar dysfunction of

**BOX 2: Environmental attributes of obsessive-compulsive disorder (OCD).**

- Changing residence—migration, joining in a new school or job, getting married or divorced
- Death of near and dear ones and other significant emotional trauma
- History of childhood physical or sexual abuse
- Following recovery after an illness
- Relationship issues such as breakup and separation
- Problem at school or work
- Economic depression
- Significant environmental changes such as COVID-19
- Life-threatening accidents of self or close relatives
- Magical thinking due to peer pressure and religious rituals

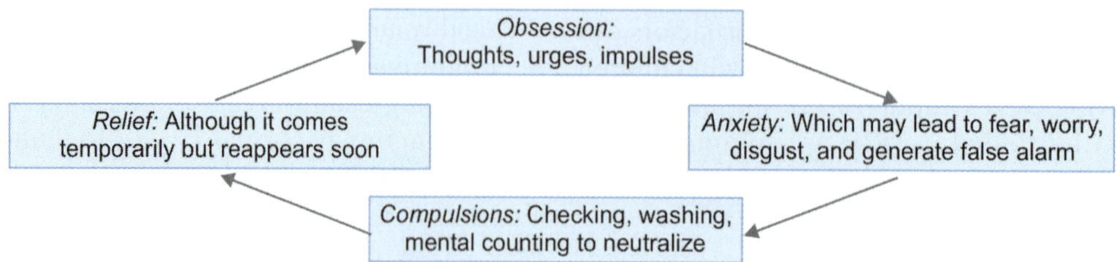


**FIG. 1:** The vicious cycle of chronology of obsessive-compulsive disorder (OCD) symptoms.

**Table 2: Neuroimaging findings in obsessive-compulsive disorder.**

| *Finding in neuroimaging* | *Region of interest (ROI)* |
|---|---|
| Stronger foci of abnormal activity | Orbitofrontal cortex (OFC), left dlPFC (dorsolateral prefrontal cortex), right premotor cortex, left STG (superior temporal gyrus), GPe (globus pallidus externa), hippocampus, right uncus |
| Weaker foci of abnormal activity | Left caudate, posterior, cingulate cortex |
| (↑) Increases activity | Orbital gyrus, ACC, head of the caudate nucleus |
| Decrease activity (hypoactivity) | mPFC (medial prefrontal cortex), posterior caudate nucleus |
| (↑) Increase activity | Precuneus and posterior cingulate cortex |
| (↓) Decrease activity | Globus pallidum, ventral anterior thalamus, posterior cortex |

executive task also involves ACC (anterior cingulate cortex) and PFC (prefrontal cortex). The involvement of OFC (orbitofrontal cortex) and dlPFC (dorsolateral prefrontal cortex) is also shared with bipolar disorder.

*Nosology*: Obsessive-compulsive and related disorders (OCRDs) are the nosology incorporated in DSM-5, which includes the following disorders:

- *Incorporated in both DSM-5 and ICD-11 [World Health Organization (WHO)]*: OCD, body dysmorphic disorder (BDD), hoarding disorder, trichotillomania (hair-pulling disorder), excoriation (skin-picking disorder)
- Incorporated in ICD only: Hypochondriasis, olfactory reference syndrome, Tourette syndrome

Obsessive-compulsive disorder was previously incorporated in the anxiety group of disorders, which has now been given due weightage and separated in DSM-5. The body dysmorphic disorder (BDD) has now been shifted from somatoform disorder to OCRD group. Similarly, trichotillomania has been incorporated in group from the previous group of impulse control disorders. Two new entries in this group of OCRDs are hoarding disorders and excoriation disorders (skin-picking disorders).

In ICD-11, this chapter also includes Tourette syndrome, a neurodevelopmental disorder, hypochondriasis (anxiety disorder), and the new entry olfactory reference syndrome.

## WHAT ARE THE DIFFERENT COMORBIDITIES OF OBSESSIVE-COMPULSIVE DISORDER?

Substance-use disorders (alcohol, cannabis, nicotine, and others), impulse-control disorders [intermittent explosive disorder, ADHD, conduct disorder, oppositional defiant disorder (ODD), etc.], mood disorders (bipolar disorder, dysthymic disorder, major depressive disorder, etc.), and anxiety disorders [separation anxiety disorder, post-traumatic stress disorder (PTSD), generalized anxiety disorder (GAD), social phobia, specific phobia, agoraphobia without panic disorder, panic disorder, etc.] are common comorbid conditions known to be associated with OCD.

## HOW TO MANAGE A CASE OF OBSESSIVE-COMPULSIVE DISORDER?

A case of OCD should be managed with a combination of pharmacotherapy and psychotherapy.

*Pharmacotherapy*: Selective serotonin reuptake inhibitors (SSRIs) require higher doses, and unlike the management of depression, the onset of action may be delayed to 8–12 weeks. The higher doses should be monitored judiciously to avoid adverse effects. Some patients fail to tolerate the doses of multiple SSRIs and may require augmentation therapy with tricyclic antidepressants (TCAs) such as clomipramine and atypical antipsychotic drugs (risperidone, aripiprazole).

*Psychotherapy*: Cognitive behavioral therapy (CBT) is a specific type of psychotherapy developed by Aaron T Beck, which is aimed to correct or change the maladaptive thoughts and schemas.

In the specific type of CBT called exposure and response prevention (ExRP), this therapy exposes the patients to disturbing thoughts, impulses, and/or images (obsessions), either in vivo or give them a real exposure. This is followed by preventing them from neutralizing these bothersome thoughts by actions, rituals, or mental imagery.

## Other Biological, Nonpharmacological Treatment

*Electroconvulsive therapy (ECT)*: In this method, electrodes are applied to the scalp, and electric shocks are delivered inside the brain through wires (brief pulse therapy). These shocks generate "micro" seizures, which help the brain to release neurotransmitters and other chemicals.

*Repetitive transcranial magnetic stimulation (rTMS)*: This method has been approved by the Food and Drug Administration (FDA) for the management of OCD in 2018. In this method, a handheld magnetic device is placed on the head, which delivers electrical impulses inside the brain and releases chemicals (serotonin), which helps to prevent obsessive thoughts.

*Neurosurgical treatment*: This may be required in intractable OCD. It is sometimes required to do surgeries such as anterior capsulotomy, tractotomy, and limbic lobotomy.

*Social care and support*: It is utmost needed by family members to provide adequate social care and support and avoid stigmatization.

*Obsessive-compulsive disorder in children and adolescents*: Childhood OCD is more common in males and is characterized by poor self-esteem, disrupted routine, difficulty in finishing homework and schoolwork, physical illness, and trouble maintaining friendships and other relationships.

## CLINICAL PEARLS

Obsessive-compulsive disorder is characterized by recurrent, unwanted, intrusive thoughts, which involves CSTC circuit in the brain having categories such as checking, contamination, symmetry and ordering, ruminations, and intrusive thoughts. OCD should be treated by combined modality of treatment: ExRP and pharmacotherapy.

## FURTHER READINGS

1. Goodman WK, Grice DE, Lapidus KA, Coffey BJ. Obsessive-compulsive disorder. Psychiatr Clin North Am. 2014;37(3):257-67.
2. Wilbur C, Bitnun A, Kronenberg S, Laxer RM, Levy DM, Logan WJ, et al. PANDAS/PANS in childhood: controversies and evidence. Paediatr Child Health. 2019;24(2):85-91.
3. Sigra S, Hesselmark E, Bejerot S. Treatment of PANDAS and PANS: a systematic review. Neurosci Biobehav Rev. 2018;86:51-65.
4. Thienemann M, Park M, Chan A, Frankovich J. Patients with abrupt early-onset OCD due to PANS tolerate lower doses of antidepressants and antipsychotics. J Psychiatr Res. 2021;135:270-8.

5. Mahjani B, Bey K, Boberg J, Burton C. Genetics of obsessive-compulsive disorder. Psychol Med. 2021;51(13):2247-59.
6. Battle DE. Diagnostic and Statistical Manual of Mental Disorders (DSM). Codas. 2013;25(2):191-2.
7. Gaebel W, Stricker J, Kerst A. Changes from ICD-10 to ICD-11 and future directions in psychiatric classification. Dialogues Clin Neurosci. 2020;22(1):7-15.
8. Leite PL, Filomensky TZ, Black DW, Silva AC. Validity and reliability of the Brazilian version of Yale-Brown obsessive-compulsive scale-shopping version (YBOCS-SV). Compr Psychiatry. 2014;55(6):1462-6.
9. Goodman WK, Storch EA, Sheth SA. Harmonizing the neurobiology and treatment of obsessive-compulsive disorder. Am J Psychiatry. 2021;178(1):17-29.
10. Grant JE, Chamberlain SR. Exploring the neurobiology of OCD: clinical implications. Psychiatr Times. 2020;2020.
11. Reid JE, Laws KR, Drummond L, Vismara M, Grancini B, Mpavaenda D, et al. Cognitive behavioural therapy with exposure and response prevention in the treatment of obsessive-compulsive disorder: a systematic review and meta-analysis of randomised controlled trials. Compr Psychiatry. 2021;106:152223.
12. Fontenelle LF, Coutinho ES, Lins-Martins NM, Fitzgerald PB, Fujiwara H, Yücel M. Electroconvulsive therapy for obsessive-compulsive disorder: a systematic review. J Clin Psychiatry. 2015;76(7):949-57.
13. Rehn S, Eslick GD, Brakoulias V. A meta-analysis of the effectiveness of different cortical targets used in repetitive transcranial magnetic stimulation (rTMS) for the treatment of obsessive-compulsive disorder (OCD). Psychiatr Q. 2018;89(3):645-65.
14. Rasmussen SA, Goodman WK. The prefrontal cortex and neurosurgical treatment for intractable OCD. Neuropsychopharmacology. 2022;47(1):349-60.
15. van Dis EAM, van Veen SC, Hagenaars MA, Batelaan NM, Bockting CLH, van den Heuvel RM, et al. Long-term outcomes of cognitive behavioral therapy for anxiety-related disorders: a systematic review and meta-analysis. JAMA Psychiatry. 2020;77(3):265-73. Erratum in: JAMA Psychiatry. 2020;77(7):768.
16. Krebs G, Heyman I. Obsessive-compulsive disorder in children and adolescents. Arch Dis Child. 2015;100(5):495-9.

CHAPTER 84

# Depression

*Ranjan Bhattacharyya*

## HOW DO YOU DEFINE DEPRESSION? HOW MUCH IS THIS PREVALENT IN THE CURRENT SCENARIO?

Depression is a common mental disorder (CMD) characterized by (1) low or depressed mood, (2) anhedonia or lack of pleasure, (3) low self-esteem, (4) inability to think or concentrate, (5) low self-esteem, (6) feelings of inappropriate guilt, (7) disturbed sleep, (8) decreased appetite, and (9) lack of energy and suicidal ideation. Globally, around 5% of adults suffer from depression. According to the World Health Organization (WHO), depression is the major contributor of global burden of diseases. WHO's Mental Health Action Plan (MHAP) 2013–2030 states that approximately 300 million (3.8%) people in the world suffer from depression. The worst outcome of depression is suicide and approximately 8 lakh people in the world die prematurely due to suicide. Suicide comes in fourth rank among the leading cause of death in 15–29 years age group. The treatment gap is huge, and around 75% people in low- and middle-income countries (LMIC) do not receive any treatment.

## WHAT ARE THE DIFFERENT TYPES OF DEPRESSIVE DISORDERS?

Mental Health Gap Initiation Program (mhGAP), an initiative by the WHO, covers priority conditions in mental health, and depression is one of them.

There are different types of depression as summarized in **Table 1**.

*Epidemiology*:

- Across the globe, 350 million people suffer from depression (WHO).
- The productive age group, 15–44 years, mostly suffers from depression, which is a leading cause of disability in this highly productive age group.
- Depression is more common in women (2:1).
- In geriatric depression, depressive symptoms become more severe.

## HOW CAN ONE CLASSIFY DEPRESSIVE DISORDERS?

The classification of depressive disorders has been summarized in **Box 1**.

**Table 1: Different types of depressive disorders.**

| *Type* | *Features* |
|---|---|
| Major depression | Long episodes of low moods or one extended episode |
| Atypical depression | Reversal of vegetative symptoms, i.e., instead of decreased sleep and appetite, the patient will experience increased sleep and appetite |
| Postpartum depression | Onset of depression within 4 weeks of childbirth |
| Catatonic depression | With features such as mutism, negativism, and rigidity |
| Seasonal affective disorder | Depressive swings coming in a particular season or month, mostly in winters (winter depression) |
| Melancholic depression | Severe depressive swig |
| Dysthymia | Less severe symptoms, lasting longer time |
| Psychotic depression | Depression with psychotic symptoms, may longitudinally convert to bipolar affective disorder |

**BOX 1: DSM-5 (Diagnostic and Statistical Manual of Mental Disorders, 5th edition) classification of depressive disorder.**

- Disruptive mood dysregulation disorder (DMDD)
- Major depressive disorder
- Persistent depressive disorder
- Premenstrual dysphoric disorder
- Substance/medication-induced depressive disorder
- Depressive disorder due to another medical condition
- Other specified depressive disorder

According to symptom severity, depressive disorders are further classified into mild, moderate, and severe types.

## WHAT IS THE ETIOLOGY OF DEPRESSION?

- *Genetic factors*: Heritable first-degree relatives are more likely to develop depression.
- *Epigenetic factors*: Early upbringing, stress in family, peer pressure, adverse childhood experiences
- *Environmental disorders* (summarized in **Flowchart 1**)
- *Biochemical factors*: Deficiencies of neurotransmitters in certain areas of brain (monoamine hypothesis; dopamine, noradrenalin, and serotonin). Different hypotheses have been postulated for the etiology of depression (biogenic amine, receptor sensitivity, serotonin only, permissive, electrolyte membrane, neuroendocrine hypothesis, etc.).
- *Endocrinological factors*: Thyroid disorders, Addison's disease, Cushing syndrome
- *Substance abuse*: Cannabis, alcohol, opioid abuse/dependence
- *Chronic medical or surgical illness*: Viral fever, type 2 diabetes mellitus, malignancy, neurological disorders (Alzheimer's disease, parkinsonism, multiple sclerosis, etc.), systemic lupus erythematosus (SLE), chronic obstructive pulmonary disease (COPD), etc.
- Iatrogenic factors/adverse effects of medications (analgesics, antihypertensives, anticonvulsants, benzodiazepine dependence, or withdrawal).

There are many physical conditions that can present or masquerade with depressive disorder. These conditions are summarized in **Box 2**.

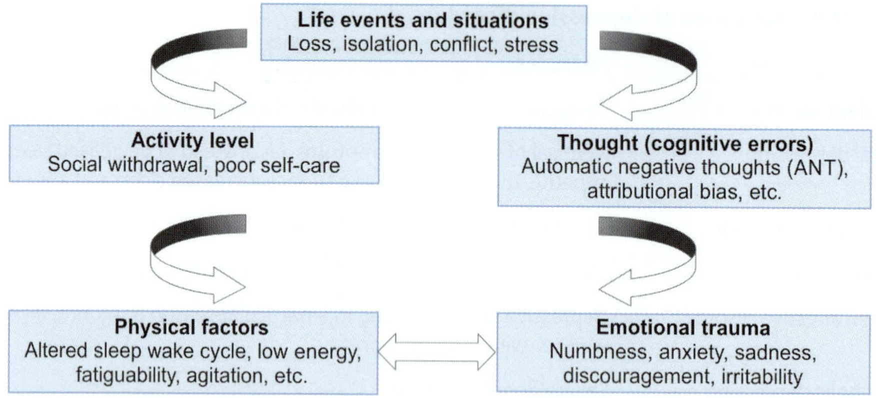


**FLOWCHART 1:** Environmental factors responsible for depression.

**BOX 2: Physical conditions presenting with depressive disorders.**

- *Cardiological*: Coronary artery diseases (CAD), hypertension, left ventricle failure, etc.
- *Neurological*: Stroke, Parkinson's disease, multiple sclerosis, head injury, meningitis, etc.
- *Endocrinological*: Hypothyroidism, hyperparathyroidism, diabetes mellitus, Cushing syndrome, etc.
- Malignancy
- Infective disorders
- *Medications/drug induced*: Steroids, beta blockers, antihypertensives, anticonvulsants, antibiotics, etc.
- *Others*: Collagen vascular diseases, chronic kidney diseases (CKD), chronic liver disease, chronic obstructive pulmonary disease (COPD)

*Stress hormones and depression*: Stress activates hypothalamic-pituitary-adrenal (HPA) axis. From adrenal gland, catecholamines and cortisols are being secreted, which in turn lead to adrenal sympathetic overactivity. Raised catecholamines are responsible for increased platelet activity and vasoconstriction acting on the endothelium of blood vessels, leading to adverse health outcomes such as myocardial ischemia and ventricular arrhythmia. On the other hand, raised cortisol leads to increased secretion of proinflammatory mediators such as interleukin (IL)-1, IL-6, and tumor necrosis factor (TNF) alpha. All these factors contribute to stress-mediated neuronal damage or apoptosis in depression.

The role of cortisol modifying the function of brain-derived neurotrophic factor (BDNF) in a functional crosstalk between stress hormones and BDNF signaling has a crucial role to play in the pathogenesis of depression.

In a nutshell, in depression, the following neurochemical abnormalities are found: (1) abnormalities in the HPA axis (nonsuppression in dexamethasone suppression test) and (2) elevated CRF levels.

## WHAT ARE THE DIFFERENT PHARMACOTHERAPEUTIC OPTIONS IN THE MANAGEMENT OF DEPRESSIVE DISORDERS?

- *Selective serotonin reuptake inhibitors (SSRI)*: Fluoxetine, fluvoxamine, sertraline, paroxetine, escitalopram
- *Serotonin and norepinephrine reuptake inhibitors (SNRI)*: Venlafaxine, duloxetine, milnacipran

- *MAO inhibitors*: Reversible (moclobemide, clorgyline); Irreversible: Isocarboxazid, iproniazid, phenelzine, tranylcypromine
- *Tricyclic antidepressants (TCAs)*: Noradrenaline (NA): Desipramine, nortriptyline, amoxapine; 5HT (serotonin) reuptake inhibitors: Imipramine, amitriptyline, doxepin, dothiepin, clomipramine
- *Atypical antidepressants*: Trazodone, mianserin, tianeptine
- *Norepinephrine and specific serotonergic antidepressant (NASSA)*: Mirtazapine
- *Norepinephrine and dopamine reuptake inhibitors (NDRI)*: Bupropion
- *Noradrenaline reuptake inhibitor (NARI)*: Reboxetine
- *Serotonin antagonist and reuptake inhibitor (SARI)*: Trazodone, nefazodone, etc.
- *Serotonin partial agonist reuptake inhibitor (SPARI)*: Vilazodone
- *Serotonin modulators*: Vortioxetine serotonin transporter (SERT) inhibition, 5HT1A full agonist; 5HT1B partial agonist; 5HT1D, 5HT3, and 5HT7 receptor full antagonist

## WHAT ARE THE ADVERSE EFFECTS OF ANTIDEPRESSANTS BASED ON THEIR RECEPTOR BLOCKING PROFILE?

- *Muscarinic receptor blockage/anticholinergic side effects*: Dry mouth, constipation, tachycardia, blurring of vision, aggravation of narrow-angle glaucoma, urinary retention, sexual dysfunction, cognitive impairment
- *Alpha-1 adrenoreceptor blockade*: Drowsiness, postural hypotension, sexual dysfunction (anorgasmia or loss of libido, erectile dysfunction, and delayed ejaculation), cognitive impairment

**Table 2: Combination therapy and augmentation strategy with antidepressants.**

| *Combination therapy* | *Augmentation strategy* |
|---|---|
| • SSRI + mirtazapine<br>• TCA + SSRI<br>• Venlafaxine + mirtazapine<br>• Bupropion + SSRI | • Atypical antipsychotics (olanzapine, quetiapine, risperidone, aripiprazole, etc.)<br>• Lithium<br>• Triiodothyronine |

(SSRI: selective serotonin reuptake inhibitor; TCA: tricyclic antidepressant)

- *Histamine H1 receptor blockade*: Weight gain, sedation
- *Membrane-stabilizing properties*: Cardiac conduction defects, cardiac arrhythmias, seizures
- *Others*: Rash, edema, raised hepatic transaminases, leukopenia, thrombocytopenia, allergic reactions

In resistant depression, some drugs are used in combination or as augmentation therapy, which are mentioned in **Table 2**.

## WHAT ARE THE OTHER BIOLOGICAL THERAPEUTIC OPTIONS IN THE MANAGEMENT OF DEPRESSION?

*Electroconvulsive therapy* (*ECT*): ECT is a fast, effective mode of biological treatment which is safe and devoid of major adverse effects. Modified ECT can be applied in pregnancy (risk of precipitated labor), suicidal patients (rapid onset), and patients presenting with catatonia (rigidity, negativity, mutism).

Other nonpharmacological, biological treatments for depression are invasive modalities such as vagus nerve stimulation

(VNS), deep brain stimulation (DBS), transcranial direct current stimulation (tDCS), and noninvasive repetitive transcranial magnetic stimulation (rTMS).

Psychological interventions are a key adjunct to the management of depressive disorders, which can be divided as first- and second-line therapies **(Table 3)**.

*Cognitive behavioral therapy* (*CBT*): CBT is an amalgamation of cognitive and behavioral therapies advocated by Aaron T Beck. In this therapy, negative automatic thoughts are challenged by alternate positive thoughts, rectifying maladaptive thought processes and cognitive errors.

**Table 3: Evidence-based psychotherapies in depressive disorders.**

| | |
|---|---|
| First line | • Cognitive behavioral therapy (CBT)<br>• Interpersonal psychotherapy (IPT) |
| Second line | • Mindfulness-based cognitive therapy<br>• Problem-solving therapy<br>• Marital and family therapy |

*Interpersonal psychotherapy* (*IPT*): In IPT, the primary goal is to identify the current trigger of the depressive episode, facilitating mourning during bereavement and building social skills.

*Other nonspecific techniques:* Relaxation exercises, deep breathing exercises, Jacobson's progressive muscular relaxation (JPMR), behavioral activation, problem-solving technique, mindfulness-based medication, improving coping skills, stress management, and supportive psychotherapy are often found to be useful and beneficial.

The management of depressive disorder is challenging in special population. The recommendations of using antidepressants in special population are summarized in **Table 4**.

The choice of antidepressants also varies depending on comorbid medical conditions, which are summarized in **Table 5**.

**Table 4: Antidepressants in special population.**

| ***Special population*** | ***Choice of antidepressant*** |
|---|---|
| *Pregnancy*: Antidepressants and CBT are recommended. Avoid antidepressants in the first trimester. There is a risk of persistent pulmonary hypertension in newborn (PPHN), neonatal withdrawal syndrome to newborn child (characterized by hypotonia, irritability, respiratory distress, tachycardia). If the lady had past response to a particular antidepressant, always consider the first antidepressant | • Sertraline<br>• Escitalopram<br>• Fluoxetine<br>(Paroxetine is an FDA category "D" drug and should be avoided) |
| Postpartum and lactation period | • Fluoxetine<br>• Sertraline<br>• Escitalopram |
| Geriatric population | • Escitalopram<br>• Sertraline<br>• Fluoxetine |
| Children and adolescent | Fluoxetine |

(CBT: cognitive behavioral therapy; FDA: Food and Drug Administration)

**Table 5: Antidepressants on comorbid medical conditions.**

| *Comorbid condition* | *Choice of antidepressant* |
|---|---|
| Ischemic heart disease (IHD) | Escitalopram, sertraline |
| Poststroke depression | Escitalopram, sertraline, mirtazapine |
| Epilepsy | Escitalopram, sertraline |
| Parkinson's disease | Escitalopram, sertraline, fluoxetine |
| Diabetes mellitus | Escitalopram, sertraline |
| Renal impairment | Escitalopram, sertraline, mirtazapine |
| Hepatic impairment | Escitalopram, sertraline, amitriptyline |

## CLINICAL PEARLS

A patient who is suffering from a major depressive disorder may present with low mood, lack of energy, multiple somatic symptoms, sleep disturbances, persistent sadness, anxiety symptoms, and suicidal thoughts. Thorough history taking and mental state examination, medical and surgical history should be enquired. A longitudinal history should be obtained to rule out bipolar disorder. According to ICD-11 description, a single-episode depressive disorder is characterized by the presence of one depressive episode without any prior history. A comprehensive action plan with pharmacotherapy, psychotherapy, and suicide risk assessment should be formulated for patients who are suffering from depressive disorder.

## FURTHER READINGS


1. Chaulagain A, Pacione L, Abdulmalik J, Hughes P, Oksana K, Chumak S, et al. WHO Mental Health Gap Action Programme Intervention Guide (mhGAP-IG): the first pre-service training study. Int J Ment Health Syst. 2020;14:47.
2. Gutiérrez-Rojas L, Porras-Segovia A, Dunne H, Andrade-González N, Cervilla JA. Prevalence and correlates of major depressive disorder: a systematic review. Braz J Psychiatry. 2020; 42(6):657-72.
3. Wu H, Xu L, Zheng Y, Shi L, Zhai L, Xu F. Application of the Delphi method in the study of depressive disorder. Front Psychiatry. 2022; 13:925610.
4. Šalamon Arčan I, Kouter K, Videtič Paska A. Depressive disorder and antidepressants from an epigenetic point of view. World J Psychiatry. 2022;12(9):1150-68.
5. Belleau EL, Treadway MT, Pizzagalli DA. The impact of stress and major depressive disorder on hippocampal and medial prefrontal cortex morphology. Biol Psychiatry. 2019;85(6): 443-53.
6. Helm K, Viol K, Weiger TM, Tass PA, Grefkes C, Del Monte D, et al. Neuronal connectivity in major depressive disorder: a systematic review. Neuropsychiatr Dis Treat. 2018;14:2715-37.
7. Wu Z, Su G, Lu W, Liu L, Zhou Z, Xie B. Clinical symptoms and their relationship with cognitive impairment in elderly patients with depressive disorder. Front Psychiatry. 2022;13:1009653.
8. Hetrick SE, Cox GR, Witt KG, Bir JJ, Merry SN. Cognitive behavioural therapy (CBT), third-wave CBT and interpersonal therapy (IPT) based interventions for preventing depression in children and adolescents. Cochrane Database Syst Rev. 2016;2016(8):CD003380.
9. Chakrabarty T, Hadjipavlou G Lam RW. Cognitive dysfunction in major depressive disorder: assessment, impact, and management. Focus (Am Psychiatr Publ). 2016;14(2): 194-206.
10. Health Quality Ontario. Psychotherapy for major depressive disorder and generalized anxiety disorder: a health technology assessment. Ont Health Technol Assess Ser. 2017;17(15):1-167.

# PART 13

# Pulmonology

# CHAPTER 85

# Cough and Expectoration

*Surya Kant, Jyoti Bajpai*

## INTRODUCTION

Cough is defined as a forced expulsive maneuver, usually against a closed glottis and which is associated with a characteristic sound. When severe, it leads to major decrement in the quality of life, with comorbidities such as incontinence, cough syncope, and dysphonia. It is one of the most common medical complaints, accounting for as many as 30 million clinical visits per year. Up to 40% of these complaints result in a referral to a pulmonologist. In Indian settings, a large proportion of patients (68.7%) with cough are treated empirically without a definite diagnosis. Worldwide, the prevalence of cough ranges from 5 to 40%. In India, the prevalence of cough in rural areas is 2.4–6% and in urban areas 1.7–5.4%. Cough is the most common single reason for primary care physician visits. It can cause profound physical and psychosocial complications; it has the potential to lead to a decrease in health-related quality of life **(Fig. 1)**.

According to the Ministry of Health Primary Care Survey 2010, cough (of varying durations) is the most common presentation, appearing in up to 25% of all general practitioner and polyclinic attendances
Chronic cough is one of the most common indications for referral to a pulmonary specialist
Careful history-taking and physical examination at the primary care level can narrow the diagnosis in many of these patients

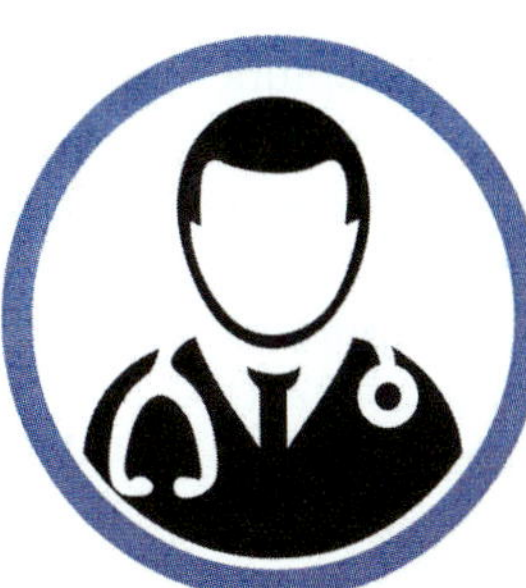

**FIG. 1:** Cough in general physician practice.

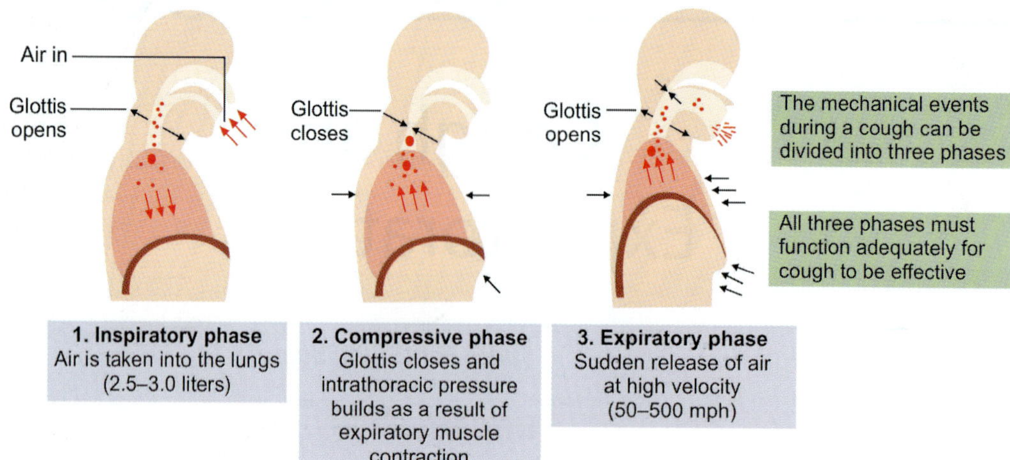


**FIG. 2:** Mechanism of cough.

## MECHANISM OF COUGH: COUGH REFLEX

There are three different phases of cough. These phases are the inspiratory phase, compressive phase, and expiratory phase **(Fig. 2)**.

The cough reflex is initiated in the upper aerodigestive tract that excites the sensory receptors, which send afferent information through neural circuits mediated by sensory neuropeptides. The integration of this neural information leads to motor commands from the brain and brainstem that make up the efferent pathway of cough.

There are intraepithelial sensory receptors that are responsible for the genesis of the cough reflex. These receptors are present in the respiratory epithelium, diaphragm, pleura, and esophagus. The most important are the rapidly adapting receptors (RAR) and the bronchial C-fiber receptors. The afferent branch of the vagus nerve, along with glossopharyngeal and phrenic nerves, is responsible for the origin of the cough reflex after these receptors are triggered. The efferents, on the other hand, supply the expiratory muscles of respiration, diaphragm, and larynx, leading to the bout of cough **(Fig. 3)**.

## CLASSIFICATION OF COUGH (FLOWCHART 1)

On the basis of the presence or absence of associated expectoration, cough is of the following two types:

1. Dry cough
2. Wet cough

Cough can also be classified into the following three types according to its duration:

1. Acute cough (<3 weeks)
2. Subacute cough (3–8 weeks)
3. Chronic cough (>8 weeks)

When chronic cough proves intractable to standard-of-care treatment, it can be referred to as refractory chronic cough (RCC). Chronic cough is now understood to be a condition of neural dysregulation. Chronic cough and RCC result in a serious, often unrecognized, disease burden.

### Acute Cough

Acute cough is defined as cough of a duration <3 weeks. Acute cough can set in due to infectious causes such as sinusitis, influenza, pneumonia, and infective bronchitis. Based on a survey of Indian patients visiting primary care clinics, upper and lower respiratory tract infections were the cause of cough in 12.2% and 8.1% of patients, respectively.

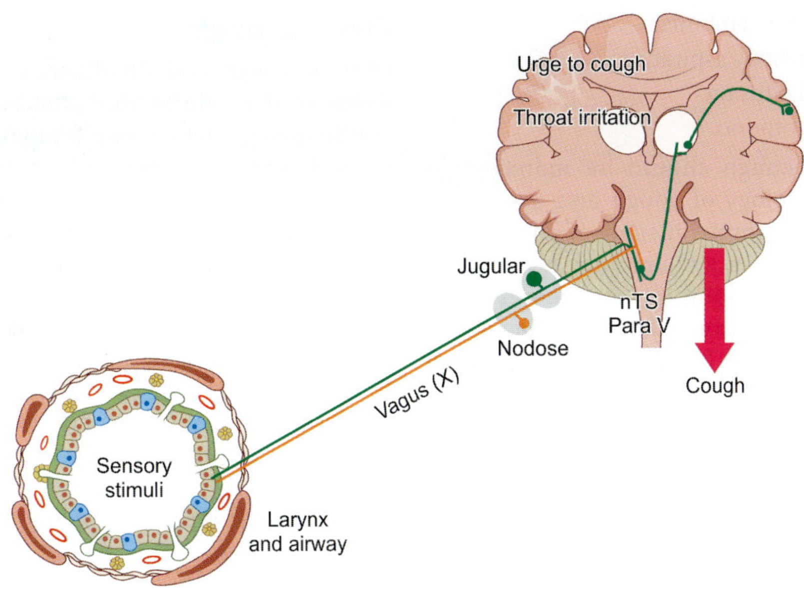


**FIG. 3:** Key elements in cough reflex—simplified flowchart.

*Note:* Vagal afferents transmit stimuli from the airways to the nucleus tractus solitarius (nTS) and paratrigeminal nucleus (para V) in the brainstem. Neuronal signals are then transmitted to the somatosensory cortex via the thalamus, causing throat irritation and the urge to cough. These sensations, if great enough, lead to cough via activation of spinal motor neurons.

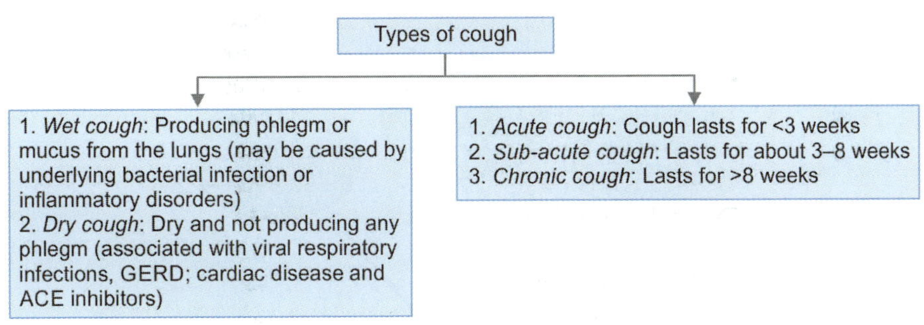


**FLOWCHART 1:** Types of cough.

(ACE: angiotensin-converting enzyme; GERD: gastroesophageal reflux disease)

In Indian settings, any cough of duration >2 weeks associated with fever, night sweats, and weight loss should prompt toward the diagnosis of tuberculosis, especially for those who are close contacts of a patient with active tuberculosis. Therefore, tuberculosis should always be ruled out before proceeding for further diagnostic workup in these patients.

Common causes responsible for an acute cough are as follows:

- Upper respiratory tract infections (bacterial or viral)
- Pneumonia
- Pulmonary tuberculosis
- Asthma
- Congestive heart failure

- Pulmonary embolism
- Foreign body aspiration
- Pleural effusion
- Pneumothorax

Acute cough should be managed as per the etiology of cough and associated signs. For example, if signs of choking are present, the acute cough may be due to a foreign body aspiration and may require urgent bronchoscopy. If it is associated with fever and coryza, it can be due to an upper respiratory tract infection. If there is marked seasonal variation in cough, the patient might be a case of allergic rhinitis/bronchial asthma. If high-grade fever, expectoration, chest pain, and hemoptysis are associated, the cause could be a pneumonia. Sometimes cardiac conditions, specifically heart failure leading to pulmonary edema, will also lead to the development of acute cough and should be promptly managed by diuretics.

Therefore, the treatment of acute cough is chiefly centered on the cause that is giving rise to the cough.

## Chronic Cough

Chronic cough is defined as a cough of 8 weeks or more duration and is a common and frequently debilitating symptom that is often viewed as an intractable problem. The main reason to classify cough on this time basis is that 3–4 weeks allows most simple infective causes of cough to have resolved by this time and identifies those children with chronic cough that might require further investigations **(Fig. 4)**. Chiefly, pulmonary causes of chronic cough are as follows:

- Chronic (nonobstructive) bronchitis and chronic obstructive pulmonary disease (COPD)
- Asthma and other eosinophilic diseases
- Lung tumors
- Infectious diseases
- Diffuse parenchymal lung disease (DPLD) (systemic diseases with diffuse lung involvement)
- Aspiration and reactive airway dysfunction syndrome (RADS)
- Bronchiectasis and cystic fibrosis

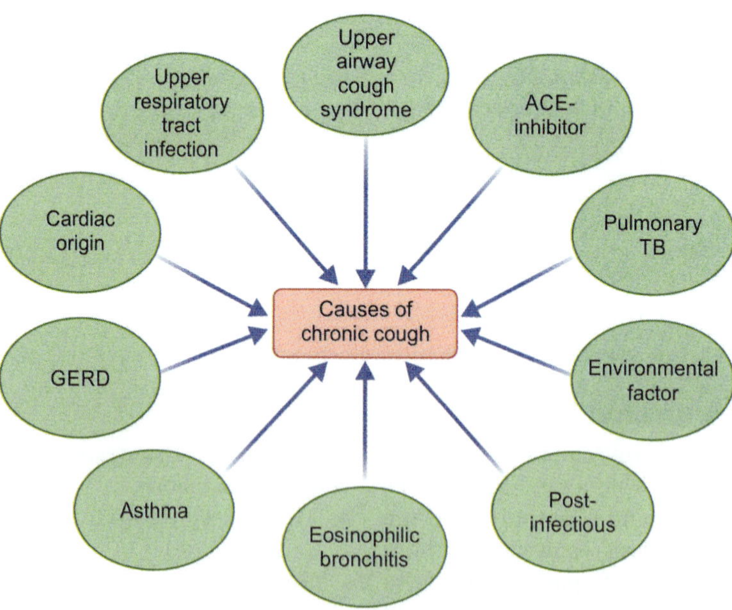


**FIG. 4:** Causes of chronic cough.

(ACE: angiotensin-converting enzyme; GERD: gastroesophageal reflux disease; TB: tuberculosis)

- Bronchomalacia
- Rare, localized disease of the tracheobronchial tree
- Drug induced
- Psychogenic cough

Cough of cardiac origin can also lead to chronic symptoms and should be suspected based on the presence of the following:

- History of cardiac illness
- Presenting symptoms such as paroxysmal nocturnal dyspnea/orthopnea

Such patients should be immediately referred to a cardiologist for further workup.

Since the list of causes leading to a chronic cough is extensive, it requires a systematic assessment.

If a patient has clinical signs and symptoms suggestive of a specific etiology such as post nasal drip (PND), gastroesophageal reflux disease (GERD), asthma, use of angiotensin-converting enzyme (ACE) inhibitors, tuberculosis, pneumonia, or COPD, then he should be treated for the same and the response should be assessed.

If the patient has no signs and symptoms that are leading to a specific diagnosis or is not responding to the treatment, but there is a strong suspicion of a pulmonary disease, then he should be further investigated in a systematic fashion according to the algorithm mentioned in **Flowchart 2**.

So, a careful clinical history may provide important diagnostic clues that allow for targeted therapeutic trials without the need for further investigations.

The smoking history and the quantity and character of sputum (if any) should be detailed in full. Chronic cough in cigarette smokers is dose-related and may be productive of mucoid or mucopurulent secretions as a result of chronic bronchitis, or it may be dry as a result of the irritant effects of cigarette smoke. Examination may reveal signs of airflow obstruction. Production of significant volumes (more than one cup per day) of sputum suggests particular pathologies. In the most common, bronchiectasis, the secretions are purulent and related to changes in posture. Examination may reveal digital clubbing, halitosis, localized or generalized coarse crepitations, or signs of airflow obstruction. Diagnosis of these causes of productive cough is usually straightforward, and strategies for intervention and treatment are well defined. Chronic dry or poorly productive cough poses a greater diagnostic challenge. A history of ACE inhibitor therapy should be sought as 15% of patients on ACE inhibitors develop dry cough soon after the commencement of therapy, and the cough usually abates with cessation of treatment, but resolution may take several months, and the cough may persist in a small minority.

Several studies have shown that in nonsmokers with normal chest radiography who are not taking ACE inhibitors, chronic cough is usually due to asthma, rhinosinusitis, or gastroesophageal reflux (GER). Symptoms suggesting these underlying diagnoses may be absent, but important clues within the history frequently go unrecognized. Abnormal physical signs are rare in patients with chronic dry cough. Wheeze, chest tightness, and dyspnea outside a paroxysm of coughing suggest asthma but may be entirely absent in cough-variant asthma (CVA). Variability from day to day and nocturnal exacerbation is suggestive. Wheeze may be audible on examination but is usually absent in CVA. Rhinosinusitis may be suggested by a history of nasal obstruction or congestion, rhinorrhea, sneezing, purulent nasal discharge, facial pain, PND (the sensation of secretions dripping down the back of the throat), or repetitive throat-clearing. Examination of the pharynx may reveal erythema, a “cobblestone” appearance of the posterior pharyngeal mucosa, or mucoid or purulent secretions dripping from the nasopharynx. Unfortunately, many pharyngeal signs and symptoms also occur in reflux disease. GER may be suggested by the presence of classic symptoms such as dyspepsia, heartburn, or waterbrash, but

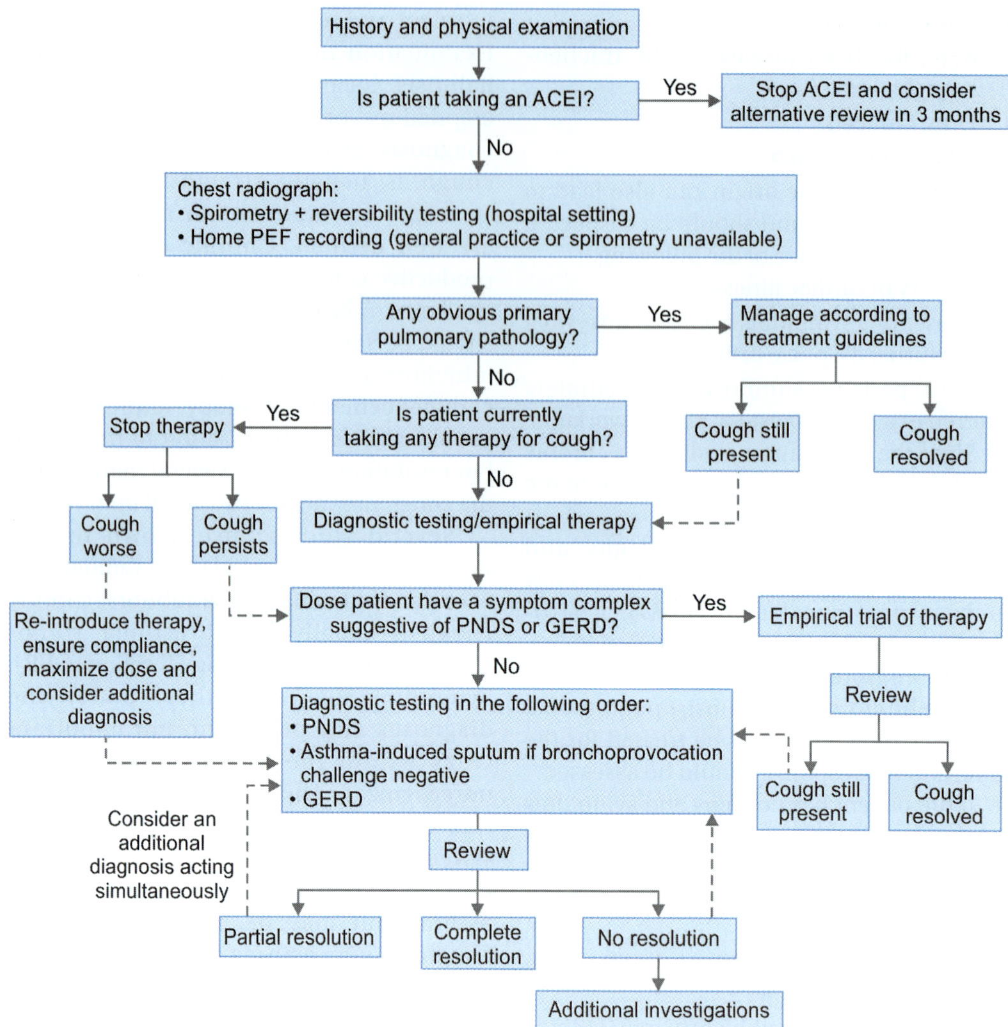


**FLOWCHART 2:** Overview of evaluation of chronic cough.

(ACEI: angiotensin-converting enzyme inhibitors; GERD: gastroesophageal reflux disease; PEF: peak expiratory flow; PNDS: postnasal drip syndrome)

symptoms such as hoarse voice, aphonia, and globus are increasingly recognized. Reflux is usually caused by transient relaxation of the low esophageal sphincter (LES). Thus, cough may occur after meals or during eating or when supine, bending, or stooping. Cough usually diminishes during sleep as the LES closes and recurs on adopting an upright posture. Talking or laughing may precipitate reflux cough since the diaphragm is an important component of the LES. GER is more common in, although not restricted to, overweight patients.

## Post-COVID Cough

Coughing is one of the most common symptoms of COVID-19. The prevalence of long-term post-COVID-19 cough, almost 1 year after COVID-19, could be considered smaller than expected. Previous meta-analyses reported a pooled prevalence of post-COVID-19 cough, ranging from 14 to 18%, at follow-ups shorter than 3 months after infection. The prevalence of long-term post-COVID-19 cough was smaller (2.5%), suggesting that maybe post-COVID-19 cough naturally decreases during the first year after SARS-CoV-2 infection. There are various mechanisms of post-COVID chronic cough, such as inflammation, epithelial damage, mucus impaction, and neuromodulatory changes (heightened cough reflex sensitivity). The approach to post-COVID cough is given in **Flowchart 3**.

Cough is also divided into wet and dry on the basis of presence or absence of expectoration.

- *Dry cough*: Not associated with expectoration
- *Wet cough*: Associated with expectoration

Characteristics of expectorated sputum often suggest the diagnosis of its cause **(Table 1)**. Chronic expectoration of large amounts of purulent and foul-smelling sputum is strongly suggestive of bronchiectasis. Sudden production of copious, sometimes blood-stained sputum in a febrile patient indicates a lung abscess. Sometimes, the color of the sputum can click the accurate diagnosis in a patient as rust-colored purulent sputum is seen in pneumococcal pneumonia, currant jelly and sticky sputum in *Klebsiella pneumoniae*, blood-tinged sputum in diseases such as tuberculosis, carcinoma lung, and pulmonary vasculitis. If the sputum is pink and frothy, it points toward the presence of pulmonary edema.

## TREATMENT

The management of patients with chronic cough can be prolonged and complex, especially in patients with multiple comorbidities requiring treatment and when the cough may ultimately be refractory to such interventions. Therefore, management includes treatment of comorbid conditions that are potentially driving chronic cough and

**Table 1: Characteristics of expectoration.**

| *Type* | *Characteristics* | *Associated pathology* |
|---|---|---|
| Purulent | Thick, yellow/green sputum | Infectious—pneumonia, bronchiectasis, and abscess |
| Mucoid | Clear, gray/white | Chronic obstructive pulmonary disease and asthma |
| Serous | Clear, frothy, can be pink | Pulmonary edema |
| Blood | Blood | Malignancy, pulmonary embolus, clotting disorders, infection |

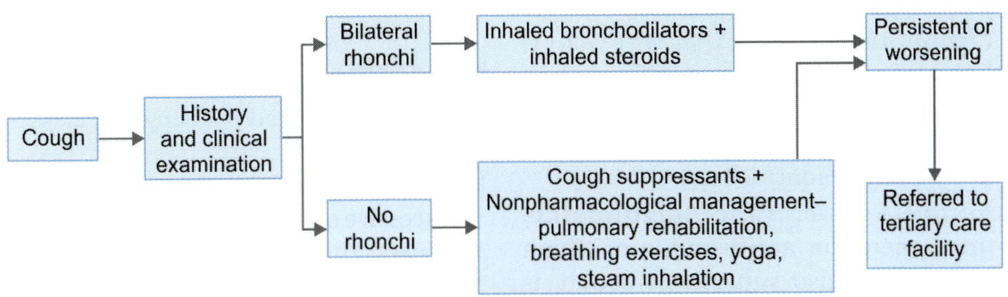


**FLOWCHART 3:** Approach to post-COVID-19 cough.

therapies directed at cough hypersensitivity in patients with refractory or unexplained cough.

## Disease-specific Therapy

For many adults with chronic cough, treatment of comorbid asthma, GERD, or nasal disease [upper airway cough syndrome (UACS)] improves their cough.

## Management of Dry Cough

Dry cough is generally managed by antitussive therapies. Antitussive therapies should be considered in patients with chronic dry cough when the cause of the increased cough reflex is unexplained, and treatment against the potential aggravating factors is not satisfactory.

For the management of dry cough, the following options are available for treatment:

- *Centrally acting opioids*: Codeine, which is given in the dose of 10–20 mg, is also effective in painful cough and additionally inhibits ciliary action, but it causes sedation. In addition to its antitussive property, codeine has analgesic and sedative effects, which may be useful in relieving painful cough.
- *Centrally acting nonopioids*: Dextromethorphan, which is actually a D-isomer of codeine itself, has no action on ciliary action as it does not cause sedation. It is given in the dose of 10–30 mg. It is nonaddictive and does not depress respiration in the usual doses. However, it has no significant analgesic or sedative properties.
- *Central as well as peripherally acting*: Levocloperastine is a novel nonopioid antitussive that acts both centrally on the cough center and on peripheral receptors in the tracheobronchial tree.
- *Antihistaminic*: Chlorpheniramine, first-generation antihistaminic, which additionally also suppresses cough, is recommended by the American College of Chest Physicians (ACCP) for the management of UACS.
- *Neurogenic cough*: Gabapentin and pregabalin are used for neurogenic cough not controlled by conventional antitussives. They cause calcium channel blockage and lead to a decrease in neurotransmitter release responsible for the genesis of cough. These are recommended in unexplained chronic cough. Gabapentin can be given in the dose of 300 mg OD, and its dose can be gradually increased (maximum dose 1,800 mg), whereas pregabalin is given at a lower dose, with the maximum dose being 300 mg/day.
- *Benzonatate*: It is a newer compound used for treating dry cough. It is peripherally acting and anesthetizes stretch receptors in the lung and pleura. It is given at a dose of 200 mg per tablet.
- *Thalidomide*: It is used mainly in cough caused due to idiopathic pulmonary fibrosis; although its mechanism is not fully understood, it is used in the dose of 100 mg OD for its anti-inflammatory and antifibrotic properties.
- *Nebulized lignocaine*: It can also be used as a resort to combat refractory cough. It is generally used in the dose of 3 mL of 4% lignocaine given thrice daily.

### *Home Remedies: Local Sialogogues*

Some natural remedies may help to relieve a cough, such as honey, ginger, acacia, glycerin, wild cherry, adequate hydration, humidification of air, steam inhalation, and demulcents (such as TurmNova lozenges).

## Management of Wet Cough

Wet cough is treated by using two classes of drugs, namely:

1. Expectorants that help to cough out the excessive secretions
2. Mucoactive agents that help in thinning out the viscous and mucoid secretion so that they can be easily coughed out

Expectorants act as irritants to the respiratory epithelium. They reduce the viscosity of respiratory secretions and finally remove them by ciliary action.

Examples of expectorants are guaifenesin, the most commonly used expectorant, potassium iodide, bromhexine hydrochloride, and ambroxol.

Mucoactive agents include three types of drugs:

1. *Mucolytic*: *N*-acetylcysteine, deoxyribonuclease (DNAase)
2. *Mucoregulators*: Glucocorticoids, macrolides, and anticholinergics
3. *Mucokinetics*: 3% NS and humidification with steam

Other than the drugs for controlling the acute bout of cough, if the patient is diagnosed with an obstructive airway disease, then specific inhaled medications in accordance with the patient's need, compliance, comfort, and affordability should be instituted as early as possible.

## FUTURE PROSPECTS

The hypothesis that adenosine triphosphate (ATP) is a neurotransmitter acting *via* specific purinergic receptors was first proposed by Geoffrey Burnstock in the 1970s. Subsequent research demonstrated that ATP is a cotransmitter in all peripheral and central nerves, leading to the investigation of purinergic receptor antagonists in a wide range of settings, including pain, overactive bladder, endometriosis, and chronic cough. The development of new potential treatments for RCC including the first-in-class P2X3 and P2X2/3 receptor antagonist gefapixant as well as more recently developed eliapixant (BAY 1817080), filapixant (BAY 1902607), sivopixant (S-600918), and agents acting on other pathways has provided new insights into the pathophysiology of RCC, including the role of P2X3 receptors in humans.

## CONCLUSION

Chronic cough is a cough that lasts for longer than 8 weeks. It is associated with significant distress and impairment in the quality of life. The three most common causes are UACS, asthma, and GERD, though many conditions, respiratory and extra-respiratory, can cause chronic cough. The initial evaluation for the patient with chronic cough relies on a thorough history and physical examination.

## CLINICAL PEARLS

- Chronic cough is a cough that lasts for longer than 8 weeks. It is associated with significant distress and impairment in the quality of life.
- The three most common causes are UACS, asthma, and GERD, though many conditions, respiratory and extra-respiratory, can cause chronic cough.
- The initial evaluation for the patient with chronic cough relies on a thorough history and physical examination.

## FURTHER READINGS

1. Shields MD, Bush A, Everard ML, McKenzie S, Primhak R. Recommendations for the assessment and management of cough in children. Thorax. 2008;63(Suppl. 3):iii1-5.
2. Apte K, Madas S, Barne M, Chhowala S, Gogtay J, Salvi S. Prevalence of cough and its associated diagnoses among 204,912 patients seen in primary care (PC) in India. Eur Respir J. 2016;48:PA864.
3. Pacheco A, Cobeta I, Wagner C. Refractory chronic cough: new perspectives in diagnosis and treatment. Arch Bronconeumol. 2013; 49(4):151-7.
4. Guleria R, Dhar R, Mahashur A, Ghoshal AG, Jindal SK, Talwar D, et al. Indian consensus on diagnosis of cough at primary care setting. J Assoc Physicians India. 2019;67(1):92-8.

5. Morice AH. The diagnosis and management of chronic cough. Eur Respir J. 2004;24(3):481-92.
6. Mahashur A. Chronic dry cough: diagnostic and management approaches. Lung India. 2015;32(1):44.
7. Kumar R, Behera D, Kant S, Menon B, Goel N, Spalgais S, et al. Post-COVID-19 respiratory management: expert panel report. Indian J Chest Dis Allied Sci. 2020;62:179-91. [Indian J Chest Dis Allied Sci. 2020;103(6):902-6.]
8. Pavord ID, Chung KF. Management of chronic cough. Lancet. 2008;371(9621):1375-84.
9. Aliprandi P, Castelli C, Bernorio S, Dell'Abate E, Carrara M. Levocloperastine in the treatment of chronic nonproductive cough: comparative efficacy versus standard antitussive agents. Drugs Exp Clin Res. 2004;30(4):133-41.
10. Li J, Ye L. Effect of pregabalin for the treatment of chronic refractory cough: a case report. Medicine. 2019;98(23):e15916.
11. Dicpinigaitis PV, Gayle YE, Solomon G, Gilbert RD. Inhibition of cough-reflex sensitivity by benzonatate and guaifenesin in acute viral cough. Respir Med. 2009;103:902-6.
12. Srivastava R, Kundu A, Pradhan D, Jyoti B, Chokotiya H, Parashar P. A comparative study to evaluate the efficacy of curcumin lozenges (TurmNova®) and intralesional corticosteroids with hyaluronidase in management of oral submucous fibrosis. J Contemp Dent Pract. 2021;22:751-5.
13. Morice A, Dicpinigaitis P, McGarvey L, Birring SS. Chronic cough: new insights and future prospects. Eur Respir Rev. 2021;30:210127.
14. Abdulqawi R, Dockry R, Holt K, Layton G, McCarthy BG, Ford AP, et al. P2X3 receptor antagonist (AF-219) in refractory chronic cough: a randomised, double-blind, placebo-controlled phase 2 study. Lancet. 2015;385:1198-205.
15. Smith JA, Kitt MM, Butera P, Smith SA, Li Y, Xu ZJ, et al. Gefapixant in two randomised dose-escalation studies in chronic cough. Eur Respir J. 2020;55:1901615.

# CHAPTER 86

# Hemoptysis

*Surya Kant, Jyoti Bajpai*

## INTRODUCTION

Hemoptysis is the expectoration of blood that originates from the lower respiratory tract. Bleeding from the upper airways is excluded from this definition. Massive hemoptysis is a potentially life-threatening emergency and requires rapid diagnosis and treatment. Although over 90% of hemoptysis are self-limiting, both the diagnosis and the treatment of massive hemoptysis are challenging.

True hemoptysis, with the source of bleeding in the airways or lungs, must be distinguished from pseudohemoptysis, where the blood originates from the upper gastrointestinal (GI) tract or the upper respiratory tract (mouth, nose, or throat). Pseudohemoptysis occurs due to infections with *Serratia marcescens*, which produces a red pigment. So, there is red expectoration, but there are no red blood cells (RBCs) in the sputum. False hemoptysis/spurious hemoptysis is bleeding from the upper aerodigestive tract (gums, nose, or pharynx). The vast majority of cases of hemoptysis occur in adults (mean age 62 years, male:female ratio 2:1); only rarely are children affected.

## SEVERITY OF HEMOPTYSIS

Hemoptysis is usually a self-limiting event, but in fewer than 5% of cases, it may be massive. It is mainly classified by the amount of blood expectorated into mild, moderate, and massive. Massive hemoptysis is either ≥500 mL of expectorated blood over a 24-hour period or bleeding at a rate ≥ 100 mL/h. A large volume of expectorated blood alone does not define massive hemoptysis; rather, an amount of blood sufficient to threaten the patient's life can be a more correct and functional definition of severe hemoptysis. Massive hemoptysis is usually a life-threatening condition with a mortality rate of >50%. Flooding of the airways with blood leads to asphyxiation, and this is usually the cause of death rather than exsanguination.

Hemoptysis should be differentiated from hematemesis as shown in **Table 1**.

## ETIOLOGY

*Two arterial vascular systems supply blood to the lungs*: Pulmonary arteries and bronchial arteries. The pulmonary arteries provide 99% of the arterial blood to the lungs and are involved in gas exchange. The bronchial arteries supply nourishment to the extra- and intrapulmonary airways. The bronchial arteries are direct branches of the aorta; hence, the blood flow is at systemic pressure, while pulmonary arteries have one-third of the systemic pressure. In cases of severe hemoptysis, the source of bleeding usually

**Table 1: Differentiation of hemoptysis from hematemesis.**

| *Hemoptysis* | *Hematemesis* |
|---|---|
| There is usually a tingling sensation in the throat prior to the episodes | Patient will usually complain of nausea and upset stomach |
| The blood is frothy and bright red | Blood is dark red, brown, and nonfrothy |
| Blood is associated with mucus | Blood is associated with food particles |
| pH will be neutral to alkaline | Blood will give an acidic pH |
| Stool examination for occult blood is usually negative | Stool is almost always positive for occult blood |
| There is history of lung disease | There is history of liver disease |
| Not associated with melena | Associated with melena |
| Patient is usually a smoker | Patient is usually an alcoholic |
| Asphyxia is possible and common | Asphyxia is unusual |

originates from bronchial vessels (in 90% of cases) and pulmonary arteries in 5% of cases.

The common causes that are to be searched for in a case of hemoptysis are given in **Table 2**.

## ANATOMY AND PATHOPHYSIOLOGY

*The lungs receive blood from two sources*: The pulmonary arteries, which are responsible for gas exchange, and the remaining capillaries. 1% is derived from the bronchial arteries. Bronchial arteries run parallel to the bronchi and branch off to supply the trachea, bronchi (peribronchial plexus), and the vasa vasorum of the pulmonary vessels. Bronchopulmonary anastomoses connect the bronchial arteries to the pulmonary arteries. The blood is drained venous from the bronchial arteries primarily through the bronchial veins into the right atrium but also through the pulmonary veins into the left atrium.

When the pulmonary arterial circulation is compromised, the secretion of neoangiogenic growth factors leads to bronchial artery proliferation.

Such impairments can be caused by the following:

- Hypoxia-induced vasoconstriction
- Thrombosis or pulmonary arterial thromboembolism
- Vasculitis is a type of autoimmune disease
- Chronic inflammatory or malignant lung disease
- Pulmonary arteriovenous fistula (e.g., Osler disease)

Because of the thinner, more fragile bronchial artery walls, the systemic arterial pressure load, and the opening of the arteries into chronically inflamed zones or neoplasms, airway ruptures and hemorrhages occur, manifesting clinically as hemoptysis. Angiographic and bronchoscopic studies, as well as measurements of expectorated blood oxygenation, have revealed that approximately 90% of hemoptysis originate in the bronchial arteries, 5% in the pulmonary arteries, and 5% in nonbronchial systemic arteries.

## APPROACH TO PATIENT

### History

The history should be directed toward the cause that is relevant to the setting as treatment is mainly treating the primary

**Table 2: Etiology of hemoptysis.**

| | |
|---|---|
| Infections | • Pulmonary tuberculosis<br>• Post-tuberculosis Rasmussen's aneurysm<br>• Pneumonia<br>• Lung abscess<br>• Bronchiectasis<br>• Fungal infections<br>• Hydatid cyst |
| Neoplasms | • Bronchogenic carcinoma<br>• Metastatic nodules<br>• Carcinoid tumor<br>• Bronchial adenoma<br>• Hamartoma |
| Cardiovascular disorders | • Mitral stenosis<br>• Pulmonary infarction from thromboembolism |
| Trauma | • Penetrating lung injury<br>• Lung contusion |
| Hematologic disorders | Blood dyscrasia |
| Autoimmune disorders | • Goodpasture syndrome<br>• Wegener's granulomatosis<br>• Small- and medium-vessel vasculitis |
| Metabolic disorders | • Uremia<br>• Liver cirrhosis |
| Vascular disorders | • Pulmonary arteriovenous malformation (PAVM)<br>• Osler–Weber–Rendu syndrome<br>• Takayasu arteritis |
| Drug induced | • Antiplatelet drugs<br>• Anticoagulant drugs<br>• Nonsteroidal anti-inflammatory drugs (NSAIDs)<br>• D-penicillamine |

cause. The color, amount of blood, and associated symptoms should be asked to determine the cause of hemoptysis and to differentiate from upper GI bleed or bleeding from the nasal tract. Old age and smoking should warrant search for malignancy. Constitutional symptoms such as fever, fatigue, malaise, and expectoration are usually seen in infectious causes. Recurrent childhood infections, recurrent sinusitis, and infertility can be associated with bronchiectasis or cystic fibrosis. Foul-smelling copious expectoration with postural variation is usually seen in lung abscess. Joint pains, skin lesions, epistaxis, hematuria, and a family history might be a clue to autoimmune disorders. Bronchogenic carcinoma might be associated with hoarseness of voice, superior vena cava (SVC) obstruction, loss of weight, and appetite. Sudden-onset chest pain and dyspnea can be a feature of pulmonary thromboembolism.

# EXAMINATION

## Physical Examination

The severity of anemia has to be assessed. Clubbing may be a feature of bronchiectasis, cystic fibrosis, lung abscess, and pulmonary arteriovenous malformation (PAVM). The oral and nasal cavities should be examined to find alternate sources of bleeding. Pedal edema might give a clue toward a cardiovascular cause. The patient might have tachypnea, tachycardia, use of accessory muscles, cyanosis, fatigue, and diaphoresis, indicating any respiratory or cardiac cause. Features of SVC obstruction are seen in malignancy, and nasal septal deformity is associated with Wegener's granulomatosis.

## Respiratory System

Auscultation of the lungs plays an important role in localizing lesions. Findings that should be kept in mind are focal wheeze and crepitations.

## Other System Examination

Auscultation of the heart will be helpful in finding murmur of mitral stenosis or mitral regurgitation, which are important causes of hemoptysis. Examination of skin helps in identifying bruising—potentially suggestive of coagulopathy, telangiectasia of Osler–Weber–Rendu, palpable purpura, or other rash suggestive of vasculitis.

# INVESTIGATIONS

## Biochemical Tests

*Hemoglobin and blood counts*: Hemoglobin levels can be low due to hemoptysis, which should be corrected either orally or parenterally depending on the degree of anemia. Leukocyte count is an important indicator of infection in conditions such as pneumonia, lung abscess, and bronchiectasis.

*Renal function tests*: Deranged urea and creatinine levels indicate conditions such as Goodpasture syndrome, Wegener's granulomatosis, and uremia. Urine microscopic examination might give clues to diagnose occult bleeding in the urinary tract and renal conditions such as vasculitis that may be a primary cause of hemoptysis.

*Bleeding profile*: Prothrombin time/international normalized ratio (PT/INR), bleeding time, and clotting time should be done to detect intrinsic clotting defects. Deranged coagulation profile due to any cause can lead to hemoptysis. They include immune thrombocytopenic purpura (ITP), disseminated intravascular coagulation (DIC), and drug use such as antiplatelets and warfarin.

## Bacteriologic

Sputum examination for acid-fast bacilli, Gram stain, and fungal elements, along with culture, should be done in suspected infective cases.

# IMAGING

## Chest X-ray

Chest X-ray (CXR) is considered the initial imaging modality for evaluating patients with hemoptysis. It is quick, inexpensive, and readily available. It can assist in lateralizing bleeding and reveal a focal or diffuse lung involvement. CXR may detect underlying parenchymal and pleural abnormalities such as mass, pneumonia, chronic lung disease, atelectasis, cavitary lesion, and alveolar opacities due to alveolar hemorrhage.

## Contrast-enhanced Computed Tomography Thorax

Since the sensitivity of CXR is not very high and all causes of hemoptysis cannot be delineated by CXR, it is essential to get a contrast-enhanced computed tomography (CECT) thorax in certain subgroups of patients. It represents a noninvasive and highly useful imaging tool in the clinical context of hemoptysis and allows a comprehensive evaluation of the lung parenchyma, airways, and thoracic vessels by using contrast material. Computed tomography (CT) may identify the bleeding site in 63–100% of patients with hemoptysis and has the ability to uncover the potential underlying causes of bleeding, such as bronchiectasis, pulmonary infections, and lung cancer.

### Computed Tomography Pulmonary Angiography

Computed tomography pulmonary angiography is important to identify the origin and course of arteries causing the bleeding. Pulmonary hemorrhage usually appears as focal or diffuse hazy consolidation or ground-glass opacity, even though thickened interlobular septa superimposed on a background of ground-glass attenuation ("crazy paving" pattern) have also been described.

### Bronchoscopy

For many years, bronchoscopy has been considered the primary method for diagnosing and localizing hemoptysis, especially if massive. Bronchoscopy, performed with either a rigid or flexible endoscope, is helpful in identifying active bleeding and for the assessment of the airways in patients with massive hemoptysis. Bronchoscopy yields additional information about endobronchial lesions, mucosal abnormality, and site for biopsy and allows samples for tissue diagnosis, microbial cultures, bronchoalveolar lavage (BAL) fluid for cell counts, cultures, and brush smears. Moreover, with bronchoscopy, cold saline solution can be instilled directly into the airways at the level of the bleeding source, if identified, and balloon inflation or laser coagulation may be used to control hemorrhage.

### Rheumatologic

Perinuclear antineutrophilic cytoplasmic antibody (p-ANCA), cytoplasmic antineutrophilic cytoplasmic antibody (c-ANCA), rheumatoid factor (RA), anticyclic citrullinated peptide (anti-CCP) are important indicators for immune-mediated diseases such as vasculitis and rheumatologic disorders.

## MANAGEMENT

### Historical Perspective

In olden days, pneumoperitoneum was created artificially by injecting air into the peritoneal cavity. This led to elevation of the diaphragm and compression of lung segments, causing suppression of bleeding by tamponade action over affected vessels. But, with the development of newer, more effective modalities of treatment and due to lack of familiarity with this procedure, it is no longer practiced and only has a historical significance **(Table 3)**.

### Management of Massive Hemoptysis

#### *Primary Management*

Management of massive hemoptysis is always an emergency. Maintenance of airway is the primary management. Oxygen saturation should be checked, and oxygen supplementation must be given. Patients with massive hemoptysis should be immediately placed into a position in which the presumed bleeding lung is in the dependent position to protect the healthy lung. Patients with massive hemoptysis are typically tachycardic and may become hypotensive. Such patients should be managed with volume resuscitation. Crystalloid intravenous fluids are generally administered first. However, blood products are an appropriate alternative in patients who are coagulopathic, anemic, and/or bleeding rapidly. Patients with massive hemoptysis may also have arrhythmias that are probably a consequence of respiratory distress and hypoxemia.

**Table 3: Initial assessment of hemoptysis.**

| *Action* | *Purpose* |
|---|---|
| Monitor the vital parameters | Registration of pulse-oximetric oxygen saturation ($SpO_2$), respiratory, and circulatory function [noninvasive blood pressure (NIBP) measurement]; assessment of risk involved in interventional procedures and medicinal treatment |
| Give oxygen | Improvement of oxygenation |
| Place the patient with the bleeding side down | Prevention of the flow of endobronchial blood into unaffected lung segments |
| Sedation/anxiolytics | Calming of the patient, facilitation of diagnostic and therapeutic measures (*Note*: Restriction of breathing activity, ability to expectorate, ability to cooperate/communicate) |
| *In massive hemoptysis*: Endotracheal or, if required, unilateral endobronchial intubation | Maintenance of gas exchange |

## Management of Cause

### *Bronchoscopy*

In patients with massive hemoptysis, after initial stabilization of the patient, bronchoscopy should be done to detect the site of bleeding and perform interventions. The various therapeutic options are balloon tamponade, cold saline lavage, topical agents such as epinephrine, vasopressin, laser therapy, and electrocautery.

## Surgical Management

Patients with unilateral, uncontrollable bleeding should be evaluated by a thoracic surgeon early. Surgical management is useful in cases where bronchoscopy fails. Typical diseases where thoracic surgery plays a role include bronchiectasis, aspergilloma, and healed tubercular lesions. The various surgeries include surgical lung resection through lobectomy and pneumonectomy. However, morbidity and mortality associated with surgical management are high.

Until the 1980s, the primary treatment for hemoptysis was surgery, which had a mortality rate of 37–42% in the emergency scenario and 7–18% in the interval between bleeding events. Recurrent hemoptysis is treated with lobectomy and pneumonectomy. It is not used when the lung parenchyma is diffusely involved; rather, a localized lesion is an indication for surgical intervention.

### *Bronchial Artery Embolization*

Bronchial artery embolization (BAE) is a safe and effective nonsurgical treatment for patients with massive hemoptysis. BAE has been extensively used in the management of hemoptysis in patients with aspergilloma. However, this approach has proved to be only temporarily effective, and recurrence of hemoptysis usually occurs because of the presence of collateral vessels in the involved area. Hence, BAE seems to be appropriate only as a "bridge" procedure in patients with massive hemoptysis until surgical resection.

## Management of Mild-moderate Hemoptysis

All patients having hemoptysis should be advised complete bed rest. The diseased side should be kept in a dependent position while lying down so that the affected blood vessels are compressed due to gravity.

Measures should be taken to suppress cough as it produces undue strain over these vessels. The commonly used cough suppressants include dextromethorphan (central cough suppression) and levocloperastine (peripheral cough suppression). Codeine preparations are no longer recommended. Hemostatic agents should be given as primary management. Tranexamic acid is an antifibrinolytic drug that prevents plasmin from binding to and degrading fibrin. Ethamsylate is a hemostatic agent that increases capillary endothelial resistance and promotes platelet adhesion. Botropase is an aqueous solution of the enzyme hemocoagulase (derived from the venom of a species of pit viper) and acts as a hemostatic drug reserved for patients with massive hemoptysis. Prophylactic antibiotics should be given to all patients with hemoptysis as blood is a good culture media. Anxiolytics are also prescribed to relieve anxiety and stress associated with hemoptysis. In addition to these general measures, adequate treatment of the primary cause should be undertaken **(Flowchart 1)**.

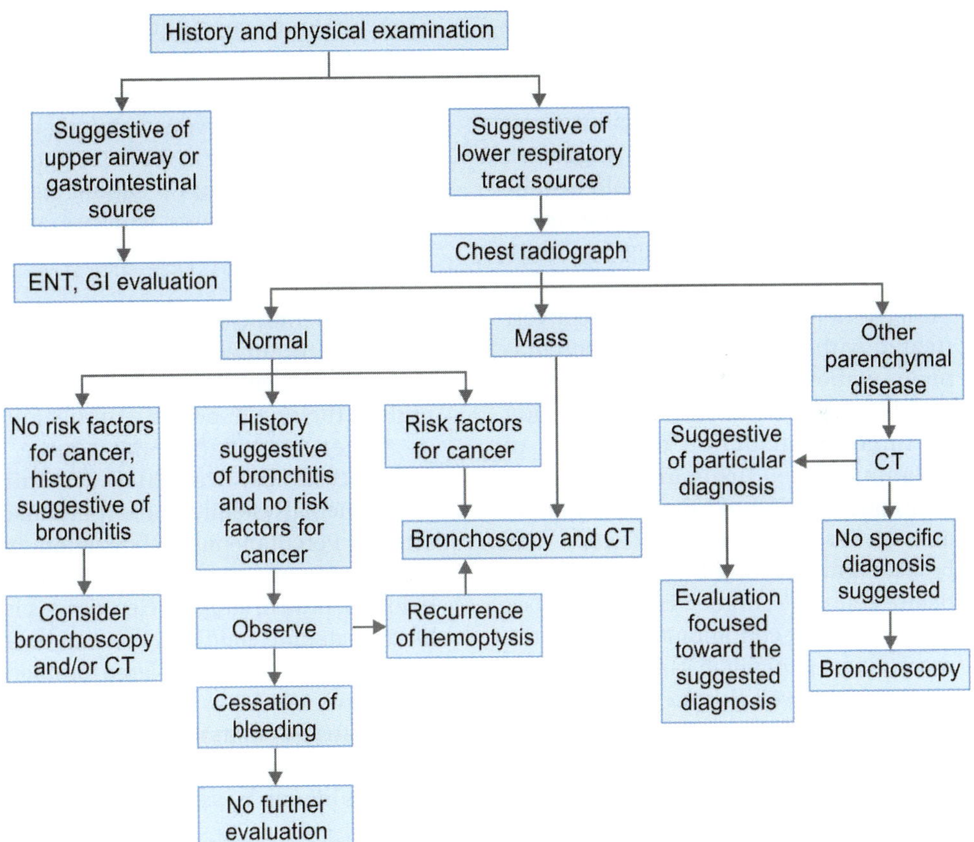


**FLOWCHART 1:** Evaluation of nonmassive hemoptysis.

(CT: computed tomography; ENT: ear, nose, and throat; GI: gastrointestinal)

*Source*: Fauci AS, Kasper D, Braunwald E, Hauser S, Longo DL, Jameson JL, et al. Harrison's Principles of Internal Medicine, 17th edition. New York: McGraw Hill Education; 2008.

## CONCLUSION

The following recommendations are the result of evidence-based consensus by the American College of Radiology Appropriateness Criteria Expert Panel on thoracic radiology:

- Initial evaluation of patients with hemoptysis should include a chest radiograph.
- Patients at high risk for malignancy (>40 years old, >40 pack-year smoking history) with negative chest radiograph, CT scan, and bronchoscopy can be followed with observation for the following 3 years. Radiography and CT are recommended imaging modalities for follow-up. Bronchoscopy may complement imaging during the period of observation.
- In patients who are at high risk for malignancy and have suspicious chest radiograph findings, CT is suggested for initial evaluation; CT should also be considered in patients who are active or ex-smokers, despite a negative chest radiograph.
- Massive hemoptysis can be effectively treated with either surgery or percutaneous embolization. Contrast-enhanced multidetector CT before embolization or surgery can define the source of hemoptysis as bronchial systemic, nonbronchialsystemic, and/orpulmonary arterial. Percutaneous embolization may be used initially to halt the hemorrhage before definitive surgery. Hemoptysis is a life-threatening condition that can be the presenting complaint in a large number of respiratory as well as systemic disorders. If the cause of hemoptysis is diagnosed in time and aggressively managed, the patient's life can be saved.

## CLINICAL PEARLS

The following recommendations are the result of evidence-based consensus by the American College of Radiology Appropriateness Criteria Expert Panel on thoracic radiology:

- Initial evaluation of patients with hemoptysis should include a chest radiograph.
- Patients at high risk for malignancy (>40 years old, >40 pack-year smoking history) with negative chest radiograph, CT scan, and bronchoscopy can be followed with observation for the following 3 years. Radiography and CT are recommended imaging modalities for follow-up. Bronchoscopy may complement imaging during the period of observation.
- In patients who are at high risk for malignancy and have suspicious chest radiograph findings, CT is suggested for initial evaluation; CT should also be considered in patients who are active or ex-smokers, despite a negative chest radiograph.
- Massive hemoptysis can be effectively treated with either surgery or percutaneous embolization. Contrast-enhanced multidetector CT before embolization or surgery can define the source of hemoptysis as bronchial systemic, nonbronchialsystemic, and/orpulmonary arterial. Percutaneous embolization may be used initially to halt the hemorrhage before definitive surgery. Hemoptysis is a life-threatening condition that can be the presenting complaint in a large number of respiratory as well as systemic disorders. If the cause of hemoptysis is diagnosed in time and aggressively managed, the patient's life can be saved.

## FURTHER READINGS

1. Jeudy J, Khan AR, Mohammed TL, Amorosa JK, Brown K, Dyer DS, et al. ACR appropriateness criteria hemoptysis. J Thorac Imaging. 2010;25:W67-9.
2. Lordan JL, Gascoigne A, Corris PA. The pulmonary physician in critical care illustrative case 7: assessment and management of massive haemoptysis. Thorax. 2003;58:814-9.
3. Ibrahim WH. Massive haemoptysis: the definition should be revised. Eur Respir J. 2008;32:1131.
4. Hirshberg B, Biran I, Glazer M, Kramer MR. Hemoptysis: etiology, evaluation, and outcome in a tertiary referral hospital. Chest. 1997;112:440-4.
5. Reisz G, Stevens D, Boutwell C, Nair V. The causes of hemoptysis revisited. A review of the etiologies of hemoptysis between 1986 and 1995. Mo Med. 1997;94:633-5.
6. Bruzzi JF, Remy-Jardin M, Delhaye D, Teisseire A, Khalil C, Remy J. Multi-detector row CT of hemoptysis. Radiographics. 2006;26:3-22.
7. Kant S, Mehra S. An interesting case of haemoptysis. Int J Pulmon Med. 2007;9(1).
8. Kant S, Verma S. Fungal ball presenting as haemoptysis. Int J Pulmon Med. 2008;10(1):1-4.
9. Chamilos G, Kontoylannis DP. Aspergillus, Candida and opportunistic mold infections of the lung. Fishman's Pulmonary Diseases and Disorders, 4th edition. New York: McGraw Hill; 2008. pp. 2291-304.
10. Chun JY, Morgan R, Belli AM. Radiological management of hemoptysis: a comprehensive review of diagnostic imaging and bronchial arterial embolization. Cardiovasc Intervent Radiol. 2010;33:240-50.
11. Kant S, Singhal S, Verma SK. Allergic bronchopulmonary aspergillosis presenting as haemoptysis: a case report. J Inter Med India. 2006;9(2):62-4.
12. Jean-Baptiste E. Clinical assessment and management of massive hemoptysis. Crit Care Med. 2000;28(5):1642-7.
13. Hsiao EI, Kirsch CM, Kagawa FT, Wehner JH, Jensen WA, Baxter RB. Utility of fiberoptic bronchoscopy before bronchial artery embolization for massive hemoptysis. AJR Am J Roentgenol. 2001;177:861-7.
14. Roebuck DJ, Barnacle AM. Haemoptysis and bronchial artery embolization in children. Paediatr Res Rev. 2008;9(2):95-104.
15. Yoon W, Kim JK, Kim YH, Chung TW, Kang HK. Bronchial and nonbronchial systemic artery embolization for life-threatening hemoptysis: a comprehensive review. Radiographics. 2002;22(6):1395-409.
16. Deffebach ME, Charan NB, Lakshminarayan S, Butler J. The bronchial circulation: small, but a vital attribute of the lung. Am Rev Respir Dis. 1987;135(2):463-81.
17. Earwood JS, Thompson TD. Hemoptysis: evaluation and management. Am Fam Physician. 2015;91(4):243-9
18. Kant S, Bajpai J, Bajaj DK, Pathak R, Rajagopal TV. Pulmonary hydatid cyst presenting with hemoptysis. Ind J Immunol Res Med. 2017;2(2):58-9.
19. Bajpai J, Bajaj DK, Kushwaha RA, Kant S, Pradhan A, Verma AK, et al. A rare cause of hemoptysis in a young female. J Med Sci. 2022;42:42-5.
20. Fartoukh M, Khoshnood B, Parrot A, Khalil A, Carette MF, Stoclin A, et al. Early prediction of in-hospital mortality of patients with hemoptysis: an approach to defining severe hemoptysis. Respiration. 2012;83:106-14.
21. Kant S. Clinical approach to hemoptysis. Clinical Methods in Respiratory Medicine. New Delhi: Jaypee Brothers Medical Publishers Pvt. Ltd; 2018. pp. 45-53.

CHAPTER 87

# Breathlessness

*Purbasha Biswas*

## INTRODUCTION

Breathlessness or dyspnea is one of the most common presenting symptoms seen by clinicians. The causes can be several, ranging from pulmonary, cardiac, anemia, obesity, and psychogenic. As causes are many and variable, it is essential to differentiate between life-threatening causes from benign ones.

## DEFINITION

The American Thoracic Society consensus statement defines dyspnea as the "subjective experience of discomfort in breathing, which consists of qualitatively distinct sensations that vary in intensity. The experience derives from interactions among multiple social, environmental, physiological, psychological, and others and induces secondary physiological and behavioral responses."

## EPIDEMIOLOGY

Dyspnea is seen in 50% of patients admitted in tertiary care hospitals under acute conditions and in 25% of patients under ambulatory settings.

## ASSESSMENT

There are a number of emerging tools that have been developed for the assessment of dyspnea. For example:

- Modified Medical Research Council (MMRC) dyspnea scale—to assess the symptoms of chronic obstructive pulmonary disease (COPD) **(Table 1)**.

**Table 1: Modified Medical Research Council classification.**

| Grade | Description |
|---|---|
| 0 | Not troubled by breathlessness except with strenuous exercise |
| 1 | Shortness of breath walking on level ground or with walking up a slight hill |
| 2 | Walks slower than peers on level ground or has to stop while walking at own pace |
| 3 | Stops to rest after walking 100 m or after walking a few minutes on level ground |
| 4 | Too breathless to leave the house or breathless with activities of daily life |

- New York Heart Association (NYHA) functional classification **(Tables 2 and 3)**.

**Table 2: New York Heart Association classification.**

| Class | Patient symptoms |
|---|---|
| I | No limitation of physical activity. Ordinary physical activity does not cause undue fatigue, palpitation, or dyspnea (shortness of breath) |
| II | Slight limitation of physical activity. Comfortable at rest. Ordinary physical activity results in fatigue, palpitation, and dyspnea (shortness of breath) |
| III | Marked limitation of physical activity. Comfortable at rest. Less than ordinary activity causes fatigue, palpitation, or dyspnea |
| IV | Unable to carry on any physical activity without discomfort. Symptoms of heart failure at rest. If any physical activity is undertaken, discomfort increases |

**Table 3: New York Heart Association subclassification.**

| Class | Objective assessment |
|---|---|
| A | No objective evidence of cardiovascular disease. No symptoms and no limitation in ordinary physical activity |
| B | Objective evidence of minimal cardio-vascular disease. Mild symptoms and slight limitation during ordinary activity. Comfortable at rest |
| C | Objective evidence of moderately severe cardiovascular disease. Marked limitation in activity due to symptoms, even during less-than-ordinary activity. Comfortable only at rest |
| D | Objective evidence of severe cardio-vascular disease. Severe limitations. Experiences symptoms even while at rest |

## CAUSES

- *Cardiac causes*:
    - Heart failure
    - Coronary artery disease
    - Arrhythmia
    - Pericarditis
    - Valvular heart disease
- *Respiratory causes*:
    - COPD
    - Asthma
    - Pneumonia
    - Acute respiratory distress syndrome (ARDS)
    - Pneumothorax
    - Pulmonary embolism
    - Pleural effusion
    - Lung cancer
- *Upper airway obstruction*:
    - Epiglottitis
    - Foreign body
    - Croup
- *Others*:
    - Anaphylactic reaction
    - Laryngeal spasm
    - Anemia
    - Metabolic acidosis

## APPROACH TO BREATHLESSNESS

The approach to breathlessness is shown in **Flowchart 1**.

## POSSIBLE PRESENTING SYMPTOMS

- *Pulmonary symptoms*:
    - Chest tightness
    - Tachypnea
    - Air hunger
    - Increased work of breathing
    - Inability to get a deep breath
- *Cardiac symptoms*:
    - Chest tightness
    - Air hunger

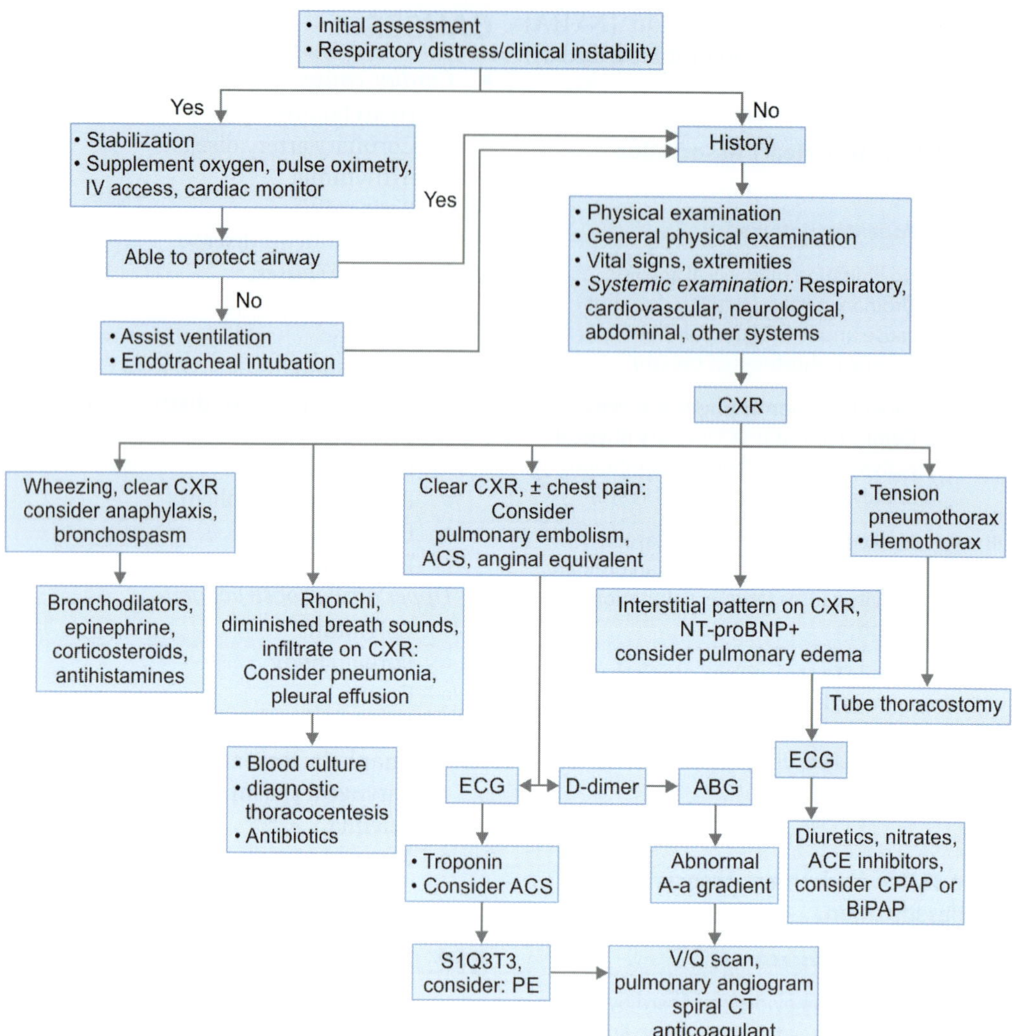


**FLOWCHART 1:** Algorithm for evaluating an adult patient presenting with acute dyspnea.[19]

(A–a: alveolar–arterial; ABG: arterial blood gas; ACE: angiotensin-converting enzyme; ACS: acute coronary syndrome; BiPAP: biphasic positive airway pressure; CPAP: continuous positive airway pressure; CT: computed tomography; CXR: chest X-ray; ECG: electrocardiogram; IV: intravenous; NT-proBNP: N-terminal pro-brain natriuretic peptide; PE: pulmonary embolism; V/Q: ventilation–perfusion ratio)

- *Others*:
  - Exertional breathlessness
  - Poor fitness
  - Anxiety

## INVESTIGATIONS

- *Pulmonary causes*:
  - Spirometry
  - Chest X-ray
  - High-resolution computed tomography (HRCT) thorax
  - D-dimer
- *Cardiac causes*:
  - Electrocardiogram (ECG)
  - ECHO
  - Brain natriuretic peptide (BNP)
  - Stress ECHO

- *Others*: Hematocrit and exclude other causes

## TREATMENT

Depending on the etiological and clinical examination, further diagnostic work-up is planned, and the patient is administered appropriate treatment.

## CONCLUSION

A detailed history, appropriate triage, clinical examination, appropriate use of laboratory investigations, and images are essential for specific evaluation and management of patients presenting with dyspnea.

## CLINICAL PEARLS

- Distinguishing cardiac from respiratory causes of dyspnea is important for treatment purposes.
- It is of utmost importance to identify acute and emergency causes for urgent intervention.
- Infections are one of the cardinal causes and should always be given priority as they are treatable condition.

## FURTHER READINGS

1. American Thoracic Society. Dyspnea. Mechanisms, assessment, and management: a consensus statement. Am J Respir Crit Care Med. 1999;159:321-40.
2. Brenner S, Güder G. The patient with dyspnea. Rational diagnostic evaluation. Herz. 2014;39:8-14.
3. Hammond EC. Some preliminary findings on physical complaints from a prospective study of 1,064,004 men and women. Am J Public Health Nations Health. 1964;54:11-23.
4. Bowden J, To T, Abernethy A, Currow D. Predictors of chronic breathlessness: a large population study. BMC Public Health. 2011; 11:33.
5. Hawthorne VM, Watt GC, Hart CL, Hole DJ, Smith GD, Gillis CR. Cardiorespiratory disease in men and women in urban Scotland: baseline characteristics of the Renfrew/Paisley (midspan) study population. Scott Med J. 1995;40:102-7.
6. Ailani RK, Ravakhah K, DiGiovine B, Jacobsen G, Tun T, Epstein D, et al. Dyspnea differentiation index: a new method for the rapid separation of cardiac vs pulmonary dyspnea. Chest. 1999;116:1100-4.

CHAPTER 88

# Chest Wall Deformities

*Purbasha Biswas*

## INTRODUCTION

Chest wall deformity (CWD) is an abnormality of the chest structure, ranging from mild to severe. These deformities occur when the cartilage that connects the ribs grows in an uneven fashion. The exact cause is not clear, but the conditions tend to run in families.

## CLASSIFICATION

The classification of CWDs is based on the morphological site of deformities, extending from the sternum to the vertebrae. This "CWDs morphological classification" divides CWDs into five types **(Table 1)**.

## OUTLINE

- Pectus excavatum
- Pectus carinatum
- Poland's syndrome
- Sternal defects
- Cleft sternum
- Ectopic cordis
- Thoracic deformities in diffuse skeletal disorders

### Pectus Excavatum

- Pectus excavatum is also called funnel chest or trichterbrust **(Fig. 1)**.
- It occurs due to the posterior depression of the sternum and costal cartilage.

**Table 1: Morphological classification of chest wall deformities.**

| *Classification* | *Deformity (anatomical site)* | *Characteristic presentation* |
|---|---|---|
| Type 1 | Sternum | Cleft sternum (±ectopia cordis), Currarino–Silvermann syndrome |
| Type 2 | Costal cartilage | Pectus excavatum, pectus carinatum |
| Type 3 | Rib | Simple complex (±syndrome) |
| Type 4 | Combined costal cartilage and ribs | Poland's syndrome VACTER syndrome |
| Type 5 | Costovertebral junction | Osteogenesis imperfecta syndromic |

*Note*: VATER syndrome/VACTERL association.

- First and second ribs and manubrium are in normal position, but lower costal cartilage and the body of the sternum are depressed.
- There is a frequent asymmetry in the depression (right > left).
- It presents at birth or within the first year of life in the majority, about 86%.
- It rarely resolves with increasing age.
- It may be associated with scoliosis (26%), asthma (5.2%), and congenital heart disease (CHD) (1.5%).

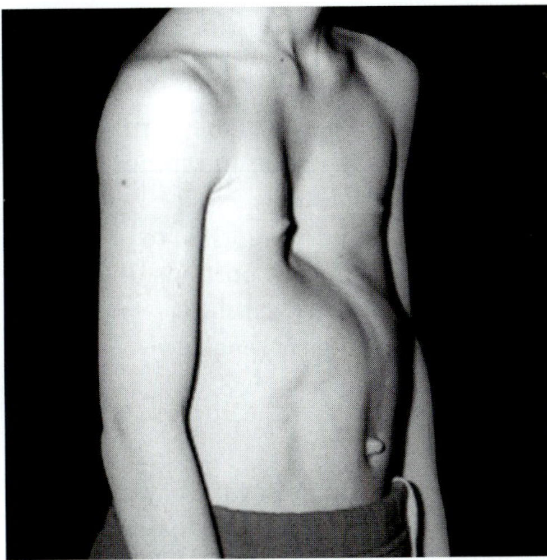

**FIG. 1:** Pectus excavatum.

## Etiology and Incidence

- It occurs in 1 in 400 live births.
- The exact etiology is unknown.
- There is a variable pattern of inheritance.
- It occurs more among boys (boys:girls = 4:1).
- It can be multifactorial.

## Symptoms

- It is well tolerated in infancy and childhood **(Figs. 2A to C)**.
- *In older children*:
  - There is pain in the area of deformed cartilage.
  - Precordial pain occurs after sustained exercise and palpitations.
  - They suffer from transient atrial arrhythmias.
  - They may have mitral valve prolapse.

## Pathophysiology

- *Cardiac and pulmonary functions*:
  - *Systolic ejection murmur (SEM)*: Closed proximity of the sternum and the pulmonary artery, results in the transmission of flow murmur.
  - *Electrocardiogram (EKG)*: Displacement and rotation of heart in the left thoracic cavity
  - Conduction blocks or arrhythmias

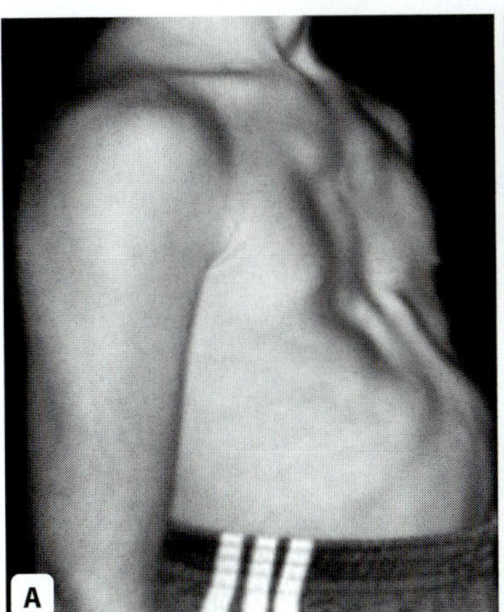


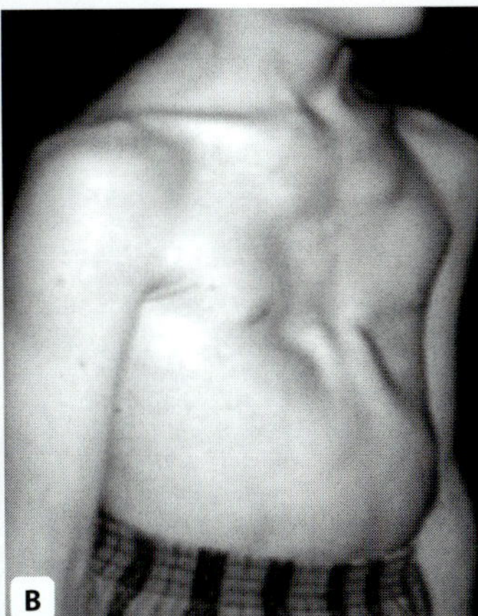


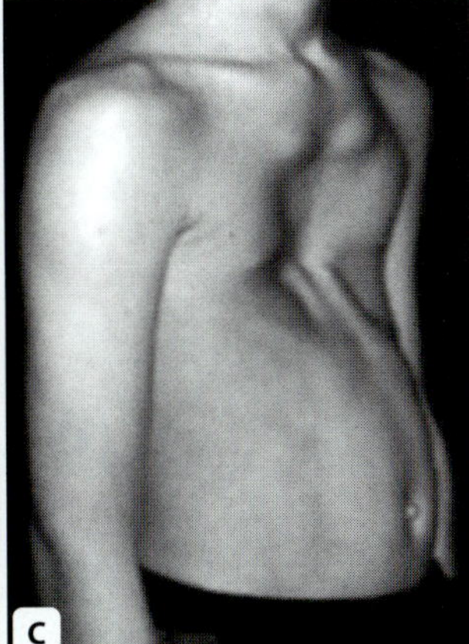


**FIGS. 2A TO C:** Grades of pectus excavatum.

- *Workup*:
  - Computed tomography (CT) scan of the chest
  - Pulmonary function test (PFT)
  - ECHO
- *Quality of life analysis postsurgery*:
  - Significant improvement:
    - Exercise tolerance
    - Shortness of breath and fatigue
- *Indications of surgery*:
  - Progressive symptoms
  - Restricted disease, decreased work production, or oxygen uptake as demonstrated by PFTs
  - CT scan shows cardiac compression or displacement.
  - Haller index > 3.25
  - Pulmonary atelectasis
  - Mitral valve prolapse, bundle branch block
  - Recurrent pectus excavatum after repair
- *Timing of surgery*:
  - Can be performed in younger children with severe exercise tolerance
  - Best deferred until after the pubertal growth spur
- *Surgical procedures* **(Figs. 3A and B)**:
  - Ravitch procedure
  - Nuss procedure
  - Haller and associates; tripod fixation
  - Judet and Jung procedure
  - Taguchi and associates

## Pectus Carinatum

- Pectus carinatum is more common in boys than girls (78:22).
- It is of a mild form at birth but often progresses during early childhood **(Figs. 4A to D)**.
- The chondromanubrial deformity is often noted at birth.
- *Treatment*: Wedge osteotomy

## Poland's Syndrome

- There is hypoplasia of the sternal head of the pectoralis major and minor muscles **(Figs. 5A to C)**.
- Normal underlying ribs to complete absence of anterior portions of the 2nd–5th ribs and costal cartilage
- *Treatment*: Surgical repair

## Cleft Sternum

- There is complete or partial separation of the sternum but a normal positioned intrathoracic heart.

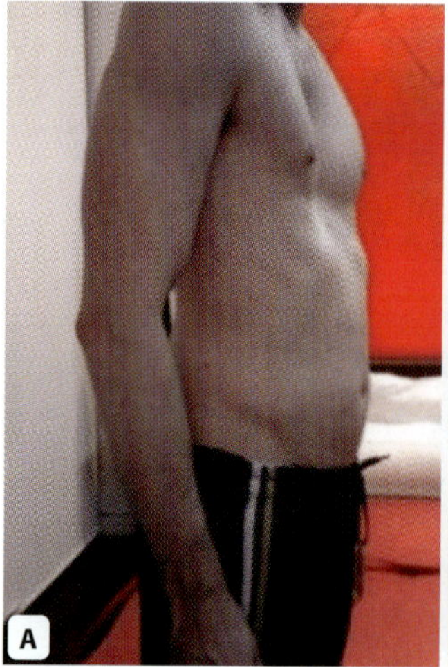


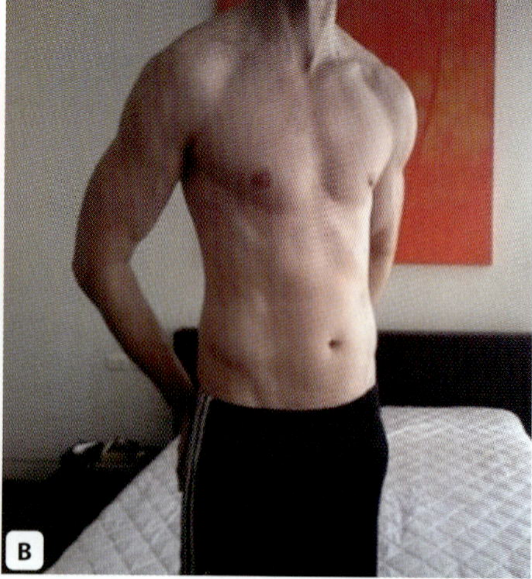


**FIGS. 3A AND B:** Pectus excavatum patient (A) 3 days before surgery and (B) 19 months post surgery.

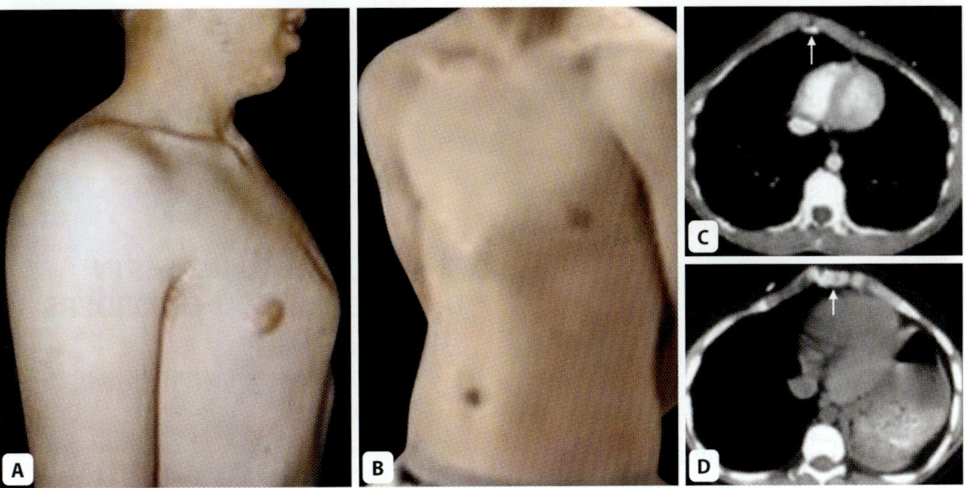

**FIGS. 4A TO D:** Pectus carinatum.

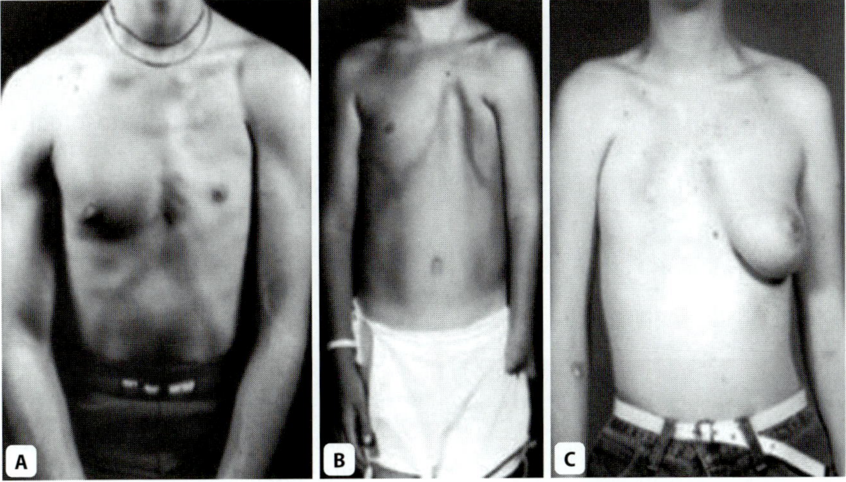

**FIGS. 5A TO C:** Poland's syndrome.

- It results from nonfusion of the sternal bars.
- Normal skin coverage is present.
- The pericardium is intact and the diaphragm is normal.
- Omphaloceles do not occur in these children.
- Dramatic increase in the deformity occurs with crying or Valsalva maneuver.
- *Treatment*: Surgical repair

## Ectopia Cordis

- *There are two types*:
  - Thoracic ectopia cordis
  - Thoracoabdominal ectopia cordis (Cantrell's pentalogy)
- *Etiology*:
  - Disruption of the amnion and chorionic layer or yolk sac
  - Chromosomal abnormalities have been reported.

### Thoracic Ectopia Cordis

- Severely deficient in the midline somatic tissues that normally cover the heart **(Fig. 6)**.
- Many attempts at primary closure fail because of the inability to mobilize adequate tissues for coverage.
- An abdominal defect is often present as well.

### Thoracoabdominal Ectopia Cordis

- Heart is covered by an omphalocele-like membrane or thin skin, which is often pigmented **(Fig. 7)**.
- *Five essential features*:
  - A cleft lower sternum
  - A half-moon-shaped anterior diaphragmatic defect resulting from lack of development of septum transversum

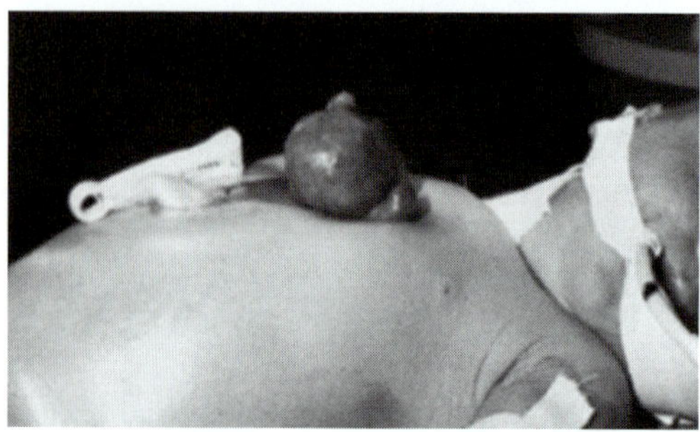

**FIG. 6:** Thoracic ectopia cordis.

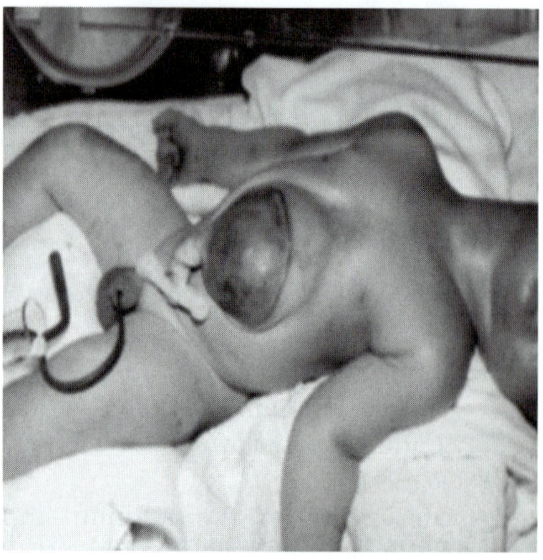

**FIG. 7:** Thoracoabdominal ectopia cordis.

  - Absence of the parietal pericardium at the diaphragmatic defect.
  - Omphalocele
  - In most patients, an intrinsic cardiac anomaly
- *Treatment*: Surgical repair

## THORACIC DEFORMITIES IN DIFFUSE SKELETAL DISORDERS

There are two types:

1. *Asphyxiating thoracic dystrophy (Jeune's syndrome)*:
   a. Narrow, rigid chest and multiple cartilage anomalies **(Figs. 8A to C)**
   b. Bell-shaped thorax and protuberant abdomen
   c. Patient dies of respiratory insufficiency early
   d. Form of osteochondrodystrophy, which has variable degrees of skeletal involvement
   e. Inherited in an autosomal recessive pattern
   f. Not associated with chromosomal abnormalities
   g. Short, stubby extremities with relatively short, wide bones
   h. Clavicles fixed and lie in elevated position
   i. Involves variable degrees of pulmonary impairment
2. *Spondylothoracic dysplasia (Jarcho-Levin syndrome)*:
   a. Autosomal recessive deformity **(Fig. 9)**
   b. Multiple vertebral and rib malformations
   c. Multiple alternating hemivertebrae in most or all of the thoracic and lumbar spine
   d. Vertebral ossification centers rarely cross the midline.
   e. Bone formation is normal.
   f. Crab-like appearance of the ribs on the chest radiograph
   g. Thoracic deformity is secondary to the spine anomaly.

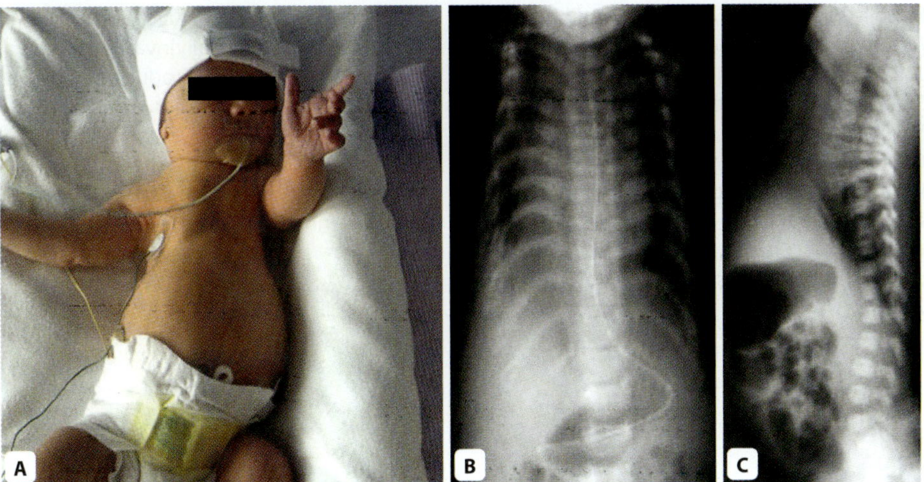


**FIGS. 8A TO C:** Asphyxiating thoracic dystrophy/Jeune's syndrome.

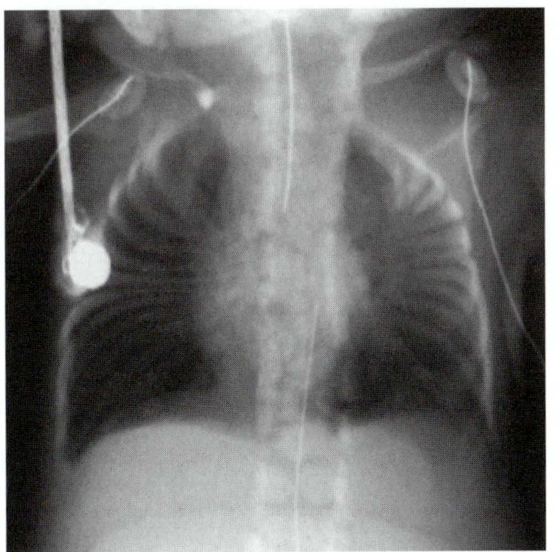

**FIG. 9:** Spondylothoracic dysplasia (Jarcho–Levin syndrome).

h. Results in close posterior approximation of origin of ribs.
i. Most infants die before 15 months.
j. One third of patients with this syndrome have associated malformations—CHD and renal anomalies.
k. No surgical efforts have been proposed and attempted.

## CLINICAL PEARLS

Chest deformities are of different types. However often they are clues to underlying disorders and it is important to be aware of associations with various inherited conditions.

## FURTHER READINGS

1. Abramson H, D'Agostino J, Wuscovi S. A 5-year experience with a minimally invasive technique for pectus carinatum repair. J Ped Surg. 2009; 44(1):118-24.
2. Bayramiçli M. Poland sendromu. Toraks Cerrahisi Bülteni. 2011;2:229-35.
3. Bouvet JP, Leveque D, Bernetieres F, Gros JJ. Vascular origin of Poland's syndrome? A comparative rheographic study of the vascularization of the arms in eight patients. Eur J Pediatr. 1978;128:17-26.
4. David TJ. Familial Poland anomaly. J Med Genet. 1982;19:293-6.
5. Haje SA, Raymundo JLP. Considerações sobre deformidades da parede torácica anterior e apresentação de tratamento conservador para as formas com componentes de protrusão. Rev Bras Ortop. 1979;14(4):167-78.

6. Pinsolle V, Chichery A, Grolleau J-L, Chavoin JP. Autologous fat injection in Poland's syndrome. JPRAS. 2008;61:784-91.
7. Shamberger RC. Chest wall deformities. In: Shields TW, LoCicero J, Ponn RB, Rusch VW (Eds). General Thoracic Surgery, Vol. 1, 6th edition. Philadelphia: Lippincott Williams and Wilkins; 2005. pp: 653-81.
8. Williams AM, Crabbe DCG. Pectus deformities of the anterior chest wall. Ped Respir Rev. 2003;4:237-42.
9. Erşen E, Demirkaya A, Kılıç B, Kara HV, Yakşi O, Alizade N, et al. Minimally invasive repair of pectus excavatum (MIRPE) in adults: is it a proper choice? Videosurg Other Mini-invasive Tech. 2016;11:98-104.
10. Kuhn MA, Nuss D. Pectus deformities. In: Mattei P (Ed). Fundamentals of Pediatric Surgery. New York: Springer; 2011. pp: 313-22.

CHAPTER 89

# Breath Sounds

*Supriya Sarkar*

## INTRODUCTION

Hippocrates first started "immediate auscultation," hearing breath sounds directly by placing the ear on the patient's chest wall. The art of auscultation was popularized by Laënnec in 1816, using rolled paper and later with a wooden tube.

The auscultation of the respiratory system is an inexpensive, noninvasive, safe, easy-to-perform, and one of the oldest diagnostic techniques. Auscultation includes the hearing of breath sounds, voice sounds, and adventitious sounds.

Three characteristics of breath sound must be carefully heard:

1. *Frequency and pitch*: Frequency is defined as waves per second, measured in hertz (Hz). Wavelengths and frequencies are inversely proportional. For a shorter wavelength, frequency will be higher and vice versa. Pitch is the perception of frequency.
2. *Amplitude and loudness*: Amplitude is the height from the mean value of the sound wave, measured in decibels (dB), and loudness is its perception.
3. *Timbre or quality*: It is the characteristic property that can differentiate two sounds of equal frequency and amplitude.

The following methods should be followed in auscultation:

- Auscultation is preferably done in quiet atmosphere, in a sitting position and after removing clothes.
- The patient must be instructed and demonstrated to take breaths deeply with open mouth. Always observe whether the patient is doing it rightly.
- Auscultate more than one breath cycle through the diaphragm of the stethoscope, starting from the apex to the base and anteriorly, axillary, and back. Sound intensity is low at the apices of the lung and increases progressively at lung bases. They are of less intensity at the back due to thick muscles.
- Start from the normal side and compare the normal side with the disease side at symmetrical points.
- Listen carefully to the three qualities of sounds.

Breath sound is produced by turbulent and vorticose airflow in the large airways. Turbulent airflow is chaotic, where particles collide with each other, and it requires high velocity, density, large irregular airway tube and Reynaud's number >2,000 whereas airflow in medium to small airways is laminar and parabolic that is usually silent. On the other hand, voice sounds are produced in the vocal cords. Low-pass filters (lungs and chest wall) filter high-frequency sounds, and there is a sharp drop in amplitude.

## ABSENT BREATH SOUND

Breath sound may be absent in pleural effusion and pneumothorax. Breath sound over the collapsed lung is classically absent, but we often hear transmitted sounds from nearby open airways.

Breath sounds can be divided into vesicular breath sound and bronchial breath sounds. The differences between them are given in **Table 1**. Different types of breath sounds are depicted in **Figure 1**.

## VESICULAR BREATH SOUND

Vesicular breath sound is a misnomer as the sound is not produced in vesicles (alveoli). The inspiratory component is produced in lobar and segmental bronchi; on the other hand, the expiratory component is originated in the more proximal airways, and as it moves away from the chest wall, it becomes fainter.

*Puerile vesicular breath sound*: It is basically a normal breath sound that is more clearly audible, for example, breath sounds in children, in thin-built persons, and in compensatory hyperinflation.

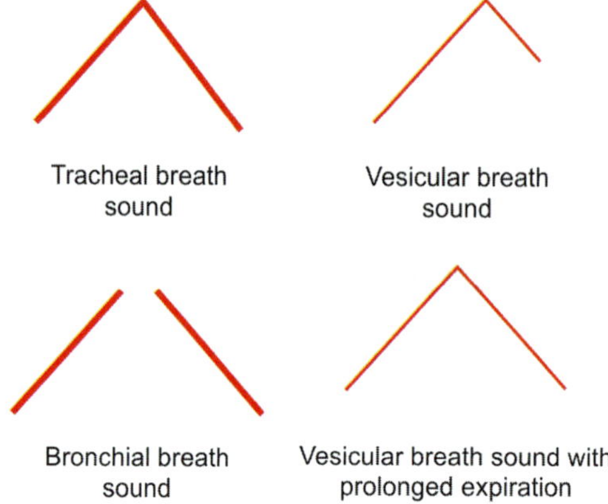


**FIG. 1:** Schematic diagram representing breath sounds.

**Table 1: The difference between vesicular and bronchial breath sounds.**

| ***Parameters*** | ***Vesicular breath sound*** | ***Bronchial breath sounds*** |
|---|---|---|
| Character of sound | Rustling, usually soft and low pitched | Blowing, loud, hollow, and high pitch |
| Gap between inspiration and expiration | Absent | There is a distinct pause between inspiration and expiration due to absent alveolar phase |
| Duration of inspiration and expiration | Inspiratory phase is longer than the expiratory phase (the ratio between them is about 2:1) | Expiratory phase is longer than the inspiratory phase or at least equal |
| Intensity and pitch | Intensity and pitch of inspiration are greater than that of expiration | Intensity and pitch of expiration are greater than that of inspiration |
| Association with vocal sounds | It is not associated with whispering pectoriloquy | It is associated with whispering pectoriloquy |
| Site where normally heard | Whole of the lungs | It is normally heard over the manubrium in the front and dorsal spine up to dorsal 3 spines in the back |
| Significance | Found over normal lung | Found over abnormal lung |

*Diminished or absent breath sound*: Intensity is reduced by weak generation (shallow breathing, airway obstruction) or decreased transmission (bulla, emphysema, pneumothorax, pleural effusion/thickening, obesity, etc.).

*Vesicular breath sound with prolonged expiration*: Expiration is as long as inspiration due to increased expiratory time. Inspiration part may be harsh. It is found in obstructive airway diseases such as asthma and chronic obstructive pulmonary disease (COPD).

## BRONCHIAL BREATH SOUND

Bronchial breath sound is high-frequency breath sounds found in conditions where the sound bypasses the filtering effect of alveoli. It is normally heard over manubrium sterni and the area between C-7 and T-3 vertebrae. The presence of whispering pectoriloquy confirms the presence of bronchial breath sound.

*Tubular bronchial*: It is a high-pitched bronchial breath sound that is found over consolidation, the upper border of pleural effusion, pulmonary fibrosis, peripheral collapse with patent bronchus, and mediastinal tumor close to a large patent bronchus.

*Cavernous bronchial*: It is a low-pitched bronchial breath sound that is found over a superficial large cavity, abscess, or bronchiectatic cavity with patent bronchi.

*Amphoric bronchial*: It is basically a low-pitched sound with high-pitched overtone having a metallic character, similar to the sound produced by blowing an empty jar (Greek word amphoreus). It is found in open pneumothorax and large (>6 cm), superficial, smooth-walled cavity with patent bronchus.

*Tracheal breath sound*: It is harsh, high-pitched, and louder sound found over the trachea. It is characterized by equality in both phases of respiration with a distinct gap in between.

*Bronchovesicular breath sound*: It is in between vesicular and bronchial breath sound in pitch and amplitude with both phases of respiration being equal. It may be found over the first and second intercostal space anteriorly and the interscapular area posteriorly.

*Cogwheel breath sound*: It is vesicular breathing with interrupted inspiratory phase found in airway obstruction by mediastinal tumor, glands, or aneurysm and in weak or nervous patients.

*Breath sound at mouth*: Breath sound audible at mouth may be found in asthma and chronic bronchitis (not in emphysema). It is often confused with stridor (a noisy inspiratory sound found in extrathoracic airway obstruction) and wheeze (a high-pitched mainly expiratory continuous sound found in intrathoracic airway obstruction).

## VOCAL RESONANCE

Voice sound is a mixture of fundamental frequency and overtones (both high- and low-frequency sound in vowels). Due to filtering effect of the lung, voice sounds are normally faintly audible. Voice sound is distinctly audible when the air in the lung is replaced by liquid or solid materials.

*Bronchophony*: It is the voice sound that is heard over consolidated lung. Bronchophony is a distinctly heard voice sound with greater clarity and intensity.

*Egophony*: When bronchophony has a nasal intonation (Ee to A) and bleating quality, it is egophony. The word egophony comes from the Greek word "ero" (goat). It is found over consolidation and the upper border of pleural effusion due to transmission of sounds through compressed lung.

*Whispering pectoriloquy*: During whispering, vocal cords do not move, resulting in a breezy sound that is faintly heard over chest wall. When it is heard distinctly and clearly, it signifies underlying lung consolidation.

# ADVENTITIOUS SOUNDS

Adventitious sounds are added respiratory sounds that are superimposed on breath sounds. They are classified into continuous adventitious sound (wheeze and rhonchi), discontinuous sound (fine and coarse crackles), squeak, pleural rub, and stridor.

## Continuous Adventitious Sound

Continuous adventitious sound lasts >250 ms. Wheezes are high-pitched continuous sounds with a dominant frequency of 400 Hz or more, and rhonchi are low-pitched continuous musical sounds with a dominant frequency of about 200 Hz or less. Wheezes are usually louder than breath sounds and more prominent over the trachea or mouth, and rhonchi are usually expiratory and better heard over the chest wall. Wheeze and rhonchi are often used interchangeably. Wheezes are heard all over the chest in asthma and COPD. Focal wheeze is found in localized airway obstruction by a foreign body, mucous plug, or tumor. Wheeze may be produced by diseases of the intrathoracic upper airway such as tracheomalacia and bronchomalacia and by extrinsic compression. Wheeze is produced by vibration or flutter of the proximal fifth to seventh generations of bronchi.

*Monophonic wheeze*: This is a single musical note having different timing of start and end. It is found in bronchial obstruction by tumor, bronchostenosis, mucus impaction, foreign, etc. Rigid obstruction causes biphasic wheeze whereas flexible obstruction causes inspiratory or expiratory wheeze depending upon the site of obstruction. Partial obstruction may rarely produce changing intensity of wheeze related to posture changes. Fixed wheeze has a long duration of constant frequency whereas random wheeze has varying frequency and duration. Monophonic wheeze in asthma is usually random.

*Polyphonic wheeze*: These are multiple musical notes, mainly expiratory, with the same timing of onset and end. They are found in dynamic obstruction of more central airway. The pitch increases at the end of expiration.

## Discontinuous Adventitious Sound

Crackles are discontinuous (25 ms or less in duration), nonmusical, explosive, and mainly inspiratory lung sounds. They are usually classified as fine and coarse crackles based on duration, loudness, pitch, and timing in the respiratory cycle, as described in **Table 2**.

Crackles signify underlying lung pathology such as fibrosis, pneumonia, COPD, pulmonary edema, interstitial lung disease (ILD), and heart failure. Fine crackles arise from small airways, medium crackles are produced by bubbling of air through mucus in small bronchi, and coarse crackles arise by bubbling of air in large bronchi or bronchiectatic lungs. Bilateral basal fine crackles are found in ILD and congestive heart failure, particularly in the early stage.

Crackles are generally classified by their relationship with the phase of respiration.

*Early inspiratory crackles*: They start at the beginning and end before mid-inspiration. They are usually coarse and found in the late stages of COPD. Crackles in COPD are produced by airway secretions in the large airway. They are gravity-independent, scanty, may be audible at mouth, and disappear after coughing.

*Late inspiratory crackles*: They start at any time after the commencement of inspiration and last till the end of inspiration. They are found in ILD, particularly idiopathic pulmonary fibrosis (IPF), desquamative interstitial pneumonia (DIP), and asbestosis.

**Table 2: Differences between fine and coarse crackles.**

| *Fine crackles* | *Coarse crackles* |
|---|---|
| Exclusively inspiratory, heard over mid to late inspiration | Generally inspiratory and may be biphasic, heard over both phases of respiration |
| Usually found in lung bases | Can be heard over any part of the thorax |
| It is short (5 ms), high pitched (about 650 Hz) and less loud sound | It is longer (15 ms), low pitched (about 350 Hz), and loud sound |
| It may be altered with body position | It is not altered with body position |
| It is not altered with coughing | It is altered with coughing |
| It is not heard at mouth | It may be heard at mouth |
| Produced by the sudden opening of small airways | Produced by air passing through vibrating (opening and closing) airways or secretions |

Their presence usually signifies subpleural fibrosis and honeycombing. They were previously described as "Velcro" crepitations.

*Expiratory crackles/biphasic crackles*: Crackles are mainly inspiratory, but sometimes they may be found during expiration. The mechanism is described as the trapped gas hypothesis. They are found in COPD, bronchiectasis, and IPF.

*Post-tussive crackles*: Crackles that appear after a bout of cough were once considered to indicate cavity in tuberculosis, lung abscess, and early pneumonia.

*Post-tussive suction*: A hissing sound produced after coughing indicates collapsible lung cavity.

### Types of Crackles Found in Different Diseases

*Crackles of bronchiectasis* are usually biphasic, loud, and coarse and found even in mild airway obstruction. They start at the beginning of inspiration, continue throughout mid-inspiration, and decline in late inspiration. Crackles may be audible at mouth. Coughing reduces crackles. *Crackles of chronic bronchitis* are early inspiratory, found only in severe airway obstruction, and are audible at mouth. *Crackles of pneumonia* are coarse and mid-inspiratory. They start in early phases and tend to be short. They tend to be end-inspiratory during the resolution phase. *Crackles of heart failure* are high-pitched late inspiratory and may extend to the expiratory phase; they are produced by the opening of narrowed airways caused by peribronchial edema. In congestive cardiac failure, crackles may be pan-inspiratory. *Crackles of IPF* are usually fine, basal, and late inspiratory, but as the disease progresses, it becomes coarser, longer, and more extensive. *Posture-induced crackles* may be found in ischemic heart disease that indicates a poor prognosis. To elicit the finding, auscultation is done over the posterior axillary line between 8th and 10th intercostal space. Firstly after positioning the patient at sitting position, then lying down at supine position, and lastly at supine position after raising patient's feet at 30° angle. If new crackles appear with a change of posture, the test is considered to be positive.

### d'Espine Sign

d'Espine sign is named after the French physician Jean Henri Adolphe d'Espine, who described a whispering sound found over the upper thoracic spinous process in trachea-bronchial lymph nodes' enlargement. Vesicular breath sounds normally heard over paraspinal areas are louder than those over the spinous process. A positive d'Espine sign means that breath sound over the spinous process is bronchial and of increased intensity than that of the paravertebral area of that level. It indicates a mass lesion/lymphadenopathy in the posterior mediastinum. Cattaneo's sign is the red spot that develops after percussion over the T1–T4 spine in d'Espine-positive patients.

### Pleural Rub

Pleural rub is a nonmusical, short, explosive, biphasic sound having a rubbing, grating, or leathery character. Classically, expiratory and inspiratory components are mirror images. The differences between the rub and crackles are depicted in **Table 3**. Rub signifies inflammation of the pleura and is usually associated with pleuritic chest pain. The presence of pleural rub usually excludes the malignant nature of pleural disease. Rarely, movements of scapula, ribs, and thoracic muscles may produce similar sound.

### Squawk

Squawk is a short (<200 ms duration), late inspiratory wheeze and is often preceded by late inspiratory crackles. It is found in fibrosis, particularly due to hypersensitivity pneumonia and bronchiolitis obliterans.

### Stridor

Stridor is a loud, musical, high-pitched sound produced by extrathoracic airway obstruction. It is primarily inspiratory sound, louder over the neck. Stridor may be found in supraglottic lesions (laryngomalacia) and vocal cord disease. it is due to turbulent flow at the narrowed upper airway. It may be biphasic in fixed upper airway obstruction like tracheal stenosis.

*Mediastinal crunch*: It is a hoarse crackling sound synchronous with systole, heard over the precordium in the presence of mediastinal emphysema.

## CONCLUSION

Careful auscultation in a quiet place after following basic principles (instruct patients, demonstrate yourselves, observe while the patient is performing, and then auscult) is an essential step in clinical medicine. Concentrate on the three qualities of breath sounds: Pitch, loudness, and quality. After auscultating breath sounds, listen for added sounds and vocal resonance. A meticulous auscultation is an essential step that not only helps in the diagnosis of diseases but also can avoid unnecessary, sometimes costly, investigations. Truly speaking, "auscultation is a poor man's investigation."

**Table 3: Difference between pleural rub and coarse crackles.**

| *Pleural rub* | *Crackles* |
|---|---|
| It is a superficial friction sound | It is an interrupted moist sound |
| It is a biphasic sound | It is usually inspiratory and may extend to expiration |
| It is localized mainly in the lateral part of the chest wall | No site predilection. Found over diseased lung |
| It is often associated with pleuritic chest pain | It is often associated with cough and expectoration |
| Pressure of the stethoscope may intensify the sound | No effect on pressing of stethoscope |
| May be palpable | It is not palpable |

## CLINICAL PEARLS

Breath sounds should be interpreted along with history and other clinical findings. As for example, bronchial breath sound with dullness indicate consolidation if mediastinum is central. The same findings with ipsilateral shifting of mediastinum indicate lung fibrosis; on the other hand, those with contralateral shifting of mediastinum indicate pleural effusion with underlying pneumonia.

The finding squawk in patient with usual interstitial pneumonia (UIP) pattern in high resolution computed tomography (HRCT) may suggest chronic hypersensitivity pneumonia.

## FURTHER READINGS

1. Forgacs P. Lung sounds. Br J Dis Chest. 1969;63: 1-12.
2. Crofton J. Physical signs in the chest. Res Medica. 1963;4:9-10.
3. Bohadana A, Izbicki G, Kraman SS. Fundamentals of lung auscultation. N Engl J Med. 2014;370:744-51.
4. Gavriely N, Nissan M, Rubin AH, Cugell DW. Spectral characteristics of chest wall breath sounds in normal subjects. Thorax. 1995;50:1292-300.
5. Forgacs P. The functional basis of pulmonary sounds. Chest. 1978;73:399-405.
6. Sánchez I, Vizcaya C. Tracheal and lung sounds repeatability in normal adults. Respir Med. 2003;97:1257-60.
7. Sarkar M, Madabhavi I, Niranjan N, Dogra M. Auscultation of the respiratory system. Ann Thorac Med. 2015;10(3):158-68.
8. Sapira JD. About egophony. Chest. 1995;108: 865-7.
9. American Thoracic Society Ad Hoc Committee on Pulmonary Nomenclature. Updated nomenclature for membership reaction. ATS News. 1977;3:5-6.
10. Forgacs P. Crackles and wheezes. Lancet. 1967;22:203-5.
11. Robertson AJ, Coope R. Rales, rhonchi, and Laennec. Lancet. 1957;2:417-23.
12. Vyshedskiy A, Alhashem RM, Paciej M, Ebril I, Rudman JJ, Fredberg R, et al. Mechanism of inspiratory and expiratory crackles. Chest. 2009;135:156-64.
13. Nath AR, Capel IH. Lung crackles in bronchiectasis. Thorax. 1980;35:694-9.
14. Piirilä P. Changes in crackle characteristics during the clinical course of pneumonia. Chest. 1992;102:176-83.
15. Piirilä P, Sovijärvi AR, Kaisla T, Rajala HM, Katila T. Crackles in patients with fibrosing alveolitis, bronchiectasis, COPD, and heart failure. Chest. 1991;99:1076-83.
16. Epler GR, Carrington CB, Gaensler EA. Crackles (rales) in the interstitial pulmonary diseases. Chest. 1978;73:333-9.
17. Deguchi F, Hirakawa S, Gotoh K, Yagi Y, Ohshima S. Prognostic significance of posturally induced crackles. Long-term follow-up of patients after recovery from acute myocardial infarction. Chest. 1993;103:1457-62.
18. Sienkiewicz TM. The clinical view of d'Espine's sign. Can Med Assoc J. 1923;13:890-2.
19. Earis JE, Marsh K, Pearson MG, Ogilvie CM. The inspiratory "squawk" in extrinsic allergic alveolitis and other pulmonary fibrosis. Thorax. 1982;37:923-6.
20. Hamman L. Mediastinal emphysema. JAMA. 1945;128:1-6.

# PART 14

# Rheumatology

CHAPTER 90

# Joint Swelling

*Udas Chandra Ghosh, Abhinaba Datta*

## WHAT IS JOINT SWELLING?

Joint swelling is one of the common complaints for which a patient may seek medical care. It can have multiple causes ranging from systemic to local. The initial role of a physician is to localize the source of the joint symptoms and to determine the possible responsible pathophysiologic process. Diagnosis may be reached with proper history and examination in most of the cases, followed by relevant investigations. Arthritis is defined as the presence of joint pain and signs of inflammation (redness, swelling, tenderness). Arthralgia is defined as the presence of only pain around a joint but no signs of inflammation.

## WHAT ARE THE CAUSES OF JOINT SWELLING?

Joints are swollen because of a number of factors:

- *Synovial effusion*: Joint fluid may be clear and acellular in association with injury, inflammatory, and cellular as in rheumatoid arthritis (RA), blood-stained as in traumatic hemarthrosis and bleeding disorders, or purulent as in pyogenic infection or acute crystal-induced synovitis.
- Bony enlargement as in osteoarthritis, Charcot joints of tabes dorsalis
- New periosteal bone depositions as in hypertrophic osteoarthropathy
- Synovial proliferation as in RA
- Rarely because of malignancy such as sarcoma

Determination of the anatomical part is often difficult but very vital. Very often, multiple factors may be contributing. The evaluation of joint pain, in terms of both the history and the physical examination findings, is best achieved through an understanding of the basic pathophysiologic types of joint disease. These include synovitis, enthesopathy, crystal deposition, infection, and structural or mechanical derangements.

*Synovitis*: The synovial membrane is the principal site of inflammation in persons with RA and many other inflammatory arthritides. It is clinically manifested as warmth, tenderness, and swelling of the soft tissues overlying the involved joint.

*Enthesitis*: It is the part where tendons and ligaments are attached to the bone. It is the principal site of seronegative arthritis.

*Crystal deposition*: The deposition of crystals in articular structures may lead to symptomatic joint disease. The responsible crystals include monosodium urate, calcium pyrophosphate dihydrate, basic calcium phosphate (including hydroxyapatite), and calcium oxalate.

*Infectious arthritis*: The synovium may become the site of acute or chronic infections related to bacterial, fungal, or viral organisms. These infections almost always arise from blood-borne organisms and may be part of a systemic infection.

*Structural or mechanical joint derangement*: Degeneration of the articular cartilage is the principal pathological feature of osteoarthritis. Trauma to the joint may also disrupt the anatomical structures.

## WHAT ARE THE POSSIBILITIES?

- *Congenital*: Achondroplasia, Fabry's disease, Down syndrome, Marfan's syndrome
- *Degenerative*: Osteoarthritis
- *Idiopathic inflammatory*: RA, spondyloarthropathy (ankylosing spondylitis, psoriatic arthritis, reactive arthritis), systemic lupus erythematosus (SLE), Sjogren syndrome, dermatomyositis, and polymyositis
- *Hematological*: Hemophilia and other bleeding disorders, leukemia, sickle cell disease
- *Infective*:
  - *Bacterial*: Staphylococcal, gonococcal, tuberculosis, syphilis, *Leptospira*, Lyme disease
  - *Viral*: Chikungunya, dengue, rubella, polio, infection mononucleosis
  - *Fungi*: Aspergillosis, *Actinomyces*, Madura foot, histoplasmosis
- *Metabolic*: Amyloidosis, gouty arthritis, hemochromatosis, Wilson disease
- *Vascular*: Granulomatosis with polyangiitis, polyarteritis nodosa
- *Neoplastic*: Sarcoma, multiple myeloma, Paget disease
- *Neuropathic*: Paraplegic syndrome, diabetic arthropathy, Charcot joints (syphilis and syringomyelia)
- *Drug induced*: Anticoagulants, corticosteroid arthropathy, serum sickness

## PATHWAY TO DIAGNOSIS

### History

- Exclude history of trauma
- The following points in history will aid in the diagnosis:
  - Articular or nonarticular involvement
  - Inflammatory or noninflammatory
  - Onset: Acute (<6 weeks) or chronic (>6 weeks)
  - Number and type of joints involved
  - Sequence of joint involvement
  - Extra-articular involvement if any
- Proper history of underlying comorbidities must be taken.
- Look for periarticular and soft-tissue rheumatism such as bursitis, tendinitis, and tenosynovitis.
- Characteristics of inflammatory joint pain include:
  - Early morning stiffness (EMS) > 30 minutes
  - Symptomatic improvement with gentle movement of the joint
  - Spontaneous flares (up and down course) are common
  - Constitutional symptoms are often present
  - Inflammatory markers [erythrocyte sedimentation rate (ESR) and C-reactive protein (CRP)] are elevated.
- *Pattern recognition of joint pain is the best marker for clinical diagnosis.*
  - *Mode of onset*:
    - Acute (<6 weeks)—rheumatic fever, gonococcal arthritis, viral arthritis
    - Chronic (>6 weeks)—RA, SLE
  - *Number of joints involved*: Monoarticular (1 joint), oligoarticular (2–3 joints), or polyarticular (4 joints or more)

- *Pattern of involvement*: Axial involvement (spine, sacroiliac, anterior chest wall, and shoulder and hip joints), appendicular involvement (peripheral joints)
- *Distribution of joint involvement*: Symmetrical or asymmetrical, small or large joints, lower limb or upper limb, involvement of any specific joint [e.g., first metatarsophalangeal joint in gout, hemarthrosis of knee joint in hemophilia, distal interphalangeal (DIP) joints of hands in osteoarthritis]
- *Order or sequence of affection*: Intermittent (gout) or progressive (classical RA), migratory (rheumatic arthritis, SLE, serum sickness), or additive (RA, reactive arthritis)
- *Extra-articular manifestations*: Constitutional symptoms, e.g., fever, rash, subcutaneous nodules, oral ulcer (SLE), uveitis or episcleritis (spondyloarthropathy), penile ulcer, nail changes (psoriasis), and Raynaud's phenomenon (scleroderma) (refer Chapter 93) **(Tables 1 to 5)**.

## Clinical Examination

- The musculoskeletal examination helps distinguish joint inflammation (e.g., RA)

**Table 1: Common causes of monoarthritis.**

| ***Acute (<6 weeks)*** | | ***Chronic (>6 weeks)*** | |
|---|---|---|---|
| ***Noninflammatory*** | ***Inflammatory*** | ***Noninflammatory*** | ***Inflammatory*** |
| • Trauma<br>• Ligament tear<br>• Meniscal tear<br>• Reflex sympathetic dystrophy<br>• Hemophilia | • Gout<br>• Pseudogout<br>• Infectious arthritis<br>• Reactive arthritis | • Osteoarthritis<br>• Osteonecrosis<br>• Neuropathic arthritis<br>• Hemochromatosis | • Psoriatic arthritis<br>• Pauciarticular JIA<br>• Indolent infection<br>• Spondyloarthropathy |

(JIA: juvenile idiopathic arthritis)

**Table 2: Common causes of polyarthritis.**

| ***Inflammatory*** | ***Noninflammatory*** |
|---|---|
| ***Acute*** | |
| • Serum sickness<br>• Acute rheumatic fever<br>• Drug-induced arthritis<br>• Early onset connective tissue disorder<br>• Viral arthritis | • Amyloid arthropathy<br>• Hemoglobinopathy |
| ***Chronic*** | |
| • Rheumatoid arthritis<br>• Polyarticular JIA<br>• Undifferentiated arthritis<br>• SLE<br>• Mixed connective tissue disorders<br>• Still's disease | • Osteoarthritis<br>• Hypothyroidism<br>• Neuropathic arthritis<br>• Metabolic arthritis<br>• Fibromyalgia |

(JIA: juvenile idiopathic arthritis; SLE: systemic lupus erythematosus)

**Table 3: Symmetrical versus asymmetrical involvement.**

| *Symmetrical* | *Asymmetrical* |
|---|---|
| • RA<br>• SLE<br>• Psoriatic arthropathy*<br>• Nodular osteoarthritis of hands<br>• JIA<br>• Hemochromatosis | • Gout<br>• Spondyloarthropathy<br>• Metabolic arthropathy |

*Psoriatic arthropathy can be symmetric or asymmetric at presentation.

(JIA: juvenile idiopathic arthritis; RA: rheumatoid arthritis; SLE: systemic lupus erythematosus)

**Table 4: Small- and large-joint involvement.***

| *Small-joint arthropathy* | *Large-joint arthropathy* |
|---|---|
| • RA<br>• SLE<br>• ReA<br>• Gout<br>• Nodular osteoarthritis<br>• Psoriasis<br>• Enteropathic arthritis | • RA<br>• ReA<br>• Ankylosing spondylitis<br>• Rheumatic arthritis<br>• Generalized osteoarthritis<br>• Psoriatic arthritis<br>• Enteropathic arthritis |

*Both large- and small-joint arthropathy: RA, spondyloarthropathy, osteoarthritis.

(RA: rheumatoid arthritis; Re A: reactive arthritis; SLE: systemic lupus erythematosus)

**Table 5: Articular versus nonarticular pain.**

| *Articular* | *Nonarticular* |
|---|---|
| • Deep or diffuse pain<br>• *Inspection*: Swelling of joint—swelling looks globular or fusiform surrounding a joint<br>• *Palpation*: Conspicuous by the presence of joint-line tenderness | • Localized pain<br>• *Inspection*: Swelling—periarticular "local" swelling around a joint<br>• *Palpation*: Tenderness is localized and usually away from joint-line margin |

from joint damage (e.g., degenerative joint disease).

- Techniques used in the musculoskeletal examination include the following:
  - Inspection
  - Palpation
  - Range of motion
- Check whether the pain is articular or not.
- *On inspection*, compare one side of the body with the other in order to detect joint abnormalities, including swelling, deformity, overlying erythema, or wasting of the periarticular musculature. Take note of joint deformities that result from the lack of full extension of a joint (e.g., flexion deformities).
- *Palpation* of the joints is used to assess for signs of inflammation (e.g., warmth, synovial hypertrophy, joint effusion, and tenderness) and signs of joint damage (e.g., bony swelling and crepitus). The examiner should palpate with enough pressure to blanch his or her thumbnail. Application of such force should not cause pain in normal joint.
- Assess *limitation of passive motion* by comparing it with the expected range of motion observed in healthy individuals

and with the range of motion in the contralateral joint.

- Assess *crepitus* by palpating the joint with one hand while moving the joint passively with the other.
- *Signs of inflammatory joint disease* include the following:
  - Synovial hypertrophy (most reliable sign)
  - Joint effusions
  - Pain with motion, particularly at the extremes of joint motion
  - Erythema and warmth
  - Limited range of motion
  - Joint tenderness
- *Signs of degenerative or mechanical joint disease* include the following:
  - Bony overgrowth of the joints (osteophytes)
  - Limited range of motion
  - Crepitus during active or passive range of motion
  - Joint deformity

## Investigations

- Screening tests for all types of inflammatory arthritis include the following:
  - ESR
  - CRP
  - Rheumatoid factor (RF) and cyclic citrullinated peptide (CCP) antibody
  - Antinuclear antibody (ANA) (if other features of SLE present)
- If septic arthritis is considered, blood culture is to be done
- Antistreptolysin O (ASO) titer for suspicion of acute rheumatic fever
- Screening tests for chronic polyarthritis include complete blood count (CBC), ESR, CRP, RF, anti-CCP, liver function test (LFT), blood sugar, serum creatinine, serum uric acid levels, and urine analysis.
- Tests for *myalgia and arthralgia* include 25-hydroxyvitamin D level, HLA-B27 (to support a diagnosis of reactive arthritis), hepatitis B and C serology testing, serum and urine protein electrophoresis (to exclude multiple myeloma), ANA and RF (if clinical features suggest RA, SLE, or another connective-tissue disease).
- For inflammatory low back pain, a magnetic resonance imaging (MRI) of sacroiliac joint and HLA-B27 is to be done (refer Chapter 91).
- Coagulation profile if hemarthrosis is suspected.
- *Plain radiography* is the least expensive imaging modality and is most useful for clarifying the nature of joint abnormalities already noted during the physical examination, such as swelling (bony vs. soft tissue), loss of motion (bony vs. soft tissue), instability (ligamentous damage vs. destruction of articular surface), and focal bony tenderness (fracture vs. osteomyelitis).
- *Musculoskeletal ultrasonography (USG)*: Ultrasonic waves are used to image soft tissues, including tendons, bursae, ligaments, and components of the joint. It can be used to differentiate articular and nonarticular pain. It can be used for joint aspiration and joint injections. USG is particularly useful in imaging of crystals in the joint (refer Chapter 92).
- *Computed tomography (CT) scan*: It can help in the following ways:
  - Assessing trauma of the spine and pelvis
  - Evaluating arthritis in axial joints (e.g., sacroiliac, atlantoaxial, and sternoclavicular)
  - Evaluating degenerative disc disease of the spine and possible disc herniations
- *MRI*: It is the best modality for sacroiliac joint imaging, spine imaging, osteomyelitis, and periarticular lesions.
- *Synovial fluid analysis* is used to broadly characterize the type of arthritis, to identify crystals, and to establish the diagnosis of septic arthritis and crystal-induced synovitis.
  - *Normal synovial fluid*: Characteristics include clear to pale yellow color, transparent clarity, and white blood

cell (WBC) count lower than 200/μL with <25% polymorphonuclear (PMN) leukocytes.
  - *Noninflammatory arthritis*: Characteristics include pale yellow color, transparent clarity, and WBC count of 200–2,000/μL with <25% PMN leukocytes.
  - *Inflammatory*: Characteristics include yellow-to-white color, translucent-to-opaque clarity, WBC count of 2,000–50,000/μL with >70% PMN leukocytes, and low viscosity; this category typifies RA and other chronic inflammatory arthritides.
  - *Septic*: Characteristics include a white-to-cream color, opaque clarity, WBC count higher than 50,000/μL with >90% PMN leukocytes, and very low viscosity.

## THERAPY

- Early recognition and prompt treatment help in preventing complications.
- Infective arthritis requires quick diagnosis and prompt antibiotics.
- Degenerative joint disease requires pain management and physiotherapy.
- Manage underlying osteoporosis.
- Manage comorbidities.
- In inflammatory arthritis, early recognition and prompt immunosuppressants prevent disease progression and deformities.
- Early treatment, even without a definitive diagnosis, may also be of benefit because the immunopathologic events mediating the disease process, as in RA, may evolve and differ in later stages from the changes in early disease.
- Nonsteroidal anti-inflammatory drugs (NSAIDs)/steroids may be used as a bridge therapy before immunosuppressant acts.

## RED FLAG SIGNS

- For acute inflammatory monoarthritis, consider septic and gouty arthritis. Both are emergencies and need to be managed immediately.
- Inflammatory polyarthritis is to be diagnosed early to prevent disease progression.
- An inflammatory type of low back pain, especially in young, is to be evaluated for axial spondyloarthropathy.
- Joint swelling, along with other features such as fever, rash, and anemia, is to be evaluated for a systemic disease such as SLE.

## CLINICAL PEARLS

- A proper history and clinical examination will help in diagnosing most of the cases.
- Always exclude emergencies (e.g., septic arthritis and gouty arthritis).
- Check inflammatory markers if history and examination are suggestive of inflammatory arthritis. Further investigations are to be done based on clinical presentation. Synovial fluid analysis may require.
- Early recognition and treatment are key to preventing joint damage.

## FURTHER READINGS

1. Loscalzo J, Fauci AS, Kasper DL, Hauser SL, Longo DL, Jameson JL, et al. Harrison's principles of Internal Medicine. 21st edition. New York: McGraw-Hill; 2022.
2. Firestein GS, Budd RC, Gabriel SE, Koretzky GA, McInnes IB, O'Dell JR. Firestein & Kelley's textbook of rheumatology. 11th edition. Philadelphia, PA: Elsevier; 2021.

CHAPTER 91

# Low Back Pain and Neck Pain

*Santanu Banerjee*

## WHAT IS LOW BACK PAIN?

Low back pain is defined as "pain and discomfort, localized below the costal margin and above the inferior gluteal folds, with or without leg pain."

It is categorized into three subtypes based on duration:

1. Acute—episode of low back pain <6 weeks
2. Subacute—between 6 and 12 weeks
3. Chronic—more than 12 weeks

## WHAT CAUSES LOW BACK PAIN?

Low back pain symptoms can derive from many potential anatomic sources, such as nerve roots, muscles, tendons, ligaments, fascial structures, bones, joints, intervertebral disc, organs within abdominal cavity, and aberrant neurological pain processing causing neuropathic pain. Low back pain can be influenced by psychological features such as stress, depression, and anxiety. Cytokines such as matrix metalloproteinases, phospholipase A2, nitric oxide, and tumor necrosis factor (TNF)-alpha are thought to attribute to the development of low back pain.

## WHAT ARE THE POSSIBILITIES?

### Causes

- *Structural defects of bone*
  - *Segmentation defects*:
    - 6 lumbar vertebrae
    - 4 lumbar vertebrae
    - Transitional lumbosacral junction
  - *Ossification defects*:
    - Spina bifida
    - Spondylosis
    - Spondylolisthesis
  - *Facet abnormalities*:
    - Asymmetry (tropism)
    - Anteroposterior (AP) lumbosacral facets
    - Increased lumbosacral angle
- *Functional defects*:
  - Lateral imbalance (leg length discrepancy, scoliosis, postural attitudes, etc.)
  - AP imbalance (pregnancy, pot belly, flexion contractures of hips and knees)
- *Infections*:
  - Staphylococcal, streptococcal
  - Tuberculosis
  - Brucellosis
  - *Salmonella* (in sickle cell disease)
- *Inflammatory*:
  - Bone and joint

    - Spondyloarthropathies, e.g., spondylitis, ankylosis, Reiter's syndrome
    - *Soft tissue*:
        - Myositis
        - Fibrositis
- *Degenerative process*:
    - Osteoarthritis (OA), osteoporosis (postmenopausal), degenerative disc disease
- *Neoplastic processes*:
    - *Primary*:
        - Multiple myeloma
        - Hemangioma
        - Giant cell tumor, eosinophilic granuloma, osteoid osteoma
        - Spinal cord tumors
    - *Metastatic*:
        - Prostrate and breast
        - Lung, kidney, thyroid, gastrointestinal tract
- *Traumatic*:
    - Compression fracture
    - Vertebral process fracture
    - Sprain and strain
    - Ruptured disc—herniation—tear of annulus fibrosus
- *Nonmusculoskeletal*:
    - *Upper abdominal*:
        - Peptic ulcer
        - Pancreatic disease
        - Retroperitoneal structure disease—lymphoma, carcinoma
        - Aortic aneurysm
    - *Lower abdominal*:
        - Inflammatory disease of colon—colitis, tumor, diverticulitis
    - *Pelvic*:
        - Urological—gynecological disease, menstrual pain, endometriosis, uterus malposition
        - Pregnancy
        - Chronic prostatitis
        - Renal disease
- *Metabolic*:
    - Osteomalacia, alkaptonuria
- Malingerer's backache
- Compensation backache
- General (miscellaneous causes)
- Idiopathic

Because of the anatomical components making up the motor spinal units, pain may be described as:

- Local pain—felt at the site of pathological processes in superficial structures
- Diffuse pain—characteristic of deep-lying tissues and has segmental distribution
- Radicular pain—as in sciatica or brachialgia
- Referred pain

# STEPS TO DIAGNOSIS

## History Taking

- Name
- Age/sex
- Marital status
- *Occupation*—heavy, moderate, sedentary (involves stooping/standing/sitting/walking/absence from work)
- Current symptoms and duration
- *Previous episodes*—(yes/no, severity, duration, treatment, when)
- *Pain (code)—CLEAR TRAP*
    - C—character
    - L—location
    - E—exacerbating factors
    - A—ameliorating factors
    - R—radiation
    - TR—time relationship
    - AP—associated phenomenon
        - Character-onset
            - Onset—sudden, gradual, while lifting, twisting, fall, pulling, injured at work, sports, bending, not apparent
            - Character—sharp, dull, aching, burning, dysthetic
        - Duration of pain and remission
        - Location—midline/paraspinal/loin to groin
        - Exacerbating factors—sitting/standing/walking/bending/cough-

ing/sneezing/during and after exercise
  - Ameliorating factors—lying down/sitting/standing/walking/analgesics/muscle relaxants/physical therapy
  - Radiation
    - ♦ First differentiate between referred pain and radiating pain
    - ♦ Referred pain does not cross the knee and is not in anatomical continuity.
    - ♦ Anterior thigh—L3/L4 root
    - ♦ Posterior gluteal, thigh, leg—L5-S1 root
    - ♦ Claudication pain—leg pain which occurs on both standing and walking and is relieved by sitting only. Vascular claudication is relieved on standing.
  - Time relationship
    - ♦ Morning stiffness in OA, rheumatoid arthritis (RA), ankylosing spondylitis
    - ♦ Night pain in tumor, infection and inflammation
    - ♦ Seasonal variation, especially in arthritis
  - Associated phenomenon
    - ♦ Numbness/weakness/stiffness/constitutional symptoms—fever, chills, weight loss, anorexia/sleep habits/menstrual history/paresthesia/sense of instability in lower extremities/cough/change in bowel or bladder habits/pattern of social and sexual activities/other joints pain
- *Past history*: Previous pain pattern/treatment history/occupational history (recent and past)/any causative episode/family history
- *Vices*: Alcohol, tobacco, smoking, others
- Family history
- *Temperament*—anxious/depressed/irritable/cooperative

## Examination of the Patient

The patient is examined in both erect and recumbent positions.

- *Standing examination*: General posture, weight, muscular development, tone, spinal curves, pelvic tilt, shortening of one limb, movements of spine (flexion, extension, lateral flexion)
- *Sitting examination*: Movements of the spine, both active and passive, and reflexes are tested.
- *Gait and posture*
  - ○ *Disc lesion*:
    - Patient has scoliosis to the same side, exaggerated in flexion, corrected in lying down and standing on contralateral leg alone.
    - Loss of lumbar lordosis
    - Threshold claudication distance after which the patient stoops or rests
  - ○ *Ankylosing spondylosis*:
    - Kyphosis
    - Patient walks while bending forward
  - ○ *Spondylolisthesis*:
    - Exaggerated lumbar lordosis
    - Protuberant abdomen
    - Tight hamstrings tilt the pelvis backward
  - ○ Obesity—exaggerated lumbar lordosis
- *Inspection*:
  - ○ Lumbar lordosis—exaggerated or obliterated
  - ○ Gibbus
  - ○ Deformity—scoliosis, kyphoscoliosis, kyphosis—location and extent
  - ○ Swelling signs of inflammation—location, site, severity, change in lying down
  - ○ Congenital deformities—neurofibromatosis, tag of skin, café au lait spots
  - ○ Step
  - ○ Sinus, scar
- Palpation
- Temperature

- *Tenderness*:
  - Midline over spinous process—tenderness should be deep. Superficial tenderness is not suggestive of spinal pathology.
  - Paraspinal region—disc prolapse, facet joint pathology, acute back strain
  - Sacroiliac joint—ankylosing spondylitis
  - Sciatic point tenderness—root pain
  - Referred tenderness to anterior thigh—high lumbar disc lesion
  - Sacral tenderness—pelvic or sacral etiology
  - Coccyx
- *Swelling*:
  - Paraspinal/iliac fossa/Petit's triangle/femoral triangle
  - Confirmation of other inspectory findings
- *Movements of spine*:
  - *First dictum*—hip movements must be prevented.
  - *Flexion*:
    - Measured by measuring tape/goniometer/extent of fingertip level to lower limb
    - Normal range—80° or fingertips 4 inches from the floor
  - *Rotation*:
    - As the lumbar spine is rotated, the spinous process of a floating segment will fail to move.
    - Normal range—45°
  - *Extension*:
    - Especially painful in spondylolisthesis and facet joint pathology
    - Normal range—20-30°
  - *Lateral bending*—30° on either side

### Examination in Lying Position

- Measurement of length and girth of limbs
- Demonstration of wasting of calf or thigh
- Range of movement of joints of the leg
- Abdominal palpation
- Rectal and prostate examination

#### Tests for Spine

- Straight leg raising (SLR) test—with the patient supine, raise the leg to the point of pain or 90°, whichever comes first. Localized pain indicates disc lesion, while radiating pain indicates sciatic radiculopathy.
- Lasegue's test
- Well leg raising test
- Femoral stretch test
- Sicard's test

#### Tests for Sacroiliac Joint

- Yeoman's test
- Sacroiliac stretch test
- Pelvic rock test
- Gaenslen's test

### Neurological Examination

#### Investigations

- Blood—hemoglobin, erythrocyte sedimentation rate (ESR), full blood count
- Blood—fasting blood sugar (FBS), uric acid, calcium, phosphorus, alkaline and acid phosphatase, prostate-specific antigen (PSA), RA factor, T3, T4, thyroid-stimulating hormone (TSH), creatinine, vitamin D3, antinuclear antibody (ANA), human leukocyte antigen (HLA) B27, serum protein electrophoresis, etc., (only when suspicion) to rule out systemic diseases
- Urine—routine examination
- Plain radiograph—AP, lateral, right and left oblique
- *Dynamic radiographic studies*:
  - AP lateral radiographs in the standing position
  - Flexion—extension and lateral bending radiographs
- Myelography—it is most useful in determining the level of pathology when it is not clear from computed tomography (CT) or magnetic resonance imaging (MRI).

- MRI—it has excellent simultaneous axial and sagittal images of soft tissues, disc structure, ligaments, muscle joints, and bone marrow.
- CT scan—to determine the condition of bones. It demonstrates the condition of lateral recesses better than myelogram and is invaluable for visualizing levels below a myelography block.
- Discography is indicated when there had been a previous negative myelogram or previous surgery or the possibility of vertebral fusion—probably now the only valid indication.
- 99Tc-diphosphonate bone scan—it is most useful as an indicator of inflammation or tumor of the spine.
- Electromyography-nerve conduction velocity (EMG-NCV) of lower limbs if neuromuscular involvement

## CONSERVATIVE TREATMENT FOR LOW BACK PAIN

The treatment decision is based on the following:

- Is there a soft-tissue syndrome, root encroachment, cauda equine encroachment, or a combination of various syndrome? Do we have an accurate diagnosis?
- Do we know the anatomical level?
- Do we know that the patient is accurately reporting the disability, or is there some medicolegal or compensation objective?
- What are the functional limitations of the patient?

Components of conservative management for low back pain:

- *Rest and controlled physical activities*:
    - Maximum bed rest advised should not be >4 days.
- *Physical therapy*:
    - Ice—used in acute pain. It decreases circulation to the area of contact, which decreases swelling and muscle spasm.
    - Heat—should not be used in the acute phase. It causes vasodilatation and increased blood flow. It decreases gamma fiber activity, muscle spindle excitability, and resting muscle tension.
    - Manipulation, mobilization, and massage-these are controversial. Manipulation should not be used in significant disc herniation and in osteopenic patients. Massage is a soothing therapy that breaks the scar tissue and stretches local muscles.
    - Exercise—it is the cornerstone of spine rehabilitation. Patients with chronic back pain are prone to deconditioning and muscle atrophy due to their restricted activity in order to avoid pain. Patients with mechanical disorders of the disc prefer extension exercises, while those with posterior component disease prefer flexion exercises.
        - William's flexion program—for strengthening abdominal muscles and reducing lumbar lordosis
        - McKenzie hyperextension program—it reduces pressure effects on the posterior annulus and nerve roots.
    - Orthosis (braces)—they stabilize the abnormal motion segment, maintain the alignment, and correct the deformity. Their routine use should be discouraged.
    - Traction
    - Drug therapy

      Patient factors to be considered before choosing medications to treat pain—type of pain, severity, duration, expected time course of resolution, coexisting medical problems, coexisting psychological problems, history of current or past chemical dependence or addiction, other

medications being taken, experience with similar medication.
    - Analgesics—non-narcotic and narcotic, nonsteroidal anti-inflammatory drugs
    - Muscle relaxants
    - Antidepressants
  - Transcutaneous electrical nerve stimulation (TENS)—originally based on gate control theory of pain
  - *Injection therapy*:
    - Trigger point infiltration
    - Epidural corticosteroids—used for patients with nerve root compression who do not respond to conservative management. Also used for patients who are poor candidates for surgical intervention.
    - Facet joint block
  - *Education*:
    - The importance of the interaction of the physician and patient education in the therapy of low back pain cannot be overlooked.

### Indications for Surgical Intervention in Low Back Pain

- Pain worsening and not relieved by conservative treatment
- Deterioration in bladder and bowel function
- Unstable fractures or collapse of the spine
- Worsening of neurological status

## RED FLAG SIGNS

Seek immediate medical attention if any of these signs or symptoms accompany low back pain:

- Saddle anesthesia or paresthesia
- Sudden or unexpected bladder or bowel dysfunction/incontinence
- Unexpected laxity of the anal sphincter
- Severe or progressive lower limb neurological deficit
- Major trauma such as road accident or fall from height
- History of cancer
- Constitutional symptoms, fever or chills
- Unexplained weight loss
- Immunocompromised patient
- Night pain that disturbs sleep
- Loss of tendon reflexes
- Upgoing plantar reflexes
- History of spine surgery in the last 12 months
- Infection

## CLINICAL PEARLS

Low back pain is a very common problem. While typically, history and physical examination are sufficient for the evaluation of back pain, the presence of red flags requires further investigation.

Imaging for adults should be part of the management of symptoms that last longer than 6 weeks with appropriate conservative management.

Early imaging in the adult population correlates with worse outcomes and more invasive treatments without a corresponding improvement in outcomes.

Care must be taken by physicians to educate their patients regarding their disease, and people should adopt preventive measures before and after the disease has developed to minimize morbidity and maximize the quality of life.

The last decade has seen a better understanding of the pathophysiology of low back pain and new management possibilities with modalities such as gene therapy, inhibition of chemical mediators of pain, and growth factors that promote spinal fusion and regeneration of disc material. New pharmacological approaches for abolishing low back pain with agents such as platelet-derived growth factor and monoclonal chimeric antibodies against TNF-alpha are being tested clinically. Future gene therapy research is likely to focus on the proper selection of the gene and delivery method so that a sufficient amount of gene is expressed in the target tissue for an appropriate time.

## NECK PAIN

Neck pain is the pain that starts in the neck and can be associated with radiating pain down one or both arms.

Neck pain can be caused by arthritis, disc degeneration, narrowing of the spinal canal, muscle inflammation, strain, or trauma. In rare cases, it may be a sign of cancer or meningitis.

Age, injury, poor posture, or diseases such as arthritis can lead to the degeneration of bones or joints, causing disc herniation or bone spurs to form. Sudden severe injury to the neck may also contribute to disc herniation, whiplash, blood vessel destruction, and vertebral injury and, in extreme cases, may result in permanent paralysis. Herniated discs or bone spurs may cause a narrowing of the spinal canal or small openings through which spinal nerve roots exit, putting pressure on the spinal cord or the nerves. Pressure on the spinal cord in the cervical region can be a serious problem because virtually all the nerves to the rest of the body have to pass through the neck to reach their final destination. Pressure on the nerve can result in numbness, pain, or weakness in the area of the arm that the nerve supplies. There may be imbalance and difficulty in walking.

Tests include blood tests, CT scan, discography, electromyography, nerve conduction studies, MRI, myelogram, and X-rays.

The treatment strategy depends mainly on identifying the location and cause of pain. Nonsurgical treatment includes pain-reducing medications, muscle relaxants, reducing physical activities, cervical collar, physiotherapy, exercises, trigger point injections, or epidural steroids.

Surgical treatment will be needed if conservative treatment is not helping, there is decrease in function due to pain, progressive neurological deterioration, or difficulty in balance or walking.

The benefits of surgery should always be weighed carefully against its risks. Although many patients report significant pain relief after surgery, there is no guarantee that surgery will help every individual. Follow-up will be on an as-needed basis or if symptoms return.

## RED FLAG SIGNS

Subjective assessments should be made to eliminate possible red flags or serious pathology such as:

- Fractures
- Instability of the vertebrae
- Coronary artery dysfunction
- Myelopathy
- Cancer
- Infection
- Visceral disorders
- Dizziness
- Diplopia
- Drop attacks
- Dysphagia
- Dysarthria
- Nystagmus
- Nausea
- Neurological symptoms

## CLINICAL PEARLS

Neck pain is a common presenting symptom in the primary care setting and causes significant disability. The broad differential diagnosis requires an efficient but global assessment. Therefore, emphasis is placed on red flags that can help in early recognition and treatment of more concerning diagnosis like traumatic injuries, infection, malignancy, vascular emergencies and other inflammatory conditions.

Accurate patient history is a critical element for appropriate diagnosis and treatment.

Physical examination findings complement diagnostic clues from history but often lack specificity to be of value independently. Imaging and electrodiagnostic tools have variable utility, especially in chronic and degenerative conditions.

Treatment of mechanical or non-neuropathic neck pain includes short term use of medications and possibly injections. However, long term data for these interventions are limited. Acupuncture or other alternative therapies may be helpful in some cases. Advanced imaging and surgical evaluation may be warranted for patients with worsening neurologic function or persistent pain but long term data are limited.

## FURTHER READINGS

1. Preuper HRS, Geertzen JHB, van Wijhe M, Boonstra AM, Molmans BHW, Dijkstra PU, et al. Do analgesics improve functioning of patients with chronic low back pain? Eur Spine J. 2014;23(4):800-6.
2. Jarvik JG, Deyo RA. Diagnostic evaluation of Low Back Pain with emphasis on imaging. Ann Intern Med. 2002;137(7):586-97.

CHAPTER 92

# Pain at the Base of the Great Toe

*Tanuka Mandal*

## ANATOMY OF THE GREAT TOE

Anatomy of the great toe is essential to analyze the causes that lie behind the pain in the base of the great toe. It consists of the bones, ligaments, muscles, and blood supply **(Fig. 1)**.

- *Bones*: The great toe consists of five bones:
  - First metatarsal
  - Proximal phalanx
  - Distal phalanx
  - Tibial sesamoid
  - Fibular sesamoid
- *Ligaments*:
  - Capsular ligaments of both the metatarsophalangeal (MTP) and the interphalangeal (IP) joints—encase the joint and hold the joint fluid
  - Plantar plates of the MTP and IP joints
  - Collateral MTP ligaments
  - Metatarso-sesamoid suspensory ligaments
  - Collateral IP ligaments
- *Muscles*:
  - *Abductor hallucis*:
    - Extends from calcaneus to the medial base of proximal phalanx
    - Abducts and aids in plantarflexion of the great toe
  - *Flexor hallucis brevis*:
    - Has medial and lateral arms in its origin as well as insertion
    - Medial tendon contains the medial sesamoid bone while the lateral sesamoid bone lies in the lateral tendon.
  - Plantarflexes the proximal phalanx of the great toe

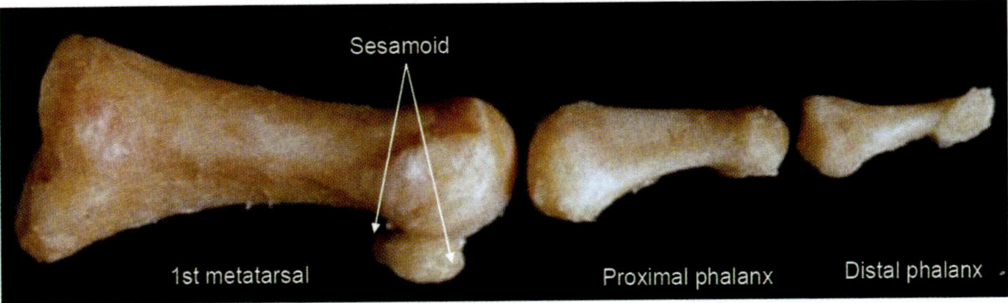


**FIG. 1:** Anatomy of the great toe.

- *Adductor hallucis*:
  - Has oblique and transverse heads
  - Adducts and plantar flexes the great toe
- *Extensor hallucis brevis*:
  - Courses obliquely from lateral to medial
  - Dorsiflexes the proximal phalanx
- *Extensor hallucis longus*:
  - Dorsiflexes the hallux at both the IP and MTP joints thereby dorsi flexing the foot.
- *Flexor hallucis longus*:
  - Plantarflexes the hallux at the IP and MTP joints, thereby plantarflexing the foot
- Blood supply—dorsalis pedis and posterior tibial artery

## WHAT CAUSES PAIN IN THE BASE OF THE GREAT TOE?

The great toe has a complex anatomy that is essential to the biomechanics of gait. Almost 20–30% of ground reactive force goes through the great toe during ambulation.

## WHAT ARE THE POSSIBILITIES?

Any deformity or inflammation in the joint space leads to pain. A few causes which may lead to pain at the base of the great toe are as follows:

- *Hallux rigidus*: It is the most common cause of pain at the base of the great toe according to the American Orthopaedic Foot and Ankle Society. It occurs due to bone spurs that affect the MTP joints. Hallux rigidus affects nearly 2.5% of people over the age of 50 years and is more commonly encountered in the female population.
- *Gout*: It is a condition in which monosodium urate monohydrate crystals are deposited in the joints. The metatarsal-phalangeal joint at the base of the big toe is most commonly affected, accounting for almost half of the cases of gout.
- *Septic arthritis*: It is painful infection in a joint secondary to an infectious etiology that reaches the joints through the bloodstream or some penetrating injury.
- *Pseudogout*: It is a condition commonly seen in young individuals in which calcium pyrophosphate dihydrate (CPPD) occurs in the joints.
- *Hemarthrosis*: It is a condition of articular bleeding that is into the joint cavity following any injury in patients suffering from bleeding disorders such as hemophilia.
- *Turf toe*: It is an injury of the connective tissue at the MTP joint that occurs during sporting activities. This form of injury happens on repetitively jumping or running on rigid surfaces such as artificial turf.
- *Sesamoiditis*: It is the inflammation of the sesamoid bones, which are located just behind the great toe. These sesamoid bones connect to tendons or are embedded in muscles. This type of inflammation is common in runners and ballet dancers.
- *Fracture*: Fracture at the base of the great toe is one of the very common findings which occurs on:
  - Kicking a hard object
  - Dropping any heavy object on the great toe
  - Performing any movement that puts too much pressure on the toes
- *Bunion*: It is the deformity of the joint at the base of the great toe, which makes the joint protrude outward and create a visible bump on the side of the foot. The great toe points in the opposite direction and overlaps onto the toe next to it. Wearing ill-fitted shoes may put further pressure onto the protruding joint leading to the formation of a bursa.

## APPROACH TO DIAGNOSIS

### History

- *Hallux rigidus*:
  - Pain while walking or running
  - Swelling at the base of the great toe
  - Pain on movement of the great toe
- *Gout*:
  - Inflammation that causes skin darkening, swelling, or warmth of the joint
  - Intense pain that occurs when a person wakes up
  - Shiny skin over the affected joint
- *Septic arthritis*:
  - Fever
  - Joint pain
  - Swelling
  - Redness
  - Warmth around the joint
- *Pseudogout*:
  - Mostly involves the knees followed by wrists and ankles
  - Swollen
  - Warm
  - Painful joints
- *Hemarthrosis*:
  - Swelling and pain around one joint
  - Bruising/discoloration of the joint
  - Warmth around the joint
- *Turf toe*:
  - History of repeated movement
  - Pain and swelling gradually develop.
  - In case of acute injury, pain may worsen over 24 hours.
- *Sesamoiditis*:
  - Trouble moving the great toe
  - Gradual buildup of pain
  - Bruising
  - Swelling
  - Pain on the ball of the foot
- *Fracture*:
  - Pain
  - Swelling
  - Discoloration with a history of external injury
- *Bunion*:
  - Swelling
  - Inflammation
  - Pain with the great toe visibly pointing inward while the joint at its base points outward.

### Investigations

- *Hallux rigidus*: X-ray of the joint shows bony abnormalities or bone spur development.
- *Gout*:
  - *Blood test*:
    - Erythrocyte sedimentation rate (ESR), C-reactive protein (CRP)—raised
    - Neutrophilic leukocytosis
    - Raised serum uric acid levels in two-thirds of patients—not essential for diagnosis
  - Demonstration of needle-shaped negatively birefringent crystals in synovial fluid by polarizing light microscopy—*gold standard*
  - *Imaging*:
    - X-ray
      - Acute gout—swelling of the affected joint
      - Chronic gout—asymmetric inflammatory erosive arthritis with soft-tissue nodules with retention of joint space
    - Ultrasonography (USG): Monosodium urate crystals may appear within synovial fluid as *snowstorm appearance* or deposited in subarticular cartilage to appear as *double contour sign*.
    - Conventional computed tomography (CT)—to visualize tophi and bone erosion
    - Dual-energy computed tomography (DECT)—to differentiate between low-density urate crystals and denser materials like calcium

    - Magnetic resonance imaging (MRI)—to visualize joint effusion, synovitis, tendon disorder, tophus, cartilage disorder, and bone edema
  - Urinary uric acid excretion—increased in 90% of patients suffering from primary gout
- *Septic arthritis*:
  - *Blood test*:
    - ESR, CRP—raised
    - Neutrophilic leukocytosis
  - Synovial fluid study—high cell count (>50,000/cu.mm) with low glucose levels
  - *Imaging*:
    - X-ray—to find associated osteomyelitis, cortical destruction, and periosteal new bone formation
    - USG—to detect joint effusion and help in aspiration
    - MRI—to evaluate musculoskeletal infection
- *Pseudogout*:
  - *Imaging*:
    - X-ray—to detect chondrocalcinosis
    - USG—to demonstrate crystal deposition in articular cartilage
    - DECT—to demonstrate CPPD crystal deposition in joints
  - Synovial fluid examination—rhomboid-shaped, intracellular crystals with weak positive birefringence
- *Hemarthrosis*:
  - *Imaging*:
    - X-ray
    - USG—to identify and characterize intra-articular fluid collections.
  - Synovial fluid examination for definitive diagnosis
- *Turf toe*:
  - *Imaging*:
    - X-ray—to rule out bone-related issues, such as a fracture
    - MRI—beneficial for people with moderate-to-severe turf toe, grade 2 or 3 injuries, or in those with deformities found in X-rays
- *Sesamoiditis*:
  - *Imaging*:
    - X-ray—to rule out bone-related issues, such as a fracture
    - MRI—to rule out any damage to nonbony structure
- *Fracture*:
  - *Imaging*:
    - X-ray—to assess the extent of the damage to the bony tissues
    - MRI—to rule out any damage to nonbony structure
- *Bunion*:
  - Diagnosed clinically
  - *Imaging*:
    - X-ray—to rule out bone-related issues, such as a fracture
    - CT scan—to identify the extent of the damage.
    - MRI—to rule out any damage to nonbony structure

## THERAPY

- *Hallux rigidus*:
  - Icing or heating
  - Nonsteroidal anti-inflammatory drugs (NSAIDs)
  - Wearing different footwear with firmer soles
  - *Surgical options*:
    - Fusing of joint
    - Removal of any bone spurs
    - Joint replacement
    - Joint resurfacing
- *Gout*:
  - Drinking plenty of fluids
  - Elevation and resting of the joint
  - Diet modification by lesser intake of alcohol, bacon, and liver, which are high in purine content.
  - *Medications*:
    - Acute gout
      - ♦ Colchicine

- NSAIDs like indomethacin—50 mg 6 hourly
- Corticosteroids—if NSAIDs and colchicine contraindicated
- Anti-interleukin—one therapy
- Chronic gout
  - Uricostatic drugs—allopurinol, febuxostat
  - Uricosuric agents—Probenecid, sulfinpyrazone, benzbromarone, lesinurad, losartan, amlodipine, fenofibrate
  - Uricolytic drugs—Uricase, rasburicase, PEGylated uricase
- *Septic arthritis*:
  - Urgent drainage of purulent joint fluid drainage
  - Initiation of empirical parenteral antibiotics
    - Linezolid/cloxacillin + cefotaxime/cefazolin + gentamicin—×2 weeks followed by oral antibiotics for another 2 weeks
- *Pseudogout*:
  - NSAIDs
  - Colchicine
  - Steroids
- *Hemarthrosis*:
  - Resting and icing the joint
  - Elevating the affected limb
  - Taking pain medications
  - Draining the blood from the joint
- *Turf toe*:
  - Stopping the repeated movement
  - Rest
  - Icing
  - Compression
  - Elevation
- *Sesamoiditis*:
  - NSAIDs
  - Steroid injections
  - Strapping, padding, or taping of toe/foot
  - Physical therapy
  - Use of custom orthopedic devices
- *Fracture*:
  - Avoiding placing weight on the toe
  - Elevation of foot
  - Icing to reduce swelling
  - Wrapping of the toe
- *Bunion*:
  - Wearing shoes that do not put extra pressure on the joint
  - Over-the-counter (OTC) bunion pads
  - NSAIDs
  - Warm soaking
  - Icing of the joint
  - Massage

## CLINICAL PEARLS

The first great toe is critically important. The amount of force that passes through the first MTP joint and great toe during normal gait varies between individuals depending on foot shape, weight, etc. However, if we consider six points of contact in the forefoot (the two sesamoids of the great toe and the second, third, fourth, and fifth metatarsal heads), then we can estimate that the great toe on average absorbs a third (2/6) of the body weight. During athletic activities such as jogging and running, these forces can approach two to three times body weight.

Processes that can affect the first MTP joint include overuse, wearing shoes that are too tight or ill-fitting, trauma, autoimmune disease, and deposition of crystals in the joint (gout, pseudogout). Thus, proper history, examination, and investigations can help us lead to the proper diagnosis and treatment of the underlying pathology.

## FURTHER READINGS

1. Patel J, Swords M. Hallux Rigidus. [Updated 2022 Sep 12]. In: StatPearls [Internet]. Treasure Island (FL): StatPearls Publishing; 2023. Available from: https://www.ncbi.nlm.nih.gov/books/NBK556019/
2. Fenando A, Rednam M, Gujarathi R, Widrich J. Gout. [Updated 2022 Dec 27]. In: StatPearls [Internet]. Treasure Island (FL): StatPearls Publishing; 2023.

3. Momodu II, Savaliya V. Septic Arthritis. [Updated 2023 Jul 3]. In: StatPearls [Internet]. Treasure Island (FL): StatPearls Publishing; 2023. Available from: https://www.ncbi.nlm.nih.gov/books/NBK538176/
4. Sidari A, Hill E. Diagnosis and Treatment of Gout and Pseudogout for Everyday Practice. Prim Care. 2018;45(2):213-36.
5. Lombardi M, Cardenas AC. Hemarthrosis. [Updated 2023 Jul 31]. In: StatPearls [Internet]. Treasure Island (FL): StatPearls Publishing; 2023.
6. Aran F, Ponnarasu S, Scott AT. Turf Toe. [Updated 2022 Oct 24]. In: StatPearls [Internet]. Treasure Island (FL): StatPearls Publishing; 2023.
7. Seder JI. Sesamoiditis. J Am Podiatry Assoc. 1974;64(6):444-6.
8. Ferrari J. Bunions. BMJ Clin Evid. 2009;2009:1112.

# CHAPTER 93

# Raynaud's Phenomenon

*Tanuka Mandal*

## WHAT IS RAYNAUD'S PHENOMENON?

Raynaud's phenomenon (RP) is an exaggerated vascular response to the digital arterial circulation triggered by cold ambient temperature and emotional stress. The patient presents with a history of excessive cold sensitivity and recurrent events of sharply demarcated pallor and/or cyanosis of fingers **(Fig. 1)**.

## WHAT CAUSES RAYNAUD'S PHENOMENON?

On cold exposure, blanching reflects digital vasospasm and cyanosis, which occurs as a result of deoxygenation of sluggishly flowing venous blood. Redness occurs as a result of reactive hyperemia as soon as the regular blood flow is restored as the temperature increases.

Normally, sympathetic stimulation is responsible for cold-induced vasoconstriction but abnormal thermoregulation is associated with a vasculopathy characterized by endothelial dysfunction and fibrotic proliferation. This leads to increased production of collagen content in the intimal layer as well as decreased vessel flexibility and ultimately obstruction of the lumen. Under such circumstances, the patients may present with superficial ulcerations to deep painful ulceration and even loss of an entire digit or limb.

## WHAT IS THE PREVALENCE OF RAYNAUD'S PHENOMENON?

Raynaud's phenomenon occurs in 3–15% of the general population—more commonly affecting females and clinical presentation appearing before the age of 20 years.

This phenomenon increases in the winters and on exposure to shifting temperatures.

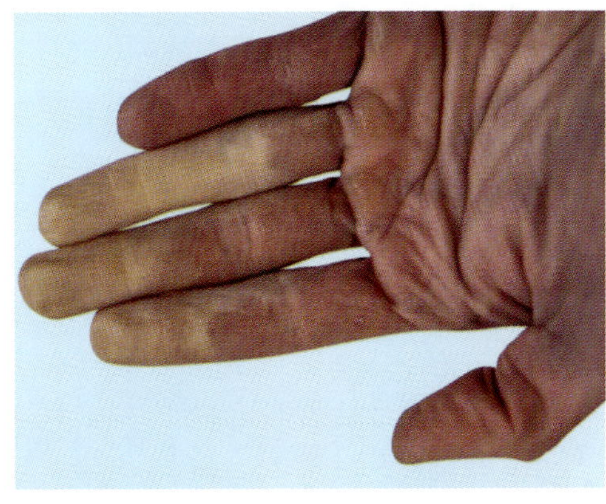

**FIG. 1:** Sharply demarcated pallor and/or cyanosis of fingers.

# WHAT ARE THE TYPES OF RAYNAUD'S PHENOMENON?

## Primary Raynaud's Phenomenon

- Not associated with any other disease process
- *Seen in patients of*:
  - Younger age groups
  - History of earlier disease onset
  - Symmetric presentation of symptoms
  - Mild-to-moderate severity of disease
  - Absence of digital ulceration
  - Normal nail fold capillary examination
- Negative antinuclear antibody (ANA) titer

## Secondary Raynaud's Phenomenon

- Associated with any other disease process such as connective tissue disorders, other rheumatic conditions, occupational trauma or certain drugs (like ergotamine derivatives or bleomycin), increased viscosity, and compressive or obstructive vascular disease

## How to Differentiate Primary and Secondary Raynaud's Phenomenon Clinically (Figs. 2A and B)?

- *Nail fold capillaroscopy*:
  - It was first discovered by Maricq and LeRoy.
  - It is done by coating the skin of the nail fold with immersion oil and then viewing the area using a bifocal dissecting microscope or an ophthalmoscope at 20–40 D.
  - An abnormal pattern of nail fold capillary vessels is found in scleroderma.
  - The abnormality progresses gradually with severity in the disease process.
  - *Primary RP*: Normal, thin, palisading capillary loops are seen.
  - *Secondary RP*: Capillary loop dilatation and dropouts are seen.

# APPROACH TO DIAGNOSIS

## History Taking

A patient presents with a history of excessive cold sensitivity and recurrent events of sharply demarcated pallor and/or cyanosis of fingers.

## Clinical Examination

- *Active RP*: Presents with coolness of distal digits with (out) a line of demarcation of skin.
- *Severe RP*: Presents with nonhealing painful digital ulceration due to critical digital ischemia.

Patients are asked to maintain a record of the duration and frequency of the attacks.

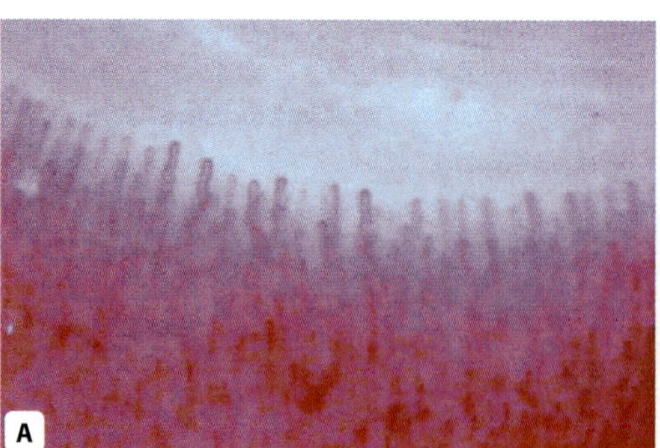


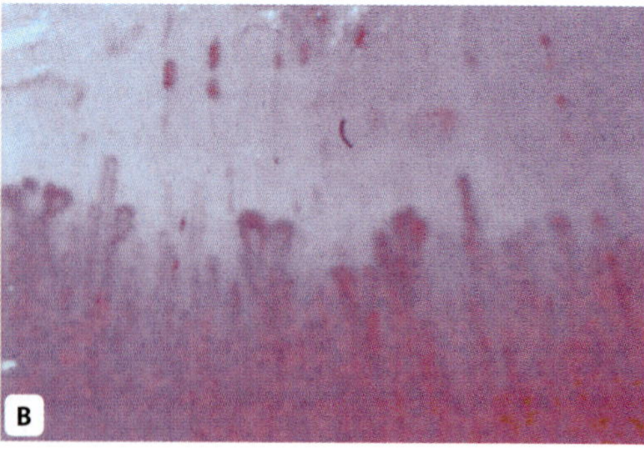


**FIGS. 2A AND B:** (A) Primary and (B) secondary Raynaud's phenomenon (RP).

*Raynaud's condition score* takes into account the impact of RP on the patient including:

- Pain
- Discomfort
- Effect on daily function

### Investigations

Although a number of tests have been used to score attacks of RP, none has been found to be practical enough to replace the clinical criteria for diagnosis and management.

Some laboratory-based measures include:

- Laser Doppler
- Thermography
- Plethysmography

In case of critical digital ischemia, assessment of correctable macrovascular disease should be performed by using:

- Arterial Doppler ultrasound
- Angiographic imaging

## RED FLAG SIGN

- Presence of nonhealing painful digital ulcerations

## THERAPY

The primary goal is to *prevent digital ischemia.*

*Nonpharmacological therapy for RP in scleroderma*:

- In order to prevent digital ischemia, maintaining warm extremities using layered clothing to maintain not only warm extremities but also a warm core body temperature
- Avoiding emotional stress to reduce sympathetic response
- Avoiding finger trauma
- Stopping smoking and other sympathomimetic drugs or migraine medications and nonselective beta-blockers

*Pharmacological therapy for RP in scleroderma*:

- *First line*: Calcium channel blockers such as nifedipine (5–10 mg three times daily), amlodipine, and nisoldipine. They work primarily by inducing arterial vasodilation by direct inhibition of the smooth muscles of the vessels. They also reduce oxidative stress and inhibit platelet activation.
- *Other drugs*:
    - *Phosphodiesterase inhibitor*:
        - Sildenafil 25–50 mg twice daily
        - Tadalafil 10–20 mg twice daily
    - Nitrates
    - *Intravenous (IV) prostaglandins*: They reduce the frequency and severity of attacks of RP. They are most helpful during periods of sustained critical ischemia. They act by their strong vasodilating effect, inhibition of platelet aggression, and enhancement of vascular function. Commonly used IV prostaglandins are:
        - Alprostadil
        - Epoprostenol
        - Iloprost
        - Treprostinil
    - Sympatholytic agents
        - Prazosin
    - *Statins*: They are thought to decrease the progression of vascular injury and prevent vascular ischemia, especially in scleroderma.

*Surgical therapy for RP in scleroderma*:

- Sympathectomy is the only viable option for patients not responding to pharmacological therapy of RP.
- Localized digital sympathectomy with lysis of perivascular fibrosis has replaced cervical sympathectomy by proving to be very effective for acute ischemia.
- Pharmacological therapy is always required along with surgical therapy to prevent any new attacks of RP.
- In the presence of any macrovascular disease, vascular surgery to reduce the occlusive process is advised.

### Treatment in Case of Critical Digital Ischemia

- Hospitalization is advised to maintain warmth, reduce any vasospastic activity, and initiate vasodilator therapy rapidly.
- IV prostaglandins for maximal vasodilatation can be used.
- Low-dose antiplatelet therapy such as aspirin can be given although the benefit has not been proven yet.
- Administration of heparin may also be considered.
- Fibrinolysis to manage acute occlusion of larger arterial vessels can be considered.
- Chemical sympathectomy of the affected digit, performed by local infiltration with lidocaine or bupivacaine
- For refractory cases only, a surgical approach to digital sympathectomy is used.

### Treatment in Case of Ischemic Digital Lesions

- Treatment with topical antibiotics and daily cleansing with soap and water
- Debridement procedures should be performed very cautiously.
- Any lesion that progresses to dry gangrene should be permitted to undergo autoamputation.
- Surgical amputation is best offered only in cases of intractable pain or deep tissue infection.

## CLINICAL PEARLS

- Raynaud's phenomenon is common in the general population and usually presents with a benign clinical course.
- It is more clinically symptomatic in scleroderma and can be associated with digital ischemia.
- Raynaud's phenomenon in scleroderma occurs due to abnormal vasomotor regulation with progressive endothelial and structural vessel disease.
- Treatment of RP includes control of excessive vasoreactivity, modification of structural vascular disease, and prevention of microthrombotic events.

## FURTHER READINGS

1. Brown S. Diagnosis and management of patients with Raynaud's phenomenon. Nurs Stand. 2012;26(46):41-6.
2. Belch J, Carlizza A, Carpentier PH, Constans J, Khan F, Wautrech JC, et al. ESVM guidelines—the diagnosis and management of Raynaud's phenomenon. Vasa. 2017;46(6):413-23.
3. Mikuls TR, Cannella AC, Moore GF, Erickson AR, Thiele GM, O'Dell JR. Rheumatology: A Color Handbook. CRC Press; 2013. p. 17.
4. Wang WH, Lai CS, Chang KP, Lee SS, Yang CC, Lin SD, et al. Peripheral sympathectomy for Raynaud's phenomenon: a salvage procedure. Kaohsiung J Med Sci. 2006;22(10):491-9.

# SECTION 2

# Medical Emergencies

# PART 15

# Emergencies

CHAPTER 94

# Shock

*Tapas Bandyopadhyay*

## INTRODUCTION

Shock is a state of cellular and tissue hypoxia due to a mismatch between the cellular demand and the circulatory supply of oxygen. It may happen due to reduced oxygen delivery, increased oxygen consumption, inadequate oxygen utilization, or a combination of the three.

The fundamental approach is to recognize the impending shock in time and restore tissue perfusion and oxygenation by successfully maintaining the circulatory pressures and simultaneously intervening against the inciting agent, e.g., controlling infection, arresting volume loss, and improving cardiac pump function.

## PATHOPHYSIOLOGY OF SHOCK

The pathophysiologic events in the various types of shock are different and complex. Shock results from a change in one or a combination of the following: Intravascular volume, myocardial function, systemic vascular resistance, or distribution of blood flow **(Fig. 1)**. Key metabolic and cellular changes leading to a shock state are as follows:

- Aerobic to anaerobic metabolism (lactic acid production and accumulation)
- Increased permeability of cell membrane
- Electrolyte and/or fluid seep in/out of the cell
- Impairment of $Na^+/K^+$-ATPase pump
- Damage to mitochondria leading to death

## COMPENSATORY MECHANISMS

- *Neurohumoral response (baroreceptor mediated)*: Increased sympathetic activity
- *Hormonal response*:
    - Renin–angiotensin system activation
    - Activation of osmoreceptors in hypothalamus
    - *Adrenal cortex*: Adrenocorticotropic hormone (ACTH) (anterior pituitary) stimulates adrenal cortex **(Flowchart 1)**.

## STAGES OF SHOCK

The stages of shock are shown in **Figure 1**.

## CLASSIFICATION OF SHOCK

The classification of shock is shown in **Flowchart 1**.

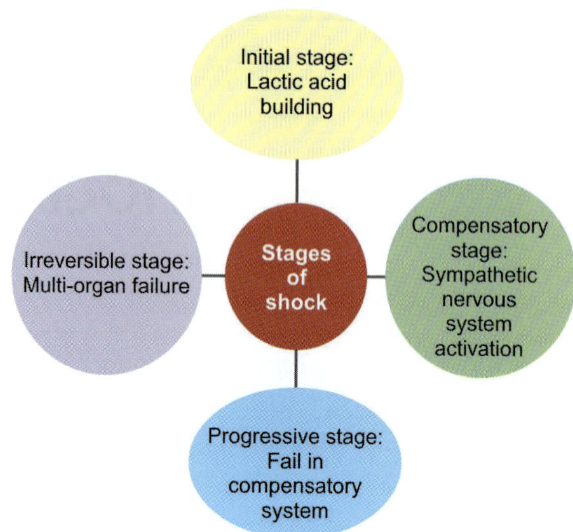


**FIG. 1:** Stages of shock.

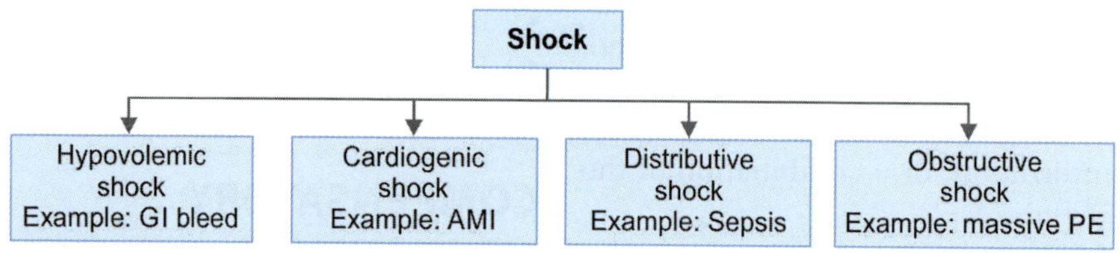


**FLOWCHART 1:** Classification of shock.

(AMI: acute myocardial infarction; GI: gastrointestinal; PE: pulmonary embolism)

## Septic Shock

Distributive shock is the most frequently encountered type of shock. Among the different types of distributive shock, septic shock comprises the majority. A relative hypovolemic state due to intense vasodilation is caused by dysregulated immune response, stimulated by a suspected or established infection. In septic shock, patients fail to improve the lactate level (<2 mmol/L) even after a fluid bolus challenge and require a vasopressor to maintain a reasonable blood pressure [mean arterial pressure (MAP) ≥ 65 mm Hg].

Sepsis is defined as a life-threatening organ dysfunction as a result of a deranged host immune response and organ dysfunction as an acute change in sequential organ failure assessment (SOFA) score of ≥2 as a result of an infectious cause. The new 2016 definition of sepsis-3 eliminates the requirement of the presence of systemic inflammatory response syndrome (SIRS) to define sepsis and removes severe sepsis from the definition and replaces it with a SOFA score of 2 points or greater secondary to the infection. Detrimental host response is a continuum ranging from sepsis to septic shock to multiorgan dysfunction syndrome (MODS).

Septic shock is associated with culture-positive bacteremia in only 30–50% of cases.

### *Diagnosis of Septic Shock*

A high index of suspicion is needed to identify subtle presentations, particularly in elderly subjects in whom typical features may not be present many times. Hence, a detailed history and careful physical examination with special attention to cardiovascular examination (e.g., blood pressure, heart rate) and pulse oximetry are indicated and are helpful in finding out the probable source of infection and assessing the severity of impairment.

Laboratory evaluation includes the following:

- Complete blood hemogram, C-reactive protein (CRP), blood biochemistry, renal and liver function, arterial blood gas analysis, coagulation profile
- Blood culture and sensitivity
- Serum procalcitonin (to differentiate bacterial from viral or fungal infection, serial procalcitonin measurement guides toward antibiotic escalation or de-escalation)
- Urine routine test, culture and sensitivity (in case of suspected urinary tract infection)
- Imaging of chest [X-ray or computed tomography (CT) scan] or abdomen or head (as indicated)
- Cerebrospinal fluid (CSF) study in case of suspected meningitis, encephalitis, or meningoencephalitis

### Quick Sequential Organ Failure Assessment Score

Sepsis-induced organ dysfunction is defined by an acute change in total SOFA score of 2 points or more secondary to infection. For screening purpose in patient of suspected sepsis, quick sequential organ failure assessment (qSOFA) has reasonable accuracy in settings outside the intensive care unit (ICU). The qSOFA is not as robust as the SOFA score as there is no laboratory test, making it a suitable tool for screening possible infection as a source of a new sepsis episode in a low-resource setting than standard ICU.

The qSOFA includes the following three criteria:

1. Altered mental status [Glasgow Coma Scale (GCS) <15]
2. Respiratory rate ≥22 breath/min
3. Systolic blood pressure (SBP) ≤100 mm Hg

The presence of two or more qSOFA points near the onset of infection was associated with a greater risk of death or prolonged ICU stay.

## *Therapeutic Approach in Septic Shock*

- *Antibiotics*: Appropriate antimicrobials should be initiated within the first hour of recognizing sepsis, after obtaining relevant samples for culture avoiding significant delay in antibiotic administration. Proper dose, duration, and frequency of antibiotics should be ensured.
- *Fluid*: The goals of resuscitation in sepsis and septic shock are to restore intravascular volume, increase oxygen delivery to tissues, and reverse organ dysfunction. A crystalloid bolus of 30 mL/kg is recommended within 3 hours of detecting severe sepsis or septic shock. Caution is to be taken against giving too much fluid, especially in patients who have limited cardiorespiratory reserve to avoid pulmonary edema, hypoxemic respiratory failure, prolonged ICU stay and time on mechanical ventilation, and even increased risk of death.

  Fluid resuscitation should be managed as follows:
  - *Rescue*: During the initial minutes to hours, fluid boluses (1- to 2-L fluid bolus of crystalloid solution) are required to reverse hypoperfusion and shock.
  - *Optimization*: During the second phase, the benefits of giving additional fluid to improve cardiac output and tissue perfusion should be weighed against potential harms.
  - *Stabilization*: During the third phase, usually 24–48 hours after the onset of septic shock, an attempt should be made to achieve a net neutral or a slightly negative fluid balance.
  - *De-escalation*: The fourth phase, marked by shock resolution and organ recovery, should trigger aggressive fluid-removal strategies.

- Hemodynamic support, e.g., inotrope and vasopressor, if hypotension refractory to fluid resuscitation
- Correct hypoxia
- To pinpoint the source of infection and source control, e.g., urinary catheter removal in case of urosepsis, incision and drainage in case of abscess along with appropriate antibiotic therapy
- Monitoring of organ function (e.g., hourly urine output) and prevention of MODS
- Ventilator support with low tidal volume in patients with acute respiratory distress syndrome (ARDS)

#### Ideal Fluid in Sepsis

The best fluid for resuscitation is still debated, but growing evidence indicates that balanced crystalloids (lactated Ringer solution, Plasma-Lyte) are associated with a lower incidence of renal injury, less need for renal replacement therapy, and lower mortality in critically ill patients. Moreover, isotonic saline is associated with hyperchloremia and metabolic acidosis, and it can reduce renal cortical blood flow.

#### Corticosteroids in Sepsis

Corticosteroids downregulate the maladaptive inflammatory response seen in sepsis and address relative adrenal insufficiency caused by adrenal suppression. They can be added as a adjunctive therapy for patients requiring higher doses of vasopressors. Current guidelines recommend hydrocortisone 200 mg/day intravenously as a continuous drip or 50-mg bolus in four divided doses for at least 3 days, based on a systematic review showing that a longer course of low-dose steroids is associated with a lower mortality rate. Steroids are stopped when vasopressors are off. There is no role of prophylactic corticosteroids in septic shock.

#### Role of Ultrasound-guided Procedures

*Source control*: Four Ds:

1. *D*rainage (e.g., lung abscess, intra-abdominal abscess, etc.)
2. *D*ebridement
3. *D*evice removal (e.g., central venous catheter, urinary catheter, shunts)
4. *D*efinitive control (usually means surgical resection)

### *Risk Factors for Sepsis*

- Age < 10 years and elderly population
- Underlying comorbidities, e.g., diabetes mellitus (DM), alcoholism, cardiopulmonary disease
- Immunocompromised state, e.g., immunosuppressive therapy, neutropenia, transplant recipient, malignancy, intravenous (IV) drug abuse
- Major surgery, trauma, burns
- Invasive procedure, e.g., intravascular device, dialysis catheter, prosthetic valves, endotracheal tubes
- Previous antibiotic therapy
- Prolonged hospital stay

The incidence of sepsis is growing exponentially in recent decades due to the following:

- Increase in life expectancy and hence increased number of elderly population
- Early and increased recognition of disease
- Immunosuppression and chemotherapy being increasingly used.
- Vast number of invasive procedures and transplants
- Increase in the use of indwelling devices.
- When the International Classification of Disease (ICD) code for sepsis was used, the incidence doubled over a 6-year period. Growing awareness and inclusion of both ICU and non-ICU patients may be another reason.

The following clinical characteristics are related to the severity of sepsis:

- Site of infection
- Type of antimicrobial therapy and timing
- Offending organisms
- Underlying disease, e.g., DM, malignancy
- Location of patient at the time of shock onset
- Advanced age and clinical evidence of organ dysfunction

Poor prognostic factors in sepsis:
- Advanced age
- Resistant organism
- Poor functional status
- Sequential organ failure despite support
- Need for vasopressor in the last 24-hour

Factors associated with higher mortality in sepsis:
- Failure of two or more organ systems at the time of sepsis
- Presence of shock
- Acidosis—pH below 7.3
- High severity of illness score

Early administration of appropriate broad-spectrum antibiotics leads to a significant reduction in mortality. Septic shock may lead to long-term sequelae in terms of neurological and cognitive function due to prolonged tissue hypoperfusion, especially in the elderly. It has a lasting effect on patients' independence and depends in large part on family support.

## Cardiogenic Shock

Cardiogenic shock is clinically defined as reduced cardiac output with tissue hypoxia in the presence of adequate intravascular volume. In the absence of a highly experienced care center, the mortality is as high as 80–90%.

Apart from tachycardia, low-volume pulse, and distant heart sounds, there are signs of hypotension (SBP < 90 mm Hg or fall in MAP by 30 mm Hg). Routine laboratory studies include the following:
- Cardiac biomarkers [e.g., creatine kinase-MB (CK-MB), troponin I, and troponin T), N-terminal pro-B-type natriuretic peptide (NT-proBNP)
- Electrocardiography (ECG)
- Two-dimensional (2D) echocardiography
- Ultrasonography (USG) to look for respiratory variation in inferior vena cava (IVC) diameter to predict fluid responsiveness
- Coronary angiography to detect coronary artery disease

### *Role of Invasive Hemodynamic Monitoring*

Pulmonary artery (PA) catheterization (Swan-Ganz catheter) is of help to differentiate different types of shock (e.g., hypovolemic, cardiogenic, or distributive). Also, in many circumstances, more than one type of shock is present and poses difficulty in assessing the contribution of each type in a given situation.
- Cardiogenic shock patients have pulmonary capillary wedge pressure (PCWP) >15 mm Hg and cardiac index (CI) <2.2 $L/min/m^2$ **(Table 1)**.
- High right filling pressure in the absence of raised PCWP correlates with right ventricular myocardial infarction (RVMI).
- In ventricular septal rupture, there is a step-up of oxygen saturation between the right atrium and the right ventricle.

### *Approach to Management of Cardiogenic Shock*

- Admission to ICU
- Fluid resuscitation

**Table 1: Differentiation of cardiogenic and distributive shock by PA catheterization.**

| | *Cardiogenic shock* | *Distributive shock* |
|---|---|---|
| RA | High (>10 mm Hg) | Low (<8 mm Hg) |
| PCWP | High (>15 mm Hg) | Low (<10 mm Hg) |
| CO (Fick) | Low (<4 L/min) | High (>7–8 L/min) |
| SVR | High (>1200 dyne × sec/$cm^5$) | Low (<800 dyne × sec/$cm^5$) |

(CO: cardiac output; PA: pulmonary artery; PCWP: pulmonary capillary wedge pressure; RA: right atrium; SVR: systemic vascular resistance)

- Pharmacologic therapy including judicious use of inotrope, e.g., norepinephrine (0.2–1.5 μg/kg/min IV infusion to maintain MAP of 60 mm Hg)
- Correction of hypokalemia, acidosis, etc.
- Invasive procedure including placement of central venous catheter for volume replacement, high-dose inotrope infusion, and central venous pressure (CVP) monitoring
- Placement of arterial line for invasive blood pressure monitoring
- Revascularization of culprit vessels by either percutaneous coronary intervention (PCI) or coronary artery bypass grafting (CABG) is the treatment of choice for cardiogenic shock due to acute myocardial infarction (AMI).
- If a coronary intervention facility is not available, then thrombolysis is the choice.
- Therapy for cardiogenic shock due to RVMI consists of fluid resuscitation. Many a time, norepinephrine is required to maintain MAP and adequate coronary artery perfusion.
- *Intra-aortic balloon pump (IABP) therapy*: In hemodynamically unstable patients, IABP sometimes may be useful to ensure adequate perfusion of compromised RV. Revascularization of the occluded artery by percutaneous transluminal coronary angioplasty (PTCA) remains the treatment of choice.

### *Predictors of Mortality in Cardiogenic Shock*

The GUSTO-1 (Global Utilization of Streptokinase and Tissue Plasminogen Activator for Occluded Coronary Arteries) trial has identified the following predictors of mortality from cardiogenic shock:

- Advanced age
- Past history of myocardial infarction
- Altered mentation
- Oliguria
- Cold clammy skin
- Echocardiographic findings such as reduced left ventricular ejection fraction (LVEF) and the presence of mitral regurgitation are independent risk factors.
- Time to reperfusion after the incidence of MI with cardiogenic shock
- RVMI
- 30% of Inferior wall MI and 10% of anterior wall MI become hemodynamically unstable but has a better prognosis than cardiogenic shock due to left ventricular (LV) failure.

### *Society for Cardiovascular Angiography and Interventions Classification of Cardiogenic Shock (Fig. 2)*

- *Stage A*: At risk
- *Stage B*: Beginning cardiogenic shock
- *Stage C*: Classic cardiogenic shock
- *Stage D*: Deteriorating/doom
- *Stage E*: Extremis

## ROLE OF SUPPORT DEVICES IN MANAGEMENT OF SHOCK

In hemodynamically unstable patients, immediate stabilization can be obtained using mechanical support devices (MCS) and options include:

- IABP therapy
- Impella device
- Extracorporeal membrane oxygenation (ECMO)

### Extracorporeal Membrane Oxygenation

Extracorporeal membrane oxygenation is a form of extracorporeal life support where an external artificial circulator carries venous blood from the patient to a gas exchange device (oxygenator) where blood becomes enriched with oxygen and has carbon dioxide removed. This blood then reenters

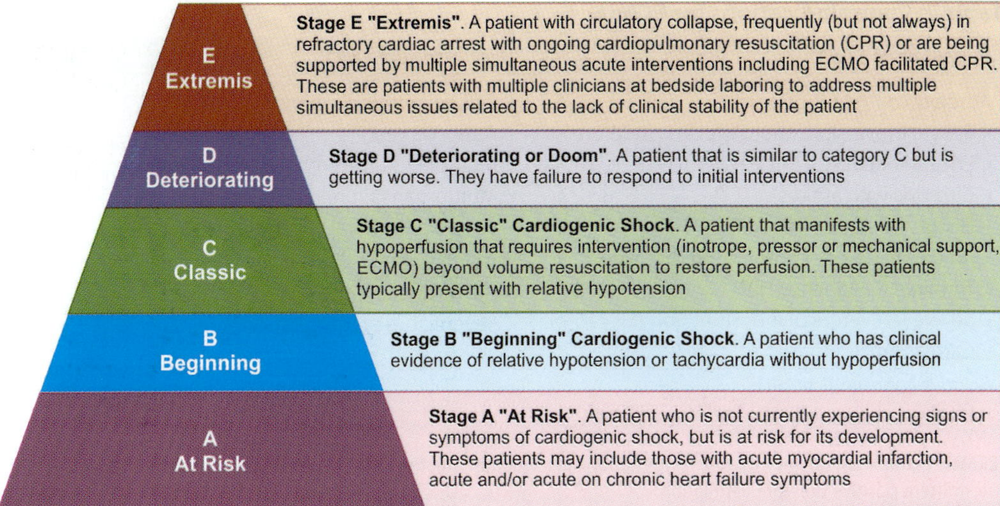


**FIG. 2:** The Society for Cardiovascular Angiography and Interventions (SCAI) classification of cardiogenic shock.

(ECMO: extracorporeal membrane oxygenation)

the patient's circulation. There are two types of ECMO:

1. *Venoarterial (VA) ECMO*:
    - Required for cardiac support, appropriate for respiratory support
    - Hemodynamics are controlled by the blood flow (pump flow plus native cardiac output) and vascular resistance.
2. *Venovenous (VV) ECMO*:
    - No hemodynamic support, preferred for respiratory support because it avoids using a major artery and avoids potential systemic embolism.
    - The patient is dependent on his own hemodynamic physiology.

### *Indications of Extracorporeal Membrane Oxygenation in Cardiogenic Shock (Venoarterial Extracorporeal Membrane Oxygenation Only)*

Typical cardiac indications include refractory low cardiac output (CI <2 L/min/m$^2$) and hypotension (SBP <90 mm Hg) despite adequate intravascular volume, high-dose inotropic agents, and IABP. Cardiogenic shock or severe cardiac failure due to any cause:

- Acute coronary syndrome
- Cardiac arrhythmic storm refractory to other measures
- Sepsis with profound cardiac depression
- Drug overdose/toxicity with profound cardiac depression
- Myocarditis
- Pulmonary embolism
- Isolated cardiac trauma
- Acute anaphylaxis

Other indications for VA ECMO for cardiac support are as follows:

- *Post cardiotomy*: Inability to wean from cardiopulmonary bypass after cardiac surgery
- *Postheart transplant*: Primary graft failure after heart or heart-lung transplantation
- *Chronic cardiomyopathy*: As a bridge to long-term ventricular assist device (VAD) support
- Periprocedural support for high-risk percutaneous cardiac intervention
- Bridge to transplantation

**Table 2: Contraindications for ECMO.**

| *Venovenous ECMO* | *Venoarterial ECMO* |
|---|---|
| *Absolute contraindications*<br>• Severe irreversible neurological condition<br>• Encephalopathy<br>• Cirrhosis with ascites<br>• History of variceal bleeding<br>• Moderate-severe chronic lung disease<br>• Terminal malignancy HIV<br>• Severe left ventricular dysfunction (EF <25%)<br>• Cardiac arrest<br>*Relative contraindications*:<br>• High pressure/high $FiO_2$ IPPV for >1 week | *Relative contraindications*<br>• Age > 65 years<br>• Multiple trauma with uncontrolled hemorrhage<br>• Multiorgan failure<br>• Severe peripheral vascular disease<br>*Absolute contraindications*:<br>• Aortic dissection<br>• Severe aortic regurgitation |

(ECMO: extracorporeal membrane oxygenation; EF: ejection fraction; HIV: human immunodeficiency virus; IPPV: intermittent positive pressure ventilation)

### *Contraindications*

Most contraindications are relative, balancing the risks of the procedure (including the risk of using valuable resources which could be used for others) versus the potential benefits **(Table 2)**.

Thus, early recognition of the type of shock and its specific management in time to prevent irreversible tissue injury is the goal. Improved devices for better monitoring such as EV1000 monitor, CytoSorb hemodialysis, Impella devices, and ECMO are acting as game changers.

## CLINICAL PEARLS

Distributive shock is the most frequently encountered type of shock in clinical practice. Among the different types of distributive shock, septic shock comprises the majority.

A high index of suspicion is needed to identify subtle presentations, particularly in elderly subjects in whom typical features may not be present many times.

Appropriate antimicrobials should be initiated within the first hour of recognizing sepsis. This has shown to improve prognosis and survival.

Balanced crystalloids (lactated Ringer solution, Plasma-Lyte) are the preferred fluids to be used in septic shock.

Corticosteroids downregulate the maladaptive inflammatory response seen in sepsis and address relative adrenal insufficiency caused by adrenal suppression. Guidelines recommend hydrocortisone 200 mg/day to be given during initial 3 days either as continuous infusion or in divided doses (50 mg qds).

Cardiogenic shock requires a well equipped facility for treatment. In the absence of a highly experienced care center, the mortality is as high as 80–90%.

Pulmonary artery (PA) catheterization (Swan-Ganz catheter) helps to differentiate between various types of shock (e.g., hypovolemic, cardiogenic, or distributive).

Mechanical support devices can be used in hemodynamically unstable patients during transport to higher center or can act as a bridge to definite treatment (cardiac transplantation).

## FURTHER READINGS


1. Rhodes A, Evans LE, Alhazzani W, Levy MM, Antonelli M, Ferrer R, et al. Surviving Sepsis Campaign: International Guidelines for Management of Sepsis and Septic Shock: 2016. Intensive Care Med. 2017;43(3):304-77.
2. Malbrain ML, Marik PE, Witters I, Cordemans C, Kirkpatrick AW, Roberts DJ, et al. Fluid overload, de-resuscitation, and outcomes in critically ill or injured patients: a systematic review with suggestions for clinical practice. Anaesthesiol Intensive Ther. 2014;46(5):361-80.
3. Seymour CW, Gesten F, Prescott HC, Friedrich ME, Iwashyna TJ, Phillips GS, et al. Time to treatment and mortality during mandated emergency care for sepsis. N Engl J Med. 2017;376(23): 2235-44.
4. Semler MW, Self WH, Wanderer JP, Ehrenfeld JM, Wang L, Byrne DW, et al; SMART Investigators and the Pragmatic Critical Care Research Group. Balanced crystalloids versus saline in critically ill adults. N Engl J Med. 2018;378(9): 829-39.
5. Krajewski ML, Raghunathan K, Paluszkiewicz SM, Schermer CR, Shaw AD. Meta-analysis of high- versus low-chloride content in perioperative and critical care fluid resuscitation. Br J Surg. 2015;102(1):24-36.
6. Rochwerg B, Oczkowski SJ, Siemieniuk RAC, Agoritsas T, Belley-Cote E, D'Aragon F, et al. Corticosteroids in sepsis: an updated systematic review and meta-analysis. Crit Care Med. 2018; 46(9):1411-20.
7. Baran DA, Grines CL, Bailey S, Burkhoff D, Hall SA, Henry TD, et al. SCAI clinical expert consensus statement on the classification of cardiogenic shock. Catheter Cardiovasc Interv. 2019;94(1):29-37.
8. Fraser JF, Shekar K, Diab S, Dunster K, Foley S, McDonald C, et al. ECMO—the clinician's view. ISBT Sci Ser. 2012;7:82-8.
9. Rochwerg B, Oczkowski SJ, Siemieniuk RAC, Agoritsas T, Belley-Cote E, D'Aragon F, et al. Corticosteroids in sepsis: an updated systematic review and meta-analysis. Crit Care Med. 2018;46(9):1411-20.

CHAPTER 95

# Acute Myocardial Infarction

*Md Hamid Ali*

## INTRODUCTION

Acute myocardial infarction (MI) is one of the leading causes of angina and death. The prevalence of the disease approaches 3 million people worldwide, with more than 1 million deaths in the United States annually. MI is the irreversible necrosis of the heart muscle. A common cause for infarction is deprivation in myocardial oxygen supply because of interruption of blood flow in atherothrombotic coronary arteries (total occlusion) as a result of plaque rupture, erosion, fissure, or coronary dissection (type I MI). The pathophysiological mechanism (partial occlusion by atherosclerosis, vasospasm, coronary dissection, oxygen supply and mismatch, other acute noncoronary trigger/illness) leading to myocardial damage is referred to as type II MI. Typical angina is characterized by (1) substernal chest pain with typical sensation, (2) chest pain provoked by exertion or emotional stress, and (3) that is relieved by rest or nitroglycerin (NTG) within minutes. Any ischemic discomfort is diagnosed as acute coronary syndrome (ACS). Among them, those showing ST elevation in electrocardiogram (ECG) are diagnosed as having ST-segment elevation myocardial infarction (STEMI). Those having no ST elevation in ECG and positive cardiac biomarkers are diagnosed as having non-ST-segment elevation myocardial infarction (NSTEMI), and negative biomarkers are diagnosed as unstable angina (UA). Acute MI is of two types, STEMI and NSTEMI. UA is similar to NSTEMI but without elevation of cardiac markers. Other important causes of chest pain to be considered in the differential diagnosis (D/D) carefully are as follows:

- *Cardiac*: Aortic dissection, pericarditis, stable ischemic heart disease (SIHD)
- *Pulmonary*: Pulmonary embolism (PE), pneumonia, spontaneous pneumothorax
- *Gastrointestinal (GIT)*: Gastroesophageal reflux disease (GERD), peptic ulcer, biliary disease, pancreatitis
- *Musculoskeletal (MSK)*: Costochondritis, cervical disk disease
- Psychological
- Preeruptive phase of herpes zoster

Acute MI causes complete closure of the coronary artery and thereby irreversible damage to the cardiac muscle. An MI may lead to the development of several complications such as impairment in diastolic and systolic function and arrhythmias. The important step of treatment is reperfusion to restore blood flow. The earlier the reperfusion (<3 hours from symptom onset), the better the prognosis. The dictum is: Time is the muscle. STEMI progresses through the following stages: Acute (7 days), healing (7–28 days), and healed (>29 days).

An MI is diagnosed when two of the following criteria are met:

- *Symptoms of ischemia*: Quality—tightness or pressure, squeezing, crushing, heavy, central precordial chest pain. It commonly occurs at rest and is more severe than angina but when it occurs during the period of activity or exertion, it does not subside with rest, unlike angina. It may radiate to the arm, jaw, and epigastrium, associated with autonomic nervous system stimulation signs—sweating and fear of impending death. Pain is deep and visceral.
- New ST-segment changes or a left bundle branch block (LBBB)
- Presence of pathological Q waves on ECG
- Presence of an intracoronary thrombus at autopsy or angiography
- Imaging study showing new regional wall motion abnormality (RWMA)

## ETIOLOGY

Decreased coronary blood flow is multi-factorial. Atherosclerotic plaques classically rupture and lead to thrombosis, contributing to acutely decreased blood flow in the coronary. Other etiologies of decreased oxygenation/myocardial ischemia include coronary artery embolism, which accounts for 2.9% of patients, cocaine-induced ischemia, coronary dissection, and coronary vasospasm **(Box 1)**.

**BOX 1: Other causes of myocardial infarction (MI).**

- Trauma
- Drug use (cocaine)
- Vasculitis
- Excess demand on the heart (hyperthyroidism, anemia)
- Coronary artery anomalies
- Aortic dissection
- Coronary artery emboli

## EPIDEMIOLOGY

Seventy percent of infarctions are due to occlusion from atherosclerotic plaques. Modifiable risk factors account for 90% in men and 94% in women **(Table 1)**.

## PATHOPHYSIOLOGY

Atherosclerotic rupture leads to an inflammatory cascade of monocytes and macrophages, thrombus formation, and platelet aggregation. This leads to decreased oxygen delivery through the coronary artery resulting in decreased oxygenation of the myocardium. The inability to produce adenosine triphosphate (ATP) in the mitochondria leads to the ischemic cascade, and therefore apoptosis (cell death) of the endocardium or MI.

## SUPPLIED AREA OF CORONARY ARTERIES

- Left anterior descending (LAD) artery
- Left circumflex (LCx)
- Right coronary artery (RCA)
- Interventricular septum, anterolateral wall, and ventricular apex
- Inferolateral wall
- Right ventricle

**Table 1: Risk factors.**

| *Nonmodifiable risk factors* | *Modifiable risk factors* |
|---|---|
| • Age<br>• Sex<br>• Family history<br>• Male pattern baldness | • Smoking<br>• Dyslipidemia<br>• Diabetes mellitus<br>• Hypertension<br>• Obesity<br>• Sedentary lifestyle<br>• Poor oral hygiene<br>• Presence of peripheral vascular disease<br>• Elevated levels of homocysteine |

## HISTOPATHOLOGY

The histology of MI changes over the time course of the disease. At time of initial event, there are no microscopic histologic changes. Under light microscopy, within 0.5–4 hours, waviness of fibers at the periphery of the tissue is seen. Glycogen is depleted. At 4–12 hours, the myocardium undergoes coagulation necrosis and edema. At 12–24 hours, the gross specimen becomes dark and mottled. There are contraction band necrosis and neutrophil predominance in histopathology. At 1–3 days, there is a loss of nuclei, and at 3–7 days, macrophages appear to remove apoptosis cells. At 7–10 days, granulation tissue appears. At 10 days and onward, there is collagen deposition. After 2 months, the myocardium is scarred.

## CARDIAC BIOMARKERS

Cardiac biomarkers are useful in the diagnosis of acute MI, specifically NSTEMI. Troponin is the most specific laboratory test and has two isoforms, I and T. Troponins peak at 12 hours and persist for 7 days. Creatinine kinase-MB (CK-MB) is also specific to the myocardium. It peaks at 10 hours; however, it normalizes within 2–3 days. Lactate dehydrogenase (LDH) peaks over 72 hours and normalizes over 10–14 hours. In clinical practice, LDH is not used to diagnose acute MI. Finally, MB has very low specificity for the myocardium and is not used clinically; it quickly rises and normalizes. High-sensitivity cardiac troponin (hs-cTn) detects MI significantly earlier. Negative hs-cTn on arrival to the emergency medical room (EMR) has a 99.4% negative predictive value. Troponin measurements are more sensitive and specific than creatine phosphokinase-MB (CPK-MB). In the American College of Cardiology/American Heart Association/European Society of Cardiology (ACC/AHA/ESC) guidelines, CPK-MB measurements are no longer recommended. Potential false-positive interpretations are as follows:

- *Cardiovascular system (CVS)*: Aortic dissection, arrhythmia, hypotension, acute congestive heart failure (CHF), takotsubo, myocarditis, hypertension (HTN), left ventricular hypertrophy (LVH), infiltrative disease, myocardial injury
- *Lung*: PE
- *GIT*: Severe GI bleeding
- *Central nervous system (CNS)*: Cerebrovascular accident (CVA), head injury
- *Hematology*: Anemia, hypoxia, thrombotic thrombocytopenic purpura (TTP)
- *Endocrine*: Diabetes mellitus (DM), hypothyroidism
- *Infection*: Sepsis, extensive burns
- *Renal*: Chronic kidney disease (CKD)

## HISTORY AND PHYSICAL EXAMINATION

The history and physical examination are often inconsistent when evaluating for acute MI. The history should focus on the onset, quality, and associated symptoms. Recent studies have found that diaphoresis, substernal chest pain >30 minutes, and bilateral arm radiating pain most often are associated with MI (STEMI) in men. Associated symptoms include:

- Light-headedness
- Anxiety
- Cough
- Choking sensation
- Diaphoresis
- Wheezing
- Irregular heart rate (HR)

*Physical examination*: Vital signs and patient's appearance, dyspnea, and diaphoresis are to be noted; lung and cardiac auscultation are to be done carefully. Anterior infarction is associated with sympathetic hyperactivity (HTN, tachycardia) and inferior infarction leads to parasympathetic overactivity (bradycardia, hypotension).

- *HR*: It may reveal tachycardia/bradycardia, atrial fibrillation (AF), or ventricular arrhythmia.

- *Heart*: It is usually quiet. Lateral displacement of apical impulse, soft S1, palpable S4, new mitral regurgitation (MR) murmur are its characteristics rupture chordae tendineae. A loud holosystolic murmur radiating to the sternum may be indicative of ventricular septal rupture.
- *Blood pressure (BP)*: It is usually high, but hypotension or 10–15 mm Hg lower than the preinfarct state in transmural MI or in shock.
- *Pulse*: Unequal pulses if the patient has an aortic dissection.
- *Jugular venous pressure (JVP)*: Neck veins may be distended, indicating right ventricular (RV) failure.
- *Chest*: Wheezing and rales are common if the patient has developed pulmonary edema; tachypnea and fever are not uncommon.
- Extremities may show edema or cyanosis and will be cold.

*Differential diagnosis of AMI*: Aortic dissection, pericarditis, acute gastritis, acute cholecystitis, asthma, esophagitis, myocarditis, pneumothorax, pulmonary embolism to be excluded in making diagnosis of AMI.

# EVALUATION

Evaluation is done by the following.

## Electrocardiogram

- Early and rapid ECG testing within 10 minutes of emergency department (ED) arrival should be employed in all patients presenting with chest pain. Women often have atypical symptoms such as abdominal pain or dizziness and may present without chest pain at all. Elderly patients more often have shortness of breath as their presenting symptom for MI. All of these presentations should prompt ECG testing as well.
- If the initial ECG is not diagnostic of STEMI but the patient remains symptomatic, and there is a high clinical suspicion for STEMI, serial ECGs at 5- to 10-minute intervals or continuous 12-lead ST-segment monitoring should be performed to detect the potential development of ST elevation.
- The ECG is highly specific for MI (95–97%), yet not sensitive (approximately 30%). Following are the options if clinically suspected patients have normal 12-lead ECG:
    - To know posterior wall myocardial infarction (PWMI) or LCx artery occlusion
    - Take leads $V_7$–$V_9$ leads
    - To know the RV infarct
    - Right-sided ECG leads (*take $V_3R$, $V_4R$*). It should be taken in IWMI to know right ventricular extension of MI or in suspected cases of RVMI
    - Criteria of AMI:
        - ACC/AHA/ESC criteria for STEMI are as follows:
            1. ST-segment elevation (STE) > 0.1 mV (1 mm) in at least 2 contiguous leads other than $V_2$ or $V_3$. In leads $V_2$ or $V_3$ the cutoff point of STE measured at J point should be ≥0.25 mV in men <40 years, ≥2 mV (2 mm) in men >40 years or ≥0.15 mV in women >40 years.
            2. New or presumably new LBBB
            3. MI criteria in the presence of LBBB: Sgarbossa criteria: (1) concordant STE ≥ 1 mm in positive QRS, (2) discordant STE ≥ 5 mm in negative QRS, and (3) concordance ST depression ≥1 mm in $V_1$–$V_3$
        - Patients with MI and right bundle branch block (RBBB) have a poor prognosis. It may be difficult to detect transmural ischemia in patients with chest pain and RBBB. Therefore, a primary percutaneous coronary intervention (PCI) strategy [emergent coronary angiography (CAG) and PCI if

indicated] should be considered when persistent ischemic symptoms occur in the presence of RBBB.
- *Isolated posterior wall infarction*: Isolated ST depression > 0.5 mm in $V_1$–$V_3$ and STE ≥ 0.5 mm in $V_7$–$V_9$
- Peaked T waves on ECG, known as "hyper acute T waves," often indicate early ischemia and will progress to ST elevation.
- The presence of ST depression ≥ 1 mm in 8 or more surface leads (inferolateral ST depression), coupled with STE in aVR and/or $V_1$, suggests multivessel ischemia or left main coronary artery obstruction, particularly if the patient presents with hemodynamic compromise.
- Most patients presenting with STEMI ultimately evolve Q waves in ECG unless there is partial or transient occlusion or rich collateral networks. Q wave is actually dependent on the volume of infarcted tissue, not by transmurality.

When present, findings of ST elevations >2 mm in 2 contiguous leads on ECG are indicative of STEMI. Often, there are reciprocal ST depressions that are visualized in opposite anatomical regions of the myocardium (e.g., anterior wall ST elevation and inferior wall ST depression and vice versa).

- Leads II, III, aVF: Inferior wall
- $V_1$, $V_2$: Septal wall
- $V_3$, $V_4$: Anterior
- I, aVL, $V_5$, $V_6$: Lateral

Electrocardiogram diagnosis of STEMI can be difficult, particularly in patients with an LBBB and pacemakers. Sgarbossa described the criteria that can assist the physician or practitioner in diagnosing STEMI in these patients. Isolated ST elevations in aVR are indicative of left main coronary artery occlusion in the appropriate clinical setting. Wellens noted deeply biphasic T waves in $V_2$, $V_3$ and found that they are often predictive of an impending proximal LAD artery occlusion, which may lead to devastating anterior wall myocardial infarction (AWMI).

Patients who present with MI may not have diagnostic ST elevation ECG abnormalities. Patients with typical chest pain should be investigated for NSTEMI with subtle abnormalities on ECG, including ST depressions and T-wave changes. Serial ECGs can be helpful here as well to look for dynamic changes. ECG without acute changes or any abnormalities is common in NSTEMI.

There are diagnostic guidelines that can assist the practitioner in determining whether further testing is useful in identifying patients with NSTEMI. Given the poor sensitivity of ECG for STEMI, troponins are almost universally used for patients with a suspicious clinical history. The HEART score has been validated and popularized. It utilizes the clinician's suspicion, patient risk factors, ECG diagnostics, and troponin level to determine the "risk level."

## Laboratory Features

- *Cardiac biomarkers*: For patients with ST elevation on the 12-lead ECG and symptoms of STEMI, reperfusion therapy should be initiated as soon as possible and reperfusion Rx don't depends on biomarker assay. Cardiac-specific troponins should be used as the optimum biomarkers for the evaluation of patients with STEMI who have coexistent skeletal muscle injury or clinical suspicion of small MI (NSTEMI or UA). hs-cTn does not have immediate value in STEMI diagnosis and management. Serial biomarker measurements can be useful to provide supportive noninvasive evidence of reperfusion of the infarct artery after fibrinolytic therapy. Serial biomarker (troponin) measurements should not be relied on to diagnose reinfarction within the first 18 hours after the onset of STEMI. Levels of cardiac troponin I (cTnI) or cardiac troponin T (cTnT) may remain elevated for 7–10 days of STEMI. In that case, CK is a good option (rises within 4–8 hours and returns to normal by 48–72 hours). CK-MB mass to CK activity >2.5 suggests myocardial origin. Although handheld bedside (point-of-care) assays may be used for a qualitative assessment of the presence of an elevated level of a serum cardiac biomarker, subsequent measurements of cardiac biomarker levels should be performed with a quantitative test **(Table 2)**.

- *Blood test*:
  - *Lipid profile*: Complete blood count (CBC)—rise of total leukocyte count (TLC) (12,000–15,000) within hours may remain elevated up to 1 week and erythrocyte sedimentation rate (ESR) may remain elevated for 1–2 weeks.
  - *Metabolic panel*: B-type natriuretic peptide (BNP) should not be ordered as a marker for MI, but it is better used to stratify risk, especially in patients with MI who develop heart failure.
  - *Renal function test*: Urea, Creatinine, eGFR, In CKD Troponin test may be false positive, RFT may be altered in cardiorenal syndrome.
  - *LFT*: It is deranged in MI with heart failure

## Cardiac Imaging

- *Cardiac angiography* is used to perform PCI or determine obstructions in the coronary vessels.
- *Portable echocardiography* is reasonable to clarify the diagnosis of STEMI and allow risk stratification of patients with chest pain on arrival at the ED, especially if the diagnosis of STEMI is confounded by LBBB or pacing, or if there is suspicion of posterior STEMI with anterior ST depressions. An echocardiogram is used to assess wall motion, degree of valve abnormality, ischemic MR, and presence of cardiac tamponade.
- *Radionuclide imaging*: Myocardial perfusion imaging (MPI) with [$^{99m}$Tc] or [$^{201}$T], which is distributed proportionately with the distribution of blood flow, will show a defect (cold spot) in transmural infarct with limitation of detection of acute infarct to chronic infarct. Radionuclide ventriculography carried out with [$^{99m}$Tc]-labeled red blood cell (RBC) is used to show wall motion abnormality and reduced ejection fraction (EF), in a patients with CAD, VHD, CHD, MI and to assess ventricular synchrony before CRT Rx.

**Table 2: Interpretation of hs-cTn with duration of pain and related necessary intervention.**

| ***A. Highly sensitive cardiac troponin (hs-cTn) < ULN*** | | |
|---|---|---|
| Pain > 6 hours | Pain free, GRACE score < 140, differential diagnosis (D/D) excluded | Discharge |
| Pain < 6 hours | Retest hs-cTn: 3 hours | |
| hs-cTn | No change | Pain free, GRACE score < 140, D/D excluded—discharge |
| hs-cTn | Change in hs-cTn | Early invasive management |
| ***B. hs-cTn > ULN*** | | |
| hs-cTn | Highly abnormal + clinical presentation | Invasive management |
| hs-cTn | Normal | Retest at: 3 hours—no change—workup D/D |

*Source*: Hatherley JD, Salmon T, Collinson PO, Khand A. Implementation of the European Society of Cardiology 0/3-hour accelerated diagnostic protocol, using high sensitive troponin T: a clinical practice evaluation of safety and effectiveness involving 3003 patients with suspected acute coronary syndromeOpen Heart 2023;10:e002366.

- *Cardiac magnetic resonance imaging (MRI)*: Gadolinium contrast with late enhancement MRI (LGE-MRI) is used to characterize myocardial tissue in MI. Bright areas of infarction appear in stark contrast to the dark areas of normal myocardium (little gadolinium enters in normal myocardium but percolates in the interstitium of myocardium).

### Chest X-ray

Patients with STEMI should have a portable chest X-ray (CXR).

## RISK SCORE CALCULATIONS

The risk score calculations are provided in **Table 3**.

## GENERAL MANAGEMENT OF ACUTE CORONARY SYNDROME

- *Oxygen*: It should be administered to patients with arterial oxygen desaturation ($SaO_2$ < 90%). It is reasonable to administer supplemental oxygen to all patients with uncomplicated STEMI during the first 6 hours.
- *NTG*: Patients with ongoing ischemic discomfort should receive sublingual NTG (0.4 mg) every 5 minutes for a total of 3 doses, after which an assessment should be made about the need for intravenous (IV) NTG. IV NTG is indicated for relief of ongoing ischemic discomfort, control of HTN, or management of pulmonary congestion. IV NTG is indicated in the following conditions:
  - Ongoing ischemic symptoms
  - Control of HTN
  - Management of pulmonary edema

  Contraindications of nitrate therapy are as follows:
  - Who have received phosphodiesterase inhibitor (within 24 hours of sildenafil or 48 hours for tadalafil)
  - Suspected RVI
  - HR < 50 or HR > 100 bpm
  - Systolic blood pressure (SBP) < 90 mm Hg (30 mm Hg below the baseline)
- *Analgesia*: Morphine sulfate (2–4 mg IV with increments of 2–8 mg IV repeated at 5- to 15-minute intervals) is the analgesic of choice for the management of pain associated with STEMI.
- *Tranquilizer*: A mild tranquilizer (usually a benzodiazepine) should be considered in anxious patients.

**Table 3: Risk score calculations.**

| ***TIMI score: Seven factors each score 1*** | |
|---|---|
| >65 years | Score 0–2 = Low risk TIMI score |
| 3 or more risk factors | Score 3–5 = Intermediate TIMI score |
| Prior coronary artery disease (CAD) | Score 6–7 = High TIMI score |
| ST deviations | Low TIMI score = 4.7–8.3% adverse effects |
| 2 or more angina episodes in 24 hours | Intermediate TIMI score = 13.2–26.2% adverse effects |
| Aspirin use within 7 days | High TIMI score = 40.9% adverse effects |
| Elevated cardiac markers | |
| ***GRACE-ACS risk model score*** | |
| *Low risk*: <108 | <1% risk of in-hospital death |
| *Intermediate*: 109–140 | 1–3% risk of in-hospital death |
| *High risk*: >140 | >3% risk of in-hospital death |

- *Antiplatelets*: Aspirin should be chewed by patients who have not taken aspirin before presentation with STEMI. The initial dose should be 150–300 mg and then 75–100 mg daily.
- *Beta-blockers (BBs)*: Oral BB therapy should be administered promptly to those patients without a contraindication, irrespective of concomitant fibrinolytic therapy or performance of primary PCI. It is reasonable to administer IV BBs promptly to STEMI patients without contraindications, especially if a tachyarrhythmia or HTN is present. *BB* therapy is mandatory in all patients with ACS. But it should not be used in the following conditions as per COMMIT/CCS-2 study:
    - Signs of heart failure
    - Evidence of low output states
    - Increased risk of heart failure—seen in the following conditions: age >70 years, SBP < 120 mm Hg, tachycardia > 110/minute, or HR < 60 bpm
    - PR interval > 0.24 seconds, 2nd degree and 3rd degree heart block, asthma, severe reactive airway disease
- *Specific therapy of STEMI* **(Flowchart 1)**:
    - *Reperfusions*: General concept—All STEMI patients should undergo rapid evaluation for reperfusion therapy and have a reperfusion strategy implemented. When ST elevation ≥2 mm in 2 contiguous precordial leads and 1 mm in 2 adjacent limb leads is present, reperfusion therapy should be seriously thought of, either primary PCI or fibrinolysis. Although the central zone of infarct is necrotic and irretrievably lost, the surrounding ischemic penumbra zone can be salvaged by the timely perfusion of infarct-related artery (IRA) and controlling the oxygen demand. Control of pain, tachycardia, CHF, and HTN can extend the window time of reperfusion.
    - *Reperfusion strategy*: The reperfusion strategy is mentioned in **Table 4**.

Primary PCI is superior to thrombolytic therapy when it can be performed in a timely manner by a skilled and experienced cardiologist and catheterization laboratory team.

*Indications of primary PCI in STEMI*:
- STEMI patients present within 12 hours.
- Those with severe heart failure or cardiogenic shock
- In patients following cardiac arrest and STE on the ECG, primary PCI is the strategy of choice.

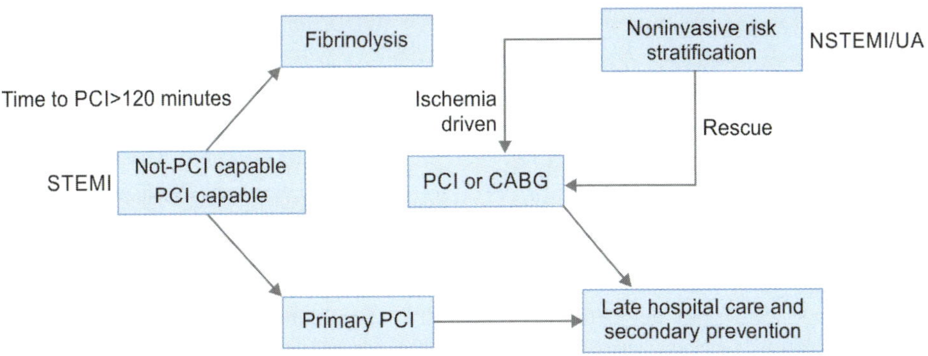


**FLOWCHART 1:** Management protocol of acute coronary syndrome (ACS) in brief with reperfusion strategy.

(CABG: coronary artery bypass grafting; PCI: percutaneous coronary intervention)

*Source*: https://doi.org/10.1093/eurheartj/ehad191

- Clinical evidence of failed fibrinolytic therapy (ST segment resolution <50% within 60–90 minutes of fibrinolytic administration)—rescue PCI
- Contraindications to thrombolytic therapy
- In the presence of hemodynamic or electrical instability, worsening ischemia, or persistent chest pain with symptoms lasting >12 hours in the presence of ECG changes
- However, there is no consensus as to whether PCI is also beneficial in patients presenting >12 hours from symptom onset in the absence of clinical and/or electrocardiographic evidence of ongoing ischemia.

For patients with significant left main disease, surgical revascularization is indicated to improve survival relative to that likely to be achieved with medical therapy. Percutaneous revascularization is a reasonable option to improve survival, compared with medical therapy, in selected patients with low-to-medium anatomic complexity of coronary artery disease and left main disease that is equally suitable for surgical or percutaneous revascularization.

*Pharmacoinvasive therapy*: Patient is sent to PCI lab after thrombolysis by fibrinolytics in non PCI capable center for catheterization. It should be done routinely within 2–24 hours of thrombolysis.

Some commonly used terminologies:
- *Door-to-balloon time (DBT)*: It is now no longer used. Nowadays, medical contact-to-device therapy (MCDT) is frequently used. The ideal goal is ≤90 minutes for PCI-capable centers; for other centers, it is 120 minutes.
- *Door in-door out (DIDO)*: PCI-not-capable center diagnoses STEMI and transfers to PCI center. The ideal goal is ≤30 minutes.

**Table 4: Reperfusion strategy.**

| | | |
|---|---|---|
| *Chest pain*: Facilitated medical center (FMC) | Non-PCI center–ECG to be done <10 minutes | Actions taken |
| | Time to PCI (FMC-Device time) ≤120 minutes-and | Send the patient to the PCI center for primary PCI strategy: Aim <90 minutes to wire crossing. Immediately transfer to PCI center for primary PCI, door in and door out (DIDO) time should be <30 minutes |
| | Time to PCI >120 minutes | *Fibrinolytic strategy*: Aim <10 minutes to lytic bolus, best to be done within 3 hours of symptom onset reperfusion by bolus fibrinolytics (TNK/rPA). Benefits may be extended up to 12 hours in special situation. Immediately transfer to PCI center after fibrinolysis for pharmaco-invasive therapy |
| *Chest pain*: FMC | *PCI center*: ECG <10 minutes (FMC device time <90 minutes) | *Primary PCI strategy*: To be done <60 minutes to wire crossing |
| Diagnostic angiogram done | For primary PCI, failed reperfusion by thrombolytics, pharmacoinvasive therapy | Go for either option as stated below:<br>• PCI<br>• CABG<br>• Medical therapy only |

(CABG: coronary artery bypass grafting; ECG: electrocardiogram; PCI: percutaneous coronary intervention)

- *Door-to-needle time (DNT)*: Time taken by a STEMI patient once he sets in EMR till the beginning of thrombolytic therapy. The generally accepted goal is ≤30 minutes.

*Primary PCI of IRA is the first choice.* New-generation drug-eluting stent (DES) of IRA is preferred over balloon angioplasty or bare metal stent (BMS). Radial access is preferred over femoral approach. Thrombus aspiration is not indicated.

*Antiplatelet cotherapy with PCI*: The ACC/AHA recommends dual antiplatelet therapy (DAPT) with either clopidogrel or ticagrelor along with aspirin. DAPT must be before PCI, preferably P2Y12 inhibitor - commonly ticagrelor - [loading dose (LD) with 180 mg then 90 mg BD] over clopidogrel (LD: 600 mg, then 75 mg/day). Prasugrel is contraindicated in a previous stroke (LD: 60 mg, then 10 mg/day). The PLATO trial suggests preferential use of ticagrelor over clopidogrel. Glycoprotein (GP) IIb-IIIa inhibitor (eptifibatide, tirofiban) may be considered (class IIb) in patients treated with an early invasive strategy with intermediate- to high-risk features in non-ST-segment elevation acute coronary syndrome (NSTE-ACS).

*Antiplatelets cotherapy with fibrinolytics*: DAPT—aspirin (the first dose of aspirin should be chewed, LD: 300 mg, then 75–100 mg/day) + P2Y12i-clopidogrel (LD: 300 mg, then 75 mg/day)

*Anticoagulant options for primary PCI* include unfractionated heparin (UFH), enoxaparin (ATOLL trial), and bivalirudin. The use of fondaparinux in the context of primary PCI was associated with potential harm.

- *UFH*: There is a large body of experience with this agent. UFH—IV bolus: 70–100 units/kg without GPIIb-IIIa inhibitor, 50–70 units/kg with GPIIb-IIIa inhibitor.
- Bivalirudin should be considered in STEMI, especially in patients at high bleeding risk. It may be given at the time of percutaneous intervention (LD: 0.75 mg/kg, then 0.175 mg/kg/h IV for 4 hours post procedure).
- *Triple antiplatelets therapy*: GPIIb/IIIa inhibitor—eptifibatide, tirofiban (LD: 25 µg/kg over 3 minutes, then 0.15 µg/kg/min IV over 18 hours). GPIIb-IIIa inhibitor may be used in STEMI patients undergoing PCI to prevent thrombotic complications, predominantly in situations of high thrombus load, reduced coronary flow, or PCI complication dissection.
- Routine postprocedural anticoagulant therapy is not indicated after primary PCI, except when there is a separate indication for either full-dose anticoagulation [due to, for instance, AF, mechanical valves, or left ventricular (LV) thrombus] or prophylactic doses for the prevention of venous thromboembolism in patients requiring prolonged bed rest.

*Antithrombotic cotherapy with fibrinolysis* (any one): UFH, enoxaparin, fondaparinux

- *UFH*: 60 units/kg IV bolus—max 4,000 units, then 12–16 units/kg/h for 24–48 hours
- *Enoxaparin*: If age <75 years, LD: 30 mg IV bolus and then 1 mg/kg SC after 15 minutes and BD; the first 2 doses should not exceed 100 mg. If age >75 years, no LD, only 0.75 mg/kg SC BD. If estimated glomerular filtration rate (eGFR) <30, LD SC OD given.
- *Fondaparinux*: 2.5 mg IV bolus in patients treated with stent thrombosis kinase (STK), then SC 24 hours after; for the period of hospitalization—maximum 8 days or revascularization

## Thrombolytic Therapy

- Fibrinolytic therapy is an important reperfusion strategy in settings where primary PCI cannot be offered in a timely manner.
- The largest absolute benefit is seen when treatment is offered <2 hours after symptom onset.

- Fibrinolytic therapy is recommended within 12 hours of symptom onset if primary PCI cannot be performed within 120 minutes from STEMI diagnosis.
- The later the patient presents (particularly after 3 hours), the more consideration should be given to transfer for primary PCI (as opposed to administering fibrinolytic therapy) because the efficacy and clinical benefit of fibrinolysis decrease as the time from symptom onset increases.
- Fibrin-specific thrombolytic (tenecteplase, alteplase, reteplase) is preferred.

*Prehospital thrombolysis*: If trained medical or paramedical staff are able to analyze the ECG on-site or to transmit the ECG to the hospital for interpretation, it is recommended to initiate fibrinolytic therapy in the prehospital setting. The aim is to start fibrinolytic therapy within 10 minutes from STEMI diagnosis.

*Pharmacoinvasive therapy*: Routinely within 2–24 hours of thrombolysis, the patient is to be shifted to the PCI laboratory after thrombolysis for catheterization. Transfer to a PCI-capable center after thrombolysis is indicated, especially if there is failed reperfusion (persistent chest pain, ST remains elevated >90 minutes), coronary reocclusion (re-elevation of ST and/or recurrent chest pain), recurrent chest pain in the early hospital stay, or positive subthreshold exercise test before discharge. Elective PCI in asymptomatic patients after thrombolysis is used less frequently. Coronary artery bypass grafting (CABG) should be reserved for those who have unsuitable coronary artery for PCI.

### Doses of Thrombolytic

- *Alteplase*: LD: 15 mg IV bolus, then 0.75 mg/kg (max: 35 mg) IV over 30 minutes and then 0.5 mg/kg (max 30 mg) IV over 60 minutes
- *Tenecteplase*: Single IV push, 30 mg if <60 kg, 35 mg if <70 kg, 40 mg if <80 kg, 45 mg if <90 kg
- *Reteplase*: 10 + 10 units IV bolus 30 minutes apart

### Contraindications of Thrombolytic Therapy

The contraindications of thrombolytic therapy are mentioned in **Table 5**.

*Complications of fibrinolytics/thrombolytics*: Allergy, hemorrhage [intracranial hemorrhage (ICH): 0.5–0.9%], which increases with age. Age > 70 years—risk rises to double.

*Noncardiac care in critical care unit (CCU)/hospital periods*:

- *Activity*: The patient should be kept on bed rest for 6–12 hours. After that, within 24 hours, the patient is allowed to sit by dangling their feet and gradually on a chair in uncomplicated cases. Three to five days before anticipating discharge, they are allowed to ambulate within the room with increasing duration.
- *Diet*: Nothing per mouth (NPM) or clear liquids in the first 4–12 hours in the fear of vomiting. Thereafter, low fat, low calorie, high fiber, rich in potassium, magnesium, and low in sodium diet is given. Take care of diabetes mellitus or hypertriglyceridemia.
- *Bowel management*: Bedside commode is preferred over bedpan. Diet rich in bulk and stool softener [dioctyl sulfosuccinate (DOSS)—200 mg/day] or laxative can be advised who remain constipated even after all previous measures.
- *Sedation*: Diazepam 5 mg or lorazepam 0.5–2 mg is given to withstand the period of inactivity and at night, for good sleep besides a quite environment.

*Duration of antithrombin therapy after thrombolytic therapy*:

- *For UFH*: 48 hours
- *For low-molecular-weight heparin (LMWH)/direct thrombin inhibitor (DTI)*: Throughout their hospitalization, up to 8 days (as per EXTRACT, CREATE, OASIS-6 studies)

**Table 5: Contraindications of thrombolytic therapy.**

| *Absolute* | *Relative* |
|---|---|
| • Any prior intracranial hemorrhage (ICH)<br>• AVM/ICSOL/malignancy<br>• CVA: Infarction within 3 months<br>• Suspected aortic dissection<br>• Active bleeding or diathesis<br>• Head injury within 3 months<br>• Intracranial or intraspinal surgery within 2 months<br>• Severe uncontrolled hypertension (unresponsive to emergency therapy)<br>• For STK: Prior treatment with STK <6 month | • TIA in the prior 6 months<br>• Oral anticoagulant therapy<br>• Active peptic ulcer<br>• Refractory hypertension < 180/110 mm Hg<br>• Advanced liver disease<br>• Infective endocarditis<br>• Pregnancy or within 1 week of postpartum<br>• Prolong resuscitation |

(AVM: arteriovenous malformation; CVA: cerebrovascular accident; ICSOL: intracranial space-occupying lesion; STK: stent thrombosis kinase; TIA: transient ischemic attack)

*NSTEMI—Non-ST-segment elevation myocardial infarction*: Caused by plaque instability with a nonocclusive thrombus or embolization with the following ECG changes:
- Persistent or transient ST depression
- T wave changes—inversion, flattening, or pseudonormalization

*HEART score*: Consisting of history, ECG, age, risk factor, troponin. Heart score ≥4 is highly suggestive of ACS. Score of 0–3 with negative troponin is not likely ACS.

Though a NSTEMI patient has lower short-term mortality risk than a STEMI patient, long-term mortality is significantly increased. After diagnosis, risk stratification is required **(see Table 6)**. A high-risk patient is treated with an early invasive strategy.

*Treatment strategy of NSTEMI*: Invasive versus conservatives as per risk stratifications:
- Very high risk—intermediate invasive (<2 hours). CAG followed by (f/b) PCI/CABG
- High risk—early invasive (<24 hours)
- Intermediate risk—invasive (<72 hours)
- Low risk—noninvasive/medical therapy (anti-ischemic and antithrombotic) initially, f/b selective invasive approach

*Non-ST-segment elevation myocardial infarction requires the following management.*

Antiplatelets—aspirin at presentation + any one of the P2Y12 inhibitors as per the situation:
- Clopidogrel
- Ticagrelor
- Prasugrel, who are proceeding to PCI
- GPIIb-IIIa inhibitor considered in bailout situations or thrombotic complications during PCI

Antianginal therapy—nitrate at presentation, anti-ischemic therapy—Beta blocker.

Anticoagulants—options include:
- UFH
- Enoxaparin
- Fondaparinux—2.5 mg SC/daily. Patients on fondaparinux undergoing PCI, a single IV bolus of UFH (70–85 IU/kg or 50–60 IU/kg concomitant with GPIIb-IIIa inhibitor) during PCI
- Bivalirudin—initiated at the time of PCI with a history of heparin-induced thrombocytopenia (HIT) as an alternative to UFH + GPIIb-IIIa inhibitor during PCI.

Thrombolytics are contraindicated in NSTEMI; they are actually harmful.

Following are the recommendations of ACS who are undergoing CABG:
- Wait at least 5 days after the last dose of clopidogrel or ticagrelor; resume after CABG for 1 year of DAPT.

**Table 6: Risk stratification.**

| *Very high risk* | *High risk* | *Intermediate risk* |
|---|---|---|
| Recurrent or ongoing chest pain, refractory pain | Rise or fall in cardiac troponin compatible with MI | DM |
| Hemodynamic instability | Dynamic ST-T changes | LVEF < 40% |
| Cardiogenic shock | GRACE score <140 | GRACE score <100–139 |
| Life-threatening arrhythmia or cardiac arrest | | Early postinfarct angina |
| Mechanical complications of MI, HF | | Prior PCI/CABG |
| Recurrent dynamic ST-T changes | | |

(CABG: coronary artery bypass grafting; DM: diabetes mellitus; HF: heart failure; LVEF: left ventricular ejection fraction; MI: myocardial infarction; PCI: percutaneous coronary intervention)

- Wait at least 7 days after the last dose of prasugrel.
- Discontinue tirofiban and eptifibatide 2–4 hours before CABG.
- Discontinue enoxaparin 12–24 hours before CABG and dose with UFH.
- Discontinue fondaparinux 24 hours before CABG and dose with UFH.
- Discontinue bivalirudin 3 hours before CABG and dose with UFH.
- For urgent CABG—clopidogrel or ticagrelor should be held for 24 hours to avoid major bleeding.

*Duration of DAPT (aspirin + clopidogrel/prasugrel/ticagrelor) treatment*: STEMI patients are to be treated with DAPT at least for 12 months irrespective of the treatment plan [PCI, CABG, thrombolysis—14 days to 12 months, guideline-directed medical therapy (GDMT)] unless they are at a high risk of bleeding (class I). In patients who are not at a high risk of bleeding or having any bleeding during these 12 months of therapy, DAPT may be continued reasonably (class IIb). In patients who are at a high risk of bleeding or having significant bleeding, DAPT may be discontinued reasonably (class IIb).

*DAPT and oral anticoagulant (OAT)*: The WOEST trial showed that double therapy [clopidogrel + vitamin K antagonist (VKA)] is superior to triple therapy (aspirin + clopidogrel + VKA). The AUGUSTUS trial showed that double therapy [P2Y12i + direct oral anticoagulant (DOAC)] is superior to triple therapy (aspirin + clopidogrel + VKA). In post-PCI patients with AF, DOAC is preferred over VKA, unless contraindicated. Clopidogrel is preferred as P2Y12i, but ticagrelor may be used reasonably in high thrombotic risk and low bleeding risk. Double therapy should be immediately considered after discharge in most cases, while triple therapy (aspirin + clopidogrel + DOAC) should only be considered in high thrombotic risk and low bleeding risk for a limited period of time (1 month).

*Triple therapy*: Aspirin + P2Y12i-clopidogrel + novel oral anticoagulant (NOAC) in patients with NSTEMI with AF/atrial flutter (AFl) for only 1 week (max: 1 month) prior to discontinuation of aspirin.

*Surgery with antiplatelets*: If cardiac and noncardiac surgeries are contemplated, ticagrelor, clopidogrel, and prasugrel should be stopped for 3, 5, and 7 days prior to the surgery, respectively, when possible.

*Clopidogrel and proton-pump inhibitor (PPI)*: There is a theoretical possibility of interaction; however, there is minimal data to suggest an effect on clinical outcome. In this regard, pantoprazole is preferable than omeprazole, which is not contraindicated.

*MINOCA*—Myocardial infarction with nonobstructive (<50% stenosis) coronary artery. Causes are as follows:

- Myocarditis
- *Epicardial coronary artery issues*: Dissection, spasm, microvascular dysfunctions
- Type II MI (oxygen supply and demand mismatch)
- PE
- *Takotsubo disease*: Stress cardiomyopathy, broken heart syndrome

*Signs of RVI*: Hypotension, distended neck veins with clear lungs. RVI is associated with 30% of inferior wall myocardial infarction (IWMI) cases. Preload reduction is detrimental in these cases. Therefore, NTG or morphine is contraindicated. Patients are treated with IV fluid and may require dopamine infusion. They need $V_3R$, $V_4R$, $V_5R$, $V_6R$ leads with STE >1 mm.

*Special consideration in ACS*: Prophylactic implantable cardioverter-defibrillator (ICD) should not be implanted in post-MI with low EF within 40 days of MI. If there is a high risk of sudden cardiac death (SCD), it can be done beyond the time limits.

*Long-term medical therapy in STEMI/NSTEMI: ABC*

- *A:*
    - *Antiplatelets*: Aspirin should be prescribed in all patients lifelong. P2Y12 inhibitor like clopidogrel is also used along with aspirin (DAPT) for 6 months to 1 year mostly; newer P2Y12 antagonist, prasugrel or ticagrelor, is more preferable than clopidogrel undergoing PCI with increased risk of bleeding.
    - *Anticoagulants*: Warfarin/DOAC for 3 months after full dose of antithrombotic therapy (LMWH/UFH) in the period of hospitalization following AWMI with severe LV dysfunction, HF, mural thrombus or AF, and previous history of embolism to prevent embolism.
    - *Angiotensin-converting enzyme inhibitor (ACEI)*: Maximum benefits are seen in high-risk patients including elderly, AWMI, low EF, and prior infarction, but short-term benefits are seen in all hemodynamically stable patients (BP > 100 mm Hg) to prevent ventricular remodeling and ventricular dysfunction and rate of reinfarction with STEMI. ACEI should be continued in large AWMI, CHF, EF < 40%, large RWMA on echocardiography, and HTN. Angiotensin receptor blocker (ARB) is used if ACEI is intolerable due to persistent cough or angioedema or has signs of HF [role of angiotensin receptor neprilysin inhibitor (ARNI)].
    - *Aldosterone antagonist* (spironolactone, eplerenone, finerenone) is used in the following conditions unless contraindicated (significant renal dysfunction—creatinine >2.5 mg/dL in men and >2.0 mg/dL in women and high potassium >5.0 mEq/L):
        - Who are on ACEI and BB and LVEF < 40%.
        - Symptomatic heart failure
        - Diabetes
- *B:* In most of the patients (usually along with ACEI) without contraindications [severe left ventricular failure (LVF), heart block, asthma, orthostatic hypotension]. In less severe HF, metoprolol succinate, carvedilol, or bisoprolol is used. Potential benefit of the use of BB gradually diminishes in those patients having excellent long-term prognosis [<55 years, no previous MI, normal LV function, no complex ventricular ectopic (VE), no angina, and expected mortality <1%/year].
- *C: Cholesterol-lowering agent*: High-intensity statin therapy is recommended, unless contraindicated by severe derangements of liver functions test or rhabdomyolysis. If the goal is not reached

with high-intensity statin, addition of ezetimibe is recommended; if even with statin and ezetimibe, low-density lipoprotein (LDL) goal < 70 mg/dL is not met, addition of PCSK9i, such as alirocumab or evolocumab, is advocated. As per the EVOPACS trial, initiation of PCSK9i at the time of hospitalization for ACS is supported.

*Complications and management*:
- New-onset MR
- Ventricular septal rupture
- LV aneurysm
- Arrhythmias
- Emboli
- Cardiogenic shock
- Pericarditis
- CHF
- RVI

*Cardiogenic shock*: End-organ hypoperfusion due to cardiac failure and the inability of the CVS to provide adequate flow to the extremities and vital organs. Clinical signs: Hypotension, oliguria, clouded sensorium, cool and mottled extremities; hemodynamic changes: SBP < 90 mm Hg for >30 minutes or MAP < 30 from baseline, cardiac index < 2.2 L/min/m$^2$, pulmonary arterial hypertension (PAH) > 15–18 mm Hg. Early reperfusion and prompt revascularization are the mainstay of therapy interpreted from the SHOCK study.

*Choice of revascularization in cardiogenic shock*: CABG is preferred in multivessel coronary artery disease (MVD). Culprit lesion only PCI is preferred over staged multivessel PCI if surgery is not an option (CULPRIT-SHOCK trial). But without cardiogenic shock, complete revascularization is the choice (COMPLETE trial).

*Percutaneous circulatory assist device (PCAD)*: The following PCADs are used for temporary support: Intra-aortic balloon pump (IABP), Impella, and TandemHeart.

*Common medical therapy in cardiogenic shock*:
- Antiplatelets
- Antithrombotic—heparin
- BB, calcium channel blocker (CCB), and vasodilators (NTG) are avoided.
- Proper oxygenation
- Low threshold for mechanical ventilation
- Antiarrhythmic therapy (IV amiodarone) is used when indicated.
- *Vasopressors support*: Lowest possible dose for the shortest possible time. Dopamine is used for mild-to-moderate shock. Norepinephrine is used for more severe shock and is superior to dopamine (SOAP study).
- Inotropic agents, such as dobutamine or milrinone, are often added to vasopressors to improve cardiac output (CO).

*Findings suggestive of postinfarct pericarditis*: Transmural infarct may develop pericarditis as early as 1 day to as late as 8 weeks post MI. Late-onset pericarditis is also called Dressler's syndrome, which is associated with fever and high ESR. Findings suggestive of pericarditis are as follows:
- Pleuritic pain
- Worse on lying down but relieved on sitting up and leaning forward (positional).
- Radiates to the trapezius ridge
- Associated with audible friction rub
- Diffuse but not focal STE
- Treated with high-dose aspirin and colchicine

*Ventricular premature beats*: These are usually treated with BB. Control the risk of ventricular tachycardia (VT) or ventricular fibrillation (VF) by keeping the serum potassium ~4.5 mmol/L and magnesium ~2.0 mmol/L; prophylactic antiarrhythmic drug (AAD) is contraindicated.

*VT and VF*: There is no role of prophylactic AAD at the initial phase of index hospitalization. But sustained VT with hemodynamically stable patients is treated with IV amiodarone (LD: 150 mg over 10–30 minutes, f/b 1 mg/min for 6 hours and then 0.5 mg/min for 18 hours or more) or less preferred agent, procainamide, is used.

*Patients with VT and hemodynamic instability*: They are treated with synchronized cardioversion (100–150 J biphasic). Unsynchronized cardioversion (100–150 J biphasic) is used immediately for VF. Nonresponders to cardioversion usually respond to cardioversion after 1 mg IV epinephrine or IV bolus of amiodarone (150 mg). One variant of VT is torsades des pointes (TdP), which is more common with hypokalemia, hypomagnesium, hypoxia, and toxic effects of other AAD. Therefore, all points are to be well taken care of. VT or VF, which develops after the first 48 hours, is associated with a poorer prognosis than earlier onset. They should undergo electrophysiology (EP) study for consideration of ICD for prevention of SCD.

*Accelerated idioventricular rhythm (AIVR)*: It is actually slow VT and occurs at the time of reperfusion. No treatment is required but close monitoring.

*Supraventricular arrhythmia (SVT)*: Sinus tachycardia is the most common. Think of secondary causes like anemia, fever, or metabolic derangements and treat the causes. But if it occurs due to sympathetic stimulation, treat with BB. AF/AFl is common due to HF and is treated with digoxin. But if no HF, consider BB, or non-dihydropyridine (DHP) CCB like—verapamil, diltiazem if BB is contraindicated to control ventricular rate. But if it persists >2 hours with HR > 120 bpm or has hemodynamic instability, go for electric cardioversion (50–100 J biphasic).

*Sinus bradycardia*: If hemodynamic instability, treat with injection atropine 0.5 mg IV. It may be repeated with 0.2 mg IV (total 2 mg) if HR < 50–60 bpm, but even after that if HR < 40 bpm, a pacemaker is the choice. Isoproterenol, ideally, is to be avoided.

*AV block and intraventricular conduction defects (IVCD)*: Mortality of AV block following AWMI (ischemic) is more than AV block with IWMI or PWMI (due to increased vagal tone and transient). Temporary RV pacing is more beneficial in inferior wall MI (IWMI) with complete heart block (CHB) and HF, marked bradycardia, and significant ventricular ectopic. IWMI with RVI dual-chamber pacing is advised if required. In all other cases, an external noninvasive pacemaker is placed on demand modes if necessary. Permanent pacing may be required in the presence of combined persistent bifascicular block and transient third-degree heart block.

*Recurrent chest pain/discomfort*: It indicates extension or reinfarction and is usually treated with prompt revascularization. Fibrinolytics are alternatives.

*Thromboembolism*: It may lead to cerebral artery embolism, leading to stroke or HTN if renal artery embolism occurs.

*Left ventricular aneurysm*: It is defined as dyskinetic or expansile wall motion. True aneurysm (contains scar tissue) is not associated with cardiac rupture in contrast to pseudoaneurysm (secondary to rupture and contains organizing thrombus). Complication occurs after 4 weeks to months after STEMI.

*Postinfarction risk stratification*:
- Identify the high-risk patients.
- Submaximal (before discharge) or symptom-limited exercise test (4–6 weeks after MI) is done to know the residual ischemia.
- MPI
- Assess EF by echocardiography or radionuclide ventriculography.
- Exercise test helps to formulate exercise prescription at home.

If angina is induced by low workload and symptomatic ventricular arrhythmia induced by exercise test, should undergo catheterization, and revascularization if required.

Before discharge, the following points are well taken care of for secondary prevention and morbidity and mortality reduction: ABCDEF:

- *A:* Antiplatelet—aspirin for lifelong and ADP P2Y12 inhibitor like ticagrelor/clopidogrel for 6–12 months
- *B:* BB and/or ACEI if high BP/LV dysfunctions
- *C:* Cholesterol-lowering agents: Statins—high intensity; if not tolerated, add ezetimibe. The strategy of quitting cigarette smoking quitting, cardiac rehabilitation, and reducing cardiac risk factors should be adopted. Take care of comorbidities.
- *D:* Diet and diabetes—dietary changes, healthy food habits
- *E:* Graded exercise and education
- *F:* Timely follow-up

# PROGNOSIS

Most death occurs prior to hospitalization. At least 5–10% of survivors die within the first 12 months after the MI, and close to 50% need hospitalization within the same year. Outcomes are good in the following:

- *Early reperfusion strategy*: Thrombolytic therapy within 30 minutes of arrival or PCI within 90 minutes
- If the EF is preserved.
- Aspirin, BBs, and ACEI started at proper time

Factors that negatively affect prognosis include:

- Diabetes
- Advanced age
- Prior MI, peripheral vascular disease (PVD), or stroke
- Delayed reperfusion
- Diminished EF (the strongest predictor)
- Presence of CHF
- Elevated C-reactive protein and BNP levels
- Depression

## Patient Education

- The patient should present to the ED as soon as possible once symptoms appear
- If no response is seen with NTG (three doses), the patient should contact the nearest health facility
- Eat a low-salt and fat-restricted diet
- Cardiac rehabilitation is to be done
- Quit smoking
- Reduce body weight if overweight
- Adhere to medications
- Abstain from alcohol
- Follow healthy lifestyle

# CLINICAL PEARLS

- Time is the equivalent of muscle
- Early revascularization by PCI is the most important step
- Early thrombolysis within 3 hours is the alternative approach to PCI
- Other therapies include: ABCDEF
  - *A:* Antiplatelet (DAPT), antithrombotic (UFH/LMWH), antianginal drug (ISDN/NTG)
  - *B:* Betablocker, BP control with ACE/ARB
  - *C:* Cholesterol high intensity statin and care of commodities (DM, dyslipidemia, smoking, alcohol)
  - *D:* Diets, stool softener
  - *E:* Evaluation by serial ECG, serial trop T/I, echocardiography, electrolytes and renal functions and risk stratification (TIMI score/GRACE score)
  - *F:* Regular follow-up is mandatory

## FURTHER READINGS

1. Alaour B, Liew F, Kaier TE. Cardiac troponin—diagnostic problems and impact on cardiovascular disease. Ann Med. 2018;50(8):655-65.
2. Scheen AJ. From atherosclerosis to atherothrombosis: from a silent chronic pathology to an acute critical event. Rev Med Liege. 2018;73(5-6):224-8.
3. Haig C, Carrick D, Carberry J, Mangion K, Maznyczka A, Wetherall K, et al. Current smoking and prognosis after acute ST-segment elevation myocardial infarction: new pathophysiological insights. JACC Cardiovasc Imaging. 2019;12(6):993-1003.
4. Niccoli G, Scalone G, Crea F. Acute myocardial infarction with no obstructive coronary atherosclerosis: mechanisms and management. Eur Heart J. 2015;36(8):475-81.
5. Lopez-Sendon J, Coma-Canella I, Alcasena S, Seoane J, Gamallo C. Electrocardiographic findings in acute right ventricular infarction: sensitivity and specificity of electrocardiographic alterations in right precordial leads V4R, V3R, V1, V2, and V3. J Am Coll Cardiol. 1985;6(6):1273-9.
6. Thygesen K, Alpert JS, Jaffe AS, Simoons ML, Chaitman BR, White HD, et al. Third universal definition of myocardial infarction. Eur Heart J. 2012;33(20):2551-67.
7. Sgarbossa EB, Pinski SL, Barbagelata A, Underwood DA, Gates KB, Topol EJ, et al. Electrocardiographic diagnosis of evolving acute myocardial infarction in the presence of left bundle-branch block. GUSTO-1 (Global Utilization of Streptokinase and Tissue Plasminogen Activator for Occluded Coronary Arteries) Investigators. N Engl J Med. 1996;334(8):481-7.
8. Widimsky P, Rohac F, Stasek J, Kala P, Rokyta R, Kuzmanov B, et al. Primary angioplasty in acute myocardial infarction with right bundle branch block: should new onset right bundle branch block be added to future guidelines as an indication for reperfusion therapy? Eur Heart J. 2012;33(1):86-95.
9. Stub D, Smith K, Bernard S, Nehme Z, Stephenson M, Bray JE, et al. Air versus oxygen in ST-segment-elevation myocardial infarction. Circulation. 2015;131(24):2143-50.
10. Madan M, Halvorsen S, Di Mario C, Tan M, Westerhout CM, Cantor WJ, et al. Relationship between time to invasive assessment and clinical outcomes of patients undergoing an early invasive strategy after fibrinolysis for ST-segment elevation myocardial infarction: a patient-level analysis of the randomized early routine invasive clinical trials. JACC Cardiovasc Interv. 2015;8(1 Pt B):166-74.
11. Nordmann AJ, Hengstler P, Harr T, Young J, Bucher HC. Clinical outcomes of primary stenting versus balloon angioplasty in patients with myocardial infarction: a meta-analysis of randomized controlled trials. Am J Med. 2004;116(4):253-62.
12. Yusuf S, Mehta SR, Chrolavicius S, Afzal R, Pogue J, Granger CB, et al. Effects of fondaparinux on mortality and reinfarction in patients with acute ST-segment elevation myocardial infarction: the OASIS-6 randomized trial. JAMA. 2006;295(13):1519-30.
13. Stone GW, Witzenbichler B, Guagliumi G, Peruga JZ, Brodie BR, Dudek D, et al. Bivalirudin during primary PCI in acute myocardial infarction. N Engl J Med. 2008;358(21):2218-30.
14. Morrison LJ, Verbeck PR, McDonald AC, Sawadsky BV, Cook DJ. Mortality and prehospital thrombolysis for acute myocardial infarction: a meta-analysis. JAMA. 2000;283(20):2686-92.
15. Hatherley JD, Salmon T, Collinson PO, Khand A. Implementation of the European Society of Cardiology 0/3-hour accelerated diagnostic protocol, using high sensitive troponin T: a clinical practice evaluation of safety and effectiveness involving 3003 patients with suspected acute coronary syndromeOpen Heart 2023;10:e002366.
16. Byrne RA, Rossello X, Coughlan JJ, Barbato E, Berry C, Chieffo A, et al; ESC Scientific Document Group. 2023 ESC Guidelines for the management of acute coronary syndromes. Eur Heart J. 2023;44(38):3720-826.

CHAPTER 96

# Left Ventricular Failure

*Md Hamid Ali*

*Heart failure (HF)*: The American College of Cardiology/American Heart Association (ACC/AHA) guidelines define HF as a complex clinical syndrome resulting from structural or functional myocardial dysfunction of ventricular filling or ejection of blood leading to dyspnea, fatigue, and fluid retention. Left ventricular failure (LVF) occurs when there is dysfunction of the left ventricle causing insufficient delivery of blood to vital body organs. It is broadly classified as follows:

- Heart failure with reduced ejection fraction (HFrEF); ejection fraction (EF): <40%
- Heart failure with midrange ejection fraction (HFmEF); EF: 41–49%
- Heart failure with preserved ejection fraction (HFpEF); EF: > 50%

*Epidemiology*: Age is a major predisposing factor of HF. The prevalence of HF increases steadily with age. The incidence of HF in men doubles with each 10-year age increase after the age of 65 years, whereas in women the incidence triples. Blacks have a higher risk of HF than Whites.

*Causes of HF are as follows*:

- Hypertension (HTN) is the most common attributable factor (M—39%, F—59%).
- The second common cause is myocardial infarction (MI) (M—34%, F—13%).

*Heart failure with reduced ejection fraction*:

- *Structural abnormalities of the heart*: Left ventricular hypertrophy (LVH), HTN-mediated organ damage (HMOD), valvular heart disease—aortic stenosis/aortic regurgitation (AS/AR), mitral regurgitation/tricuspid regurgitation (MR/TR), uncontrolled arrhythmia (tachycardiomyopathy), myocarditis, congenital heart disease—intracardiac shunts, and dilated cardiomyopathy (DCM)
- *Toxic cardiomyopathy*: Chemotherapy—daunorubicin, immunotherapy drugs—hydroxychloroquine (HCQ), alcohol, cocaine
- Coronary artery disease (CAD), acute coronary syndrome (ACS)
- *Autoimmune disease*: Lupus myocarditis, giant cell myocarditis
- *Other triggering factors*: Diabetes mellitus (DM), HTN, infections—Chagas, human immunodeficiency virus (HIV), renal dysfunctions
- Nonadherence

*Heart failure with preserved ejection fraction*—with impaired ventricular filling—restrictive cardiomyopathies: Amyloidosis, sarcoidosis, hemochromatosis, endomyocardial fibroelastosis, radiation therapy and constrictive pericarditis, hypertrophic cardiomyopathy (HCM), obesity, CAD, valvular disease—AS/mitral stenosis (MS)

*High-output HF*: Thyrotoxicosis, anemia, beriberi, cirrhosis, arteriovenous (AV) shunt, chronic lung disease

*Precipitating factors*: Anemia, infection, thyrotoxicosis, arrhythmia, worsening renal or hepatic failure, uncontrolled HTN, MI, ischemic heart disease (IHD), drug/toxin use—nonsteroidal anti-inflammatory drugs (NSAIDs), calcium channel blocker (CCB), inadequate dose of diuretics, alcohol, excessive use of sodium and water; nonadherence of medication is an important factor.

Stages of HF:
- *Stage A*: No structural heart disease (SHD), at risk of HF
- *Stage B*: SHD but no symptoms at present
- *Stage C*: SHD with past or present symptoms
- *Stage D*: Refractory HF

## FRAMINGHAM DIAGNOSTIC CRITERIA FOR HEART FAILURE

The presence of two major criteria or one major and two minor criteria is required to make the diagnosis of HF with relatively low specificity.

*Major criteria*: Acute pulmonary edema, cardiomegaly, hepatojugular reflex, neck vein distention, paroxysmal nocturnal dyspnea (PND) or orthopnea, pulmonary rales, third heart sound (S3 gallop), weight loss of 4.5 kg or more in 5 days in response to treatment, central venous pressure > 16 cm of water, radiographic cardiomegaly.

*Minor criteria*: Ankle edema, dyspnea on exertion, hepatomegaly, nocturnal cough, pleural effusion, tachycardia [heart rate (HR) >120 beats/min], a decrease in vital capacity by one-third of the maximal value recorded

*New York Heart Association (NYHA) functional classification (FC) is as follows*:
- *Class I*: No limitation of ordinary physical activity
- *Class II*: Somewhat limited inability to exercise, symptoms onset at ordinary activity
- *Class III*: Marked limitation of physical activity, dyspnea with minimal activity
- *Class IV*: Unable to do any physical activity, dyspnea at rest

*Acute decompensated heart failure (ADHF)* is a clinical syndrome of worsening signs/symptoms of HF requiring hospitalization or other unscheduled medical care.

*Clinical phenotypes of ADHF*:
- Hypertensive HF
- Decompensated HF
- Cardiogenic shock/advanced HF

*Pathophysiology*: Many compensatory mechanisms that activated at the initial stage of HF perpetuate disease progression. Myocardium responds to adaptive or maladaptive changes. All remodeling stimuli (wall stress, cytokines, neurohormonal, oxidative stress) cause myocyte hypertrophy and altered interstitial matrix leading to ventricular enlargement, which again increases the wall stress and a vicious cycle goes on. All remodeling stimuli also cause fetal gene expression, altered calcium handling protein, and apoptosis, which predispose to systolic or diastolic dysfunction leading to increased wall stress. In this way, the vicious cycle continues.
- A decrease in cardiac output (CO) stimulates the neuroendocrine system with a release of epinephrine, norepinephrine, endothelin-1 (ET-1), and vasopressin. They cause vasoconstriction leading to increased afterload. An increase in afterload and myocardial contractility with impaired myocardial relaxation leads to increased myocardial oxygen demand eventually leading to myocardial cell death and apoptosis. This perpetuating cycle

of increased neurohumoral stimulation and maladaptive hemodynamic and myocardial responses continues.

- A decrease in CO also stimulates the renin–angiotensin–aldosterone system (RAAS), leading to increased salt and water retention, along with increased vasoconstriction, direct myocardial toxicity, electrolyte and renal dysfunction, baroreceptor dysfunction, and cardiac arrhythmia. This ultimately causes remodeling at the tissue level including atherosclerosis. This further contributes to the maladaptive mechanisms.
- In addition to this, the RAAS system releases angiotensin II, which has been shown to increase myocardial cellular hypertrophy and interstitial fibrosis.
- In HFpEF, there is a decrease in myocardial relaxation and an increase in the stiffness of the ventricle due to an increase in ventricular afterload. This perpetuates a similar maladaptive hemodynamic compensation and leads to progressive HF.
- Sodium-glucose cotransporter-2 (SGLT-2): In HF, SGLT-2 contributes to sodium and water retention, endothelial dysfunctions, abnormal myocardial metabolism, and impaired calcium handling. So there is a role of SGLT-2 inhibitor (SGLT-2i) in HF irrespective of diabetes status.
- *Cyclic guanosine monophosphate (cGMP)*: In HF, cGMP is reduced, leading to endothelial dysfunction. It suggests the role of oral guanylate cyclase stimulator in the management of HF.
- *Vasodilatory hormones*: Many counter-regulatory hormones including atrial natriuretic peptide (ANP), B-type natriuretic peptide (BNP), prostaglandin E (PGE), prostacyclin (PGI), bradykinin, adrenomedullin, and nitric oxide are upregulated. ANP and BNP cause vasodilation of systemic and pulmonary circulation through guanylate cyclase stimulation, increased sodium and water excretion, inhibition of renin and aldosterone, and baroreceptor stimulation. But natriuretics and bradykinin are destroyed by neprilysin. Therefore, there is a role of angiotensin receptor-neprilysin inhibitor (ARNI).
- *Dyssynchrony and electrical instability*: Left bundle branch block (LBBB) or intraventricular conduction delay (IVCD) causes abnormal ventricular contraction. So there is a role of cardiac resynchronized therapy (CRT)/biventricular pacing. Atrial fibrillation (AF) with inadequate rate control and multiple premature ventricular contractions (PVCs) contributes to HF. Besides this, direct effect on the heart, abnormal rhythm, and tachycardia causes increased wall stress, neurohormonal stimulation, and inflammation.
- Secondary distortion of the mitral valve (MV) leading to MR contributes to the progression of HF by various mechanisms; therefore, there is a role of treatment of distorted MV by the transcatheter technique.
- *Cardiorenal interactions*: HF causes dysfunctions of vital organ such as kidney and liver. Heart and kidney interaction causes increased circulatory volume, worsening of symptoms, and progression of HF. This is called cardiorenal syndrome.
- Splanchnic congestion causes portal vein distension and activation of hepatorenal and splenorenal reflexes, which ultimately causes renal vasoconstriction and perpetuates HF. So there is a role of venous decongestion and ultrafiltration in selected cases.
- Gut congestion and altered microbial composition stimulate the chronic state of inflammation and immune system dysregulation in various ways [lipopolysaccharides (LPS), macrophage activation, increased cytokines—interleukin 1 (IL-1), IL-6, tumor necrosis factor-alpha (TNF-α)], which causes cardiac cachexia.

*Left ventricular failure hypotension—increased sympathetic nervous system (SNS) activation*:
- Increased HR—increased $O_2$ demand—decreased ventricular filling—decreased CO later on
- Direct myocardial toxicity
- RAAS activation
- Vasoconstriction—increased wall stress—increased $O_2$ demand
- All lead to ventricular remodeling.

*Left ventricular failure—decrease renal perfusion—RAAS activation*:
- Increased Na and water reabsorption
- Increased vasoconstriction
- Interstitial fibrosis
- Increased myocardial remodeling

*Neurohormonal activation*:
- Release of ANP, BNP, N-terminal pro-B-type natriuretic peptide (NT-proBNP)—they cause vasodilatation, dieresis, and Na excretion, but they are readily destroyed by neprilysin enzymes (role of ARNI).
- *Cytokine activation*: Role of anticytokine?
- *Oxidative stress*: Role of antioxidant?
- *Apoptosis*: Antiapoptotic therapy?
- *Altered gene expression*: Role of gene therapy?

*Pathophysiological mechanism*:
- *Myocardial*: Reduced CO, left ventricular diastolic dysfunction (LVDD), MR, tachycardia, myocardial injury
- *Renal*: $Na^+$ and fluid retention, acute kidney injury (AKI), RAAS activation
- *Vascular*: Endothelial dysfunction, increased arterial stiffness, vasoconstriction, volume redistribution, capillary leakage
- *Neurohormonal*: RAAS activation, SNS stimulation, oxidative stress, inflammation
- Finally, all lead to congestion and end-organ damages/dysfunctions and vice versa.

*Initial clinical assessments*: Check posture, pulse, blood pressure (BP), temperature, jugular venous pressure (JVP), hepatomegaly, ascites, and edema.
- When a patient enters the clinic, observe for shortness of breath on exertion (SOBE) in mild-to-moderate HF and check for 6-minute walk test (6MWT) to assess cardiopulmonary reserve if necessary. In severe HF, patients remain upright anxious, diaphoretic, and pallor due to anemia or low CO. Assess dyspnea and cardiac cachexia.
- Ask for fatigue and PND. PND is defined as episodes of shortness of breath that awakens the patients from sleep after prolonged recumbency with feelings of anxiety and suffocation that get relieved by ≥30 minutes in an upright position. PND is often associated with coughing and wheezing often called cardiac asthma. Assess for dyspnea level by NYHA classification.
- Oxygen saturation ($SpO_2$) may give erroneous results because of poor perfusion due to HF. Be cautious about nail polish.
- *Posture*: Inability to lie down without dyspnea. The patient remains sited. Orthopnea is defined as dyspnea at a recumbent position within 1–2 minutes of lying down due to increased venous return, increased work of breathing (WOB) because of decreased lung compliance, or due to elevation of diaphragm because of ascites or hepatomegaly.
- *Pattern of breathing*: Periodic breathing like—Cheyne-Stokes breathing due to increased sensitivity of respiratory center to arterial oxygen pressure ($PaO_2$) and prolonged circulatory time, suggestive of HF. Central sleep apnea may be found.
- Cool extremities and cyanosis and sweating in severe HF.
- *Temperature*: Low-grade fever due to cytokine activation is seen in acute severe HF.

- *HR*:
    - Tachycardia is usually a sign of shock, but if the patient is getting beta-blockers (BBs), there may not be such increments of HR. A normal HR *does not* rule out shock in an HF patient.
    - AF is a surrogate marker of suspicious HF. Irregularly irregular pulse with pulse deficit >10 suggests AF. Pulse deficit is <10 in multiple ectopics.
    - Check for other arrhythmias.
    - Pulsus alternans—an alternating strong and weak pulse due to incomplete recovery and accentuation of P2
- *BP*:
    - Hypotension is more common among HFrEF patients and can be a sign of poor perfusion and even shock.
    - HTN may be an exacerbating factor for HF. Therefore, control of BP with vasodilation/afterload reduction is very much helpful for HF management.
    - *Pulse pressure*: A narrow pulse pressure is a sign of a low output state. Lower pulse pressure is associated with increased mortality in HFrEF patients.
- *Temperature*: If increased, it suggests that infections are the precipitating factor.
- *JVP*:
    - Used to determine the intracardiac filling pressure, which is a marker for left ventricular (LV) preload
    - *There are two ways to check*:
        (i) Position the patient upright at 90°. If JVP is seen above the clavicle, then it is obvious that the patient has elevated intracardiac pressures.
        (ii) Position the bed at 45° and assess how high the jugular venous distention (JVD) is above the sternal angle in centimeter. Then add 5 mm to it to get the actual JVP in centimeter of $H_2O$. If it is above 8 mm, it indicates high filling pressure or increased JVP.
    - TR can cause JVD elevation in the absence of elevated cardiac filling pressures; prominent V waves and Y descent are seen in significant TR.
    - Kussmaul's sign increased JVP in inspiration, seen in severe biventricular failure.
    - Arterial pulsation and venous pulsation should be differentiated when assessing JVD.
        - Check the radial pulse. Venous pulsation should have two upstrokes for every pulsation felt in the wrist. If it correlates 1:1, it may be arterial.
        - Hepatojugular reflex: Increased fullness of the pulsation on application of abdominal pressure, especially in liver bed for 15–30 seconds, drops down abruptly on releasing the abdominal pressure. It is positive in HF.
- *Abdomen*: Hepatomegaly is seen due to venous congestion. Tenderness due to stretching of liver capsule and soft liver is very much suggestive of acute right HF [congestive cardiac failure (CCF)]. Tenderness disappears later on. Pulsatile liver is seen in severe TR. Mild degree of ascites is very common in CCF but massive ascites indicate other causes—chronic liver disease (CLD) with portal hypertension (PHT) and constrictive pericarditis. Chronic hepatic congestion may cause cardiac cirrhosis.
- *Pedal edema* is highly suggestive of HF. It is present in severe HF and indicates that a substantial degree of volume overload is present. Pedal edema may be absent in chronic HF in young adults. Unilateral edema is very unlikely; it indicates other causes such as deep vein thrombosis (DVT), lymphedema, and filariasis. Anasarca—generalized edema of leg, scrotum, and abdominal wall—may be seen rarely in chronic HF.
- *Palpation*: Apical impulse is displaced down and out in DCM, but sustained

in AS. Parasternal lift/heave is seen in biventricular HF or right HF. Palpable third heart sound may be found.

- *Auscultation*:
  - Accentuation of P2 or loud P2 is found in pulmonary arterial hypertension (PAH).
  - Presence of an S3/S4 or gallop rhythm is a specific sign of overload in HF. An S3 gallop is the most significant and early finding associated with HF. It is also found in HFpEF due to HTN.
  - S3/S4 or gallop rhythm is a sign of HF.
  - *Murmur*: MR or TR murmur is seen in decompensated DCM. New-onset murmur or change of character of murmur indicates infective endocarditis as the cause.
  - Lung auscultation reveals pulmonary rales at the lung bases initially and then gradually spreads upward as the severity of HF increases. Wheezing may be present in acute decompensated HF. Frothy and blood-tinged sputum may be seen in severe HF. Absence of rales does not exclude pulmonary congestion. Crackles and rales are neither sensitive nor specific for pulmonary edema in chronic HF. Decreased breath sound may be seen bilaterally due to pleural effusion commonly. If it is unilateral, it is right-sided.

## INITIAL LABORATORY WORKUP

- *Routine blood tests*: Check for anemia [hemoglobin (Hb%)]; iron deficiency—ferritin, renal dysfunction—renal function test (RFT), and liver dysfunction—liver function test (LFT) are needed to find the cause and/or severity.
- *Role of biomarkers in HF*: Symptoms and signs are sufficient in young patients to diagnose HF. But it is difficult in the elderly, especially with comorbidities such as chronic obstructive pulmonary disease (COPD). In those cases, we need biomarkers or other investigations.
  - *BNP*: Serum BNP or NT-proBNP levels can aid in differentiating cardiac from noncardiac causes of dyspnea in patients with ambiguous presentations.
  - BNP is an independent predictor of increased LV end-diastolic pressure, and it is used for assessing mortality risk in patients with HF. BNP levels correlate with NYHA classification, and the utility is primarily as a marker to assess treatment efficacy.
  - Predischarge natriuretic peptide levels are strong predictors of the risk of death and hospital readmission in patients with HF. Elevated BNP (>900 pg/mL in people aged > 50 years, >450 pg/mL in those aged < 50 years) supports HF diagnosis; cutoff BNP >100 had a positive predictive value of 79% and a negative predictive value of 89% and <100 makes congestive heart failure (CHF) less likely. Assess the trend.
  - Some factors increase or decrease the BNP
    - BNP levels are usually lower in obese patients with HF.
    - Patients with chronic kidney disease (CKD), sepsis, elderly people and AF tend to have elevated BNP levels.
    - Neprilysin inhibitors (e.g., sacubitril + valsartan) can cause elevated BNPs but decreased NT-proBNP levels, which reflects an improved hemodynamic state.
- *Troponins*:
  - Particularly for patients with impending shock or ACS is the precipitating cause of shock.
  - In patients with an acute MI who developed cardiogenic shock, early revascularization lowers 6-month mortality.

- *Sodium*:
    - Low sodium on admission is a predictor of both all-cause mortality and cardiovascular (CV) mortality for patients admitted with an HF exacerbation (OPTIME-CHF trial).
    - A drop in Na levels of >3 mEq/L was associated with increased mortality.
    - The risk of death was particularly worse for Na <125 mEq/L in HF exacerbations.
- *Creatinine*:
    - Elevation compared to baseline on admission is usually a sign of cardiorenal syndrome from elevated renal venous congestion. Manage with diuretics.
    - If the elevation occurs during diuresis, it may not be due to renal injury.
    - Assess the cause of elevations of creatinine.
    - For small elevations secondary to diuresis in a patient who is clinically improving, the best course of management may be continuing diuresis if no other cause of the elevated creatinine is found.
- Complete blood count (CBC)—to look for anemia or infection as the precipitating factor.
- Capillary blood glucose/fasting blood sugar/postprandial blood sugar (CBG/FBS/PPBS)—to exclude diabetes.
- LFT—may reveal elevations of liver enzymes due to venous congestion
- *Other workups*:
    - *Chest X-ray (CXR) posteroanterior (PA) view*—findings indicative of CHF on chest radiographs include enlarged cardiac silhouette cardiomegaly [(CTR) > 50%], edema at the lung bases, and vascular congestion. In florid HF, Kerley B lines may be seen on chest radiographs. The absence of these findings in patients with clinical features of HF does not rule out CHF.
    - *Electrocardiogram (ECG)* may give an indication of ACS, CAD, or precipitating arrhythmia—AF, frequent ventricular premature contraction (VPC).
    - *Echocardiography (Echo)*—it can assess for systolic and diastolic dysfunction and help elucidate the presence of focal wall motion abnormalities or valvular pathology. Transesophageal echocardiography (TEE) is an alternative for severe obesity, pregnancy, or mechanical ventilation.
        - Global hypokinesia with dilated all four chambers suggests DCM.
        - Regional wall motion abnormality (RWMA)—CAD [ischemic cardiomyopathy (ICM)]
        - Dilated right atrium (RA) and right ventricle (RV) suggest PAH and cor pulmonale.
        - Dilated left atrium (LA) and RV with MR suggests restrictive cardiomyopathy (RCM).
        - Septal hypertrophy with (PW) thickness > 13 mm and PW/septal thickness > 1.5, with dynamic outflow tract obstruction with systolic anterior motion (SAM), suggests hypertrophic cardiomyopathy (HCM).
    - *Ultrasound (USG) whole abdomen*—dilated inferior vena cava (IVC)/bilateral mild pleural effusion is suggestive of HF.
    - *Cardiac magnetic resonance imaging (CMRI)*—computed tomography (CT) and magnetic resonance imaging (MRI) in patients with HF are used principally for the diagnosis of congenital cardiac abnormalities. CMRI is also the gold standard test for evaluating right ventricular function.
        - Helpful to evaluate biventricular EF with tissue characteristics with

late gadolinium enhancement (LGE)
    - Sensitive tests for infiltrative cardiomyopathy with characteristic LGE, fibrosis/scar
    - Assessment of myocardial viability in ICM
    - To evaluate myocarditis, arrhythmogenic right ventricular dysplasia (ARVD)
  - *Nuclear imaging*:
    - Radionuclide ventriculography can quantify left ventricular ejection fraction (LVEF).
    - Ischemia and viability detection
  - *Coronary angiography (CAG)*: Invasive or CT angiogram to detect CAD
  - *Endomyocardial biopsy (EMB)* in suspected cases of infiltrative myocardial disease
  - *ECG-gated myocardial perfusion imaging* is another diagnostic tool for assessing EF, regional wall motion, and regional wall thickening.

*Treatment goals*: Improve symptoms of congestion, optimize volume status, identify and treat the triggers, optimize chronic oral therapy, minimize side effects, select the patients for revascularization, and educate the patients about modifications of medicines and disease management.

# MAINSTAY OF THERAPY—ANGIOTENSIN-CONVERTING ENZYME INHIBITOR/ ANGIOTENSIN RECEPTOR BLOCKER/ANGIOTENSIN RECEPTOR-NEPRILYSIN INHIBITOR, BETA-BLOCKER, AND DIURETICS

- Angiotensin-converting enzyme inhibitor (ACEI)/angiotensin receptor blocker (ARB)/ARNI
- BB
- *Cholesterol-lowering agent*: CORONA trial and GISSI-HF trial demonstrated no benefit in HF other than other indications like CAD, dyslipidemia, atherosclerotic cardiovascular disease (ASCVD), peripheral artery disease (PAD), and DM.
- *Diuretics*: Loop diuretic, potassium-sparing diuretic—mineralocorticoid receptor antagonist (MRA), SGLT-2i: dapagliflozin/empagliflozin, digoxin, and dilator-vasodilator
- Evaluation by ECG, Echo, and electrolytes
- Follow-up on a regular basis

## Angiotensin-converting Enzyme Inhibitor/Angiotensin Receptor Blocker/Angiotensin Receptor-neprilysin Inhibitor

The primary combination therapy for HFrEF includes diuretics, a renin–angiotensin system inhibitor (such as ARNI, ACEI, or ARBs), and a BB. The combination therapy of ARB + ARNI significantly reduced CV death and HF hospitalizations when compared to ACEI alone.

- *Complete RAAS blockade*: Though it is theoretically promising, a study on VALLIANT (captopril + valsartan) and ATMOSPHERE (enalapril + aliskiren) trials showed an increased risk of hyperkalemia, worsening of renal function, and other adverse outcomes. Therefore, a combination of ACEI and ARB is discouraged.
- *ARNI*: PARADIGM-HF study definitely proves the efficacy of ARNI (sacubitril + valsartan) in HFrEF to reduce CV mortality, hospitalization for heart failure (HHF) in comparison to enalapril (ACEI). PARAGON-HF trial marginally failed to prove the efficacy of ARNI in HFpEF, but ARNI may be used in subsets of patients in midrange EF and women to get improvement in quality of life (QOL), NYHA class, and renal benefits. PIONEER-HF study proved the superiority of ARNI over enalapril when added at the time of

discharge of ADHF patients in terms of greater reduction of natriuretic peptide and lower rates of composite death and HHF at 8 weeks.

- *How to initiate ARNI?*: In place of ARB, ARNI is to be started at the time of scheduled ARB dose. In place of ACEI, ARNI is to be started after 36 hours of ACEI use to avoid a higher risk of angioedema. Start with 50 mg BD and then gradually build up the dose to 200 mg BD.
- They are often hold due to elevated creatinine on admission or during diuresis; patients are then discharged without them.
  - Continuation or resumption of these medications prior to discharge to be done. These medications are important for improving lifetime morbidity and mortality.
  - It may be reasonable to consider continuing ACE/ARB or decreasing the dose in patients who have only a mild AKI.
  - The combination of hydralazine and nitrate is an alternative to an angiotensin system blocker for primary therapy if ACEI, ARNI, and ARB therapies are contraindicated.

## Beta-blockers

- In HF exacerbations, BBs should be continued unless the patient is in cardiogenic shock. Altered mental status or somnolence, cool and/or clammy extremities, livedo reticularis, low BP or pulse pressure, tachycardic or thready radial pulse can all suggest cardiogenic shock. Guideline-directed medical therapy (GDMT) suggests keeping the resting HR < 70–75 beats/min and BP in the normal to low normal range.
- Decreasing or discontinuing BBs is associated with increased mortality.
- If a patient's BB is discontinued during an HF exacerbation, they are less likely to be on it, even *months* after follow-up.
- Observational data suggests improved outcomes in HF patients discharged on BBs compared to those who are not.
- CCB—verapamil and diltiazem are contraindicated. Amlodipine and felodipine safely reduce BP but do not have an effect on morbidity, mortality, or QOL.
- *Ivabradine* selectively inhibits the funny current (I-f) in the sinoatrial node. According to the AHA/ACC, ivabradine is indicated in patients with persistently symptomatic HF and an EF of ≤35% in sinus rhythm (SR). The resting HR should be >70 beats/min despite goal-directed BB therapy.

*Sequence of administration of ACEI/ARB and BB*: CIBIS-III trial proved that outcome does not vary on the sequence of administration: ACEI first or BB. The basic point is that an optimally titrated dose of ACEI and BB in a timely manner improves mortality.

*High dose or low dose of ACEI and BB?*: ATLAS (ACEI), HEALL (ARB), and MOCHA (BB) trials consistently favor the higher dose in terms of lower death and lower HHF.

*Time for uptitration*: In the absence of symptoms of hypotension, i.e., (fatigue and dizziness) uptitration is to be done every 2 weeks in stable ambulatory patients as tolerated.

## Diuretics

Because of their potent effect on renal excretion of sodium, loop diuretics are preferred over thiazide diuretics, which are commonly used with loop diuretics for refractory volume overload. Frequent dose adjustment is necessary. Those who do not respond to furosemide at high doses, torsemide and bumetanide are offered. They have greater oral bioavailability. Dosing should be minimized as possible to avoid neurohormonal activations.

- Various clinicians' practices range from starting with 2–2.5 times the patient's home diuretic dose to using 1 mg/kg intravenous (IV).

- *Thresholds and ceiling*: Loop diuretics have a threshold dose below which they do not have much effect. Loop diuretics also are considered to have a "ceiling" dose, and doses above that will not cause a significant increase in diuresis.
- *Dose adjustment*
  - A *"good" dose of a loop diuretic* will result in excretion of 250 mEq (~6 g) of Na in about 2–3 L of urine.
  - Increase the dose if the patient does not have an adequate response to the dose.
  - Increase the frequency of administration if the patient has an adequate response to the dose but 24-hour urine output (UOP) is not sufficient.
  - A *spot urine sodium* can be checked if unsure about the effectiveness of diuresis based on questionable Is/Os and inability to do accurate weights. If spot urine Na > 100 mEq/L, the dose was effective. If significantly lower, you may need to increase the dose.

### Furosemide Drip

- As per the DOSE (Diuretic Optimization Strategies Evaluation) trial, it has not been proven to improve symptoms or length of stay in a typical HF patient.
- Reasonable to consider for diuretic-resistant patients
- Results of the DOSE trial support the aggressive approach to volume overload though renal functions, electrolytes, and volume status need to be monitored diligently to avoid more chance of renal dysfunctions [cardiorenal syndrome (CRS)].

In warm and wet patients, rapid diuresis is okay in a patient who can hemodynamically tolerate it. The clinical condition of the patient will guide therapy.

### Mineralocorticoid Receptor Antagonists

Mineralocorticoid receptor antagonistss are indicated in patients with NYHA FC II to IV and an LVEF of ≤35% in addition to ACEI and BB. It is also indicated in symptomatic HF after an MI and an LVEF of <40%. Spironolactone helps with long-term remodeling and potassium-sparing properties. High creatinine and hyperkalemia become the concern points to be taken care of during therapy. RALES study with spironolactone proved its efficacy. Eplerenone is studied in class II symptoms. As it lacks the antiandrogenic effects (gynecomastia, erectile dysfunctions, diminished libido) of spironolactone, it may be an alternative if sexual dysfunction is experienced with the use of spironolactone.

### Other Diuretics: For Additional Volume Removal

- *Thiazide and thiazide-like diuretics*: Addition of a thiazide diuretic to a loop diuretic can lead to improved diuresis in a diuretic-resistant patient.
  - They act on the distal convoluted tubule, working downstream of furosemide, which can help augment diuresis.
  - Hydrochlorothiazide and chlorthalidone are reasonable options. Metolazone may be used rarely.
  - Be cautious as thiazides can cause significant laboratory abnormalities, particularly potassium and magnesium.
  - Check electrolytes twice daily, especially if metolazone is used.
  - Metolazone can be effective for a few days, so it does not need to be dosed daily. Typical dose ranges from 5 to 20 mg. Typically, start with 5 mg and add an extra dose if needed.
- *Diuresis in COPD*:
  - Can start retaining $CO_2$ to compensate for the metabolic alkalosis that diuresis causes.

  - Can lead to dangerously elevated $PCO_2$.
  - Aggressive chloride repletion can be used to help prevent this.
- *Chloride depletion metabolic alkalosis*:
  - Aggressive diuresis will lead to more chloride depletion and hypokalemia, which decreases pendrin's ability to remove bicarbonate.
  - Therefore, decreased activity of pendrin in aggressive diuresis will worsen the chloride depletion metabolic alkalosis and result in elevated bicarbonate.
  - If the patient can tolerate it, consider adding spironolactone to help with hypokalemia.
  - Give KCl to help the chloride depletion state.
- *Ultrafiltration*: CARRESS-HF trial proved its efficacy in ADHF with worsening renal function. It is another option for volume removal.
  - Usually, it will only be done after diuresis fails; however, there are exceptions.
  - If a patient is on a very large dose of diuretics and is very volume overloaded, one can consider going straight to ultrafiltration.
  - A decision to do ultrafiltration in this situation is often stylistic and determined in conjunction with the HF specialist and nephrologist.

## Vasodilator Therapy

Rapid reduction of preload and afterload helps the patients to get relief from dyspnea due to pulmonary edema, low CO, and high systemic vascular resistance. Nitroglycerine (NTG), isosorbide dinitrate (IDN), isosorbide mononitrate (IMN), sodium nitroprusside, nesiritide, and serelaxin are vasodilators. ASCEND-HF and RELAX-AHF-2 failed to prove the mortality benefits of nesiritide and serelaxin, respectively. They are not commonly used. Vasodilators are rarely used in the following scenario. Acute decompensated heart failure with concomitant HTN and pulmonary edema do not respond sufficiently enough to IV diuretics (They responds preferably to NTG and nitroprusside).

*Alternative vasodilator*: Fixed-dose combinations of nitrate and hydralazine: Hydralazine causes arterial vasodilatation and nitrates, which transforms into NO (stimulate cGMP production) and induce arterial and venous vasodilatation. This combination therapy provides a survival benefit to a lesser extent than ACEI. It is used in patients with chronic HF, especially in HFrEF unable to tolerate ACEI/ARB therapy due to hyperkalemia or renal insufficiency. A-HeFT trial also showed benefit along with ACE and BB with decreased adherence.

## Inotrope Therapy: Dopamine/Dobutamine/Milrinone

Though theoretically promising, practical data (milrinone in OPTIME-CHF, dopamine in ROSE-AHF trial) did not support its use in majority of patients. It is still used in few patients of cardiogenic shock with severe end-organ dysfunction for short-term stabilization for waiting for the definitive therapy is available. Low-dose dopamine (renal dose) does not appear to provide an incremental advantage over IV diuretic therapy (ROSE-AHF trial). Milrinone may provide additional benefits to those patients receiving BB who are admitted for HF. Long-term safety is not proved in HF. REVIVE II and SURVIVE trials with a novel calcium sensitizer, levosimendan, were not promising.

## Sodium-glucose Cotransporter-2 Inhibitor

The DAPA-HF and EMPEROR-REDUCED trials proved the efficacy of SGLT-2i in the management of HFrEF.

2021 American Diabetes Association (ADA) guidelines recommend considering SGLT-2i (dapagliflozin/empagliflozin) therapy in all patients with diabetes and HF regardless of baseline HbA1c. Consider SGLT-2i in patients with HFrEF and NYHA class II or III in addition to optimal medical treatment (OMT) with an ACEI/ARNI, a BB, and an MRA for patients with HFrEF regardless of diabetes status. 2021 ACC Expert Consensus suggests consideration for use in NYHA class IV as well. Diuretic dose may be reduced. Therapy with SGLT-2i may increase the risk of recurrent genital fungal infections. A small reduction in estimated glomerular filtration rate (eGFR) following initiation is expected and is reversible and should not lead to premature discontinuation of the drug. DELIVER and EMPEROR-PRESERVED assessed the efficacy in HFpEF.

*Digoxin*:
Digoxin is a mild ionotropic, it attenuates baroreceptor activity, and is sympathoinhibitory. It may be considered in symptomatic patients in SR despite adequate goal-directed therapy to reduce the all-cause rate of hospitalizations, but its role is limited in females (DIG trial). A low dose is sufficient enough. The dose may be reduced in higher doses and therapeutic level is to be checked if higher doses are used. It is mainly used in AF.

*Hydralazine and IDN*:
- They should be considered in self-identified Black patients with LVEF < 35% or with an LVEF < 45% combined with a dilated left ventricle in NYHA class III/IV despite treatment with an ACEI (or ARNI), a BB, and an MRA to reduce the risk of HF hospitalization and death.
- They may be considered in patients with symptomatic HFrEF who cannot tolerate any of an ACEI, an ARB, or an ARNI (or they are contraindicated) to reduce the risk of death.
- Target doses of heart failure medications from clinical trials see **Box 1**.

**BOX 1: Starting dose and target dose range consecutively.**

*ACEI*
- Captopril 6.25 to 50 mg TID
- Enalapril 2.5 to 10–20 mg BID
- Lisinopril 2.5–5 to 20–35 mg OD
- Ramipril 2.5 to 5 mg BID

*MRA*
- Eplerenone 25 to 50 mg OD
- Spironolactone 25 to 50 mg OD

*Other agents*
- Ivabradine 5 to 7.5 mg BID
- Vericiguat 2.5 to 10 mg OD
- Digoxin 0.25 to 0.50 mg OD
- Hydralazine/isosorbide dinitrate 37.5/20 to 75/40 mg TID

*Beta-blockers*
- Bisoprolol 1.25 to 10 mg OD
- Carvedilol 3.125 to 25 mg BID
- Metoprolol succinate 12.5–25 to 200 mg/day
- Nebivolol 1.25 to 10 mg OD

*SGLT-2 inhibitor*
- Dapagliflozin 10 to 10 mg OD
- Empagliflozin 10 to 10 mg OD

*ARB*
- Losartan 50 to 150 mg OD
- Valsartan 40 to 160 mg BID
- Telmisartan 40 to 80 mg OD
- Olmesartan 20–40 mg OD

(ACEI: angiotensin-converting enzyme inhibitor; ARB: angiotensin receptor blocker; MRA: mineralocorticoid receptor antagonist; SGLT-2: sodium-glucose cotransporter-2)

*Source*: https://www.ncbi.nlm.nih.gov/pmc/articles/PMC6528811/table/T4/?report=objectonly

## Anticoagulation

Heart failure is a hypercoagulable state, but routine use of oral anticoagulant (OAC) is discouraged by WARCEF trial other than following indications to prevent stroke or pulmonary embolism (PE).
- AF with prior cardioembolic stroke
- In severe LV dysfunction with echocardiographic evidence of LV thrombus

## Cardiac Rhythm Management for Heart Failure with Reduced Ejection Fraction: Device Therapy

- Implantable cardiac defibrillator (ICD) is indicated in the following conditions:
  - DCM with prior sustained ventricular arrhythmia or survivors of cardiac arrest, hemodynamically unstable sustained (VT)
  - In nonischemic cardiomyopathy LVEF ≤ 35% and NYHA II/III even on at least 90 days of GDMT and life expectancy >1 year.
  - Syncope with induced sustained VT/(VF) on electrophysiological (EP) study
  - SHD with sustained VT
  - EF < 35%, 40 days after MI, NYHA II/III
  - LVEF ≤ 30% and 40 days after MI, NYHA I
- CRT is also called biventricular pacing. It is indicated in the following conditions:
  - LVEF < 35% in normal SR with LBBB and QRES > 150 ms on GDMT and NYHA FC II, III, or ambulatory IV symptoms
  - May be considered in LVEF < 35% in LBBB with QRS 120–149 ms

## Cardiac Contractility Modulator

Cardiac contractility modulator (CCM) involves nonexcitatory stimulus to the RV septal wall during the absolute refractory period to augment the subsequent contraction. It mostly benefits the symptomatic patients (EF 25–45%) with narrow QRS who are not eligible for CRT.

- *Extracorporeal membrane oxygenation (ECMO):* In rare situations
- *Advanced HF: The following pattern is found*:
  - More than two HHF
  - CRS
  - Cardiac cachexia
  - Intolerance to BB due to worsening HF or hypotension
  - Frequent systolic blood pressure (SBP) < 90 mm Hg
  - NYHA IV
  - Progressive decline in Na, K < 133 mEq/L
  - Need to escalate diuretic therapy > 160 mg of furosemide.
  - Frequent need of ICD
- *Diet:*
  - *Fluid*: Restrict fluid intake to 1–2 L in advance HF or stage D HF, especially in patients with hyponatremia < 130, or fluid retentions difficult to control despite high-dose diuretics and sodium retentions.
  - *Sodium restriction*: 2–3 g/day. <2 g in severe HF. Salt substitute is not generally recommended. In most of the cases, KCl is used as a substitute of NaCl; if at all permitted, K level is to be carefully monitored, especially along with ACEI/ARB and in renal disease.
  - Stool softener, preferably to be added at night.
- *Exercise training program may be beneficial (HF-ACTION study)*
- *Evaluation* by ECG, Echo, and electrolytes is mandatory for successful management of HF in the long run.
- *Follow-up*: Routine and dedicated follow-up to uptitrate or downtitrate the medication; to know the adverse reaction and alteration of metabolic and biochemical panels is very much necessary for the reduction of HHF.
- *Gene-based therapy*: Cellular and gene-based therapy are promising but initial studies (CUPD) are not conclusive. More randomized controlled trials (RCTs) are needed to conclude.
- *Heart transplantation*: This is indicated in the following conditions:
  - Severe HF stage D, with poor short-term prognosis with GDMT requiring continuous ionotropic therapy and or mechanical support [intra-aortic

balloon pump (IABP), left ventricular assist device (LVAD), ECMO]
  - Refractory angina despite GDMT is not amenable to revascularization with a poor short-term prognosis.
  - RCM or HCM with NYHA III or IV
  - Refractory or recurrent arrhythmia despite GDMT or device therapy
  - Complex congenital heart disease with progressive HF even with GDMT
  - Unresectable low-grade tumor confined to the heart without metastasis
- *I-f channel inhibitor*:
  - Ivabradine should be considered in symptomatic patients with LVEF < 35%, in SR and a resting HR > 70 beats/min despite treatment with an evidence-based dose of BB (or maximum tolerated dose below that), ACEI (or ARNI), and MRA to reduce the risk of HF hospitalization and CV death.
  - *Ivabradine* should be considered in symptomatic patients with LVEF < 35%, in SR and a resting HR > 70 beats/min who are unable to tolerate or have contraindications for a BB to reduce the risk of HF hospitalization and CV death. Patients should also receive an ACEI (or ARNI) and an MRA.
- *Inflammatory marker reduction*: Anti-inflammatory therapy is not promising in RCT (ACLAIM-HF). Only in the CANTOS study using Canakinumab-anti IL-1β in post-MI with elevated high-sensitivity C-reactive protein (hsCRP) associated with a reduction in HHF. However, efficacy in established HF is yet to be proved.
- ICD—already discussed in device therapy
- K should be checked periodically.
- *Lower extremity therapy* by graded external pneumatic compression at higher pressure may be effective in mild-to-moderate HF.
- Long-term monitoring of all clinical parameters including HR, BP, $SpO_2$, and daily weight
- Morphine is used in ADHF with severe pulmonary edema and hypoxia. Oxygen and noninvasive ventilation [NIV—bilevel positive airway pressure (BiPAP), continuous positive airway pressure (CPAP)] are also required.
- *Micronutrients*: Thiamine and selenium supplementation may be beneficial in chronic HF, especially in malnutrition and prolonged diuretic therapy.
- *Novel therapy*:
  - *Adenosine receptor antagonist*: Rolofylline (PROTECT trial) failed to provide any CV or renal benefits.
  - *Vericiguat* is an oral agent that stimulates soluble guanyl cyclase (sGC) that stimulates cGMP and NO pathways. NO is a potent vasodilator. VICTORIA trial proved its effects on the reduction of HHF. It was recently approved by the Food and Drug Administration (FDA) in 2021 to reduce the risk of mortality and HF hospitalizations in adults admitted with HF exacerbation who have chronic symptomatic HF and an EF of < 45%.
  - *Myosin activator*: Omecamtiv mecarbil is a myosin activator which prolongs the contraction without increasing the force of contraction. Beneficial effects have been proved by COSMIC-HF trial initially and GALACTIC-HF trial later on.
  - *Fish oil*: Omega 3 polyunsaturated fatty acid (PUFA) is associated with a modest clinical improvement (GISSI-HF).
- Oxygen therapy in ADHF
- *Optimization of risk factors*: It is also important to address potential triggers for HF exacerbation once the diagnosis of HF is made. Drugs that should be avoided in patients with HF include NSAIDs, CCBs except vasoselective CCBs, and most antiarrhythmic drugs (AADs) (except those in class III). Comorbid conditions like diabetes, sleep

apnea, obesity, depression should be taken care.

- *Poor prognostic factors*: Male sex, advanced age, DM, CKD, CAD, depression, hyponatremia, hyperuricemia, elevated biomarkers and neurohormones, persistent tachycardia, widened QRS/LBBB, AF, PVC, VT, reduced EF, LVH, increased LV mass, LVDD, PAH, advanced NYHA, decreased exercise capacity, hypotension, prior history of HHF, elevated BNP/NT-proBNP, elevated troponin T/I
- *Prognosis*: The mortality rate following hospitalization for HF is estimated at around 10% at 30 days, 22% at 1 year, and 42% at 5 years. This can increase to >50% for patients with NYHA class IV, stage D HF. *Ottawa Heart Failure Risk Score*: It is a useful tool for prognosis determination in patients with HF who present to the emergency department with symptoms of HF. A score of 1–2 is considered a moderate risk, a score of 3–4 is considered a high risk, and a score of 5 or higher is considered a very high risk. Most of the patients die from advanced HF or sudden cardiac death.
- QOL should be considered along with laboratory parameters.
- Referral to HF specialist to be considered in the following conditions: I NEED HELP (see the **Box 2**)

**BOX 2: I NEED HELP.**

I—IV inotropes
N—NYHA IIIb/IV, persistently elevated BNP
E—End-organ dysfunctions
E—EF < 35%
D—Defibrillator shock
H—Hospitalizations > 1
E—Edema despite escalating inotropes
L—Low SBP < 90 mm Hg
P—Progressive intolerance or down titration of medications

- *Statins*: Routine use of statins in nonischemic HF other than genuine indications of statin has been proved not effective to improve clinical outcome (CORONA trial, GISSI-HF trial).
- *Surgical therapy*: In selected cases only after proper GDMT as the last resort like
- Coronary artery bypass grafting (CABG) is considered in ICM with multivessels CAD. Revascularization is mostly indicated in patients with ongoing chest pain and LV failure.
- *Surgical ventricular restoration (SVR)*: Infarct exclusion to remodel the LV by reshaping it surgically in patients with ICM and LV anterior wall dysfunction. External mesh-like net attached around the heart is another procedure but does not provide clinical benefits.
- *Surgical mitral valve repair (MVR)* may be considered in functional or secondary MR due to HFrEF, symptomatic even after GDMT and CRT. The COAPT study supports it, but the MITRA-FR trial did not support surgical MVR.
- *Specialized interventions of refractory stage D HF:*
    - HFrEF: Mechanical circulatory support (MCS) (LVAD or ECMO) or cardiac transplantation
    - HFpEF: Cardiac transplantation, few patients may get the benefit of MCS
- *Implantable devices specific for HF*: Implantable pulmonary artery (PA) (PA monitoring), transcatheter edge-to-edge clipping of the MV in secondary mitral incompetence, interatrial shunt device to dynamically decompress LA
- Transfer of ADHF patients to intensive cardiac care unit (ICCU)
- Utilization of cost-effective therapy is the keyword of success.
- *Vaptan*: EVEREST trial failed to prove any benefit of selective vasopressin-2 antagonist, tolvaptan, in regard to mortality or HF-related morbidity. It is indicated in HF with volume overload

and hyponatremia to get short-term symptomatic improvement.

- *When to discharge?*
  *Discharge criteria*:
  - Based on clinical judgments, not by laboratory parameter
  - Exacerbating factors well addressed
  - Near-optimal volume status attained
  - IV to oral therapy done at least for 24 hours.
  - GDMT achieved
  - Education of patient and patient party
  - Schedule follow-up within 7–10 days post discharge.
- *WOB*: Avoid physical and mental stress to avoid increased WOB.
- To yield a best clinical outcome, treat the patients not the parameters only, think of A to Z during HF therapy.

*Differential diagnosis*: Diseases that may present with clinical features of volume overload and/or dyspnea are in the differential for HF. These include acute renal failure, acute respiratory distress syndrome (ARDS), cirrhosis, pulmonary fibrosis, nephrotic syndrome, and PE.

*Complications*:

- *Clinical complications*: Decreased QOL, decreased functional capacity, unintentional weight loss (cardiac cachexia), renal dysfunction (cardiorenal disease), and liver dysfunction (hepatic congestion)
- Adverse cardiac events include valvular dysfunction with DCM, MI, and ventricular arrhythmias. Sudden cardiac death is a potential complication for patients with HFrEF and requires primary prevention with ICD placement.
- Complications of the treatment for HF include renal failure, hypotension, and recurrent nosocomial infections due to frequent hospitalizations and central venous access.
- *Cardiogenic shock*: Inotropic therapy, usually catecholamines, MCS-IABP, percutaneous ventricular assist device (VAD), and ultrafiltration, is the mainstay of therapy.
- *CRS* Worsening of renal function (rise of creatinine > 0.3 mg/dL from baseline) during hospitalization for ADHF. It is associated with poor outcome. Improvement of CRS is dictated by cardiac and vascular decongestion. As per CARRESS-HF study, ultrafiltration in addition to diuretics is not superior and safer.
- *Treatment of chronic HFpEF (HF symptoms—dyspnea, orthopnea with LVEF ≥ 50%)*: Current therapy does not improve mortality or hospitalization.
  The following measures are taken:
  - Control of HTN
  - Control of ventricular rate in AF
  - Correction of CAD by revascularization
  - BBs if prior MI, HTN, AF
  - ACE/ARB if HTN, DM, ASCVD
  - ARNI in EF < 57%, female sex
  - Diuretics should be used to control volume overload and pulmonary congestion. They must be of judicious use.
  - MRA in elevated BNP or HHF within 1 year; eGFR must be >30 mL/min, creatinine <2.5 mg/dL, potassium <5.0 mEq/L
  - Non-DHP CCB in AF to control rate, HTN (amlodipine may be considered)
  - No role of nitrate or phosphodiesterase inhibitor

*Some specific types of HF*:

- Takotsubo cardiomyopathy—stress induced—reversible
- Tachycardia-induced cardiomyopathy—AF, atrial flutter (AFl), PVC > 10% of heartbeats
- Toxin-mediated cardiomyopathy—alcohol

- Peripartum cardiomyopathy—HF in the last trimester or within 6 weeks of delivery. Risk factors such as pregnancy, multiparity, eclampsia, aged mother, and ACEI are contraindicated in HF therapy.
- DCM—no RWMA, global hypokinesia. Mostly presents with HFrEF.
- RCM—HFpEF, Kussmaul's sign (increase JVP with respiration), ECG—low or normal voltage but Echo shows increased LV thickness, LVH without HTN/AS, known risk factors for infiltrative cardiomyopathy like amyloidosis, sarcoidosis, hypereosinophilia, and diabetic cardiomyopathy. History of recent down titration of antihypertensive therapy is also suggestive of RCM. Common features with constrictive pericarditis are prominent Y descent, dip and plateau, or square root sign on RV pressure but different in the following parameters: PAH > 50 mm Hg, diastolic pressure difference of LV and RV > 5 mm Hg, RV diastolic to systolic pressure ratio <1:3. On Echo, myocardium appears brighter with sparkling or grainy appearance, tissue velocity and longitudinal strain are severely reduced, and there is intolerance of BB, ACEI/ARB/ARNI, or digoxin. Cardiac CT or MRI is preferred over EMB. The patient is treated with judicious use of diuretics with MRA.
- HCM—voltage criteria (Lyon Sokolow criteria—SV1 + RV5/6 ≥35) with prominent q waves seen in ECG. On Echo, asymmetrical LVH with diastolic wall thickness ≥ 15 mm, septal to PW thickness ratio ≥ 1:3 in asymmetric septal hypertrophy (ASH), LV end-diastolic dimension (LVEDD) < 45 mm, LA-enlarged, impaired relaxation, positive family history. Mostly presents with dyspnea, angina, and syncope. The following medications are generally to be avoided—preload-reducing agents—diuretics and nitrates, afterload-reducing agents—ACEI/ARB, CCB, and NTG. Positive ionotropic agents—digoxin, dobutamine, phosphodiesterase inhibitor—milrinone. Preferred agents are BB, non-DHP CCB, class I AAD with negative ionotropic effects—disopyramide and inhibitor of cardiac myocyte ATPase inhibitor—mavacamten. Nonpharmacological therapy—septal myectomy, alcohol septal ablation (ASA), dual chamber pacing in elderly and who are not candidates of myectomy or ASA, an ICD in high-risk patients SCD (FH-SCD, massive LVH, unexplained syncope, apical aneurysm, EF > 50%) and to the survivors of SCD.

## CLINICAL PEARLS

- Involvement of pericardium, myocardium and endocardium of heart can lead to left heart failure.
- Common etiologies are-CAD, HTN, DM, smoking, alcohol, obesity, sedentary lifestyle.
- Thereby, insufficient delivery of blood/$O_2$ to the vital organ occurs.
- HF classified as HFrEF < 40%, HFmEF 41–49%, HFpEF > 50%.
- More common in the elderly, HFpEF is more common in women as opposed to HFrEF.
- After proper physical examination, evaluation by ECG, ECHO and biomarkers are necessary.
- The four pillars of heart failure management after Diuretics for volume over load are: (1) ACE/ARB/ARNI, (2) BB, (3) SGLT-2i, (4) MRA.
- For HFpEF, the therapy depends on the underlying cause and contributing factors like control of HTN, DM, revascularization in ischemic cardiomyopathy, control of arrhythmia
- Mortality if significantly high in males, HFrEF>HFpEF, low EF, high NT-proBNP, anemia, low sodium, renal failure, low BP, high pulse rate.

# FURTHER READINGS

1. Nussbaumerová B, Rosolová H. Diagnosis of heart failure: the new classification of heart failure. Vnitr Lek. 2018;64(9):847-51.
2. Ziaeian B, Fonarow GC. Epidemiology and aetiology of heart failure. Nat Rev Cardiol. 2016;13(6):368-78.
3. King M, Kingery J, Casey B. Diagnosis and evaluation of heart failure. Am Fam Physician. 2012;85(12):1161-8.
4. CONSENSUS Trial Study Group. Effects of enalapril on mortality in severe congestive heart failure. Results of the Cooperative North Scandinavian Enalapril Survival Study (CONSENSUS). N Engl J Med. 1987;316(23): 1429-35.
5. Kemp CD, Conte JV. The pathophysiology of heart failure. Cardiovasc Pathol. 2012;21(5): 365-71.
6. Obokata M, Reddy YNV, Borlaug BA. Diastolic dysfunction and heart failure with preserved ejection fraction: understanding mechanisms by using noninvasive methods. JACC Cardiovasc Imaging. 2020;13(1 Pt 2):245-57.
7. Ali AS, Rybicki BA, Alam M, Wulbrecht N, Richer-Cornish K, Khaja F, et al. Clinical predictors of heart failure in patients with first acute myocardial infarction. Am Heart J. 1999;138(6 Pt 1):1133-9.
8. Yancy CW, Jessup M, Bozkurt B, Butler J, Casey DE, Colvin MM, et al. 2017 ACC/AHA/HFSA focused update of the 2013 ACCF/AHA guideline for the management of heart failure: a report of the American College of Cardiology/American Heart Association Task Force on Clinical Practice Guidelines and the Heart Failure Society of America. J Am Coll Cardiol. 2017;70(6):776-803.
9. Klein L, O'Connor CM, Leimberger JD, Gattis-Stough W, Piña IL, Felker GM, et al. Lower serum sodium is associated with increased short-term mortality in hospitalized patients with worsening heart failure: results from the Outcomes of a Prospective Trial of Intravenous Milrinone for Exacerbations of Chronic Heart Failure (OPTIME-CHF) study. Circulation. 2005; 111(19):2454-60.
10. Jain S, Londono FJ, Segers P, Gillebert TC, De Buyzere M, Chirinos JA. MRI assessment of diastolic and systolic intraventricular pressure gradients in heart failure. Curr Heart Fail Rep. 2016;13(1):37-46.
11. Bhatt AS, Vaduganathan M, Claggett BL, Liu J, Packer M, Desai AS, et al. Effect of sacubitril/valsartan vs. enalapril on changes in heart failure therapies over time: the PARADIGM-HF trial. Eur J Heart Fail. 2021;23(9):1518-24.
12. Ferdinand KC, Elkayam U, Mancini D, Ofili E, Piña I, Anand I, et al. Use of isosorbide dinitrate and hydralazine in African-Americans with heart failure 9 years after the African-American Heart Failure Trial. Am J Cardiol. 2014;114(1):151-9.
13. Imamura T, Narang N. Comment on: Efficacy of early initiation of ivabradine treatment in patients with acute heart failure: rationale and design of SHIFT-AHF trial. ESC Heart Fail. 2021;8(2):1725-6.
14. Beygui F, Cayla G, Roule V, Roubille F, Delarche N, Silvain J, et al. Early aldosterone blockade in acute myocardial infarction: the ALBATROSS randomized clinical trial. J Am Coll Cardiol. 2016;67(16):1917-27.
15. Yancy CW, Jessup M, Bozkurt B, Butler J, Casey DE, Drazner MH, et al. 2013 ACCF/AHA guideline for the management of heart failure: a report of the American College of Cardiology Foundation/American Heart Association Task Force on Practice Guidelines. J Am Coll Cardiol. 2013;62(16):e147-239.
16. Ezekowitz JA, Zheng Y, Cohen-Solal A, Melenovský V, Escobedo J, Butler J, et al. Hemoglobin and clinical outcomes in the Vericiguat Global Study in Patients with Heart Failure and Reduced Ejection Fraction (VICTORIA). Circulation. 2021;144(18):1489-99.
17. van der Meer P, Gaggin HK, Dec GW. ACC/AHA versus ESC guidelines on heart failure: JACC guideline comparison. J Am Coll Cardiol. 2019;73(21):2756-68.
18. Lucas C, Johnson W, Hamilton MA, Fonarow GC, Woo MA, Flavell CM, et al. Freedom from congestion predicts good survival despite previous class IV symptoms of heart failure. Am Heart J. 2000;140(6):840-7.
19. Ilieșiu AM, Hodorogea AS. Treatment of heart failure with preserved ejection fraction. Adv Exp Med Biol. 2018;1067:67-87.

# CHAPTER 97

# Acute Diarrhea

*Md Hamid Ali*

## INTRODUCTION

Diarrhea is still a major problem in Southeast Asia with high morbidity and mortality, particularly among children under 5 years of age. The diarrhea episode in rural population is 85.4%; 39% of them are children under 5 years of age. The most common enteropathogens found in all countries are rotavirus followed by enterotoxigenic *Escherichia coli* (ETEC), *Vibrio* species, *Salmonella* species, *Shigella* species, and *Campylobacter*. Poor breastfeeding, socioeconomic sociocultural condition, and environmental sanitation also have a great role in the causation of disease, morbidity, and mortality.

## WHAT IS DIARRHEA?

Diarrhea is loose motions three or more times loose or watery stool per day.

### Classification of Diarrhea

- *Acute*: <7 days
- *Persistent*: 7–14 days
- *Chronic*: >14 days

#### *Classification of Acute Diarrhea*

- *Infectious*:
    - Noninflammatory
        - Viral: Rotavirus, adenovirus, norovirus
        - Protozoal: *Giardia* (*Cryptosporidium*, *Cyclospora* in immunocompromised)
        - Bacterial
            - Preformed toxin: *Staphylococcus aureus*, *Bacillus cereus*, *Clostridium perfringens*
            - Enterotoxin production: ETEC, *Vibrio cholerae* colonize in the small intestine and produce toxin to cause secretory diarrhea
    - Inflammatory
        - Viral: *Cytomegalovirus*
        - Protozoal: *Entamoeba histolytica*
        - Bacterial:
            - Cytotoxin production: Enterohemorrhagic *E. coli* (EHEC), *Clostridium difficile*
            - Mucosal invasion: *Shigella*, *Salmonella*, enteroinvasive *E. coli* (EIEC), chlamydia, *Campylobacter jejuni*, *Yersinia*, *Listeria monocytogenes*, *Neisseria gonorrhoeae*

*Mode of transmission*: Acute diarrheal diseases are usually transmitted by contaminated hands or ingestion of contaminated food or drinks.

*Incubation period*: This period is usually from a few hours to 5 days after exposure for bacterial diarrhea and 1–3 days for viral diarrhea.

- *Noninfectious*:
    - Food allergy
    - Drug induced: Cocaine, antibiotic-associated diarrhea, chemotherapy, colchicine, endocrine disorders—hyperthyroidism, adrenocortical insufficiency, carcinoid tumors, medullary thyroid cancer
    - Gastrointestinal: Gastrinoma, vasoactive intestinal peptide tumor (VIPoma), Zollinger-Ellison syndrome, ulcerative colitis, Crohn's disease, irritable bowel syndrome, celiac disease, lactose intolerance, ischemic colitis, colorectal cancer, short bowel syndrome

## Signs of Medically Important Diarrhea

- *Signs of inflammatory diarrhea*: High fever > 101°F, severe abdominal pain, especially in >50 years of age, bloody stool, white blood cell (WBC) > 15,000/µL
- Profuse watery diarrhea with severe dehydration
- Pus in stool
- Duration > 3 days
- Advanced age > 70 years
- Immunocompromised state—acquired immunodeficiency syndrome (AIDS)/post-transplant

## Symptoms Other than Diarrhea

- Mainly depends on the degree of dehydration—increased thirst, irritability, restlessness, drowsiness, convulsion, coma
- Nausea, vomiting
- *Abdominal symptoms*: Pain in abdomen, tenderness, tenesmus in inflammatory cases
- *Systemic features*: Fever in infectious cases

## Complications

- Prerenal failure
- Electrolyte imbalance, metabolic acidosis (cholera)
- Paralytic ileus
- Acute tubular necrosis
- Hemolytic uremic syndrome (HUS) associated with *Campylobacter* species, Shiga toxin-producing *E. coli* [HUS, thrombotic thrombocytopenic purpura (TTP)]. Antibiotic increases the chance.
- Hemorrhagic colitis in Shiga toxin-producing *E. coli*—6–22%
- Miller Fisher syndrome—variant of Guillain-Barré syndrome in *Campylobacter* species
- Cardiovascular complications—rarely occur in *Campylobacter* fetus like endocarditis, pericarditis, and thrombophlebitis.
- Pseudoappendicitis syndrome—may occur in *C. jejuni, Yersinia.*
- Toxic megacolon

*Diagnosis*: Mostly clinical but rarely need some investigations to detect etiology.

### *When to Suspect?*

- *From history*:
    - Community outbreaks—viral or common food source
    - Family members affected—infectious origin
    - Ingestion of improperly stored or prepared food indicates food poisoning.
    - Voluminous diarrhea and rice water stool are suggestive of cholera. When a child older than 5 years develops severe dehydration from acute watery diarrhea (usually with vomiting), there is suspicion of cholera.
    - Pregnancy—increased chance of listeriosis
    - Exposure to impurified water (swimming)—may indicate *Giardia, Cryptosporidium.*
    - Recent travel history—traveler's diarrhea
    - Prolong administration of broad spectrum

- Risk of human immunodeficiency virus (HIV)-AIDS-associated diarrhea
- Diarrhea persisting for >14 days is not attributable to bacterial pathogen.
- Infectious diarrhea should be separated from ulcerative colitis, which may have fever, pain abdomen, and bloody diarrhea.
- Flu-like illness may be associated with *Campylobacter*.
- Afebrile, abdominal pain with bloody diarrhea—Shiga toxin-producing *E. coli*
- Bloody stools—*Salmonella, Shigella, Campylobacter*, Shiga toxin-producing *E. coli, C. difficile, E. histolytica, Yersinia*
- Fried rice ingestion—*B. cereus*
- Raw ground beef or seed sprouts—Shiga toxin-producing *E. coli* (e.g., *E. coli* O157:H7)
- Raw milk—*Salmonella, Campylobacter*, Shiga toxin-producing *E. coli, Listeria*
- Undercooked beef, pork, or poultry—*S. aureus, Clostridium perfringens, Salmonella, Listeria* (beef, pork, poultry), Shiga toxin-producing *E. coli* (beef and pork), *B. cereus* (beef and pork), *Yersinia* (beef and pork), *Campylobacter* (poultry)
- Hospital admission—antibiotic therapy-induced *C. difficile*
- AIDS—*Cryptosporidium*, microsporidia, *Isospora, Cytomegalovirus, Mycobacterium avium* intracellulare complex, *Listeria*
- Persistent diarrhea with weight loss—*Giardia, Cryptosporidium, Cyclospora*, malignancy
- Rectal pain or proctitis—*Campylobacter, Salmonella, Shigella, E. histolytica, C. difficile, Giardia*
- Several persons with common food exposure have acute onset of symptoms—food poisoning with preformed toxins. Onset of symptoms within 6 hours: *Staphylococcus, B. cereus* (typically causes vomiting). Onset of symptoms within 8–16 hours: *C. perfringens* type A (typically causes diarrhea).

## Physical Assessment

- Degree of dehydration by checking pulse, blood pressure (BP), urine output, skin elasticity, capillary refilling, and mental status.
- Severe dehydration—two of the following signs should be present: (1) Lethargy or unconsciousness, (2) sunken eyes, (3) unable to drink, and (4) skin pinch goes back slowly longer than 2 seconds.
- Some (Mild to moderate) dehydration—two of the following signs should be present: (1) Restlessness/irritability, (2) sunken eyes, (3) able to drink or drinking eagerly, and (4) skin pinch goes back very slowly less than 2 seconds.
- Abdominal examination—for tenderness or peritonitis, this may be present in ETEC, *C. difficile*.
- How to differentiate the small bowel diarrhea from large bowel diarrhea? See the **Table 1**.

## Investigations

Ninety percent of noninflammatory diarrhea presents with self-limiting mild illness and responds well with mostly oral rehydration solution (ORS)/antidiarrheal agent. Diagnostic investigations are unnecessary. It is done only in the following conditions:

- If the signs of medically important diarrhea are present.
- Illness persists for >7 days/worsens.
- Systemic illness

### *List of Tests*

- Drop of stool with methylene blue in slides with a cover slip under a microscope
- Fecal leukocytes
- Stool culture/stool for viral pathogen
- Stool for *C. difficile* toxin assay—if there is recent hospitalization/antibiotic

**Table 1: Differences of small-bowel diarrhea and large-bowel diarrhea.**

| *Parameter* | *Small bowel diarrhea 90%* | *Large bowel diarrhea <10%* |
|---|---|---|
| Inflammation | Noninflammatory | Inflammatory |
| Stool character | Watery | Semi-formed, mixed with mucous and blood |
| Frequency of stool | Infrequent | Frequent |
| Tenesmus | Usually absent | Often present |
| Fever | Usually absent | Often present |
| Symptoms | Abdominal cramp, bloating | Pain and tenderness in the lower abdomen |
| Systemic signs | Usually absent | Often present |
| Stool culture | Usually not required | May be required |

- Stool for ova, parasite, cyst (O/P/C) if diarrhea >10 days or HIV infection
- Serotyping of Shiga toxin-producing *E. coli*—in case of bloody stool
- Blood sugar, HIV, complete blood count
- Blood for sodium, potassium, and arterial blood gas analysis, urea, creatinine to detect complications

## Management

- *Recommendations for dietary management of acute diarrhea*:
  - Frequent tea, beverages, easily digested foods—soup, bananas, rice, toast, etc.
  - To avoid high-fiber foods, fats, milk products, caffeine, alcohol, coarse fruits and vegetables
  - Breastfeeding should be continued uninterrupted even during rehydration with ORS.
  - Household foods should be offered during diarrhea, in small quantities but frequently at least once every 2–3 hours.
- *Management of dehydration*: Rehydration is the most effective treatment. In majority of cases, no other treatment is required.
  - ORS containing glucose, sodium, potassium, chloride, and bicarbonate/citrate is indicated in patients who can take it orally at the rate of 50–100 mL/kg/day, depending on the degree of dehydration (about 5 mL/kg/h).
  - Intravenous fluid—Ringer's lactate is preferred—give 100 mL/kg Ringer's lactate solution if IV channel couldn't be done-Fluid can be given through NG Tube (or, if not available, normal saline).

Diarrhea treatment plan:

- *Diarrhea treatment plan A*: For mild or no dehydration. To treat diarrhea at home: Prevention of dehydration is the main motto with home-based foods, fluids, and ORS.
  - Give extra fluid (as much as the child will take).
  - Give zinc supplements, especially in children.
  - Give the recommended amount of ORS in the clinic over a 4-hour period.
- *Diarrhea treatment plan B*: For moderate dehydration—strategy in between plans A and C. More focus is given on ORS for rehydration. If the patient deteriorates, start intravenous (IV) fluid immediately. If the patient can drink, give ORS by mouth while the drip is set up. Give 100 mL/kg Ringer's lactate solution (or, if not available, normal saline), divided as follows: Like treatment plan C.
- *Diarrhea treatment plan C*: For severe dehydration: 100 mL/kg IV fluid should

**Table 2: Intravenous fluid therapy in severe dehydration.**

| *Age* | *First give 30 mL/kg in* | *Then give 70 mL/kg in* |
|---|---|---|
| <12 months old | 1 hour* | 5 hours |
| Older children/adults | 30 minutes* | 2.5 hours |

*Repeat once if radial pulse is still very weak or not detectable. Reassess every 1–2 hours. If hydration status is not improving, give the IV more rapidly.

be given, for details of administration see **Table 2**.

- To be repeated once if the radial pulse is still very weak or not detectable. Reassess every 1–2 hours. If the hydration status is not improving, give the IV more rapidly. Also give ORS (about 5 mL/kg/h) as soon as the patient can drink: Reassess after 3 hours. Classify dehydration. Then choose the appropriate plan (A, B, or C) to continue.

- *Drug therapy in acute diarrhea*:
  - *Antimotility agent*: Loperamide 4 mg stat and 2 mg after each loose stool (max—16 mg/24 h)
  - Contraindicated in case of bloody diarrhea, fever, or systemic toxicity
  - *Bismuth sulfate*: 30 mL four times daily in traveler's diarrhea
  - *Anticholinergic agents*: Diphenoxylate contraindicated in acute diarrhea, especially in bloody stool

*Antimicrobial drugs (including antibiotics)*: Empiric antimicrobial drugs are not required for the treatment of majority of cases of acute diarrhea because these are caused by viral agents or by *E. coli* that acts by elaborating enterotoxins (ETEC). Antibiotic increases the chances of HUS. Clinical studies have shown that antibiotic therapy does not offer any significant clinical benefit even in inflammatory diarrhea.

### Antibiotics Indicated if there are Signs of Medically Important Diarrhea

Antimicrobial agents are used in the following specific clinical indications:

- Bacterial infection-specific antibiotics
- *E. histolytica, Giardia* metronidazole/tinidazole and/or paromomycin
- Traveler's diarrhea—single dose of fluoroquinolones (FQs)—ciprofloxacin 750, levofloxacin 500, ofloxacin 400 mg BD-1 day in invasive disease characterized by fever, systemic toxicity, bloody diarrhea. Azithromycin 1 g is alternative to FQ. Rifaximin 200 mg TID for 3 days in noninvasive diarrhea.

### Other Nonspecific Therapy

- *Prebiotics/probiotics*—probiotics work by stimulating the immune system and competing for binding sites on intestinal epithelial cells. Their use in children with acute diarrhea is associated with reduced severity and duration of illness (an average of about one less day of illness).
- *Zinc*: Dose of zinc (20 mg tab) to give—
  - Up to 6 months—10 mg (0.5 tab) per day for 14 days
  - >6 months—20 mg (1 tab) per day for 14 days
- *Oral vitamin A*: Given if associated with measles at once and again the next day: 200,000 units/dose for age 12 months to 5 years, 100,000 units for age 6 months to 12 months, and 50,000 units for age <6 months.

### Treatment of Complications

- Appropriate management of electrolyte imbalance such as hyponatremia, hypokalemia, HUS, convulsions, and acute kidney injury (AKI).

## Prevention

Maintenance of good personal hygiene, food hygiene, and environmental hygiene—hand washing, safe food preparation, and access to clean water—is a key factor in preventing diarrheal illness. Public health interventions to promote hand washing alone can reduce the incidence of diarrhea by about one-third. Vaccine development remains a high priority for disease prevention, particularly for those in the developing world. Effective and safe vaccines exist for rotavirus, typhoid fever, and cholera.

## CLINICAL PEARLS

- Mostly caused by virus, rarely *Shigella, Salmonella, Vibrio cholerae, E. coli,* etc.
- Assess for signs of dehydration by: duration, blood in stool, body weight—pre-illness and post illness, general condition (thirst, restless, irritable, lethargic), sunken eyes, offering fluid, skin pinching of abdominal wall, pulse, BP, dryness of mucous membrane, tongue.
- Classify the dehydration as clinical or as % of weight loss: mild dehydration—3%, moderate dehydration—6%, severe dehydration—9%.
- Management depends on the degree of dehydration: First restore circulatory volume, then find cause.
- Total fluids to be given = replacement fluid + maintenance fluid + ongoing loss (200 mL/loose stool).
- The first and most important Rx is rehydration either by oral (ORS—50 mL/kg in the first 4 hours for mild-to-moderate dehydration or IV fluid for severe dehydration).
- Monitor rehydration status by pulse, BP, and urine output (most useful clinically).
- Antibiotic is required rarely in infective diarrhea or bloody diarrhea (FQ-3 days/CFT-3–5 days).
- Suspect cholera if ADD presents with rapid onset severe dehydration.
- Doxycycline-300 mg or azithromycin-1 g or ciprofloxacin-1 g stat in cholera.
- Administer zinc in children >6 months: 20 mg/day for 14 days.
- Role of prebiotic and probiotics in antibiotic associated diarrhea.
- Administer vitamin A 2 lakhs unit for 2 days in ADD with measles.

## FURTHER READINGS

1. Guerrant RL, Van Gilder T, Steiner TS, Thielman NM, Slutsker L, Tauxe RV, et al. Practice guidelines for the management of infectious diarrhea. Clin Infect Dis. 2001;32(3):331-51.
2. Aranda-Michel J, Giannella RA. Acute diarrhea: a practical review. Am J Med. 1999;106(6):670-6.
3. Turgeon DK, Fritsche TR. Laboratory approaches to infectious diarrhea. Gastroenterol Clin North Am. 2001;30(3):693-707.
4. Thielman NM, Guerrant RL. Clinical practice. Acute infectious diarrhea. N Engl J Med. 2004; 350(1):38-47.
5. Ilnyckyj A. Clinical evaluation and management of acute infectious diarrhea in adults. Gastroenterol Clin North Am. 2001;30(3):599-609.
6. Hahn S, Kim Y, Garner P. Reduced osmolarity oral rehydration solution for treating dehydration due to diarrhoea in children: systematic review. BMJ. 2001;323(7304):81-5.
7. Gadewar S, Fasano A. Current concepts in the evaluation, diagnosis and management of acute infectious diarrhea. Curr Opin Pharmacol. 2005;5(6):559-65.
8. Wong CS, Jelacic S, Habeeb RL, Watkins SL, Tarr PI. The risk of the hemolytic-uremic syndrome after antibiotic treatment of *Escherichia coli* O157:H7 infections. N Engl J Med. 2000; 342(26):1930-6.
9. McMahan ZH, DuPont HL. Review article: the history of acute infectious diarrhoea management—from poorly focused empiricism to fluid therapy and modern pharmacotherapy. Aliment Pharmacol Ther. 2007;25(7):759-69.

10. Allen SJ, Martinez EG, Gregorio GV, Dans LF. Probiotics for treating acute infectious diarrhoea. Cochrane Database Syst Rev. 2010;(11): CD003048.
11. Bhutta ZA, Bird SM, Black RE, Brown KH, Gardner JM, Hidayat A, et al. Therapeutic effects of oral zinc in acute and persistent diarrhea in children in developing countries: pooled analysis of randomized controlled trials. Am J Clin Nutr. 2000;72(6):1516-22.
12. Alam NH, Yunus M, Faruque AS, Gyr N, Sattar S, Parvin S, et al. Symptomatic hyponatremia during treatment of dehydrating diarrheal disease with reduced osmolarity oral rehydration solution. JAMA. 2006;296(5):567-73.
13. Ejemot RI, Ehiri JE, Meremikwu MM, Critchley JA. Hand washing for preventing diarrhoea. Cochrane Database Syst Rev. 2008;(1):CD004265.

CHAPTER 98

# Hypertensive Emergency

*Md Hamid Ali*

## INTRODUCTION

*Definition*: A hypertensive emergency is an acute, marked elevation in blood pressure (BP) [systolic blood pressure (SBP) >220 mm Hg or diastolic blood pressure (DBP) > 120 mm Hg] that is associated with signs of target-organ damage (TOD). End organs commonly affected are: Lung—pulmonary edema, heart-cardiac ischemia, eye-retinal changes, brain—neurologic deficits, kidney—acute renal failure (ARF), large artery—aortic dissection, and eclampsia. Presence of end-organ damage is more important than a specific value of BP (usually, the SBP is >180 mm Hg and/or the DBP is >120 mm Hg).

*Management principle*: It is "treat the patients, not the number." The basic principle of the necessity of emergency treatment of hypertensive patients is the presence of end-organ damage or TOD. Hypertensive emergency patients with TOD require urgent admission for close monitoring and to initiate intravenous (IV) therapy to reach the targeted BP within a time frame, especially with acute worsening of organ function to limit extension or promote regression of acute hypertension-mediated organ damage (HMOD). On the contrast hypertensive urgency patients without TOD and stable, require BP reduction over hours or days by oral therapy and usually discharged after a short period of observation and careful outpatient follow up is mandatory. Balances should be maintained between the benefits of BP reduction and the risk of lethal reduction of end-organ perfusion.

*Type of drug and rapidity to bring the BP*: The type of TOD is the principal factor of the choice of treatment, target BP, and timeframe by which BP should be lowered depending on which organ has been damaged.

*Malignant hypertension*: It is used to describe a hypertensive emergency coexisting with high BP values (often >200/120 mm Hg) and the following conditions:

- *Eyes*: Advanced retinopathy (retinal hemorrhages, cotton wools spots, and/or papilledema)
- *Kidneys*: Deteriorating renal functions with proteinuria
- *Brain*: Hypertensive encephalopathy
- Thrombotic microangiopathy (TMA)

The term malignant hypertension was coined because of limited survival in these patients at a time when treatment of hypertension was not yet possible. Nowadays, malignant hypertension is obsolete. The preferred term could be "acute hypertensive microangiopathy" because of microcirculatory damage, which is the pathological hallmark of malignant hypertension.

*Examples of hypertensive emergencies are as follows*:

- Hypertensive encephalopathy
- Severe hypertension in patients with intracranial hemorrhage and acute stroke
- Severe preeclampsia and eclampsia
- Acute coronary syndrome
- Cardiogenic pulmonary edema
- Acute aortic disease
- Scleroderma renal crisis (SRC)
- Cocaine/amphetamine-induced
- Pheochromocytoma
- Malignant hypertension with TMA/ARF
- Sympathetic crashing acute pulmonary edema (SCAPE)
- Pain including postoperative, anxiety
- Withdrawal from alcohol, benzodiazepine, clonidine
- *Drugs*: Cyclosporine, tacrolimus, erythropoietin, antiangiogenic therapy
- Posterior reversible encephalopathy syndrome (PRES)

Blood pressure can be affected by a myriad of factors. Before initiation of antihypertensives, consider some simple interventions, which may be highly effective in reducing the BP. Interventions which may rapidly reduce the BP are as follows:

- *Pain*: Treat with appropriate analgesia.
- *Agitation*: Treat with antipsychotics or dexmedetomidine.
- *Volume overload*: Treat with diuresis or dialysis.
- *Alcohol withdrawal*: Phenobarbital
- *Urinary retention*: Foley catheter

## Hypertensive Encephalopathy

Hypertensive encephalopathy is a hypertensive emergency characterized by severe hypertension and one or more of the following: Seizures, lethargy, cortical blindness and coma, and in the absence of an alternative explanation.

## Hypertensive Retinopathy in Malignant Hypertension

Characterized by flame-shaped hemorrhages, cotton wool spots (grade III) with the presence of papilledema (grade IV). These changes, if present bilaterally, are highly specific. The presence of advanced hypertensive retinopathy (grade III/IV) is associated with much higher renin-angiotensin system (RAS) activation and more pronounced HMOD in other areas compared with patients without these retinal lesions, despite comparable BP values.

## Thrombotic Microangiopathy

It is suspected when severe BP elevation coincides with Coombs-negative hemolysis (elevated lactic dehydrogenase levels, unmeasurable haptoglobin, or schistocytes) and thrombocytopenia in the absence of another plausible cause and improvement with BP-lowering therapy.

- Other causes of TMA such as thrombotic thrombocytopenic purpura (TTP) and hemolytic uremic syndrome (HUS) should also be considered.
- TMA associated with malignant hypertension is usually less severe compared with other causes. It is associated with only moderate thrombocytopenia and few schistocytes present in a peripheral blood smear.
- Severe BP elevation with advanced retinopathy is usually sufficient to establish the diagnosis of TMA.
- The activity of the von Willebrand factor cleaving protease, ADAMTS13, may be needed to discriminate TTP (low levels) from TMA (usually normal).
- BP-lowering treatment will usually improve TMA associated with malignant hypertension within 24–48 hours.

### Sympathetic Crashing Acute Pulmonary Edema

Sympathetic crashing acute pulmonary edema (SCAPE) is also known as flash pulmonary edema (FPE): Risk factors and associations of FPE are: Elderly > 65 years, preexisting heart failure, previous episodes of SCAPE, and renal artery stenosis. It is a relatively abrupt onset of shortness of breath and rapidly (over minutes to hours) develops into life-threatening pulmonary edema. Patients are restless, diaphoretic, and hypoxic and have tachycardia and marked hypertension, suggesting elevated sympathetic activity. Echocardiography shows ejection fraction >0.5, suggesting worsening of diastolic dysfunction. Initial treatment includes nitroglycerin (NTG), noninvasive ventilation (NIV), diuretics, and morphine. It is different from acute congestive heart failure (CHF) exacerbation or hypotensive cardiogenic shock, which does not have a sympathetic overdrive. Patients need rapid intervention. They are generally more fluid-depleted despite "wet" lungs; therefore, overzealous diuretic therapy should be avoided.

### Scleroderma Renal Crisis

Scleroderma renal crisis is a life-threatening complication of scleroderma, most commonly of diffuse variety (10–25%), and presence of anti-ribonucleic acid (RNA) polymerase III antibodies, corticosteroid therapy in doses >15 mg/day. It presents with an abrupt onset of severe hypertension accompanied by rapidly progressive renal failure, hypertensive encephalopathy, CHF, and/or microangiopathic hemolytic anemia. The basic pathogenesis is the stimulation of RAS.

### Posterior Reversible Encephalopathy Syndrome

Posterior reversible encephalopathy syndrome is a reversible, vasogenic edema, which occurs predominantly in the posterior brain. PRES is less commonly known as "reversible posterior leukoencephalopathy syndrome" (RPLS). It is a clinicoradiologic diagnosis. PRES often occurs in the context of a hypertensive emergency, *preeclampsia/eclampsia*, acute glomerulonephritis, Guillain–Barré syndrome with autonomic instability. 25% of patients may not have hypertension. It usually presents with encephalopathy, seizures, headache, and visual loss. The hallmark findings of *vasogenic edema* are invariably seen in magnetic resonance imaging (MRI) [where it appears as hyperintensity on T2/fluid-attenuated inversion recovery (FLAIR)]. Edema tends to occur in a bilateral pattern within the white matter, centered at the watershed areas between vascular territories: Most commonly, parieto-occipital (50%), superior frontal sulcus (25%).

The term *hypertensive urgency* has been previously used to refer to situations where very high BP values, usually >180/110 mm Hg, but acute hypertension-mediated TOD is absent.

This also means that the term hypertensive crisis that includes hypertensive urgencies and emergencies becomes obsolete.

## ETIOLOGY

Majority of hypertensive emergencies occur in the following patients:

- Already diagnosed with chronic hypertension
- Noncompliance with antihypertensive medications (AHMs)
- Uses of sympathomimetics
- Secondary causes of hypertension

These lead to a rapid rise in BP beyond the body's innate autoregulation capacity. The rate of rise of BP from baseline is the more important contributor. That is why chronic hypertension tolerates high BP without any symptoms or TOD than acutely elevated high BP.

## EPIDEMIOLOGY

About 1–2% of hypertension will have a hypertensive crisis.

## PATHOPHYSIOLOGY

The mechanical stress leads to endothelial damage and a pro-inflammatory response. Exposure of blood to the subendothelium leads to increased vascular permeability, coagulation activation, platelet activation, and the formation of a fibrin network, thereby reducting blood flow to the target organ. It also causes intravascular hemolysis as a result of trapping and destruction of erythrocytes within the fibrin network. Severe uncontrolled hypertension causes RAS activation, increase in (renal) vascular resistance, and autoregulatory failure. All these lead to TOD.

## HISTOPATHOLOGY

Fibrinoid necrosis of renal arteries is a classic feature of malignant hypertension. Pathologically, it is associated with diffuse necrotizing vasculitis, arteriolar thrombi, and fibrin deposition in the arteriolar wall.

## HISTORY AND PHYSICAL

Symptoms usually depend on the organ involved. Common symptoms are as follows:

- Headache
- Dizziness
- Altered mental status
- Shortness of breath
- Chest pain
- Decreased urine output
- Vomiting
- Changes in vision

Similarly, exam findings also vary depending on the specific target organ mostly affected.

- *CVS examination* may reveal rales, engorged jugular venous pressure (JVP), and edema, and extra heart sounds may be noted. In the event of a very rapid onset of hypertension such as sympathomimetic cocaine abuse or renal artery stenosis, marked dyspnea in the absence of peripheral edema due to FPE may be seen.
- *CNS examination*: Altered mental status, visual problem, ataxia or other cerebellar dysfunction, aphasia, or unilateral numbness or weakness
- *Eye exam* is mandatory, which may reveal papilledema as well as exudates and flame-shaped hemorrhages.
- *Kidneys*: ARF may also result in signs of pulmonary edema or peripheral edema.
- *Pregnancy*: Eclampsia may lead to convulsion and coma in pregnancy.

## EVALUATION

*Routine tests depend on symptoms and signs*:

- *Routine tests*: Hemoglobin and/or hematocrit, platelet count, peripheral smear to look for schistocytes
- Fasting blood glucose and/or glycated hemoglobin (HbA1c)
- *Blood lipids*: Total cholesterol, low-density lipoprotein cholesterol (LDL-C), high-density lipoprotein cholesterol (HDL-C), triglycerides
- *Renal function test*: Creatininie, urea, eGFR. Urine analysis: Protein, RBC, liver function tests
- Blood potassium and sodium, uric acid
- Cardiac enzymes, brain natriuretic peptide (BNP)
- Chest X-ray (CXR) posteroanterior (PA) view: Widening of mediastinum in aortic dissection, pulmonary edema
- 12-lead electrocardiography (ECG) in angina arrhythmia, left ventricular hypertrophy (LVH)
- Ultrasonography (USG) of the renal system to exclude secondary causes
- Echocardiography to look for cardiac structural disease

- Computed tomography (CT) angiography of chest or abdomen to exclude aortic dissection
- CT scan head

*Approach to hypertensive emergency*: Symptomatic severe BP elevation:

- Search for acute HMOD.
- Presence of HMOD? If no, it is uncontrolled hypertension.
- Presence of HMOD? If yes - positive, it is diagnosed as hypertensive emergency.

Need treatment according to organ damage and symptoms.

# TREATMENT/MANAGEMENT

*Optimal pharmacotherapy* depends on the specific organ involved, and acute lowering of BP is the mainstay of therapy. The goal is to lower the mean arterial pressure (MAP) by 20–25% in the first 1–2 hours. The drugs should be rapid-acting and easily titratable. IV drugs such as labetalol, esmolol, nicardipine, NTG, and sodium nitroprusside are typically effective options.

*Management principle*: There is a general agreement that patients without acute HMOD usually can be treated with oral BP-lowering medication or alterations of their current BP-lowering medication. A controlled BP reduction to safer levels without risk of hypotension should be the therapeutic goal. Once the decision of administering pharmacotherapy is taken, an observation period of at least 2 hours is suggested to evaluate BP-lowering efficacy and safety.

*The rapidity and amount of BP reduction*, as well as the type of BP-lowering therapy, mainly rely on the clinical scenario. Urgent BP lowering is necessary in patients with pulmonary edema and acute aortic dissection; in contrast, BP-lowering therapy is generally withheld in patients with ischemic stroke. Whether BP should be acutely lowered in patients presenting with severe hypertension and acute intracranial hemorrhage is still a subject of debate. Though there are differences in opinion, most hypertensive emergencies could be managed with either labetalol or nicardipine.

## Malignant Hypertension and Hypertensive Encephalopathy: Management

Activation of RAS is highly variable; therefore, angiotensin-converting enzyme inhibitors (ACEI) have an unpredictable response. Sodium nitroprusside, labetalol, nicardipine, and urapidil are all safe and effective. Fenoldopam, a short-acting selective dopamine-1 agonist, and clevidipine, an ultra-short-acting calcium-channel blocker for IV use, are alternative options for severe hypertension with limited availability. In hypertensive emergency, administration of ACEI must be started at a very low dose and IV saline infusion could be thought of to correct precipitous BP falls if necessary.

## Management of Specific Types of Hypertensive Emergency

### *Hypertensive Encephalopathy*

Labetalol is preferred over nitroprusside as it maintains cerebral blood flow relatively well and does not increase intracranial pressure. Nitroprusside and nicardipine can alternatively be used for this type of emergency.

### *Acute Ischemic and Hemorrhagic Stroke*

In ischemic stroke, acute BP reduction within the first 5–7 days is associated with adverse neurological outcome. Acute transient BP elevations that persist for days to weeks are frequently seen after stroke. Aggressive BP reduction should be avoided.

- If BP is very high (>220/120 mm Hg), BP-lowering therapy is indicated. It is probably safe to lower MAP by 15% in the first 24 hours of stroke, ischemic or hemorrhagic.

- *Ischemic stroke*: If BP > 180/105 mm Hg, it is probably safe to lower MAP by 15% within 1–2 hours if there is a concomitant condition such as acute coronary event, acute heart failure, aortic dissection, or presence of end-organ damage.
- For acute ischemic stroke and an indication for thrombolytic therapy, lowering BP to <185 mm Hg systolic and 110 mm Hg diastolic is recommended before thrombolysis is given and maintained at SBP lower than 180 mm Hg and DBP lower than 105 mm Hg for the first 24 hours.
- *Intracerebral hemorrhage (ICH)*: Acute BP-lowering treatment to SBP < 140 mm Hg in patients with intracerebral hemorrhage reduces intracranial hematoma volume and has a (borderline) significant effect in improving functional outcome in INTERACT (Intensive Blood Pressure Reduction in Acute Cerebral Hemorrhage Trial)-2, while ATACH-2 (Antihypertensive Treatment of Acute Cerebral Hemorrhage II) failed to show any benefit of acute BP-lowering treatment. Therefore, it is preferable to keep the SBP < 180 mm Hg or MAP < 130 mm Hg if intracranial tension (ICT) is increased. If ICT is normal, keep MAP < 110 mm Hg (SBP < 160 mm Hg) in the initial period. Extreme vigilance is necessary to prevent hypotension, which causes decreased cerebral perfusion pressure.
- For neurologically stable patients with BP > 140/90 mm Hg, starting or restarting antihypertensive therapy after the first 24 hours to improve long-term BP control is reasonable.
- *Subarachnoid hemorrhage (SAH)*: Management of hypertension is controversial. If MAP > 130 mm Hg, cautious reduction of BP reduction is helpful (SBP below 160 mm Hg). Nimodipine is used to prevent delayed ischemic neurodeficit, not for acute hypertension. Nicardipine, labetalol, or esmolol is preferred.

## ACUTE CORONARY ARTERY EVENTS

In case severe hypertension is associated with acute coronary syndrome (cardiac ischemia or myocardial infarction), afterload needs to be reduced without an increase in heart rate in order to decrease myocardial oxygen demand without jeopardizing diastolic filling time.

- Both NTG and labetalol have been used to lower BP in patients with an acute coronary event. Immediately reduce SBP to <140 mm Hg.
- Sodium nitroprusside decreases regional blood flow in patients with coronary abnormalities and increases myocardial damage after acute myocardial infarction.
- *Additional beta-blockade* may be indicated for patients receiving NTG, especially if tachycardia is present. Urapidil may be a good alternative for the management of hypertension in patients with myocardial ischemia with limited availability. Metoprolol may be used for heart rate control but not for BP control.

### Acute Cardiogenic Pulmonary Edema

- In patients with acute pulmonary edema caused by hypertensive heart failure, both NTG and sodium nitroprusside can be used as they will optimize preload and decrease afterload. Immediately reduce SBP to <140 mm Hg.
- Nitroprusside is the drug of choice as it will acutely lower ventricular pre- and afterload.
- NTG may be a good alternative, although high doses (>200 mg/min) may be required to achieve the desired BP-lowering effect.
- *Urapidil* gives a better BP reduction and improvement of arterial oxygen content without reflex tachycardia in comparison to NTG.

- *Noninvasive continuous positive airway pressure* may be of additional benefit as it acutely reduces pulmonary edema and venous return.
- *Loop diuretics*: Concomitant administration of it decreases volume overload and helps to further lower BP.

## Acute Aortic Disease (Dissection or Rupture)

- Lower the BP to as low as organs will allow, with close monitoring of the patient's mental status, which actually acts as a guide of antihypertensive therapy.
- SBP and heart rate need to be immediately reduced to 120 mm Hg or lower and 60 bpm or less to reduce aortic wall stress and disease progression.
- Beta-blockers (BBs) are therefore considered first-line treatment. Esmolol can be used together with ultra-short-acting vasodilating agents such as nitroprusside or clevidipine or nicardipine.
- Use of nitroprusside is infrequent due to its rapid and profound hypotension, tachyphylaxis, and potential for cyanide toxicity.
- Nicardipine with the addition of a BB would also be a reasonable choice.

## Eclampsia and Severe Preeclampsia

- There are two patients to consider at a single time. The first-line therapy is magnesium sulfate, administered as a 4–6 g loading dose followed by 1–2 g/h infusion. Monitor urine output, deep tendon reflexes, and respiratory status.
- In patients with eclampsia or severe preeclampsia, BP-lowering therapy is thought of next to IV magnesium sulfate and delivery needs to be considered after the maternal condition has stabilized.
- In preeclampsia with severe features, delivery is recommended if >34 weeks, but expectant management may be considered if <34 weeks if the mother becomes stabilized.
- Indications of delivery in preeclampsia if <34 weeks: If unremitting symptoms, laboratory abnormalities and refractory hypertension persists even after medical therapy.
- The consensus is to lower SBP and DBP <160/105 mm Hg to prevent acute hypertensive complications in the mother. High BP should be reduced slowly to avoid hypotension in the mother and reduced blood flow to the fetus.
- Both labetalol and nicardipine have shown to be safe and effective for the treatment of severe preeclampsia. BBs—labetalol—may be used as an adjunctive therapy if BP remains above target, SBP is higher than 160 mm Hg.
- Monitoring of fetal heart rate is mandatory. The cumulative dose of labetalol should not exceed 800 mg/24 h to prevent fetal bradycardia.
- Timely institution of oral BP-lowering therapy (e.g., methyldopa or long-acting nifedipine) or dose adaptation may help to improve BP control and reduces the risk of fetal bradycardia in case labetalol is used.
- Treatment with hydralazine is not widely practiced and not recommended because of associated adverse perinatal outcomes if other alternatives are available. Besides this, hydralazine having a delayed onset of action, prolonged duration, and unpredictable hypotensive effects is not the primary choice of therapy.
- Nitroprusside is contraindicated because it carries the risk of fetal cyanide toxicity.
- The entire patient needs close monitoring in a critical care setting.

# SPECIFIC SITUATIONS

- *Methamphetamine and cocaine toxicity*: It causes autonomic hyperreactivity
  - Treatment with benzodiazepines should be initiated first.

- Phentolamine, a competitive alpha-blocking agent, is used for BP reduction if necessary or nicardipine or nitroprusside can be considered.
- Alternatively, clonidine can be used, which, apart from its sympathicolytic action, also has sedative effects.
- *NTG*: In case of coronary ischemia, treatment with NTG and aspirin is recommended next to benzodiazepines.
- *Percutaneous coronary intervention (PCI)*: In high-risk patients with (non-) ST-segment elevation myocardial infarction
- *Nondihydropyridine (non-DHP) calcium channel blocking agents*, such as diltiazem and verapamil, can be used to treat patients with tachyarrhythmias under close ECG monitoring.
- Beta-blocking agents (including labetalol) are relatively contraindicated because they do not seem to be effective in reducing coronary vasoconstriction.

- *Pheochromocytoma*: The basic pathogenesis is adrenergic overstimulation.
  - Treatment with labetalol has been associated with acceleration of hypertension in individual cases.
  - Phentolamine, nitroprusside, and urapidil have been successfully used in the perioperative management of pheochromocytoma.
  - Nicardipine may also be a good alternative.
- *SCAPE*: Initiate NIV at $cmH_2O$ of positive end-expiratory pressure (PEEP). Initiate NTG bolus 500–1,000 µg IV over 2 minutes, then start infusion @ 100 µg/minute and uptitrate to 400 µg/minute until the goal is reached. Then downtitrate to 100 µg/minute. If clinical improvement occurs, taper off NTG and NIV.
- *SRC*: Start with short-acting ACEI such as captopril and rapidly titrate the dose to lower SBP by about 20 mm Hg in 24 hours and reaching goal BP of 120/70 mm Hg within 72 hours. Once BP is at goal and dose is stabilized, substitute by long-acting ACEI. If target BP is not achieved with maximum doses of ACEI, a DHP calcium channel blocker can be added. Diuretics are usually not used to avoid stimulation of RAS.
- *In patients with a hypertensive emergency elicited by cytotoxic or antiangiogenic drugs*: Withhold the offending agent until BP control is achieved with antihypertensive agents. Alternative agents, dose adjustments, and follow-up are needed.
- *PRES*: MAP should be lowered by approximately 20–25% within 1–2 hours. A MAP target of 105–125 mm Hg is often reasonable, although this may need to be personalized. *Calcium channel blocking agents* are preferable to reduce the risk of vasospasm. IV agents are initially preferred: Nicardipine infusion or clevidipine infusion. Oral calcium channel blockers may subsequently be utilized: Nifedipine extended-release (ER). NTG should be avoided as this may aggravate PRES. Levetiracetam can be used for seizure control. Treat *hypomagnesemia* or hypervolemia if present. The recovery rate is excellent but it takes some days.
- *Malignant hypertension with or without ARF*: Within several hours, reduce MAP by 20–25% by using labetalol or nicardipine. Nitroprusside and urapidil are the alternative choices.
- *Perioperative hypertensive emergency*: It is defined as BP > 160/90 mm Hg or more or SBP elevation > 20% of the preoperative value and that persists for >15 minutes. Nitroprusside, NTG, clevidipine, nicardipine, or esmolol are the preferred choices. Target the perioperative BP within 20% of the baseline value. Perioperative BBs are the first choice for cardiovascular (CV) surgery. But do not initiate BB in the first time before operation. Discontinue ACEI or angiotensin receptor blocker (ARB) in preoperative hypertensive before elective surgery.

*Postacute care: IV to per oral (PO) transition*:

- When does the patient meet the IV to PO conversion? If BP is at goal (for medical patients, <160/100 for 6 hours, for cardiovascular patients, SBP < 120 for 24 hours, for stroke, MAP < 15–20% of presentation for 24 hours) BP does not vary >15%, and eating or taking other medications without nausea, vomiting, or gastrointestinal (GI) disturbances or gastric residual volume (GRV) <150–250 mL, then conversion may be tried. But if criteria are not met, then continue IV therapy and reevaluate at 24 hours if previously there was no history of hypertension. If previous hypertension was there and was on multiple AHM, restart 1–2 outpatient department (OPD) medicines for hypertension in an attempt to avoid prolonged use of IV therapy.
- *From IV to oral therapy*: After a suitable period, usually 8–24 hours of target BP control in intensive care unit (ICU), oral medications are started and initial IV therapy is gradually tapered to a minimum dose and oral dose is administered. Discontinue IV over 1–2 hours and titrate oral dose upward to maintain goal BP. Another option for the transition from IV to oral—initiate low-dose oral agents and titrate oral dose upward as the IV dose is slowly reduced.
- *Oral therapy options*: Choose the agent as of IV class. Restart the same or part of preadmission regimen.
- Evaluation of common forms of secondary hypertension should be evaluated.
- High-quality outpatient follow-up is mandatory for long-term improvement of morbidity and mortality.

*Most common mistakes*: Overdiagnosis of hypertensive emergency without TOD. Treatment of hypertensive emergency too aggressively and dropping the BP too much and too rapidly are other common mistake. Another common mistake is trying to transition from an antihypertensive infusion to an oral agent that takes a long time to have any effect (e.g., amlodipine).

Details of drug therapy in hypertensive crisis see **Table 1**.

## PROGNOSIS

In the past, hypertensive emergencies were frequently associated with kidney impairment, myocardial infarction, stroke, or death. With more awareness and better control of BP, mortality has decreased significantly in the past three decades. However, after the acute treatment, strict control of BP is vital if one wants to lower morbidity and mortality. Unfortunately, the overall long-term prognosis of patients with hypertensive emergencies is guarded. A significant number of these patients may develop adverse cardiac events or a stroke within 12 months.

*Complications*: Renal failure, vision loss, myocardial infarction, eclampsia, stroke

## PATIENT EDUCATION

- Ask the patients to maintain strict adherence with antihypertensive therapy.
- Low sodium diet and weight losses are recommended.
- Controlled bed rest for the period of high BP

*Summary of guidelines*: The management of hypertensive emergencies is mainly based on consensus from clinical experience, observations, and comparisons on intermediate outcomes. The initial goal is to decrease the MAP by approximately 20% within 1–2 hours. If compelling conditions such as aortic dissection, eclampsia, pheochromocytoma crisis are present, lower BP <140 mm Hg during the first hour and to below <120 mm Hg if aortic dissection is there. If compelling conditions are absent, decrease the MAP by maximum 20% within 1–2 hours. If this reduction is tolerated, then decrease the MAP to approximately

**Table 1: Some points about specific antihypertensive therapy.**

| *Name of drugs* | *Dose* | *Indications* | *Contraindications* | *Cautions* |
|---|---|---|---|---|
| Labetalol | 20 mg IV—bolus Then 20–80 mg IV q10 minutes to a total dose of 300 mg, OR Constant infusion @ 0.5–2 mg/min | Most hypertensive emergency, including pregnancy-induced HTN, CVA, CAD, hypertensive encephalopathy, postoperative HTN | Asthma, COPD, 2nd or 3rd-degree heart block, CCF, HF, bradycardia | Labetalol should not be used prior to alpha-blocker in pheochromocytoma, cocaine or methamphetamine overdose Avoid in acute decompensated HF |
| Esmolol | LD: 500 μg IV over 1 minute, then 25–50 μg/kg/min, increased up to 300 μg/kg/min | Perioperative HTN, aortic dissection | Bronchospasm, first-degree heart block | Avoid in acute decompensated HF |
| Enalaprilat | 1.25–5 mg q6h IV | LVF | Renal failure, pregnancy, rarely used now | Precipitous fall in pressure in high-renin state, headache, dizziness |
| Nicardipine | 5–15 mg/h infusion, max up to 30 mg/h | Most hypertensive emergency including pregnancy | Acute HF | Caution with coronary ischemia |
| Nitroglycerin (glyceryl trinitrate) | 10–100 μg/h infusion | Used as an adjunct therapy in ACS, acute pulmonary edema | Avoid in CVA | Reflex tachycardia, headache, vomiting, flushing can happen, tolerance may develop |
| Nitroprusside | 0.25–10 μg/kg/min as IV infusion | Due to its toxicity, it is now rarely used if alternatives are available | AMI, CAD, CVA, increased ICT, AKI, hepatic impairment | Due to its toxicity (decreased cerebral blood flow and coronary flow cyanide toxicity), it is now rarely used |
| Phentolamine | 5–15 mg IV q5–15 minutes | Pheochromocytoma, cocaine overdose | | Tachycardia, flushing, headache, N/V |
| Clevidipine | 1–2 mg/h infusion with rapid titration to 4–6 mg/h max up to 21 mg/h | Hypertensive emergency including postoperative HTN | | May cause AF, allergy |
| Fenoldopam | 0.1 μg/kg/min titrate up to 1.6 μg/kg/min | Most hypertensive emergencies | Use caution with glaucoma or increased ICT | Tachycardia, flushing, N/V may occur |

(ACS: acute coronary syndrome; AF: atrial fibrillation; AKI: acute kidney injury; AMI: acute myocardial infarction; CAD: coronary artery disease; CCF: congestive cardiac failure; COPD: chronic obstructive pulmonary disease; CVA: cerebrovascular accident; HF: heart failure; HTN: hypertension; IV: intravenous; LD: loading dose; LVF: left ventricular failure)

125 mm Hg (~160/110 mm Hg) over the next 2–6 hours. The BP may further be gradually decreased over a period of days as tolerated to normal levels. For a patient with chronic hypertension (chronic kidney disease with hypertension), a more gradual approach to lowering the BP may be wise. In chronic hypertension, BP target should be well above the patient's baseline value. For acute development of hypertension (e.g., postoperatively or due to an acute ingestion), more rapid reduction of BP is more practical. Treatment with vasodilation may cause hypotension (due to unmasking of their hypovolemia due to hypertension natriuresis). Stabilizing these patients may require volume administration. In ICH, reduction may be tried SBP <160–140 mm Hg avoiding hypotension and cerebral hypoperfusion. Assess for target organ injury and start parenteral medications as needed. If the patient has an acute emergency such as aortic dissection, lower the BP to below 140–120 mm Hg in the first hour. With no organ damage, lower the BP by 15–25% over days.

## CLINICAL PEARLS

- A hypertensive emergency is an acute and marked rise in BP (mostly >180/120 mm Hg but absolute vale is not very important) associated with signs of TOD: These include pulmonary edema, cardiac ischemia, neurodeficit, ARF, eclampsia, aortic dissection.
- Non-compliance, use of sympathomimetics drugs and secondary hypertension is the common cause.
- Careful history taking and physical examination ophthalmoscopy is helpful in making the diagnosis.
- Evaluation by ECG, ECHO, CXR, and basic metabolic panel (BMP) and urine REME ACR is very important to know TOD. Continuous monitoring of BP, TOD and pharmacotherapy is the management goal depends on gradual reduction of BP, MAP reduction by 20–25% within the first 1–2 hours.
- IV vasoactive drugs like labetalol, esmolol, nicardipine and nitroglycerine are typically effective options.
- But if there is no compelling indication, then gradual reduction of BP (MAP) by 25% in the first hour, then to 160/100 mm Hg over the next 2–6 hours, then gradually to normal over a few (2) days.
- But if there is compelling indication, like aortic dissection, eclampsia, Pheochromocytoma crisis, lower the SBP below 140 mm Hg in the first hours and to below 120 and pulse around 60/in ischemic CVA: BP is not to be reduced if not eligible for thrombolysis, unless >220/120 or >180/110 mm Hg if associated with cardiac ischemia, aortic dissection, ARF or HF for 3 days or in hemorrhagic CVA <6 hours of onset lower BP <140/90 mm Hg to reduce hematoma expansion.
- Eclampsia and severe preeclampsia/HELLP: Immediately reduce SBP to <160 mm Hg and DBP to <105.
- Acute cardiogenic pulmonary edema/acute coronary events: Immediately reduce SBP to <140.
- Hypertensive encephalopathy: Immediately reduce MAP by 20–25%.

## FURTHER READINGS

1. Tocci G, Figliuzzi I, Presta V, Miceli F, Citoni B, Coluccia R, et al. Therapeutic approach to hypertension urgencies and emergencies during acute coronary syndrome. High Blood Press Cardiovasc Prev. 2018;25(3):253-9.
2. Paini A, Aggiusti C, Bertacchini F, Agabiti Rosei C, Maruelli G, Arnoldi C, et al. Definitions and epidemiological aspects of hypertensive urgencies and emergencies. High Blood Press Cardiovasc Prev. 2018;25(3):241-4.

3. Viera AJ. Hypertension update: hypertensive emergency and asymptomatic severe hypertension. FP Essent. 2018;469:16-9.
4. Salvetti M, Paini A, Bertacchini F, Stassaldi D, Aggiusti C, Agabiti Rosei C, et al. Acute blood pressure elevation: therapeutic approach. Pharmacol Res. 2018;130:180-90.
5. Chiariello M, Gold HK, Leinbach RC, Davis MA, Maroko PR. Comparison between the effects of nitroprusside and nitroglycerin on ischemic injury during acute myocardial infarction. Circulation. 1976;54:766-73.
6. Gregorini L, Marco J, Palombo C, Kozàkovà M, Anguissola GB, Cassagneau B, et al. Postischemic left ventricular dysfunction is abolished by alpha-adrenergic blocking agents. J Am Coll Cardiol. 1998;31:992-1001.
7. Schreiber W, Woisetschläger C, Binder M, Kaff A, Raab H, Hirschl MM. The nitura study–effect of nitroglycerin or urapidil on hemodynamic, metabolic and respiratory parameters in hypertensive patients with pulmonary edema. Intensive Care Med. 1998;24:557-63.
8. Ulici A, Jancik J, Lam TS, Reidt S, Calcaterra D, Cole JB. Clevidipine versus sodium nitroprusside in acute aortic dissection: a retrospective chart review. Am J Emerg Med. 2017;35:1514-8.
9. American College of Obstetricians and Gynecologists, Task Force on Hypertension in Pregnancy. Hypertension in pregnancy. Report of the American College of Obstetricians and Gynecologists' Task Force on Hypertension in Pregnancy. Obstet Gynecol. 2013;122: 1122-31.
10. Duley L, Henderson-Smart DJ, Meher S. Drugs for treatment of very high blood pressure during pregnancy. Cochrane Database Syst Rev. 2006;(3):CD001449.
11. Briggs RS, Birtwell AJ, Pohl JE. Hypertensive response to labetalol in phaeochromocytoma. Lancet. 1978;1:1045-6.
12. Tauzin-Fin P, Sesay M, Gosse P, Ballanger P. Effects of perioperative alpha1 block on haemodynamic control during laparoscopic surgery for phaeochromocytoma. Br J Anaesth. 2004;92:512-7.
13. van den Born BJ, van der Hoeven NV, Groot E, Lenting PJ, Meijers JC, Levi M, et al. Association between thrombotic microangiopathy and reduced ADAMTS13 activity in malignant hypertension. Hypertension. 2008;51:862-6.
14. Martínez-Díaz AM, Palazón-Bru A, Folgado-de la Rosa DM, Ramírez-Prado D, Navarro-Juan M, Pérez-Ramírez N, et al. A one-year risk score to predict all-cause mortality in hypertensive inpatients. Eur J Intern Med. 2019;59:77-83.

CHAPTER 99

# Diabetic Coma

*Shambo Samrat Samajdar*

## WHAT IS DIABETIC COMA?

Acute hyperglycemic or hypoglycemic episodes in both type 1 and type 2 diabetes mellitus patients as a result of metabolic complications of diabetes mellitus, leading to life-threatening unconsciousness which is reversible with timely appropriate interventions, are designated as diabetic coma. Diabetic ketoacidosis (DKA) and hyperglycemic hyperosmolar state (HHS) are two important acute hyperglycemic episodes associated with coma, and severe hypoglycemia associated with unconsciousness comes under the broad heading of diabetic coma. In this chapter, we discuss acute hyperglycemic complications of diabetes—DKA and HHS. Severe hypoglycemia is discussed in Chapter 102.

Hyperglycemia, ketonemia, and large anion gap metabolic acidosis make up the biochemical triad of DKA. The terms "hyperglycemic hyperosmolar nonketotic state" and "hyperglycemic hyperosmolar nonketotic coma" have been replaced with "hyperglycemic hyperosmolar state" to emphasize that (1) the HHS may include moderate to variable degrees of clinical ketosis detected by the nitroprusside method and (2) alterations in consciousness may frequently be present without coma. Since it takes 1/10 as much insulin to inhibit lipolysis as it does to promote glucose utilization, while DKA is a condition of almost complete insulinopenia, there is enough insulin in HHS to prevent ketogenesis and lipolysis but not enough to trigger glucose uptake.

## WHAT CAUSES DIABETIC KETOACIDOSIS AND HYPERGLYCEMIC HYPEROSMOLAR STATE?

The underlying pathogeneses in cases of DKA and HHS are as follows:

- As a result of reduced insulin secretion (DKA) or ineffective action of insulin in HHS, the net effective action of circulating insulin would be reduced.
- Counter-regulatory hormones, such as glucagon, catecholamines, cortisol, and growth hormone, are elevated and result in increased hepatic glucose production and impaired glucose utilization in peripheral tissues.
- Osmotic diuresis associated with glycosuria causes dehydration and dyselectrolytemia.
- Additionally, increased gluconeogenesis, lipolysis, and ketogenesis, as well as reduced glycolysis, are characteristics of DKA.

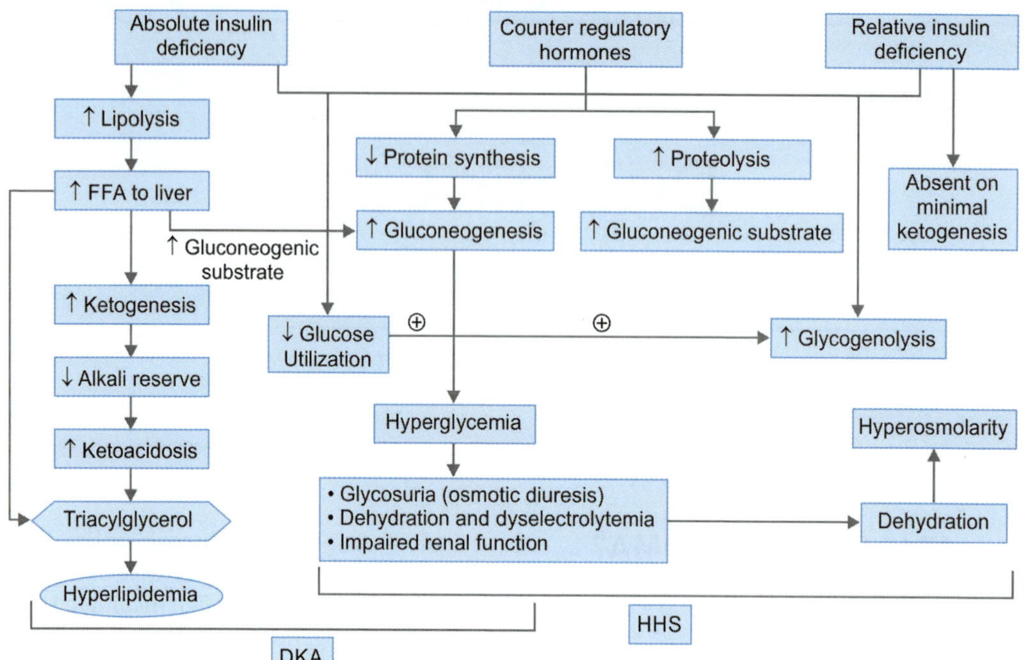


**FLOWCHART 1:** Pathogenesis for diabetic ketoacidosis (DKA) and hyperglycemic hyperosmolar state (HHS). (↑: increase, ↓: decrease, FFA: free fatty acid)

**Flowchart 1** describes briefly the pathogenesis of HHS and DKA. The absence of or an insufficient insulin regimen and infections are the two most frequent causes that can lead to the development of DKA or HHS. Myocardial infarction, cerebrovascular accidents, pulmonary embolism, pancreatitis, alcohol usage, and illicit drug use are additional precipitating factors. DKA or HHS may be triggered by medications such as corticosteroids, thiazide diuretics, sympathomimetic drugs (dobutamine and terbutaline), sodium-glucose cotransporter-2 (SGLT-2) inhibitors (canagliflozin, dapagliflozin, and empagliflozin), immune checkpoint inhibitors (ipilimumab, nivolumab, pembrolizumab), and second-generation antipsychotics.

## WHAT ARE THE POSSIBILITIES? (DIFFERENTIAL DIAGNOSIS)

There are a few conditions such as starvation or high-fat intake, lactic acidosis, uremic acidosis, alcoholic acidosis, especially in the presence of starvation, salicylate intoxication, methanol or ethylene glycol intoxication, isopropyl alcohol injection, hypoglycemic coma, and rhabdomyolysis that need to be considered as differential diagnosis. Hyperglycemia and presence of glycosuria can establish the diagnosis of DKA or HHS, excluding other differentials. **Figure 1** depicts the triad of hyperglycemia, ketosis, and metabolic acidosis associated with DKA and what are the different conditions that can present as each component of this triad.

## PATH TO DIAGNOSIS

- *Symptoms and signs*: Usually, within a few hours of the precipitating incident, DKA progresses rapidly. However, HHS development is insidious and may take days to weeks to manifest. Polyuria, polyphagia, polydipsia, weight loss, weakness, and physical indicators of depleted intravascular volume,

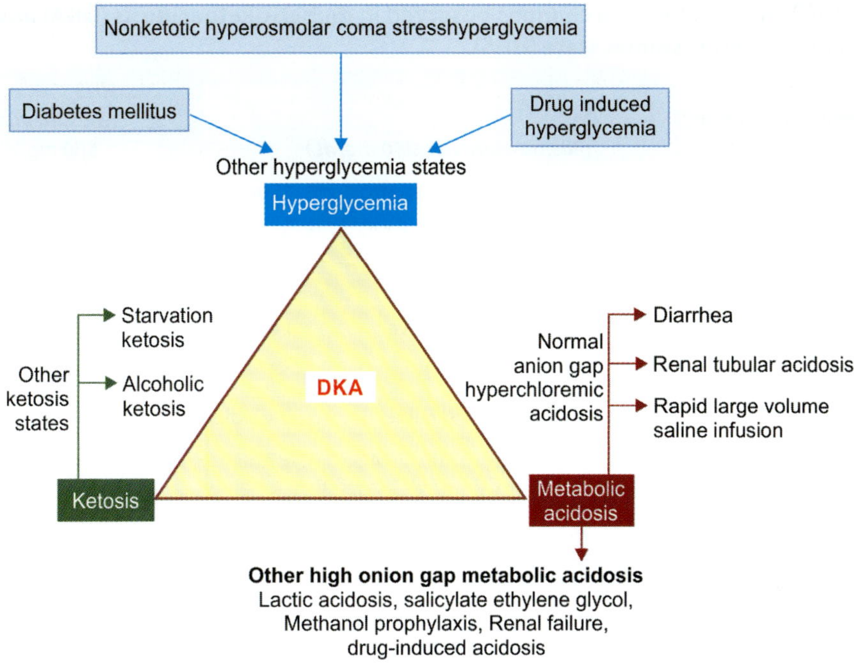


**FIG. 1:** Triad of diabetic ketoacidosis (DKA) and other conditions mimicking each component of the triad.

such as poor skin turgor, dry buccal mucosa, tachycardia, sunken eyeballs, hypotension, and shock in severe instances, are most prevalent clinical manifestations of DKA and HHS caused by hyperglycemia. Patients presenting with euglycemic DKA, particularly those on SGLT-2 inhibitors, may first appear with nonspecific symptoms such as weakness and malaise rather than polydipsia and polyuria. Ketosis and acidosis are the causes of Kussmaul respiration, acetone breath, nausea, vomiting, and abdominal discomfort, all of which are more common in DKA. In 50–75% of instances, abdominal discomfort, which coincides with the degree of acidosis, may be severe enough to be misdiagnosed with acute abdomen. Therefore, it is important to examine DKA as a cause of acute abdomen when acidosis is present. Even if an infection is present, patients often have normal body temperatures or moderate hypothermia. So, in the absence of a fever, a thorough investigation for an infection source should be carried out. Mental status alterations in DKA are less common than in HHS. Neurological condition in individuals with DKA can range from complete alertness to a deep lethargy and coma.

- *Laboratory investigations*: Urine ketones by dipstick, plasma glucose, blood urea nitrogen, serum creatinine, serum ketones, and electrolytes with calculated anion gap, osmolality, urinalysis, arterial blood gases, and complete hemogram should all be determined during the initial laboratory evaluation of patients with suspected DKA or HHS. If necessary, a chest X-ray, an electrocardiogram, blood, urine, or sputum cultures, and other tests should also be carried out. Glycated hemoglobin (HbA1c) may be helpful in separating acute metabolic decompensation from chronic hyper-glycemia of uncontrolled diabetes in a patient with previously well-controlled

**Table 1: Different biochemical changes observed in diabetic ketoacidosis (DKA) and hyperglycemic hyperosmolar state (HHS).**

| ***Biochemical changes in DKA and HHS*** | ***DKA (plasma glucose > 250 mg/dL)*** | | | ***HHS (plasma glucose > 500 mg/dL)*** |
|---|---|---|---|---|
| Biochemistry | Mild | Moderate | Severe | |
| Sodium bicarbonate (mEq/L) | 15–18 | 10–15 | <10 | >18 |
| Urine ketone* | Positive | Positive | Positive | Small |
| Serum ketone* | Positive | Positive | Positive | Small |
| Anion gap† | >10 | >12 | >12 | Variable |
| Serum osmolality‡ (effective) | Variable | Variable | Variable | >320 mOsm/kg |
| Arterial pH | 7.25–7.30 | 7.00–7.24 | <7.00 | >7.30 |
| Mental status | Alert | Alert/drowsy | Stupor/coma | Stupor/coma |

*Measurement via nitroprusside reaction method.

†Anion gap = [measured $Na^+$ – (measured $Cl^-$ + measured $HCO_3^-$) mEq/L].

‡Effective serum osmolality = 2 [measured Na (mEq/L) + glucose (mg/dL)/18].

diabetes. **Table 1** elaborates different biochemical changes observed in DKA and HHS. Depending on the degree of metabolic acidosis and the existence of an altered mental status, DKA can be categorized as mild, moderate, or severe. As per recent studies, 25–30% cases of hyperglycemic crisis present with both DKA and HHS. In general, HHS patients present with pH > 7.30, bicarbonate level > 20 mEq/L, and negative ketone bodies in plasma and urine. Nevertheless, a few of them could have ketonemia. There is a positive linear correlation between serum osmolarity, pH, and mental obtundation according to several research studies. Beta-hydroxybutyrate (β-OHB) of ≥3.8 mmol/L estimated by a highly sensitive and specific assay is extremely useful for diagnosing DKA. The diagnosis of DKA in the presence of concomitant underlying chronic metabolic acidosis or mixed acid-base disorders among CKD stage 4–5 patients is typically supported by an anion gap of >20 mEq/L. According to the 2009 publication by the American Diabetes Association (ADA), "euglycemic DKA" is manifested by features such as metabolic acidosis, increased total body ketone concentration, and blood glucose levels below 250 mg/dL. It is observed in up to 10% of patients with DKA and is primarily linked to pathological states that have low glycogen reserves and/or higher rates of glucosuria, such as pregnancy, liver disorders, and alcohol use. Euglycemic DKA is a well-known adverse effect of SGLT-2 inhibitors. If significant anion gap metabolic acidosis is evident in a diabetic patient being treated with SGLT-2 inhibitors, DKA must be ruled out whether or not hyperglycemia is present. However, in those who have enough glycogen stores to sustain hyperglycemia even in the presence of increased glucosuria, an SGLT-2 inhibitor can also be linked to hyperglycemic DKA.

Due to glucose-mediated osmotic diuresis, which causes the body to lose more water than electrolytes, there is a significant water deficit in those with DKA and HHS. Although there has been a lot of water loss, the serum sodium level during admission is often low. Because of insulinopenia in cases of DKA and HHS, blood glucose is prevented from entering the cells. During hyperglycemic crises, glucose forces water to move from within cells to outside cells by its osmotic effectiveness. This results in decrease in sodium concentration—dilutional or hyperosmolar hyponatremia. The corrected serum sodium concentration in hyperglycemic crisis patients should be estimated by adding 2.4 mmol/L per 100 mg/dL rise in serum glucose concentration to the observed serum sodium concentration (when serum glucose concentration is >100 mg/dL). Hypertriglyceridemia presented as a secondary complication to uncontrolled diabetes needs to be considered in the background of hyponatremia. Although concomitant symptoms such as diarrhea and vomiting can also increase sodium losses, osmotic diuresis and ketonuria can enhance sodium deficit through urinary losses. Extracellular fluid volume can contract as a result of overall sodium loss, and signs of intravascular volume depletion may also appear. Due to insulin deficit, volume loss, and potassium shift from intracellular to extracellular compartments in response to acidosis, serum potassium levels may be high upon arrival of patients in emergency. However, urinary potassium losses via osmotic diuresis and excretion of ketones are typically present, leading to a total body potassium deficit. The initial serum potassium level is in most time either low or normal, which could be fatal. If potassium is not quickly replenished after starting insulin therapy, which results in the transfer of potassium into cells, hypokalemia might be lethal. Although phosphorus depletion in DKA is ubiquitous, it might be low, normal, or high at admission, much like with potassium. Leukocytosis is common in DKA or HHS, but in case of ongoing leukocytosis (>25,000/μL), persisting infections and further detailed investigations are required. Hypertriglyceridemia is found in almost all DKA patients and many HHS patients. Elevated amylase and lipase are seen in 16–25% DKA patients. A nonpancreatic tissue such as parotid gland is the major source of amylase in DKA.

## TREATMENT

While managing patients with hyperglycemic crises, we need to consider the following principles of therapy: (1) Enhancement of tissue perfusion and improvement of circulation, (2) progressive reductions in serum osmolality and glucose, (3) electrolyte imbalance correction, and (4) early recognition and promptly treating comorbid causative factors.

- *Management of DKA*: After starting insulin treatment and intravenous (IV) fluid replacement, the cause of the episode of DKA should be found and promptly addressed. A nasogastric tube should be placed to avoid aspiration of gastric contents if the patient is vomiting or showing signs of neurological instability. Careful monitoring and regular evaluation to make sure the patient and the metabolic derangements are improving are essential for the effective treatment of DKA. Chronological changes in vital signs, fluid intake and output, and laboratory results as a result of insulin administration should all be documented on a thorough flow sheet.

  Replacement of the sodium and free water deficit is done throughout the course of the first 24 hours following the initial bolus of normal saline or lactated Ringer's (fluid deficit is often 3–5 L). Depending on the determined volume deficit, IV fluids should be changed to lactated Ringer's or 0.45% saline once hemodynamic stability and acceptable urine output have been attained. Later on, in the course of DKA, the tendency for hyperchloremia is lessened by switching to 0.45% saline or by utilizing lactated Ringer's. Short-acting regular insulin (0.1 units/kg) is typically given as an IV bolus right after, and following therapy should maintain steady and appropriate levels of circulating insulin. In patients with severe or difficult DKA, IV administration is often preferable (0.1 units/kg of regular insulin per hour), since it assures fast dispersion and enables modulation of the infusion rate as the patient responds to treatment. If regular IV insulin is decided, it should be administered until the acidosis clears up and the patient's metabolism is stable. The rate of insulin infusion can be reduced (to 0.02–0.1 units/kg/h) if the acidosis and insulin resistance associated with DKA improve. In order to simplify the transition to an outpatient insulin regimen and shorten hospital stay, long-acting insulin should be delivered together with subcutaneous (SC) short-acting insulin as soon as the patient begins eating. When delivering long-acting insulin via the SC method, it is essential to keep up the insulin infusion or SC until appropriate insulin levels are reached. In this transition phase, even brief intervals of insufficient insulin treatment might cause DKA to return. Due to insulin-mediated glucose elimination, decreased hepatic glucose release, and rehydration, hyperglycemia typically improves at a rate of 50–100 mg/dL each hour. Rehydration decreases catecholamines, improves glucose excretion from the urine, and increases intravascular volume. The volume expansion is mostly responsible for the plasma glucose fall within the first 1–2 hours, which may be more rapid. When the plasma glucose level goes to 200–250 mg/dL, glucose should be added to the 0.45% saline infusion to keep the level between 150 and 200 mg/dL, and the insulin infusion should be kept going at a lower rate to limit ketogenesis. Cerebral edema may occur sooner if the serum glucose is corrected more quickly. As insulin decreases lipolysis, boosts peripheral ketone body use, inhibits hepatic ketone body synthesis, and encourages bicarbonate regeneration, ketoacidosis starts to clear up.

Compared to hyperglycemia, acidosis and ketosis recover more slowly. The anion gap will equalize (but not bicarbonate) when serum chloride rises. Following a successful course of therapy, a hyperchloremic acidosis [serum bicarbonate of 15–18 mmol/L (15–18 mEq/L)] is common. This condition progressively disappears as the kidneys produce new bicarbonate and eliminate chloride. DKA causes a depletion of potassium reserves [estimated deficit: 3–5 mmol/kg (3–5 mEq/kg)]. In patients receiving insulin and fluids, hypokalemia can arise for a variety of reasons. These include potassium entrance into cells mediated by insulin, potassium entry into cells facilitated by acidosis resolution, and potassium salts of organic acids lost by urine. So as soon as sufficient urine production and a normal serum potassium level are noted, potassium repletion should start. Potassium replacement should be postponed until the serum potassium level returns to normal if it was initially high. It is normal to provide 20–40 mEq of potassium to each liter of IV fluid; however, extra potassium supplements could also be necessary. Potassium phosphate or acetate can be used in place of the chloride salt in order to deliver less chloride. The objective is to keep the serum potassium level at or above 3.5 mmol/L (3.5 mEq/L). Despite a deficiency in bicarbonate, bicarbonate supplementation is typically not required. In fact, theoretical reasoning implies that quick acidosis reversal and the injection of bicarbonate may compromise cardiac function, decrease tissue oxygenation, and worsen hypokalemia. The majority of clinical studies' findings do not support the regular replenishment of bicarbonate, and a study of children indicated that bicarbonate usage was linked to a higher risk of cerebral edema. However, sodium bicarbonate [50 mmol (mEq/L) in 200 mL of sterile water with 10 mEq/L KCl per hour] may be supplied for the first 2 hours until the pH is >7.0 in the case of severe acidosis (arterial pH < 7.0). Increased glucose consumption may cause hypophosphatemia, although randomized clinical trials have not shown that phosphate supplementation is helpful in DKA. The serum calcium should be checked, and phosphate supplementation should be suggested if the serum phosphate is <1 mg/dL. During DKA treatment, hypomagnesemia may occur and may also call for supplements. **Flowchart 2** describe a protocol for managing hyperglycemic crisis.

- *Management of HHS*: Both HHS and DKA include hyperglycemia and volume depletion as key characteristics. As a result, the treatment for these illnesses includes a number of components. Careful observation of the patient's hydration state, laboratory results, and insulin infusion rate is essential for both illnesses. The presence and treatment of underlying or triggering issues should be pursued vigorously. Due to the illness's

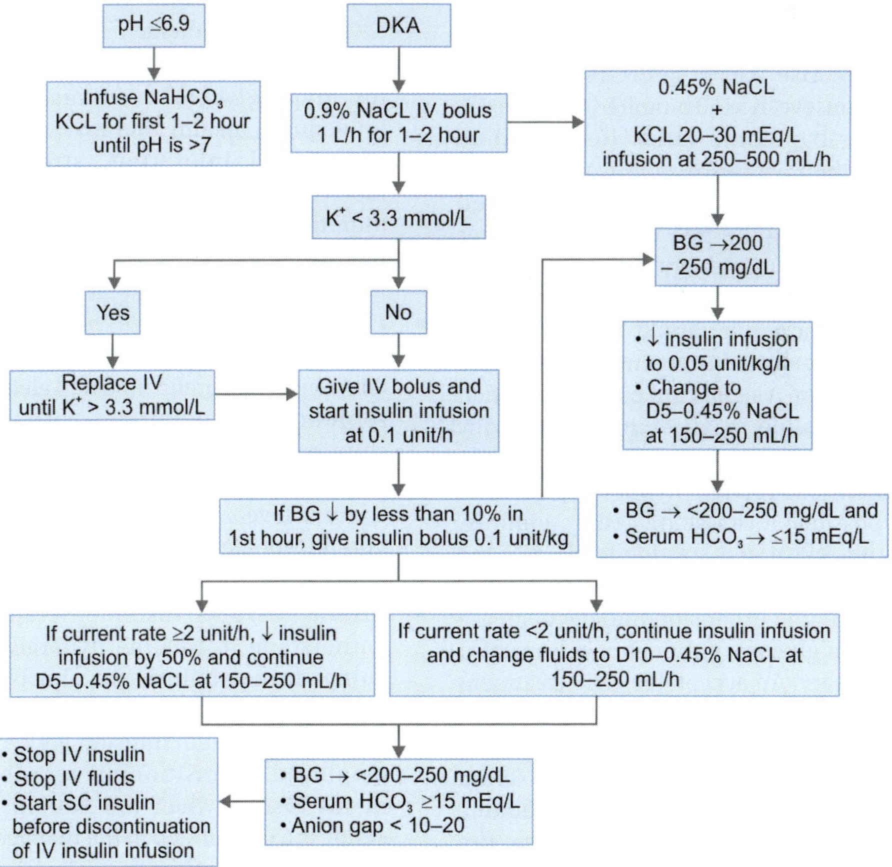


**FLOWCHART 2:** Protocol for diabetic ketoacidosis (DKA) management.

(BG: blood glucose; IV: intravenous)

extended duration in HHS, fluid losses and dehydration are typically more severe than in DKA. The patient with HHS is often older, more prone to experiencing changes in mental state and more likely to experience a life-threatening triggering event with coexisting conditions. HHS has a significantly greater fatality rate than DKA, even with appropriate therapy (up to 15% in certain clinical studies). Fluid replenishment (1–3 L of 0.9% normal saline throughout the first 2–3 hours) should first stabilize the patient's hemodynamic condition. The velocity of reversal of the hyperosmolar state must weigh the necessity for free water replenishment with the possibility that a too quick reverse may damage neurologic function since the fluid deficit in HHS accumulates over a period of days to weeks. Use 0.45% saline if the serum sodium level is >150 mmol/L (150 mEq/L). Using hypotonic fluids [0.45% saline first, then 5% dextrose in water (D5W)], the IV fluid administration is focused on restoring the free water deficit after hemodynamic stability has been attained. It is often required to replenish potassium, and the amount should be determined by frequent measurements of the serum potassium. A significant potassium deficit and possible magnesium insufficiency can occur in diuretic-using individuals. Treatment-related hypophosphatemia is possible; it can be treated by administering KPO4 and starting feeding of the patient. Similar to DKA, rehydration and volume expansion initially decrease plasma glucose, although insulin is also necessary. An acceptable HHS treatment plan starts with a 0.1 unit/kg IV insulin bolus and continues insulin infusion with 0.1 unit/kg IV per hour. If the serum glucose level does not decrease, double the insulin infusion rate. When the plasma glucose falls to 11.1–13.9 mmol/L (200–250 mg/dL), as in DKA, glucose should be given to the IV fluid, and the rate of insulin infusion should be lowered to 0.02–0.1 unit/kg/h. Until the patient is able to switch to a SC insulin regimen and has started eating again, the insulin infusion should be maintained.

## CLINICAL PEARLS

- *Differentiating DKA and HHS*: Hyperglycemic coma encompasses DKA and HHS. DKA is characterized by ketonemia, acidosis, and pronounced symptoms like acetone breath, while HHS presents with high blood glucose and severe dehydration but minimal ketosis. Distinguishing between the two is crucial for accurate management.
- *Precipitating factors*: Common triggers for hyperglycemic comas include inadequate insulin therapy, infections, myocardial infarction, stroke, and medications like corticosteroids, thiazide diuretics, and certain SGLT-2 inhibitors. Identifying and addressing these triggers is essential in treatment.
- *Fluid and electrolyte management*: Effective management of hyperglycemic coma involves careful fluid and electrolyte repletion. Rehydration with saline solutions is crucial, especially in HHS, but should be adjusted based on serum sodium levels. Additionally, potassium and phosphate supplementation may be necessary to correct imbalances.
- *Insulin therapy*: Insulin therapy is a cornerstone in treating hyperglycemic coma. Initial boluses of short-acting insulin followed by continuous intravenous (IV) insulin infusion are typically employed. Transitioning to subcutaneous insulin when the patient starts eating is a critical step in the management process.

- *Caution with bicarbonate*: Bicarbonate supplementation is generally not recommended in hyperglycemic comas, even in cases of severe acidosis. Rapid correction of acidosis with bicarbonate can have adverse effects on cardiac function and tissue oxygenation. It's vital to monitor acidosis and make adjustments cautiously.

## FURTHER READINGS


1. Kitabchi AE, Wall BM. Diabetic ketoacidosis. Med Clin North Am. 1995;79(1):9-37.
2. Samajdar SS, Dasgupta S, Mukherjee S, Tripathi SK, Joshi SR. Incretin mimetics in the Indian context: revisiting exenatide. Bengal Physician J. 2022;9(2):51-4.
3. Kitabchi AE, Umpierrez GE, Miles JM, Fisher JN. Hyperglycemic crises in adult patients with diabetes. Diabetes Care. 2009;32(7):1335-43.
4. Gosmanov AR, Gosmanova EO, Kitabchi AE. Hyperglycemic crises: diabetic ketoacidosis and hyperglycemic hyperosmolar state. In: Feingold KR, Anawalt B, Boyce A, et al. (Eds). Endotext [Internet]. South Dartmouth (MA): MDText.com, Inc.; 2000. [online] Available from https://www.ncbi.nlm.nih.gov/books/NBK279052/. [Last accessed September, 2023].
5. Handelsman Y, Henry RR, Bloomgarden ZT, Dagogo-Jack S, DeFronzo RA, Einhorn D, et al. American Association of Clinical Endocrinologists and American College of Endocrinology position statement on the association of SGLT-2 inhibitors and diabetic ketoacidosis. Endocr Pract. 2016;22(6):753-62.
6. Spasovski G, Vanholder R, Allolio B, Annane D, Ball S, Bichet D, et al. Clinical practice guideline on diagnosis and treatment of hyponatraemia. Nephrol Dial Transplant. 2014;29(Suppl. 2): i1-39.
7. Adrogue HJ, Lederer ED, Suki WN, Eknoyan G. Determinants of plasma potassium levels in diabetic ketoacidosis. Medicine (Baltimore). 1986;65(3):163-72.
8. Wilson HK, Keuer SP, Lea AS, Boyd 3rd AE, Eknoyan G. Phosphate therapy in diabetic ketoacidosis. Arch Intern Med. 1982;142(3): 517-20.
9. Slovis CM, Mork VG, Slovis RJ, Bain RP. Diabetic ketoacidosis and infection: leukocyte count and differential as early predictors of serious infection. Am J Emerg Med. 1987;5(1):1-5.
10. Vinicor F, Lehrner LM, Karn RC, Merritt AD. Hyperamylasemia in diabetic ketoacidosis: sources and significance. Ann Intern Med. 1979;91(2):200-4.
11. Yadav D, Nair S, Norkus EP, Pitchumoni CS. Nonspecific hyperamylasemia and hyperlipasemia in diabetic ketoacidosis: incidence and correlation with biochemical abnormalities. Am J Gastroenterol. 2000;95(11):3123-8.
12. Jameson J, Fauci AS, Kasper DL, Hauser SL, Longo DL, Loscalzo J (Eds). Harrison's Principles of Internal Medicine, 20th edition. New York: McGraw Hill; 2018. [online] Available from https://accessmedicine.mhmedical.com/content.aspx?bookid=2129§ionid=159213747. [Last accessed September, 2023].

CHAPTER 100

# Hypoglycemia

*Shambo Samrat Samajdar, Sougata Sarkar,
Saibal Das, Shashank R Joshi*

## INTRODUCTION

Hypoglycemia is the most common drug-related morbidity that diabetics suffer from. Strict glycemic control to prevent microvascular complications often endangers patients at risk of developing hypoglycemia. Undetected and untreated hypoglycemia may lead to fatal outcomes, including death. Elderly patients, especially those who have longstanding diabetic autonomic neuropathy and take drugs that mask the hypoglycemic symptoms, are at risk. The prevalence of hypoglycemia is high among diabetic patients. According to a study by Shriraam et al., 78.1% of people with type 2 diabetes mellitus (T2DM) had at least one symptom that was relieved by consuming glucose.

## WHAT IS HYPOGLYCEMIA?

Whipple's triad can be used to describe hypoglycemia. In the presence of features such as (1) signs and symptoms of hypoglycemia, (2) a low plasma glucose concentration determined by a precise technique, and (3) relief from symptoms following an increase in plasma glucose, we can establish the diagnosis of hypoglycemia. In general, the lower limit of fasting plasma glucose concentration is around 70 mg/dL. In normal circumstances, situations such as long after a meal, during pregnancy, and during prolonged fasting (>24 hours), the venous glucose level reaches below the lower limit of normal. Hypoglycemia can also be brought on by different conditions, such as severe organ failure, sepsis, inanition, hormone deficits, noncell tumors, insulinomas, alcoholism, and previous stomach surgery. Insulin and drugs that promote insulin secretion are most commonly associated with hypoglycemia. Any patient who experiences confusion-like episodes, an altered level of consciousness, or a seizure should be evaluated for hypoglycemia. Severe hypoglycemia can result in substantial morbidity. During and after the first hypoglycemic episode, death risk is raised.

## WHAT CAUSES HYPOGLYCEMIA?

On the basis of relative or absolute insulin excess, the traditional risk factors for hypoglycemia in diabetes are determined. In **Table 1**, different risk factors for hypoglycemia have been depicted. Proinflammatory, procoagulant, and proatherothrombotic responses are stimulated by hypoglycemia. These reactions augment intravascular coagulation, decrease fibrinolytic balance

**Table 1: Risk factors for hypoglycemia.**

| *Risk* | *Example* |
|---|---|
| Insulin (or insulin secretagogue) | Doses are excessive, ill-timed, or of the wrong type, wrong dose exposure |
| Exogenous glucose influx is reduced | During an overnight fast, periods of temporary fasting, or after missed meals or snacks |
| Increased insulin-independent glucose utilization | Exercise |
| Sensitivity to insulin is increased | Improved glycemic control, in the middle of the night, after exercise, or with increased fitness or weight loss |
| Endogenous glucose production is reduced | Alcohol ingestion |
| Insulin clearance is reduced | Renal failure |

(raise plasminogen activator inhibitor-1), and enhance platelet aggregation. In healthy, type 1 diabetes mellitus (T1DM), and T2DM people, hypoglycemia also decreases protective nitric oxide-mediated arterial vasodilator responses.

Under physiological circumstances, glucose serves as the brain's essential metabolic fuel source. The brain needs a constant supply of glucose from the arterial circulation since it cannot produce glucose or store more than a few minutes' worth in glycogen. Blood to brain glucose transfer decreases as arterial plasma glucose concentrations fall below the physiological range, making it difficult for the brain to maintain energy metabolism and function. Hypoglycemia is often avoided or treated quickly due to a wide range of integrated glucose counterregulatory systems.

Despite large variation in exogenous glucose delivery from meals and in endogenous glucose utilization, such as by exercise, plasma glucose concentrations are typically maintained within a relatively narrow range—roughly 70–110 mg/dL in the fasting state, with temporary higher excursions after a meal. Plasma glucose levels are kept steady between meals and when fasting by endogenous glucose synthesis, hepatic glycogenolysis, and hepatic (and renal) gluconeogenesis. Although hepatic glycogen stores are typically adequate to maintain plasma glucose levels for 8 hours or more, this time frame can be shortened if activity increases the body's need for glucose or if sickness or starvation causes the body's glycogen stores to be depleted. **Flowchart 1** depicts glucose counter-regulation physiology. How the human body normally prevents or corrects hypoglycemia has been described here. The essential insulin and glucagon counterregulatory responses, as well as the stimulation of sympathoadrenal outflow, are compromised in insulin-deficient diabetes. Increased platelet aggregation, reduced fibrinolytic balance by increase in plasminogen activator inhibitor-1, and increased intravascular coagulation are important contributors in related pathogenesis and progression of complications in the background of hypoglycemia.

The limiting element in the glycemic control of diabetes mellitus is hypoglycemia. First of all, it increases morbidity and frequently recurs in persons with T1DM and advanced T2DM. Second, it prevents stark realization of the recognized microvascular advantages of glycemic management and maintenance of euglycemia across a lifetime of diabetes. Third, it results in hypoglycemia-associated autonomic failure, which includes the clinical syndromes of

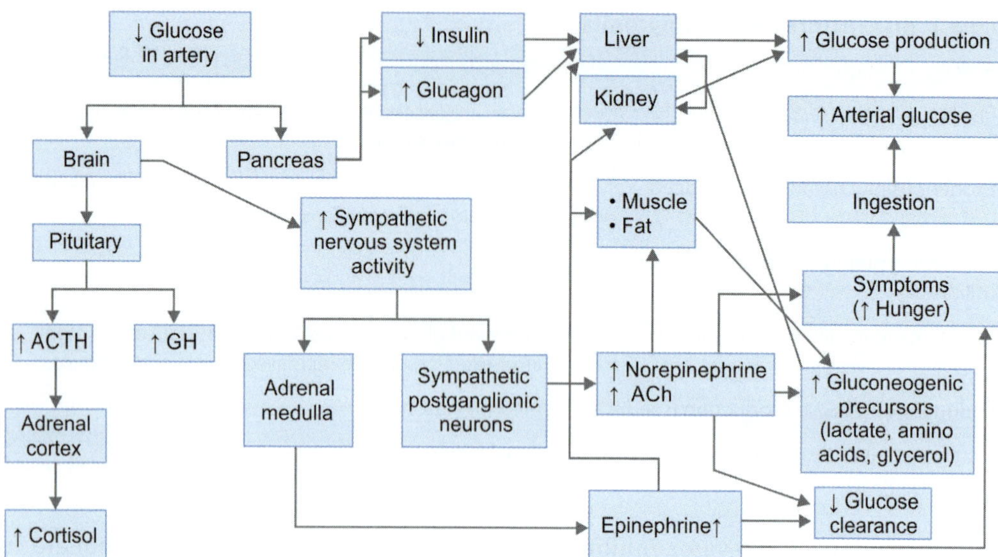


**FLOWCHART 1:** Glucose counter-regulation physiology: Prevention or correction or hypoglycemia.

(ACTH: adrenocorticotropic hormone, GH: growth hormone, ACh: acetylcholine, ↑: increase, ↓: decrease)

impaired glucose counterregulation and hypoglycemia unawareness, and this creates a vicious cycle of recurrent hypoglycemia.

The clinical syndrome of hypoglycemia unawareness, or loss of the warning adrenergic and cholinergic symptomatology that previously allowed the patient to recognize developing hypoglycemia and, as a result, to abort the episode by ingesting carbohydrates, is brought on by the attenuated sympathoadrenal response (primarily the reduced sympathetic neural response) to hypoglycemia. The risk of severe iatrogenic hypoglycemia in affected individuals receiving aggressive glycemic treatment for their diabetes is raised sixfold.

## WHAT ARE THE POSSIBILITIES?

Hypoglycemia in the background of diabetes is commonly associated with drug-host interactions and impaired counterregulatory hormone physiology. Medication history needs to be taken carefully to find out the cause in the presence or absence of diabetes. Other causes such as critical illnesses, hormone deficiency, or nonislet cell tumor hypoglycemia need to be explored. The attention should switch to potential endogenous hyperinsulinism or unintentional, covert, or even malicious hypoglycemia if none of these etiologic elements are present and the patient appears to be in good health. In **Table 2**, a few important considerations have been discussed.

## PATH TO DIAGNOSIS

Patients with typical symptoms, those who also exhibit disorientation, altered levels of awareness, or seizures, as well as those who present in clinical settings where hypoglycemia is known to occur, are all considered to have the condition. When feasible, blood should be collected prior to the delivery of glucose so that a low plasma glucose concentration may be documented. Whipple's triad must be met for hypoglycemia to be convincingly documented. Therefore, a symptomatic episode is the optimal opportunity to evaluate the plasma glucose

**Table 2: Possibilities while exploring hypoglycemia.**

| *Cause* | *Example* |
|---|---|
| Drugs | Insulin and insulin secretagogues, ethanol, uncommon: Angiotensin-converting enzyme inhibitors and angiotensin receptor antagonists, β-adrenergic receptor antagonists, quinolone antibiotics, indomethacin, quinine, and sulfonamides |
| Critical illness | Renal, hepatic, or cardiac failure; toxic hepatitis; sepsis; starvation |
| Hormone deficiencies | Primary adrenocortical failure (Addison's disease) or hypopituitarism; chronic cortisol deficiency; growth hormone deficiency in young children |
| Non-β-cell tumors | Large mesenchymal or epithelial tumors (e.g., hepatomas, adrenocortical carcinomas, carcinoids) |
| Endogenous hyperinsulinism | β-cell tumor (insulinoma); antibody to insulin or to the insulin receptor; ectopic insulin secretion |
| Inborn errors of metabolism | • *Fasting hypoglycemia*: Glycogen storage disease (GSD) of types 0, I, III, and IV and Fanconi–Bickel syndrome<br>• *Postprandial hypoglycemia*: Glucokinase, SUR1, and Kir6.2 potassium channel mutations; congenital disorders of glycosylation |
| Exercise-induced hypoglycemia | Following exercise results in hyperinsulinemia by increased activity of monocarboxylate transporter 1 in β cells |

level. Hypoglycemia is ruled out as the source of the symptoms by a normal glucose level. If the symptoms go away once the glucose level is elevated, a low glucose level proves that hypoglycemia is the source of the symptoms.

A plausible hypoglycemic cause in a patient with confirmed hypoglycemia may frequently be determined from the history, physical examination, and relevant laboratory results. Even in the absence of a known usage of a relevant substance, drugs, especially medications used to treat diabetes or alcohol, should be the first thing to be considered due to the possibility of covert, unintentional, or malicious drug administration. Given the high level of suspicion, evidence of a relevant critical disease that can be pursued for diagnostic purposes, though rarely, a non-β-cell tumor and hormone deficiencies are additional factors that require immediate attention. The diagnostic approach is to evaluate the patient as just stated and check for Whipple's triad both during and after an episode of hypoglycemia when the history implies prior hypoglycemia and no probable explanation is obvious. On the other hand, a noticeably low plasma glucose concentration recorded in a patient without associated symptoms raises the probability of an artifact, even though it cannot be excluded (pseudohypoglycemia).

## TREATMENT

Urgent recognition and treatment initiation are the key to optimizing outcome in hypoglycemic patients. Oral therapy with glucose tablets or drinks, candies, or food that contains glucose is suitable if the patient is able and willing. A recommended starting dosage of glucose is between 15 and 20 g. Parenteral treatment is required if the patient is unable or unwilling (due to neuroglycopenia) to consume carbohydrate orally. Following a 25 g intravenous (IV) glucose infusion, a glucose infusion should be maintained by serial plasma glucose readings. Subcutaneous (SC) or intramuscular (IM) glucagon (1.0 mg in adults) can be utilized instead of IV treatment, especially in T1DM patients. Due to its ability to induce the release of insulin, glucagon is less effective in T2DM. In sulfonylurea-induced hypoglycemia, the somatostatin analog octreotide can be administered to inhibit insulin secretion. Patients should be advised to eat as soon as it is practicable in order to replenish glycogen reserves because these medications only momentarily elevate plasma glucose concentrations.

Patients on insulin infusion developing hypoglycemia [blood glucose (BG) <70 mg/dL] need stoppage of infusion, and a calculated dose of 25% dextrose should be infused immediately. Calculated dose in mL = (100 – BG) × 0.8 (BG – value of BG in mg/dL)

One example of calculating dose of 25% dextrose is as follows: if BG = 40 mg/dL, the patient requires [(100 – 40) × 0.8] = 60 × 0.8 = 48 mL of 25% dextrose IV and BG should be checked after a 15-minute interval. The patient needs repeat dose of 25% dextrose as per BG value. If BG > 70 mg/dL, check BG at 30-minute interval till BG rises >90 mg/dL. If BG > 90 mg/dL, check BG hourly, and if BG > 140 mg/dL, restart insulin infusion at 50% of previous rate.

## CONCLUSION

Rational glucose-lowering drug therapy by balancing risk versus benefit, assured adherence to medications, and food habit with regular monitoring (self and office) of glucose are essential steps to reduce the risk of hyper- as well as hypoglycemia in a patient.

## CLINICAL PEARLS

- Whipple's triad can be used to describe hypoglycemia: (1) Signs and symptoms of hypoglycemia, (2) a low plasma glucose concentration determined by a precise technique, and (3) relief from symptoms following an increase in plasma glucose.
- On the basis of relative or absolute insulin excess, the traditional risk factors for hypoglycemia in diabetes are determined.
- Deranged integrated glucose counter-regulatory systems are crucial issues behind the development of hypoglycemia.
- Urgent diagnosis and prompt management are two most important steps. A recommended starting dosage of glucose is between 15 and 20 g for those who are able to eat. Other patients required a calculated dose of 25% dextrose.

## FURTHER READINGS

1. Shriraam V, Mahadevan S, Anitharani M, Jagadeesh NS, Kurup SB, Vidya TA, et al. Reported hypoglycemia in type 2 diabetes mellitus patients: prevalence and practices-a hospital-based study. Indian J Endocrinol Metab. 2017;21:148-53.
2. Cryer PE, Davis SN. Hypoglycemia. In: Jameson J, Fauci AS, Kasper DL, Hauser SL, Longo DL, Loscalzo J (Eds). Harrison's Principles of Internal Medicine, 20th edition. New York: McGraw Hill; 2018.
3. Mathew P, Thoppil D. Hypoglycemia. StatPearls [Internet]. Treasure Island (FL): StatPearls Publishing; 2022.
4. Samajdar SS, Dasgupta S, Tripathi SK, Joshi SR. Management of hyperglycemia in in-hospital COVID-19 patients: a review. Bengal Phys J. 2020;7(2):31-4.

CHAPTER 101

# Pulmonary Thromboembolism

*Boudhayan Das Munshi*

## DEFINITION

Pulmonary thromboembolism (PTE) refers to the obstruction of the pulmonary artery or its branches by a thrombus that originated elsewhere in the body.

Based on the timeline of onset, it is of three types: Acute, subacute, and chronic.

1. *Acute*: Symptoms and signs develop immediately after obstruction of pulmonary vessels.
2. *Subacute*: Symptoms and signs develop within days and weeks of obstruction of pulmonary vessels.
3. *Chronic*: Symptoms of pulmonary hypertension develop over several years.

Based on hemodynamic instability, it is of three types: Low risk, intermediate risk, and high risk.

1. *High risk*: It is also called as "massive" PTE. It is associated with hemodynamic instability.
2. *Intermediate risk*: It is also called as "submassive" PTE. There is no hemodynamic instability; however, right ventricular strain pattern is present.
3. *Low risk*: There is neither hemodynamic instability nor right ventricular strain pattern.

Hemodynamically unstable PTE is characterized by hypotension:

- Systolic blood pressure <90 mm Hg
- Drop in systolic blood pressure from baseline by ≥40 mm Hg for >15 minutes
- Hypotension that needs vasopressors or inotropic support and cannot be explained by sepsis, arrhythmia, left ventricular dysfunction from acute myocardial infarction

Hemodynamically unstable PTE is usually caused by a massive PTE, but it can also be due to a small PTE in the background of a cardiopulmonary disease.

Hemodynamically stable PTE can be symptomatic or asymptomatic.

Based on the anatomic location, PTE can be classified as saddle, lobar, segmental, and subsegmental.

Saddle PTE is located at the bifurcation of the main pulmonary artery, often extending into the right and left main pulmonary arteries.

The thrombi that are smaller and located in the peripheral segmental or subsegmental branches are more likely to cause pulmonary infarction and pleuritis.

## WHEN TO SUSPECT?—CLINICAL CLUES IN HISTORY AND EXAMINATION

Risk factors for PTE/VTE (venous thromboembolism)—inherited or acquired

- Inherited thrombophilia—genetic
  - Factor V Leiden mutation
  - Prothrombin gene mutation (20210A)
  - Protein C deficiency
  - Protein S deficiency
  - Antithrombin deficiency
- Other
  - Presence of a central venous catheter
  - Malignancy
  - Surgery, especially orthopedic
  - Trauma
  - Immobilization
  - Pregnancy
  - Oral contraceptives
  - Hormone replacement therapy
  - Certain cancer therapies (tamoxifen, thalidomide, lenalidomide, asparaginase)
  - Heart failure
  - Congenital heart disease
  - Antiphospholipid syndrome
  - Older age (>65 years)
  - Obesity
  - Severe liver disease
  - *Myeloproliferative neoplasms*: Polycythemia vera, essential thrombocythemia
  - Paroxysmal nocturnal hemoglobinuria
  - Inflammatory bowel disease
  - Nephrotic syndrome

The symptoms of acute PTE:

- *Dyspnea*: Acute and severe episodes may happen in central pulmonary embolism (PE), while it is often mild and transient in peripheral small PE
- Chest pain
- Cough
- Features related to deep vein thrombosis (DVT)
  - Pain, redness, and swelling of the affected part of the lower limbs (usually below the knees)
  - Limb edema may be unilateral or bilateral if the thrombus is extending to pelvic veins, red and hot skin with dilated veins and tenderness

The validated clinical prediction rules used to estimate the pretest probability of PE and to interpret test results are:

- Well's scoring system
- Modified Well's scoring system
- Revised Geneva scoring system
- Simplified revised Geneva score
- Pulmonary embolism rule-out criteria (PERC)

**Table 1** shows the Well's criteria and modified Well's criteria: Clinical assessment for PE.

The other prediction score used is the Geneva score **(Table 2)**. It is a clinical prediction rule used in determining the pretest probability of PE based on a patient's risk factors and clinical findings. It is nearly as accurate as the Well's score and is less reliant on the experience of the doctor applying the rule.

*Pulmonary embolism rule-out criteria* includes the following:

- Age ≥50 years
- Heart rate ≥100 beats/min
- Arterial oxygen saturation ($SaO_2$) on room air <95%
- Venous thromboembolism
- Recent (<28 days) trauma or surgery
- Unilateral leg swelling
- Hemoptysis
- Oral hormone use

Pulmonary embolism workup is not required in the following situations:

- None of the above eight conditions are met.
- Very low pretest probability (<15%)

Pulmonary embolism rule-out criteria evaluation is considered positive if any of the above conditions are met.

**Table 1: Well's criteria and modified Well's criteria: Clinical assessment for pulmonary embolism (PE).**

| *Risk factors* | *Points* |
|---|---|
| Clinical symptoms of DVT (leg swelling, pain with palpation) | 3.0 |
| Other diagnosis less likely than pulmonary embolism | 3.0 |
| Heart rate >100 beats/min | 1.5 |
| Immobilization (≥3 days) or surgery in the previous 4 weeks | 1.5 |
| Previous DVT/PE | 1.5 |
| Hemoptysis | 1.0 |
| Malignancy | 1.0 |
| ***Probability*** | ***Score*** |
| *Traditional clinical probability assessment* (*Wells criteria*) | |
| High | >6.0 |
| Moderate | 2.0–6.0 |
| Low | <2.0 |
| *Simplified clinical probability assessment* (*modified Wells criteria*) | |
| PE likely | >4.0 |
| PE unlikely | ≤4.0 |

(DVT: deep vein thrombosis)

**Table 2: Geneva score.**

| *Risk factors* | *Points* |
|---|---|
| Age older than 65 years | 1 |
| Previous DVT or pulmonary embolism | 3 |
| Surgery (under general anesthesia) or fracture (of the lower limbs) within 1 month | 2 |
| Active malignant condition (solid or hematologic, currently active or considered cured <1 year) | |
| ***Symptoms*** | |
| Unilateral lower limb pain | 3 |
| Hemoptysis | 2 |
| ***Clinical signs*** | |
| Heart rate 75–94 beats/min | 3 |
| Heart rate ≥95 beats/min | 5 |
| Pain on lower limb deep venous palpation and unilateral edema | 4 |
| ***Clinical probability*** | ***Score*** |
| Low | 0–3 |
| Intermediate | 4–10 |
| High | ≥11 |

(DVT: deep vein thrombosis)

## Hemodynamic Stability versus Instability

It is important to assess at the outset whether the PTE is associated with hemodynamic stability or instability. Hemodynamic instability is defined by presence of cardiac arrest, obstructive shock, or persistent hypotension.

Central or extensive PE may manifest as hemodynamic instability. Syncope is associated with a greater degree of hemodynamic compromise and right ventricular dysfunction.

Distal emboli may cause pulmonary infarction, irritation of the pleura, and chest pain.

Complications of PTE include recurrent thrombosis, chronic thromboembolic pulmonary hypertension (CTEPH), and death.

Recurrent thrombosis depends on the adequacy of therapeutic anticoagulation and the clinical nature of the embolic event (provoked, unprovoked).

Chronic thromboembolic pulmonary hypertension is considered as a late complication.

Early mortality is death in the first week following PTE. It is due to shock and recurrent thromboembolism. However, most deaths in PTE are multifactorial and due to preexisting comorbidities.

# HOW TO MANAGE?—INVESTIGATIONS AND TREATMENT

## Investigations

- D-dimer: The D-dimer cutoff values depend on the pretest probability of PTE. A concentration below the cutoff value excludes PTE—
  - If the pretest probability is low, the cutoff value is 1 mg/L.
  - If the pretest probability is moderate, the cutoff values are:
    - 0.5 mg/L for people below 50 years of age
      (age/100) mg/L for people of 50 or more years (e.g., 0.6 mg/L for people of 60 years)
- Cardiac biomarkers [troponin, N-terminal prohormone of brain natriuretic peptide (NT-proBNP)]: Right ventricular microinfarction leads to elevated troponins, while myocardial stretch causes elevated NT-proBNP levels.
- *Electrocardiography (ECG)*: In severe PTE, features suggestive of right ventricular strain—inversion of T waves in leads $V_1$-$V_4$, a QR pattern in $V_1$, S1Q3T3 pattern, incomplete/complete right bundle branch block
- *Echocardiography*: In significant PTE, right ventricular dilatation, right ventricular dysfunction/hypokinesia, or pulmonary hypertension. To visualize the thrombus, transesophageal echocardiography is preferred over transthoracic echocardiography.
- Chest X-ray—usually nonspecific. It is usually done to rule out other causes of dyspnea.
- Lung ventilation/perfusion scans (V/Q planar scan, V/Q SPECT): It is not easily available though.
- Multidetector computed tomography pulmonary angiography (CTPA) is the method of choice for imaging the pulmonary vasculature. Pulmonary arteries till the subsegmental level can be adequately visualized with CTPA.
- Invasive pulmonary angiography is considered the gold standard for the diagnosis of PTE.

## Treatment

Any patient in whom PTE is suspected should be admitted and monitored. The initial monitoring will include assessment of the vital signs to determine whether the patient is hemodynamically stable or not. It is imperative to provide adequate oxygenation and stabilize the patient. Once PTE is confirmed, the mainstay of treatment is anticoagulation. Other enlisted modalities of treatment include thrombolysis, inferior vena cava (IVC) filters, and embolectomy **(Flowchart 1)**.

There are two stages of managing PTE:

1. Suspected stage
2. Confirmed stage

*Suspected stage*: Patients with suspected PTE should undergo initial stabilization while clinical evaluation and confirmatory diagnostic testing are going on.

Treatment algorithm for hemodynamically stable patients with suspected PTE is shown in **Flowchart 2**.

Treatment algorithm for hemodynamically unstable patients with suspected PTE is shown in **Flowchart 3**.

## *Anticoagulation*

### Agents Used

- *Injectable agents*: Unfractionated heparin (UFH), low molecular weight heparin (LMWH), fondaparinux
- *Oral agents*
    - Vitamin K antagonists (VKAs): Warfarin
    - Direct oral anticoagulants:
        - Direct oral thrombin inhibitor: Dabigatran
        - Direct oral factor Xa inhibitors: Rivaroxaban, apixaban, edoxaban

Advantages of LMWH over UFH include a lower risk of inducing major bleeding, heparin-induced thrombocytopenia (HIT), and nonrequirement of monitoring of anti-Xa levels.

Fondaparinux is suitable for patients with heparin allergy and for the treatment of HIT.

### Risk Factors for Bleeding with Anticoagulation

(1) Age > 65 years, (2) age > 75 years, (3) previous bleeding, (4) cancer, (5) metastatic cancer, (6) renal failure, (7) liver failure, (8) thrombocytopenia, (9) previous stroke, (10) diabetes, (11) anemia, (12) poor anticoagulant control, (13) comorbidity and reduced functional capacity, (14) recent surgery, (15) frequent falls, (16) alcohol abuse

Categorization of risk of bleeding:

- Low risk (0 risk factors)
- Moderate risk (1 risk factor)
- High risk (≥2 risk factors)

The increase in bleeding associated with a risk factor will vary with (1) severity of the risk factor (e.g., location and extent of metastatic disease, platelet count), (2) temporal relationships (e.g., interval from surgery or

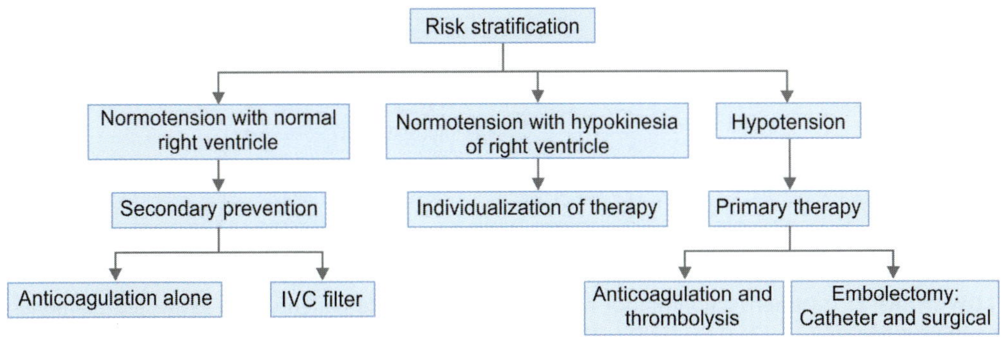


**FLOWCHART 1:** Risk stratification in pulmonary thromboembolism (PTE).

(IVC: inferior vena cava)

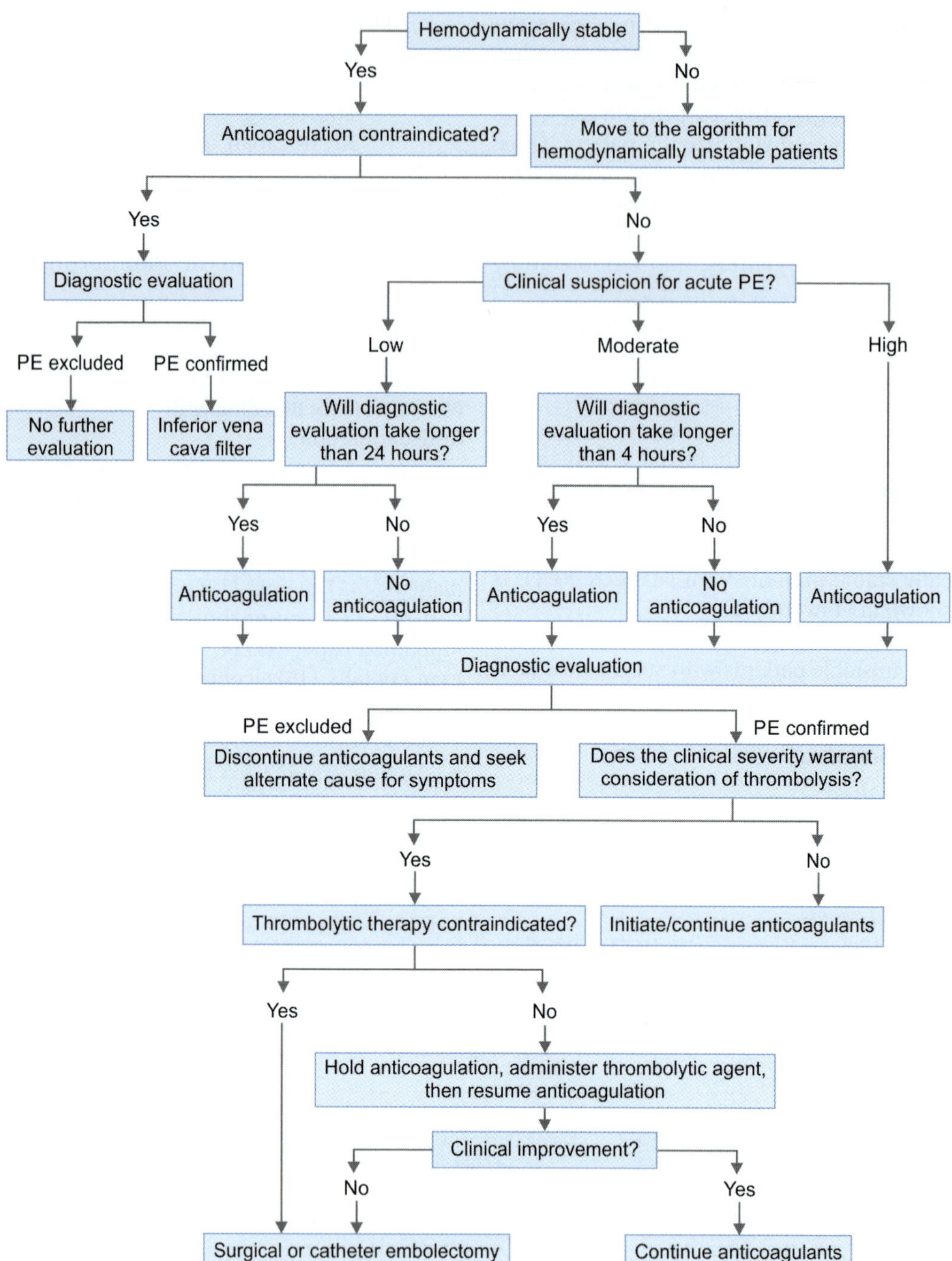


**FLOWCHART 2:** Treatment algorithm for hemodynamically stable patients with suspected pulmonary thromboembolism.

(PE: pulmonary embolism)

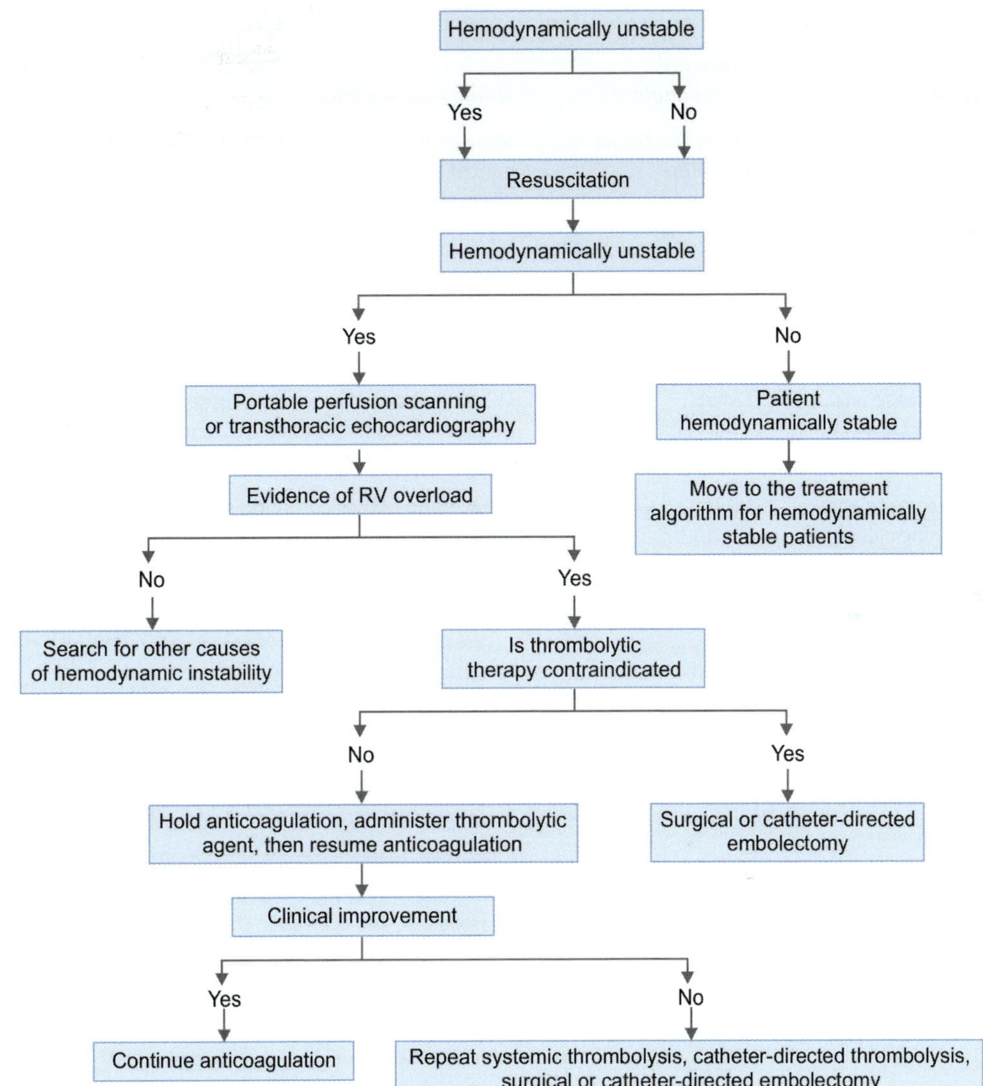


**FLOWCHART 3:** Treatment algorithm for hemodynamically unstable patients with suspected pulmonary thromboembolism.

(PE: pulmonary embolism; RV: right ventricle)

a previous bleeding episode), and (3) how effectively a previous cause of bleeding was corrected [e.g., upper gastrointestinal (GI) bleeding].

The preferred choice of anticoagulant in specific clinical scenarios is enumerated in **Table 3**.

Recommendations regarding the duration of anticoagulation therapy is shown **Table 4**.

### *Thrombolytic Therapy*

The American Society of Hematology 2020 guidelines recommend using thrombolytic therapy followed by anticoagulation over anticoagulation alone in patients with PTE and hemodynamic compromise. In patients in whom thrombolysis is considered appropriate, systemic thrombolysis is preferred over catheter-directed thrombolysis.

**Table 3: Preferred choice of anticoagulant in specific clinical scenarios.**

| *Factor* | *Preferred anticoagulant* | *Qualifying remarks* |
|---|---|---|
| Cancer | LMWH, factor Xa inhibitors | More so if: Just diagnosed, extensive VTE, metastatic cancer, very symptomatic; vomiting; on cancer chemotherapy |
| Initial parenteral therapy to be avoided | Rivaroxaban; apixaban | VKA, dabigatran, and edoxaban require initial parenteral therapy |
| Once daily oral therapy preferred | Rivaroxaban; edoxaban; VKA | |
| Liver disease and coagulopathy | LMWH | DOACs contraindicated if INR raised because of liver disease; VKA difficult to control and INR may not reflect antithrombotic effect |
| Renal disease and creatinine clearance <30 mL/min | VKA | DOACs and LMWH contraindicated with severe renal impairment. However, dosing of some DOACs can be renally adjusted, although adjustment varies with different levels of renal impairment depending on the DOAC |
| Coronary artery disease | VKA, rivaroxaban, apixaban, edoxaban | Coronary artery events appear to occur more often with dabigatran than with VKA. This has not been seen with the other DOACs, and they have demonstrated efficacy for coronary artery disease. Antiplatelet therapy should be avoided if possible in patients on anticoagulants because of increased bleeding |
| Dyspepsia or history of GI bleeding | VKA, apixaban | Dabigatran increased dyspepsia. Dabigatran, rivaroxaban, and edoxaban may be associated with more GI bleeding than VKA |
| Poor compliance | VKA | INR monitoring can help to detect problems. However, some patients may be more compliant with a DOAC because it is less complex |
| Thrombolytic therapy use | UFH infusion | Greater experience with its use in patients treated with thrombolytic therapy |
| Reversal agent needed | VKA, UFH, DOACS | Reversal agents for DOACS may not be universally readily available |
| Pregnancy or pregnancy risk | LMWH | Potential for other agents to cross the placenta |
| Cost, coverage, licensing | Varies among regions and with individual circumstances | |

(DOACs: direct oral anticoagulants; GI: gastrointestinal; INR: international normalized ratio; LMWH: low molecular weight heparin; UFH: unfractionated heparin; VKA: vitamin K-dependent antagonist; VTE: venous thromboembolism)

**Table 4: Recommendations regarding the duration of anticoagulation therapy.**

| *Indication* | *Duration* |
|---|---|
| Presence of transient risk factors such as recent surgery, trauma, pregnancy, immobility, use of oral contraceptives, or hormone replacement therapy in the first episode of thrombosis | 3 months |
| First episode of unprovoked thrombosis | 3–6 months |
| A patient of active carcinoma, antiphospholipid syndrome, protein C or S deficiency, factor V Leiden, etc., presenting with first episode of thrombosis | Lifelong |
| Recurrent unprovoked thrombosis | Lifelong |
| First life-threatening thrombosis without risk factor | Lifelong |

**Table 5: Thrombolytic therapy in patients with acute pulmonary thromboembolism.**

| *Drug* | *Dosing* |
|---|---|
| Recombinant tissue plasminogen activator | • 100 mg total dose<br>• 10 mg of 100 mg as bolus dose<br>• Remaining 90 mg by constant rate infusion over 2 hours |
| Urokinase | 4,400 IU/kg as a loading dose over 10 minutes, followed by 4,400 IU/kg/h over 12–24 hours |
| Streptokinase | 2.5 lakh IU loading dose over 30 minutes followed by 1 lakh IU over next 12–24 hours |

Thrombolytic therapy in patients with acute PTE is shown **Table 5**.

#### Contraindications to Thrombolysis

Absolute:
- History of hemorrhagic stroke
- Ischemic stroke in previous 6 months
- Major trauma, surgery, or head injury in previous 3 weeks

Relative:
- Transient ischemic attack in previous 6 months
- Oral anticoagulation
- Pregnancy or first postpartum meeting

### *Inferior Vena Cava Filter*

Indicated in those with high risk of DVT or PE and anticoagulant therapy is contraindicated.

### Other Treatment Modalities: Alternatives to Thrombolysis

- Percutaneous mechanical fragmentation of the embolus with a catheter
- Local thrombolytic therapy
- Surgical embolectomy

### *Follow-up*

Patients with PTE treated with unfractionated heparin or warfarin should be monitored for laboratory evidence of therapeutic efficacy.

## CLINICAL PEARLS

Symptoms of chest pain and dyspnea in appropriate clinical setting, especially with conditions that increase the risk of venous thromboembolism, should raise the suspicion of PTE.

Depending upon the presence or absence of hemodynamic instability as manifested by cardiac arrest, persistent hypotension, or obstructive shock, the decision regarding management must be decided.

Investigations such as blood D-dimer estimation, ECG, echocardiography, ventilation/perfusion (V/Q) scan form the initial investigation modalities. However, multidetector CTPA is the noninvasive investigation of choice, while invasive pulmonary angiography is the gold standard diagnostic tool for PTE.

Treatment options include anticoagulation, thrombolysis—systemic or catheter mediated, IVC filter, or surgical embolectomy.

## FURTHER READINGS

1. Rogers MA, Levine DA, Blumberg N, Flanders SA, Chopra V, Langa KM. Triggers of hospitalization for venous thromboembolism. Circulation. 2012;01;125(17):2092-9.
2. Anderson FA, Spencer FA. Risk factors for venous thromboembolism. Circulation. 2003; 107(23 Suppl 1):I9-16.
3. Blom JW, Doggen CJ, Osanto S, Rosendaal FR. Malignancies, prothrombotic mutations, and the risk of venous thrombosis. JAMA. 2005; 293(6):715-22.
4. Kucher N, Goldhaber SZ. Management of massive pulmonary embolism. Circulation. 2005;112(2):e28-32.

CHAPTER 102

# Tension Pneumothorax

*Boudhayan Das Munshi, Sudip Ghosh, Onkar Awadhiya, Monidipa Ghosh*

## DEFINITION

Air in the pleural space is termed pneumothorax.

Tension pneumothorax is a severe form of pneumothorax where the air accumulates and gets trapped within the pleural space under positive pressure, displaces mediastinal structures, and compromises cardiopulmonary function.

It is considered a life-threatening condition. So, this emergency must be identified early in order to save precious lives, as it is associated with hemodynamic instability and respiratory distress.

It is said to be present when the intrapleural pressure exceeds atmospheric pressure throughout expiration and often during inspiration as well. Most tension pneumothoraces occur in patients who are receiving positive-pressure ventilation, either from mechanical ventilation or during resuscitation. If the patient is not receiving positive-pressure ventilation, then the mechanism by which a tension pneumothorax develops is probably related to some type of one-way valve process in which the valve is open during inspiration and closed during expiration. During inspiration, owing to the action of the respiratory muscles, the pleural pressure becomes negative and air moves from the alveoli into the pleural space. Then, during expiration, with the respiratory muscles relaxed, the pleural pressure becomes positive. A one-way valve mechanism must be implicated; otherwise, on expiration, when the pleural pressure is positive with respect to the alveolar pressure, gas would flow from the pleural space into the alveoli, and no positive pressure would develop in the pleural space.

## CAUSES

- Idiopathic spontaneous pneumothorax
- Open pneumothorax
- Conversion of spontaneous pneumothorax
- Traumatic

### Iatrogenic

- Central venous catheterization in the internal jugular or subclavian vein
- Positive-pressure ventilation leading to barotrauma
- Lung biopsy
- Percutaneous tracheostomy
- Thoracocentesis
- Pacemaker insertion
- Bronchoscopy
- Cardiopulmonary resuscitation
- Intercostal nerve block

## Noniatrogenic

- Penetrating or blunt trauma
- Rib fracture
- Diving or flying

# WHEN TO SUSPECT?

## Clinical Clues in History and Examination

Pneumothorax can be asymptomatic or symptomatic. However, tension pneumothorax presents with striking clinical features as it is an emergency. Though it can evolve from spontaneous pneumothorax, it commonly occurs in patients on mechanical ventilation or during cardiopulmonary resuscitation. If difficulty is encountered in the ventilation of a patient during cardiopulmonary resuscitation or if a patient has electromechanical dissociation, a tension pneumothorax should also be suspected. Patients with unrecognized pneumothoraces who are receiving mechanical ventilation are those most likely to develop a tension pneumothorax.

*General physical examination*:

- Altered mental status
- Hypotension (decrease in blood pressure)
- Tachycardia (increase in heart rate)
- *Possible other findings*: Cyanosis, jugular venous distension

*Inspection*:

- Increased respiratory rate
- Reduced movement of the chest wall on the affected side
- Retraction of the chest wall on the affected side
- Use of accessory muscles of respiration
- Deviation of the trachea to the opposite side

*Palpation*:

- Reduced tactile fremitus on the affected side
- Deviation of the trachea to the opposite side

*Percussion*:

- Hyperresonant on the affected side

*Auscultation*:

- Decreased or absent breath sounds on the affected side
- Reduced vocal fremitus

In severe cases, if the diagnosis is delayed or missed, then patients may present with acute respiratory failure or cardiac arrest.

## Complications

Complications can arise due to the underlying primary disease process, tension pneumothorax, or tube thoracostomy used as the treatment modality.
They include:

- Death
- Respiratory failure or arrest
- Cardiac arrest
- Hemothorax
- Bronchopulmonary fistula
- Pneumopericardium
- Pneumoperitoneum
- Empyema
- Pyopneumothorax
- Skin infection and pain at the site of tube thoracostomy
- Damage to the neurovascular bundle during tube thoracostomy

*Clinical re-evaluation*:

- Chest pain or hemoptysis perimenstrually in a young woman with or without a history of endometriosis might suggest catamenial pneumothorax.
- A family history of pneumothorax may suggest inheritable disorders such as alpha-1 antitrypsin deficiency or Birt-Hogg-Dubé syndrome and rarely Marfan or Ehlers-Danlos syndrome.
- A personal or family history of renal cancer may also support Birt-Hogg-Dubé syndrome.
- A history of travel (e.g., to regions where tuberculosis is endemic) or reason to suspect an underlying human immune

deficiency disorder may be sought in those with a possible infectious reason for pneumothorax.

- A joint and skin examination may reveal dry eye and joint disease suggestive of Sjögren's syndrome (which can be complicated by lung cysts), joint hypermobility or hyperextensible skin consistent with Ehlers-Danlos syndrome, or pectus carinatum and disproportionate tall stature to suggest Marfan syndrome.
- A detailed drug history or track marks may suggest illicit drug use or identify immunosuppressant drugs not previously suspected as an etiology of pneumothorax.
- A history of weight loss or sweats may suggest occult malignancy.
- A detailed social history may identify recent air travel or scuba diving as a hobby.
- Any lucencies or nodules on chest radiography (CXR) in a young smoking male or nonsmoking female should prompt computed tomography (CT) chest imaging to look for evidence of Langerhans cell histiocytosis (LCH), subpleural blebs, or lymphangioleiomyomatosis (LAM).
- Cysts identified on CT should prompt a diagnostic evaluation for cystic lung disorders.

## HOW TO MANAGE?

### Investigations and Treatment

Tension pneumothorax is a medical emergency. So, in patients with hemodynamic instability and respiratory distress, patients can undergo an urgent ultrasonography (USG) of the chest if available. USG has a higher sensitivity than the traditional upright anteroposterior CXR for the detection of pneumothorax. If the patient is hemodynamically stable, then CXR may be performed initially.

The following findings on USG are suggestive of pneumothorax:

- Absence of lung sliding
- Absence of comet tail artifact

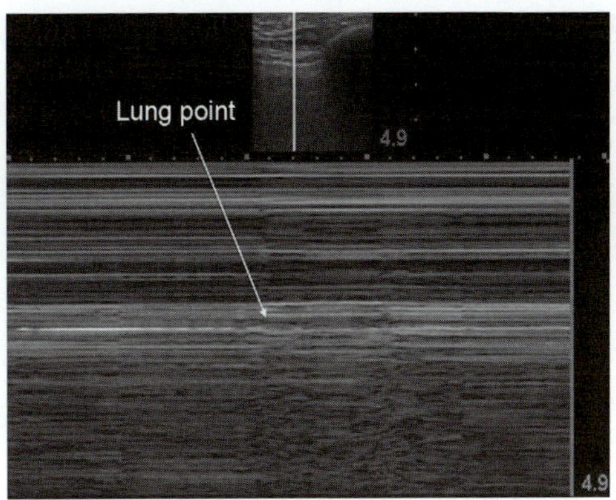


**FIG. 1:** Presence of lung point on USG Thorax.

- Presence of lung point **(Fig. 1)**
- A line pattern on B mode. On the M mode, the seashore sign is replaced by the barcode sign **(Fig. 2)**.

As larger pneumothoraces are more likely to require thoracostomy, it is important to determine the size of the pneumothorax. The location of the lung point may assist in determining the size of the pneumothorax. If a lack of lung sliding is visualized anteriorly, the probe can progressively be moved to more lateral and posterior positions on the chest wall searching for the location of the lung-point. The more lateral or posterior the 'lung-point sign' is identified, the larger the pneumothorax. Therefore, if the 'lung-point sign' is seen in an anterior location on the chest wall, the pneumothorax is relatively small. The lung point sign had an overall sensitivity of 66% and a specificity of 100%. Keep in mind that the sensitivity may be low because in large pneumothoraces, the lungs are so collapsed that there is no point when the inflated lung is in contact with the parietal pleura.

#### *Chest X-ray*

Pneumothorax is seen as an area of increased lucency. It tends to be larger in tension pneumothorax and results in relative lucency of the entire hemithorax. There may be associated mass effect on the diaphragm,

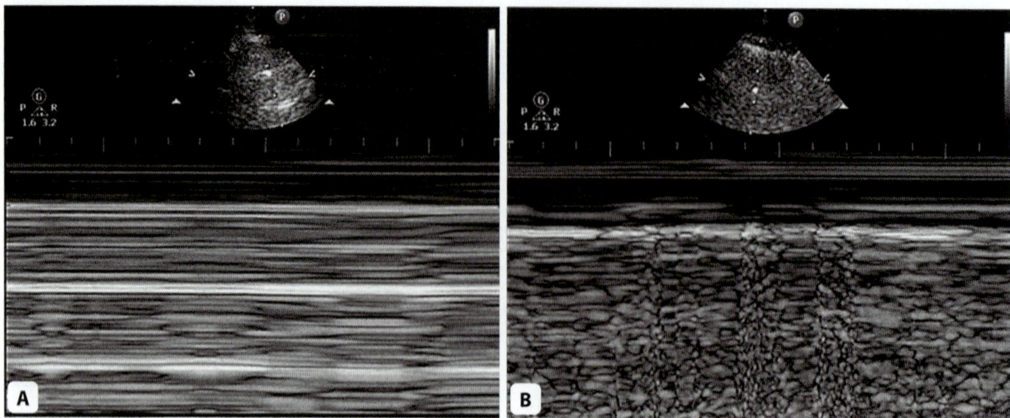


**FIGS. 2A AND B:** TUS with M-Modus showing the absence of lung sliding. (A) "Barcode sign" with pneumothorax) and presence of lung sliding; (B) "Seashore-sign", no pneumothorax. The difference could be noted in the M-Modus-parts below the star-marked white line, that reflects a regular (B) or missing sliding pleural line, leading to repetitive horizontal lines in the case of a pneumothorax in part (A).

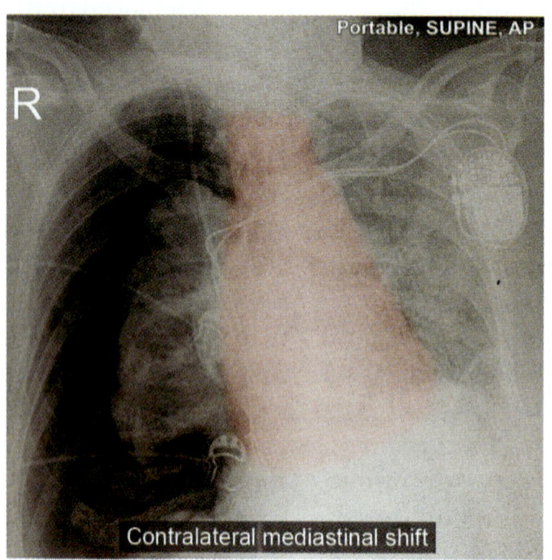


**FIG. 3:** Mediastinal shift.

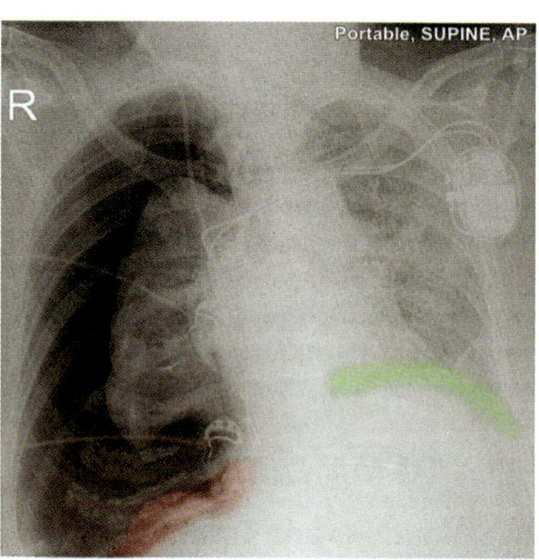


**FIG. 4:** Hemidiaphragm depression.

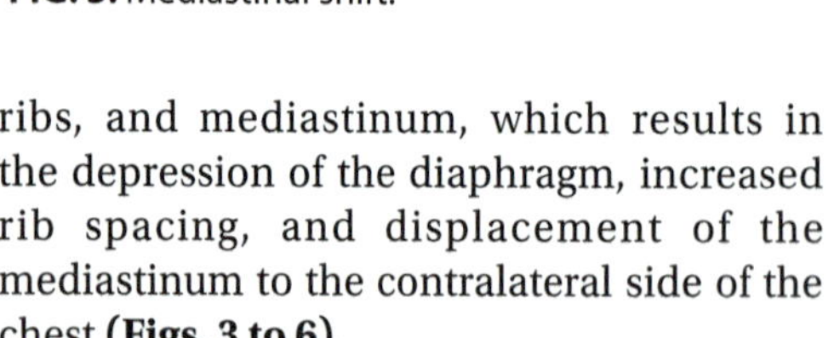

ribs, and mediastinum, which results in the depression of the diaphragm, increased rib spacing, and displacement of the mediastinum to the contralateral side of the chest **(Figs. 3 to 6)**.

### *Computed Tomography Scan of the Chest*

It is the best modality for determining the presence, size, and location of pneumothorax. It is used when chest X-ray is unclear. However, it is not recommended for routine use **(Fig. 7)**.

- A young smoking male may reveal subpleural blebs, nodules, or cysts consistent with LCH.
- A young nonsmoking female may reveal cysts consistent with LAM or pleural and parenchymal abnormalities that suggest thoracic endometriosis.
- A cigarette smoker of over 20 pack-years, marijuana smoker, or user of illicit drugs

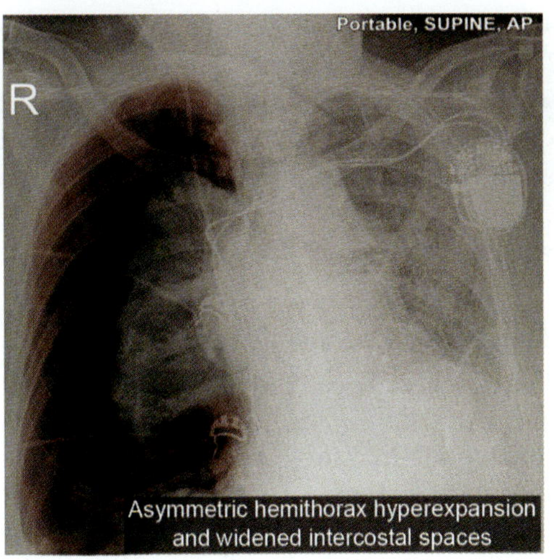


**FIG. 5:** Hemithorax hyperexpansion.

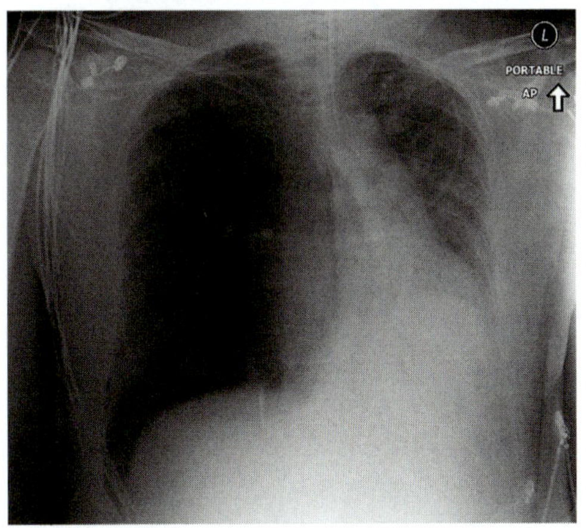


**FIG. 6:** Right-sided tension pneumothorax.

may reveal emphysema, bullous disease, or malignancy.

- A young adult with a family history of pneumothorax, skin lesions, or kidney tumors may reveal lung cysts consistent with Birt-Hogg-Dubé syndrome.
- Patients with a history of previous pneumothorax or prolonged air leak on chest tube drainage where chest CT may reveal underlying cysts or other pathologies that may prompt additional testing.

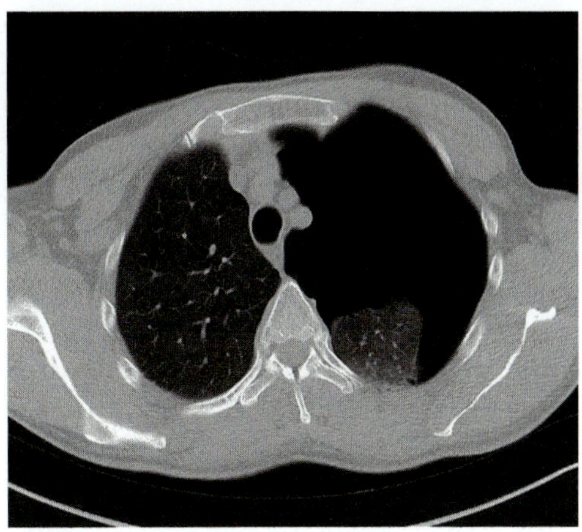

**FIG. 7:** Computed tomography scan of the chest showing tension pneumothorax.

- Patients with unusual etiologies for pneumothorax (e.g., drugs, anorexia, exercise) in whom more serious pathologies need to be excluded.
- Patients with ongoing air leak and/or requiring surgery (as preoperative workup)

Pulmonary function tests do not have much of a role in the diagnosis or during the treatment of pneumothorax. However, they can be performed after recovery when the underlying lung disease needs to be detected. They should be performed only in stable patients and are not helpful in those in whom a chest tube is in place or in whom pleurodesis has been recently performed.

## *Treatment*

Tension pneumothorax is a medical emergency.

Although the diagnosis of tension pneumothorax can be established radiographically by demonstrating severe contralateral mediastinal shift and ipsilateral diaphragmatic depression, valuable time should not be wasted on radiologic studies because the clinical situation and the physical findings are usually sufficient to establish the diagnosis.

When the diagnosis is suspected, the patient should immediately be given a high concentration of supplemental oxygen to combat hypoxia.

Then, the elevated pressure in the pleural space must be eliminated. Optimally, this is done with a silicon catheter such as that advocated for thoracentesis. Ideally, the catheter should be attached to a three-way stopcock and a 50-mL syringe partially filled with sterile saline solution. After the catheter is inserted into the pleural space, it is connected through the three-way stopcock to the syringe. Then, the stopcock is opened to the syringe, and the plunger is withdrawn. A rush of air bubbling outward through the fluid in the syringe establishes the diagnosis of tension pneumothorax.

If a tension pneumothorax is confirmed, the catheter should be left in place and in communication with the atmosphere until air ceases to exit through the syringe. Additional air can be withdrawn from the pleural space with the syringe and the three-way stopcock.

There have been instances reported where 16-gauge cannulae were insufficient in the drainage of air from tension pneumothorax.

If a tension pneumothorax is present, preparations should be made for the immediate insertion of a large chest tube. If no bubbles escape from the syringe, the patient does not have a tension pneumothorax and the catheter should be withdrawn from the pleural space.

In recent years, some emergency medical services have begun performing needle thoracostomies prehospital in patients suspected of having a tension pneumothorax. The outpatient use of needle thoracostomy is controversial, and its utilization varies markedly from region to region.

For performing the procedure, a quick revision of the surface anatomy of the lungs is necessary:

- Lungs extend from about 2 cm above the clavicle down to the 6th rib in the midclavicular line and the 8th rib in the midaxillary line.
- The oblique fissure goes from the 6th rib midclavicular line to T3 in the back.
- The horizontal fissure (only on the right) starts at the 4th rib at the sternum and then meets the oblique fissure at the 5th rib in the midaxillary line.
- The pleura generally is two ribs below.

### *Chest Tube Insertion Procedure*

Insert a chest tube in the *4th* or *5th* intercostal space in the *anterior axillary line*. When making the incision, make it one rib below the intercostal space where you want to insert the tube. Also, remember to go *above the rib* as the neurovascular bundles travel along the underside of the ribs.

### *Needle Decompression Procedure*

These are used in a pinch when a patient is suspected to have a tension pneumothorax and needs immediate decompression. A 14- or 16-gauge needle is inserted above the 2nd or 3rd rib in the midclavicular line **(Fig. 8)**.

## CLINICAL PEARLS

- Tension pneumothorax is an emergency that needs to be identified and treated promptly.
- The associated hemodynamic instability and the accompanying respiratory distress should prompt immediate management.
- Clinical features include altered mental status, hypotension, tachycardia, tachypnoea, reduced movement, retraction of the chest wall on the affected side, use of accessory muscles of respiration and deviation of the trachea to the opposite side, with reduced tactile fremitus on the affected side, hyper-resonant note on affected side, and decreased/absent breath sounds on the affected side.
- Complications include death, respiratory failure or arrest, cardiac arrest, hemothorax, bronchopulmonary fistula, pneumopericardium, pneumoperi-

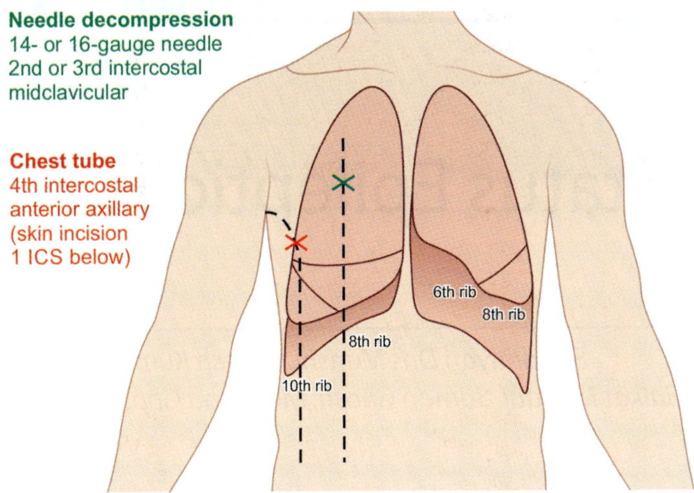


**FIG. 8:** Needle decompression procedure and Intercostal chest tube drainage in tension pneumothorax.[7]

(ICS: intercostal space).

toneum, empyema, pyopneumothorax, skin infection, pain at the site of tube thoracostomy, and damage to the neurovascular bundle during tube thoracostomy.

- Imaging such as chest X-ray, bedside USG, and CT chest can be useful diagnostics.
- Immediate needle decompression or chest tube drainage are the life-saving treatment modalities.

## FURTHER READINGS

1. Pneumothorax in adults: Epidemiology and etiology - UpToDate [Internet]. [cited 2023 Sep 28]. Available from: https://www.uptodate.com/contents/pneumothorax-in-adults-epidemiology-and-etiology.
2. Lung Point Sign and Pneumothorax | Emory School of Medicine [Internet]. [cited 2023 Sep 28]. Available from: https://med.emory.edu/departments/emergency-medicine/sections/ultrasound/case-of-the-month/lung/lung-point.html.
3. Eisenmann S, Winantea J, Karpf-Wissel R, Funke F, Stenzel E, Taube C, et al. Thoracic Ultrasound for Immediate Exclusion of Pneumothorax after Interventional Bronchoscopy. J Clin Med. 2020;9(5):1486.
4. Botz B. Radiopaedia. [cited 2023 Sep 28]. Tension pneumothorax (annotated signs) | Radiology Case | Radiopaedia.org. Available from: https://radiopaedia.org/cases/tension-pneumothorax-annotated-signs.
5. Radiopaedia [Internet]. [cited 2023 Sep 28]. Playlist "Trauma chest" by Rachel Robinson. Available from: https://radiopaedia.org/play/54627/entry/968789/case/23278/presentation.
6. Jones J. Radiopaedia. [cited 2023 Sep 28]. Tension pneumothorax (summary) | Radiology Reference Article | Radiopaedia.org. Available from: https://radiopaedia.org/articles/tension-pneumothorax-summary.
7. Lung surface anatomy and chest tubes vs needle decompression|Sketchy Medicine [Internet]. [cited 2023 Sep 28]. Available from: https://sketchymedicine.com/2012/04/lung-surface-anatomy-and-chest-tubes-vs-needle-decompression/.
8. Lee, YC Gary. "UpToDate." Www.uptodate.com, 20 Sept. 2023, www.uptodate.com/contents/clinical-presentation-and-diagnosis-of-pneumothorax?search=tension%20pneumothorax&source=search_result&selectedTitle=1~114&usage_type=default&display_rank=1.

CHAPTER 103

# Status Epilepticus

*Boudhayan Das Munshi, Rakesh Kumar, Saikat Mondal, Suman Ghosh, Monidipa Ghosh*

## DEFINITION

Status epilepticus is a condition resulting from either the failure of the mechanisms responsible for seizure termination or from the initiation of mechanisms that lead to abnormally prolonged seizures. It is a condition that can have long-term consequences, including neuronal death, neuronal injury, and alteration of neuronal networks, depending on the type and duration of seizures.

The temporal threshold that defines an abnormally prolonged seizure depends on the type of seizure.

For convulsive status epilepticus (CSE), the threshold is 5 minutes.

For nonconvulsive status epilepticus (NCSE), the threshold is 10 minutes.

In patients with baseline coma or encephalopathy, NCSE was recently defined by the American Clinical Neurophysiology Society (ACNS) as ictal activity constituting >20% of an hour of recording (i.e., >12 minutes).

Common causes in adults:

- *Acute structural brain injury*:
  - Stroke
  - Head trauma
  - Subarachnoid hemorrhage
  - Cerebral anoxia or hypoxia
- *Infection*:
  - Encephalitis
  - Meningitis
  - Abscess
- Brain tumor
- *Remote or long-standing structural brain injury*:
  - Prior head injury or neurosurgery
  - Perinatal cerebral ischemia
  - Cortical malformations
  - Arteriovenous malformations
  - Low-grade brain tumors
- Antiseizure medication nonadherence or discontinuation in patients with prior epilepsy
- Withdrawal syndromes associated with the discontinuation of alcohol, barbiturates, or benzodiazepines
- *Metabolic abnormalities*:
  - Hypoglycemia
  - Hepatic encephalopathy
  - Uremia
  - Hyponatremia
  - Hyperglycemia
  - Hypocalcemia
  - Hypomagnesemia
- Sepsis
- *Use of, or overdose with, drugs that lower the seizure threshold*:
  - Theophylline
  - Carbapenems (e.g., imipenem)
  - High-dose penicillin G
  - Cefepime

- Quinolone antibiotics
- Metronidazole
- Isoniazid
- Tricyclic antidepressants
- Bupropion
- Lithium
- Clozapine
- Flumazenil
- Cyclosporine
- Lidocaine
- Bupivacaine
- Metrizamide
- Dalfampridine
- Phenothiazines, especially at higher doses

- *Autoimmune causes*:
    - Autoimmune encephalitis—autoantibodies directed against neuronal proteins [e.g., antileucine-rich glioma inactivated 1 (LG1) protein, *N*-methyl-D-aspartate (NMDA) receptor, alpha-amino-3-hydroxy-5-methyl-4-isoxazolepropionic acid (AMPA) receptor, B1 subunit of the gamma-aminobutyric acid B (GABA B) receptor]
    - Multiple sclerosis
    - Adult-onset Rasmussen's encephalitis
    - Hashimoto's encephalitis
    - Lupus vasculitis

## WHEN TO SUSPECT?

Recognition of generalized tonic-clonic seizures (GTCS)

*Step 1*: History taking and physical examination.

Triggering events include fever, lack of sleep, menstrual period, stress, strong emotions, strenuous exercise, flashing of light, and loud music.

*Aura or prodrome*: Subtle changes in mood, cognition, and headache. They help to localize the site of origin of the seizures. It indicates a focal onset of seizure instead of a generalized seizure. There can be staring spells suggestive of absence seizures or early morning myoclonic jerks. The presence of multiple seizure types can indicate the presence of epilepsy or a particular epileptic syndrome.

Generalized tonic-clonic seizure begins with an abrupt loss of consciousness without any aura. The tonic phase occurs with generalized stiffening of the body, with or without cyanosis. This is followed by clonic jerking. Next appears the postictal sleepiness, agitation, and confusion.

On physical examination, there might be a postictal state of confusion, somnolence, headache, personality, and mood changes. Examination of the oral mucosa can reveal lateral tongue bites. Bruises and scrapes over the body can be seen after an episode of seizure. Back pain can present with vertebral compression fracture. Meningeal inflammation can present with nuchal rigidity and metabolic disorder can present with asterixis. Asymmetry or focal weakness can indicate focal seizures. Neurocutaneous syndromes, e.g., neurofibromatosis, tuberous sclerosis, and Sturge–Weber syndrome, can present with varied skin manifestations. Urinary incontinence can be a manifestation of GTCS.

After 30–45 minutes, the signs become increasingly subtle. Patients may have only mild clonic movements of only the fingers or fine, rapid movements of the eyes. This may be accompanied by episodes of dilated pupils, hypertension, and tachycardia.

Presentations include:

- Generalized CSE
- Focal motor status epilepticus

Focal motor status epilepticus has clinical manifestations depending on the epileptogenic area of the brain. It may be characterized by focal jerking activity of a limb progression along the homunculus "Jacksonian march" or widespread but unilateral jerking muscle activity with or without impaired consciousness.

## WHY IS GENERALIZED CONVULSIVE STATUS EPILEPTICUS AN EMERGENCY?

Prolonged seizures can lead to hyperthermia, cardiorespiratory dysfunction, and metabolic abnormalities, which in turn can lead to irreversible neuronal injury.

Central nervous system (CNS) injury can occur when electrographic seizures in a patient are paralyzed with neuromuscular blockade.

So, early recognition of generalized convulsive status epilepticus (GCSE) and the institution of early therapy are essential in minimizing neurologic insult.

## HOW TO MANAGE?

### Investigations

One of the goals of the management of status epilepticus is to identify the possible underlying cause for status epilepticus.

As soon as the patient enters the emergency department, simultaneous evaluation for the underlying etiology must continue alongside the ongoing treatment. The following investigations may be done:

- Plasma glucose or point-of-care capillary blood glucose to rule out hypoglycemia
- Serum electrolytes including sodium, potassium, calcium, magnesium, and phosphorus
- Serum urea and creatinine
- Complete blood count
- Liver function tests
- Toxicology screen using samples of urine and blood
- Serology and autoantibodies
- Thyroid function tests
- Serum lactate
- *Imaging*:
    - Computed tomography (CT) scan of the brain
    - Magnetic resonance imaging (MRI) of the brain
    - Positron emission tomography (PET) scan
- Electrocardiogram (ECG)
- Continuous electroencephalogram (EEG) monitoring
- Arterial blood gas analysis
- Lumbar puncture for cerebrospinal fluid (CSF) analysis

A CT scan of the brain is usually done in the emergency room as it is comparatively easier to perform and less time-consuming than MRI. However, MRI of the brain may be more useful in finding the underlying structural cause.

Lumbar puncture for CSF analysis can be done in patients suspected of having CNS infection or leptomeningeal metastasis from malignancy.

*Electroencephalogram*: Generalized slowing, lateralized periodic discharges (LPDs), background voltage attenuation, burst suppression, and focal slowing.

*Generalized convulsive status epilepticus* is an emergency. NCSE is considered less urgent than GCSE as the accompanying metabolic derangements are less severe. However, ongoing focal seizure activity is associated with cellular injury in the region of the seizure focus. So, it should be treated promptly like GCSE.

### Phases of Status Epilepticus

- *Impending and early status epilepticus*: 5–30 minutes
- *Established and early refractory status epilepticus (RSE)*: 30 minutes to 48 hours
- *Late RSE*: >48 hours

### Convulsive Status Epilepticus (Flowchart 1)

The major goals of treatment include:

- Circulation, airway, and breathing (CAB) to be established and maintained
- Prompt stoppage of seizures and prevention of brain injury

- Identification and treatment of life-threatening causes of status epilepticus such as structural brain lesions, encephalitis, meningitis, sepsis, and trauma:
  - In-hospital management starts with the establishment of immediate intravenous (IV) access.
  - Prompt administration of anti-seizure medications must occur simultaneously with immediate supportive care.
  - Proper positioning of the head to maintain an open airway (rapid-sequence intubation may be required at any point during management if oxygenation or ventilation is impaired)
    - Patients with continuous generalized CSE should be monitored *continuously for*:
      - ♦ Heart rate
      - ♦ Heart rhythm
      - ♦ Breathing
      - ♦ Pulse oximetry for oxygen saturation
    - *Intermittently for*:
      - ♦ Blood pressure
      - ♦ Temperature

However, it should be noted that continuous motor activity might interfere with the ability of electronic monitors to correctly record the readings. Thus, simultaneous clinical assessment of pulse, breathing, and color to detect shock, apnea, or cyanosis must continue at periodic intervals.

## Management Strategies at Different Stages for Termination of Seizures

The drugs with their dosing used at various stages include **(Table 1)**:

- *Impending and early status epilepticus*:
  - *IV benzodiazepines*:
    - Lorazepam (LZP)
    - Midazolam (MDZ)
    - Clonazepam (CLZ)
    - Diazepam
  - *IV antiseizure drugs*:
    - Phenytoin/fosphenytoin (PHT)
    - Valproic acid (VPA)
    - Levetiracetam (LEV)
- *Established and early RSE*:
  - IV MDZ
  - IV propofol (PRO)
- *Late refractory status epilepticus*:
  - Pentobarbital (PTB)
  - *Other medications*:
    - Lidocaine
    - Verapamil
    - Magnesium
    - Ketogenic diet
    - Immunomodulation
  - *Other anesthetics*:
    - Isoflurane
    - Desflurane
    - Ketamine
  - *Other approaches*:
    - Surgery
    - Vagus nerve stimulation (VNS)
    - Responsive neurostimulation (RNS)
    - Repetitive transcranial magnetic stimulation (rTMS)
    - Electroconvulsive therapy (ECT)
    - Hypothermia

### *Correction of Metabolic Disturbances*

- If hypoglycemia is detected on initial capillary blood glucose screening, it should be corrected using 25% 100 mL dextrose immediately. Glucagon may be administered intramuscularly (IM) or intraosseously (IO) for nonresponders.
- Thiamine 100 mg IV dose may be administered.
- Electrolyte disturbances, if any, should be corrected immediately.

### *Indications for Immediate Endotracheal Intubation and Mechanical Ventilation*

- Hypoxemia
- Apnea
- Unmaintainable airway

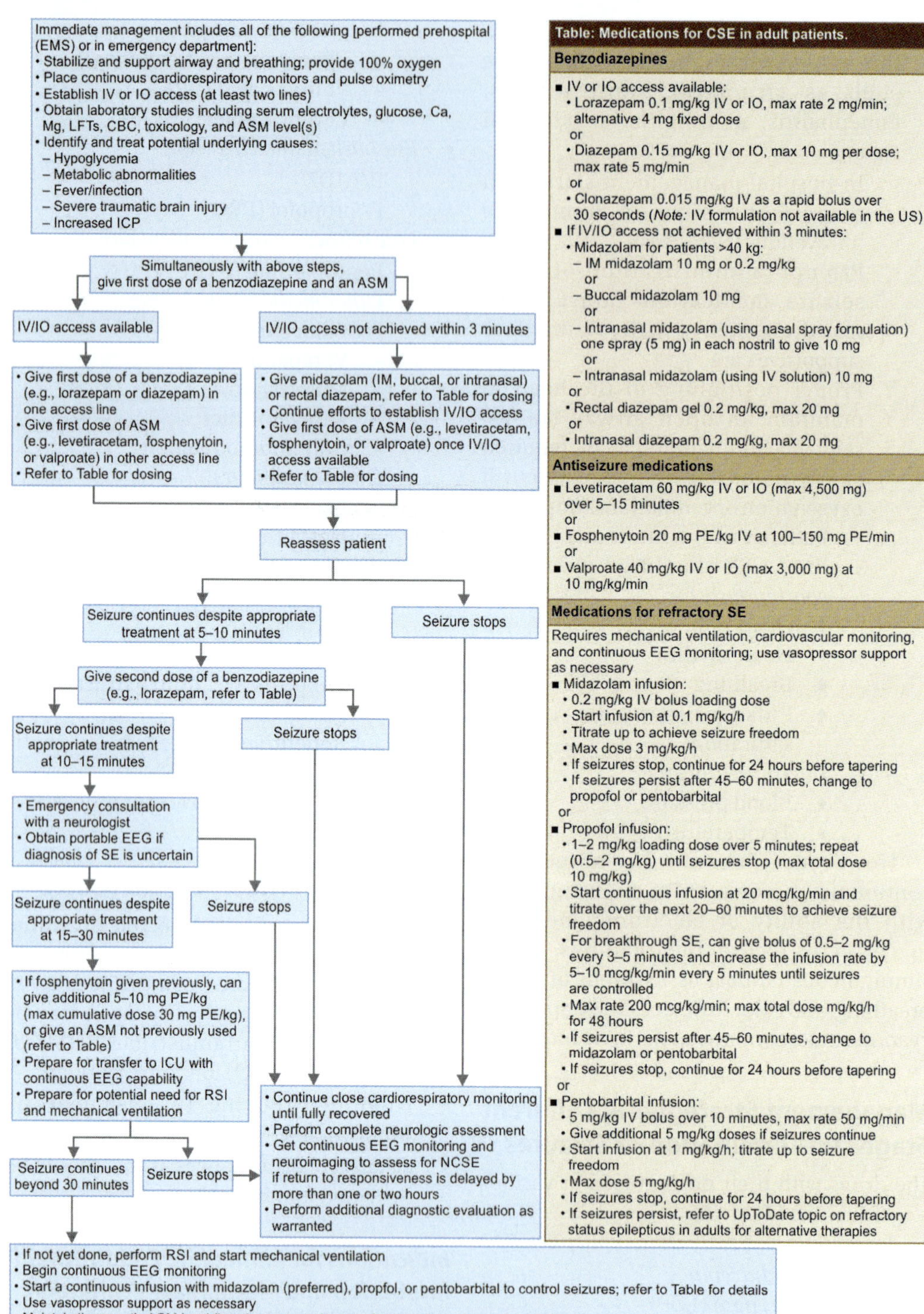


| Table: Medications for CSE in adult patients. |
|---|
| **Benzodiazepines** |
| ■ IV or IO access available:<br>• Lorazepam 0.1 mg/kg IV or IO, max rate 2 mg/min; alternative 4 mg fixed dose<br>or<br>• Diazepam 0.15 mg/kg IV or IO, max 10 mg per dose; max rate 5 mg/min<br>or<br>• Clonazepam 0.015 mg/kg IV as a rapid bolus over 30 seconds (*Note:* IV formulation not available in the US)<br>■ If IV/IO access not achieved within 3 minutes:<br>• Midazolam for patients >40 kg:<br>– IM midazolam 10 mg or 0.2 mg/kg<br>or<br>– Buccal midazolam 10 mg<br>or<br>– Intranasal midazolam (using nasal spray formulation) one spray (5 mg) in each nostril to give 10 mg<br>or<br>– Intranasal midazolam (using IV solution) 10 mg<br>or<br>• Rectal diazepam gel 0.2 mg/kg, max 20 mg<br>or<br>• Intranasal diazepam 0.2 mg/kg, max 20 mg |
| **Antiseizure medications** |
| ■ Levetiracetam 60 mg/kg IV or IO (max 4,500 mg) over 5–15 minutes<br>or<br>■ Fosphenytoin 20 mg PE/kg IV at 100–150 mg PE/min<br>or<br>■ Valproate 40 mg/kg IV or IO (max 3,000 mg) at 10 mg/kg/min |
| **Medications for refractory SE** |
| Requires mechanical ventilation, cardiovascular monitoring, and continuous EEG monitoring; use vasopressor support as necessary<br>■ Midazolam infusion:<br>• 0.2 mg/kg IV bolus loading dose<br>• Start infusion at 0.1 mg/kg/h<br>• Titrate up to achieve seizure freedom<br>• Max dose 3 mg/kg/h<br>• If seizures stop, continue for 24 hours before tapering<br>• If seizures persist after 45–60 minutes, change to propofol or pentobarbital<br>or<br>■ Propofol infusion:<br>• 1–2 mg/kg loading dose over 5 minutes; repeat (0.5–2 mg/kg) until seizures stop (max total dose 10 mg/kg)<br>• Start continuous infusion at 20 mcg/kg/min and titrate over the next 20–60 minutes to achieve seizure freedom<br>• For breakthrough SE, can give bolus of 0.5–2 mg/kg every 3–5 minutes and increase the infusion rate by 5–10 mcg/kg/min every 5 minutes until seizures are controlled<br>• Max rate 200 mcg/kg/min; max total dose mg/kg/h for 48 hours<br>• If seizures persist after 45–60 minutes, change to midazolam or pentobarbital<br>• If seizures stop, continue for 24 hours before tapering<br>or<br>■ Pentobarbital infusion:<br>• 5 mg/kg IV bolus over 10 minutes, max rate 50 mg/min<br>• Give additional 5 mg/kg doses if seizures continue<br>• Start infusion at 1 mg/kg/h; titrate up to seizure freedom<br>• Max dose 5 mg/kg/h<br>• If seizures stop, continue for 24 hours before tapering<br>• If seizures persist, refer to UpToDate topic on refractory status epilepticus in adults for alternative therapies |

**FLOWCHART 1:** Approach to the treatment of convulsive status epilepticus in adults.

(ASM: antiseizure medication; CBC: complete blood count; CSE: convulsive status epilepticus; EEG: electroencephalogram; EMS: emergency medical services; ICP: intracranial pressure; ICU: intensive care unit; IM: intramuscular; IO: intraosseous; IV: intravenous; LFT: liver function test; LP: lumbar puncture; NCSE: nonconvulsive status epilepticus; PE: phenytoin equivalents; RSE: refractory status epilepticus; RSI: rapid sequence endotracheal intubation; SE: status epilepticus)

- Status epilepticus lasting ≥ 30 minutes
- To allow urgent brain imaging (e.g., in patients with basilar territory stroke or preceding trauma)

The agents used for induction include:

- PRO
- Etomidate
- MDZ

It is essential to continuously monitor seizure activity using EEG and administer antiseizure medications irrespective of the induction agent used.

## Treatment of Nonconvulsive Status Epilepticus

In critically ill comatose patients, there is considerable controversy about whether to treat NCSE as aggressively as CSE. In all patients with NCSE, a concerted effort should be made to diagnose and treat seizures as quickly as possible but with minimal sedation, trying to avoid inducing or prolonging coma and intubation.

For patients presenting with NCSE, treatment with an IV benzodiazepine under closely monitored conditions with continuous EEG, combined with an IV noncoma-inducing antiseizure medication, is recommended. Dosing is lower than that used for CSE, with repeat doses given as needed.

The likelihood of success with the initial pharmacologic treatment of NCSE varies according to the subtype of NCSE. Absence status epilepticus and focal status epilepticus without impairment of consciousness usually have a good response to treatment without the need for aggressive coma-inducing anesthetics. Focal status epilepticus with impairment of consciousness (but without coma) typically has a good response to initial therapy, although clinical improvement may be delayed. In contrast, NCSE in coma, which can develop de novo or after CSE, may be refractory to multiple initial therapies and require intubation and coma-inducing anesthetic agents.

A typical initial regimen is LZP 2–4 mg combined with any one of the following antiseizure medications:

- Fosphenytoin [15 mg phenytoin equivalents (PE)/kg at a maximum rate of 150 mg PE/min; maximum dose 2,000 mg]
- Valproate (30 mg/kg IV at a maximum rate of 5 mg/kg/min; maximum cumulative dose after reloading of 4,000 mg)
- LEV (40 mg/kg IV bolus, maximum 4,500 mg, over 15 minutes)
- Lacosamide (200 mg IV bolus over 15 minutes)

Note that doses used for NCSE are lower than those used for CSE as there is time to give a lower dose, assess the acute response, and give more if needed; in CSE, there is no time for this, and the full loading doses should be given immediately.

Therapy for NCSE should be administered under close clinical supervision and with continuous EEG monitoring in most cases. In patients with preexisting epilepsy, optimization of antiseizure medications currently utilized may be of value, especially when nonadherence to the outpatient regimen is suspected.

If NCSE persists after IV doses are given, repeat doses can be given without significant delay (within minutes) of any of the above at the same or lower dose.

Ambulatory patients with NCSE, usually with a history of epilepsy, have a good prognosis, whereas acutely ill, stuporous, or comatose patients with NCSE have a poorer prognosis. RSE, which is usually nonconvulsive, is associated with a mortality rate of up to 50%. Poor outcomes are driven primarily by the underlying acute process associated with NCSE rather than the seizures themselves, although prolonged nonconvulsive seizure activity may cause secondary neuronal injury and worse outcomes, especially in those with acute brain injury **(Table 1)**.

**Table 1: Summary of interventions for status epilepticus with their dosages.**

| | *Initial dose* | *Reloading dose* | *Maintenance dose* |
|---|---|---|---|
| ***Parenteral benzodiazepine choices (initial regimen)*** | | | |
| Lorazepam | 2–4 mg IV bolus up to 2 mg/min | 2–4 mg IV | N/A |
| Diazepam | 5–10 mg IV bolus up to 5 mg/min | 5–10 mg IV | N/A |
| Midazolam | 5–10 mg IV or IM | 5–10 mg IV or IM | N/A |
| ***Nonsedating antiseizure choices (initial regimen)*** | | | |
| Phenytoin | 15 mg/kg IV (up to 50 mg/min) | 10–15 mg/kg up to a maximum cumulative dose of 30 mg/kg | 5–7 mg/kg/day orally/IV, divided every 8 hours |
| Fosphenytoin | 15 mg PE/kg IV (up to 150 mg PE/min) | 10 mg PE/kg up to a maximum cumulative dose of 25–30 mg/kg | 5–7 mg PE/kg/day IV, divided every 8 hours |
| Valproate | 30 mg/kg IV (up to 5 mg/kg/min) | 20 mg/kg up to a maximum cumulative dose of 4,000 mg | 30–60 mg/kg/day orally/IV, divided every 6–12 hours |
| Levetiracetam | 40 mg/kg IV (up to 5 mg/kg/min, typically given over 15 minutes, maximum 4,500 mg) | 1,000–2,000 mg up to a maximum cumulative dose of 4,500 mg | 2–4 g/day orally/IV, divided every 6–12 hours |
| Lacosamide | 200 mg IV (over 15 minutes) | 200 mg IV | 200–600 mg/day orally/IV, divided every 12 hours |
| ***Potential oral or nasogastric add-on nonanesthetic options*** | | | |
| Topiramate | 100 mg orally every 12 hours | N/A | 300–800 mg/day orally, divided every 8–12 hours |
| Gabapentin | 300 mg orally every 8 hours | N/A | 1,800–3,600 mg/day orally, divided every 6–8 hours |
| Pregabalin | 75 mg orally every 12 hours | N/A | 150–600 mg/day orally, divided every 8–12 hours |
| Clobazam | 10–20 mg orally every 12 hours | N/A | Up to 60 mg/day orally, divided every 12 hours |
| Perampanel | 6–12 mg orally every 24 hours | N/A | Up to 12 mg orally every 24 hours |
| Oxcarbazepine | 300–600 mg orally every 12 hours | N/A | Up to 2,400 mg/day orally, divided every 12 hours |
| Carbamazepine | 300–800 mg orally in two to four divided doses (product dependent) | N/A | Up to 1,600 mg/day orally, divided every 12 hours (tablets) or every 6 hours (liquid) |

*Continued*

*Continued*

| | ***Initial dose*** | ***Reloading dose*** | ***Maintenance dose*** |
|---|---|---|---|
| Vigabatrin | 500–750 mg orally every 12 hours | N/A | Up to 3,000 mg/day orally, divided every 12 hours |
| ***Continuous infusion anesthetic options in critically ill mechanically ventilated patients*** | | | |
| Midazolam | 0.2 mg/kg IV (up to 2 mg/min) every 5 minutes until seizures controlled or maximum dose of 2 mg/kg; followed by continuous infusion | N/A | 0.05–2.9 mg/kg/h continuous IV infusion |
| Propofol | 1–2 mg/kg IV every 5 minutes until seizures controlled or maximum dose 10 mg/kg; followed by continuous infusion | N/A | 1.8–12 mg/kg/h continuous IV infusion (limit to 5 mg/kg/h for treatment > 48 hours) |
| Pentobarbital | 5 mg/kg IV (up to 50 mg/min) every 5 minutes until seizures controlled up to a maximum of 25 mg/kg; followed by continuous infusion | N/A | 0.5–10 mg/kg/h continuous IV infusion |
| Ketamine | 1.5 mg/kg IV every 5 minutes until seizures controlled or up to a maximum dose of 4.5 mg/kg; followed by continuous infusion | N/A | 1.2–7.5 mg/kg/h continuous IV infusion |
| ***Other potential treatments*** | | | |
| Ketogenic diet | | | |
| Methylprednisolone | 1 g/day for 3 days | N/A | 1 mg/kg/day and then taper |
| IVIG | 0.4 g/kg/day for 5 days | N/A | N/A |
| Plasma exchange | | | |
| Hypothermia | | | |
| Electroconvulsive therapy | | | |

(IM: intramuscular; IV: intravenous; IVIG: intravenous immunoglobulin; PE: phenytoin equivalent)

## DIFFERENTIAL DIAGNOSIS

- Acute intoxication
- Brain hypoxia
- Encephalopathy of toxic and metabolic origin
- Ischemic stroke (basilar artery)
- Trauma

## CLINICAL PEARLS

- Status epilepticus is a medical emergency that can be convulsive (generalized or focal motor) or nonconvulsive.
- Prolonged seizures in generalized CSE can lead to hyperthermia, metabolic disturbances, and cardiorespiratory dysfunction which can lead to irreversible neuronal injury.
- Causes include structural, metabolic, e.g., hypoglycemia, inflammation, infections, stroke, drugs, and tumors, e.g., noncompliance to medications.
- Phases of status epilepticus include (1) impending and early status epilepticus: 5–30 minutes, (2) established and early RSE: 30 minutes to 48 hours, and (3) late RSE: >48 hours.
- Generalized CSE is characterized by triggering factors followed by aura or premonitory symptoms, followed by GTCS and postictal state.
- It is essential to identify correctable causes such as hypoglycemia and dyselectrolytemia and correct them immediately.
- Maintenance of CAB constitutes the initial steps.
- Treatment options include drugs, such as benzodiazepines, and antiseizure medications, such as LEV, PHT, and valproate.
- Refractory seizures will require general anesthetic agents such as ketamine, PRO, MDZ, and PTB.
- Emergent therapies include the ketogenic diet and ECT.
- Nonconvulsive status epilepticus requires lower dosages of medications than CSE.

## FURTHER READINGS

1. Guidelines for Epidemiologic Studies on Epilepsy. 1993. Epilepsia: Wiley Online Library [Internet]. [cited 2023 Dec 17]. Available from: https://onlinelibrary.wiley.com/doi/epdf/10.1111/j.1528-1157.1993.tb00433.x
2. The history of status epilepticus and its treatment. Neligan. 2009. Epilepsia: Wiley Online Library [Internet]. [cited 2023 Dec 17]. Available from: https://onlinelibrary.wiley.com/doi/full/10.1111/j.1528-1167.2009.02040.x
3. Trinka E, Höfler J, Zerbs A. Causes of status epilepticus. Epilepsia. 2012;53(s4):127-38.
4. Betjemann JP, Josephson SA, Lowenstein DH, Guterman EL. Emergency Medical Services Protocols for Generalized Convulsive Status Epilepticus. JAMA. 2019;321(12):1216-7.
5. Khoueiry M, Alvarez V. Status epilepticus in adults: a clinically oriented review of etiologies, diagnostic challenges, and therapeutic advances. Clin Epileptol. 2023;36(4):288-97.
6. Treatment of CSE in adults - UpToDate [Internet]. [cited 2023 Dec 17]. Available from: https://www.uptodate.com/contents/image?imageKey=NEURO%2F74649&source=graphics_gallery&topicKey=96933.
7. Nonconvulsive status epilepticus: Treatment and prognosis - UpToDate [Internet]. [cited 2023 Dec 17]. Available from: https://www.uptodate.com/contents/nonconvulsive-status-epilepticus-treatment-and-prognosis?search=nonconvulsive%20status%20epilepticus&source=search_result&selectedTitle=2~67&usage_type=default&display_rank=2

CHAPTER 104

# Scorpionism: A Lethal Sting to a Battle Won

*Apu Adhikary*

*"An untrampled scorpion troubles no one."*

**—Paolo Bacigalupi**

## INTRODUCTION

Scorpion bite accounts for a substantial number of hospitalizations, deaths, and a significant financial burden, mostly to people living in rural communities. It is especially prevalent in tropical as well as subtropical countries such as South Africa, Saudi Arabia, and India. Older studies from South India quote a staggering mortality of 3–22% in pediatric population. Nowadays, we have newer insight into the pathophysiology and effects of scorpion sting, but still, the mortality is high (33.3–100%) when complications such as myocarditis, acute pulmonary edema, and encephalopathy set in. Early use of prazosin and antivenom, however, can change the game with a surprisingly lower mortality rate.

## COMMON SPECIES AND HABITAT

Venomous scorpions are mostly those from the family Buthidae except *Hemiscorpius lepturus*. Most reported scorpion bites that are symptomatic belong to "Buthus" (Mediterranean Spain to the Middle East), "Parabuthus" (Western and Southern Africa), "Hottentotta" (South Africa to South East Asia), "Tityus" (Central America, South America, and the Caribbean), "Liurus" (Northern Africa and the Middle East), "Androctonus" (Northern Africa to Southeast Asia), "Centruroides" (Southern United States, Mexico, Central America, and the Caribbean), and "Mesobuthus" (throughout Asia).

In India, 2 species among 86 are most commonly described. Envenomation following stings from *Mesobuthus tamulus* (Indian red scorpion) accounts for the majority of cases in Western India, while *Heterometrus bengalensis* is usually reported from the eastern parts of the country. *Palamneus swammerdami* is also responsible for significant morbidity.

Scorpions are nocturnal arachnids that are mostly found in hot and dry habitats although some species of scorpions are also seen in wet, marshy lands and forest areas. They are resistant to extremes of environmental conditions and can adapt to almost any habitat. In the morning hours, scorpions hide in covered places such as cracks, crevices, open shoes, and even coat pockets, thereby exposing a person to the venomous sting. The venomous scorpion seems to have weak and thin pincers and thin bodies with a fat tail. The bulbous terminal part of the segmented tail contains a pair of poison-secreting glands with sharp curved stinger **(Fig. 1)**.

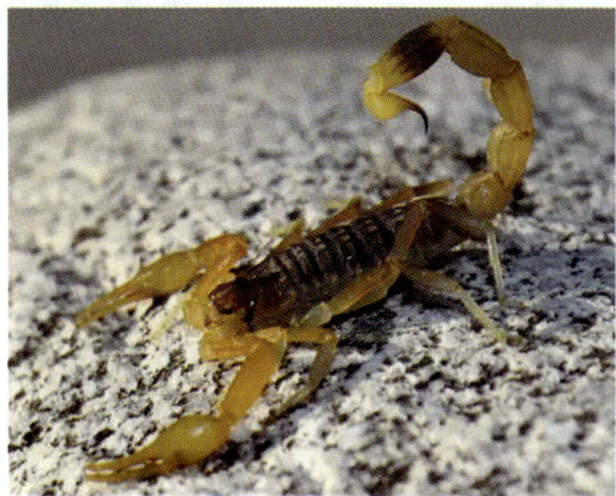

**FIG. 1:** Scorpion.

## THE VENOM—NATURE AND ACTION

Scorpion venom is species-specific, but most contain short-chained neurotoxic peptides. Along with that, there is a variable mixture of hyaluronidase, trypsinogen activator, and serotonin. It acts on the cell membrane ion channels, such as the sodium channel (activation) and calcium-dependent potassium channel (inhibition), thus precipitating the dreaded autonomic storm. The alpha and beta toxins are the major toxins responsible for clinical manifestations, which act on the sodium channel. Others include the scyllatoxin and charybdotoxin acting on the potassium channel. Apart from these, scorpion venom also has an agonist effect on the alpha sympathetic receptor causing hypertension, tachycardia, and other cardiovascular morbidities. Some studies also report a raised angiotensinogen I level.

### Clinical Features

The clinical features depend on geographical distribution. For instance, cardiac complications dominate in India, Mexico, and Brazil, whereas neurological complications dominate in the United States. Hemolysis is often the presenting complication in South Africa. In a large study done on Indian pediatric patients with scorpion (red scorpion) stings, the progression of symptoms was chiefly divided into relatively benign, potentially dangerous, and invariably fatal. Benign symptoms usually include nonprogressive but often excruciating pain at the sting site. Life-threatening symptoms start as local pain, paresthesia, vomiting, sweating, lacrimation, cool limbs, and priapism but rapidly progress to tachycardia, hypertension, myocardial dysfunction, arrhythmia, pulmonary edema, and shock within 48 hours. Complications that are invariably fatal include encephalopathy, seizures, hemiparesis, aphasia, cerebral hemorrhages, disseminated intravascular coagulation (DIC), or respiratory failure.

#### *Local Effect*

Severe pain at the sting site is always the presenting feature associated with shooting up of blood pressure, fall in heart rate, and sweating. There is a paradoxical relation to severity of pain and sting severity. Dry sting or nonvenomous stings often present with excruciating pain and tenderness with the so-called tap sign, which can be elicited as severe tenderness and withdrawal on lightly touching the sting area. More venomous bites are associated with increased levels of circulating catecholamines, which cause vasoconstriction and hence a milder pain. For the same reason, pain increases during the recovery phase as levels of circulatory catecholamines fall. Local edema and vasoconstriction make it difficult for lidocaine to penetrate the sting site.

#### *Effect on Myocardium*

Suppression of the secretory system of insulin as a consequence of a strong alpha stimulation ultimately leads to myocardial dysfunction. Multiple mechanisms have been proposed, including hyperglycemia, hyperkalemia, free radical, and free fatty acid deposition in the myocardium. Ultimately, this leads to a condition of acute myocarditis.

### Effect on Nervous System

Encephalopathy and convulsions have been documented to be the effect of direct action of toxin. Fibrin deposition secondary to DIC may explain hemiparesis and cerebral infarction in some patients. Uncontrolled hypertension, secondary to sympathetic stimulation, can cause the rupture of unprotected perforating arteries and consequently cerebral bleeds.

### Effect on Other Organ Systems

Toxins of certain species of scorpions (*Tityus* species) have been known to cause acute lung injury, with the mechanism being diffuse microthrombi formation. Rarely, transaminitis progressing to hepatic necrosis, pancreatitis, hemolysis with secondary acute renal failure, and even cutaneous changes such as erythema are reported after scorpion sting.

### Systemic Inflammatory Response Syndrome

Systemic inflammatory response syndrome is reported with stings from *Tityus serrulatus.* Interleukin (IL)1beta, IL6, and tumor necrosis factor (TNF)-alpha are found to be increased in these patients along with inducible nitric oxide synthase (iNOS), with levels correlating with clinical severity.

### Autonomic Storm

Autonomic storm occurs due to overlapping cholinergic and adrenergic stimulation. Features of cholinergic crisis, including sweating and "ropy salivation," can be seen for 6–13 hours, along with vomiting and priapism. Sweating is often so profuse that it has been monikered "skin diarrhea." Hypotension and bradycardia can occur in 1–2 hours.

Hypertension and tachycardia are the major adrenergic features with an "ashen pallor skin." Early in the course, the sympathetic alpha stimulation also produces mydriasis or dilated pupil poorly reactive to light. Hypertension lasts for 4–48 hours, while tachycardia persists for a longer period of 24–72 hours. Patients mainly present with a holocranial headache, perioral tingling sensations, and mild chest pain or discomfort. External manifestations of uncontrolled hypertension may be evident as apical bulge, parasternal lift, gallop rhythm, and even a papillary muscle dysfunction state producing a faint apical systolic murmur of lower grade. In children, confusion, oculogyric crisis, puffy face and eyes, and finally drowsiness and stupor, with or without convulsions, are often the clinical manifestations seen. Ultimately, this leads to myocardial dysfunction manifested by delayed hypotension (4–48 hours) and pulmonary edema, which may occur within 30 minutes in severe cases. On examination, in a patient who presents with acute-onset shortness of breath with cyanosis, we find a rapid thready pulse, low blood pressure, increased respiratory rate, gallop rhythm, systolic murmur, bilateral fine crepitations, and cold extremities. In Indian studies, as many as 19–20% of children have been shown to progress to pulmonary edema after venomous scorpion sting.

A condition called catecholamine exhaustion may lead to warm skin with low blood pressure during the recovery phase.

### Death

The majority of deaths are due to fatal ventricular tachycardia, which may be as early as 30 minutes after a scorpion sting. Pulmonary edema also has a major role in mortality. A significant proportion of deaths due to scorpion bite can be attributed to low-level awareness, both on the part of the population and healthcare professionals, with delayed transport adding to the burden. However, intensive care units, vasodilators, prazosin, and antivenom, if available, have reduced the fatality rate, which was as high as 20–25% in the latter half of the twentieth century, to a significantly lower percentage (<1%).

## INVESTIGATION FINDINGS IN SCORPION ENVENOMATION

Interlobular septal thickening, pulmonary vascular congestion, and the "bat-wing shadow" of pulmonary edema may be found in the chest roentgenogram.

Multiple electrocardiographic changes have been reported in venomous scorpion sting due to underlying myocardial dysfunction. The most numerously seen are widened QR complex, left ventricular hypertrophy (LVH) voltage criteria, ST elevation in lateral limb leads, and tall peaked T waves in precordial leads $V_{2-6}$. Low voltage complexes and left anterior fascicular block (LAFB) herald a graver prognosis. Atrial arrhythmias, nonsustained ventricular arrhythmias, and a variety of conduction defects often become evident in the electrocardiogram (ECG).

Echocardiography usually reveals left ventricular dilatation and left ventricular systolic dysfunction, with or without regional wall motion abnormality **(Fig. 2)**.

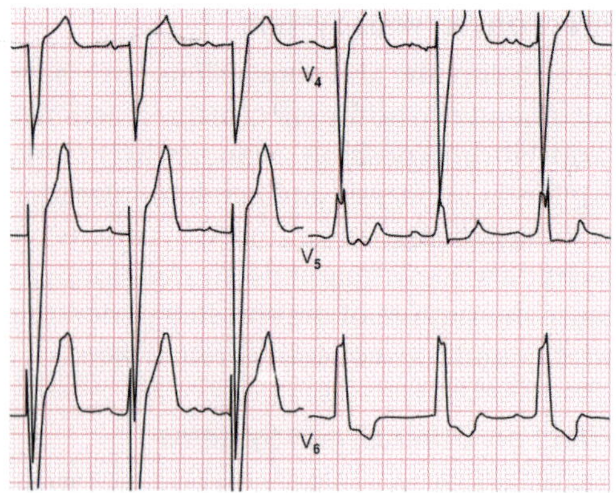


**FIG. 2:** Left ventricular dilatation and left ventricular systolic dysfunction on echocardiography.

## TREATMENT IN A CASE OF VENOMOUS SCORPION STING

### Antivenom

Recently, a pharmaceutical company in Mumbai has introduced a nonspecific F(ab)2 scorpion antivenom (SAV), which is being used mostly in the southern parts of India since 2002. It is shown to be active against Indian red scorpion or *M. tamulus.* Blood levels of toxin, as well as neurological symptoms, have shown significant improvement following antivenom use. We administer the SAV as an intravenous solution as soon as possible after a scorpion sting. Predose skin testing is not done usually. Generally, 30 mL of the antitoxin is used for a standard red scorpion sting, which can inject up to 1.5 mg of venom.

### Prazosin

A phosphodiesterase inhibitor, prazosin reduces the preload as well as left ventricular impedance and counteracts the unopposed alpha-stimulating (alpha 1) effect of a scorpion sting, thereby acting as a physiological antidote to the venom action. It also, via cyclic guanosine monophosphate (cGMP) and endothelial nitric oxide synthase (eNOS), counteracts vasoconstriction, thereby reducing peripheral vascular resistance. Prazosin has been shown to cause miraculous improvement in cases of severe envenomation and significantly reduce mortality not only in India but also in other endemic areas. It is a cheap drug that is easily available even in rural areas. A large study from South India has shown that antivenom plus prazosin use can successfully reduce the dose requirement of prazosin when used alone. The recommended dose of prazosin is 30 μg/kg, available in 1 mg/5 mg tablets. Caution should be advised regarding the "first dose effect" of prazosin, especially in the pediatric age group.

### Other Modalities

Fluid and electrolyte balance is to be maintained in case of severe vomiting, sweating, and salivation.

Initial pain may be managed by benzodiazepines. Diazepam is widely used in children with excruciating pain following a scorpion sting. Other medications shown to be beneficial are nonsteroidal anti-inflammatory drugs (NSAIDs), topical or injectable xylocaine, and rarely streptomycin for nerve block. Local ice pack application can also give relief to the pain and swelling of a recent sting.

Vasodilation with nitroprusside 0.3–5 mg/kg/min may be required in massive life-threatening pulmonary edema with hypertension. However, isolazine, nitrates, etc., can cause reflex tachycardia and exacerbate an increased myocardial oxygen demand. Glyceryl trinitrate (GTN) infusion at 5 mg/min has been used as an alternative to nitroprusside.

Angiotensinogen-converting enzyme (ACE) inhibitor captopril has been used in pulmonary edema.

Dobutamine (5–15 mg/kg/min), invasive as well as noninvasive positive-pressure ventilation, can also be used in pulmonary edema and myocardial dysfunction.

Insulin, along with bicarbonate and alpha blockade, has been shown to be of some use in reversing electrocardiographic changes.

### Modalities which are Ineffective or Potentially Harmful

Morphine should be avoided in pulmonary edema as it worsens dysrhythmia.

A combination of pethidine, promethazine, and chlorpromazine was used under the moniker "lytic cocktail," but it was shown that whatever alpha-blocking effect is there it is neutralized if not overcome by pethidine, which increases the lethality of the venom and causes respiratory depression.

Steroids were not found to be beneficial. In some reports, they accelerate the necrotizing action of catecholamines on the myocardium.

Atropine further worsens tachycardia and hypertension.

Nifedipine also causes tachycardia and reduced myocardial contractility, precipitating heart failure and acute pulmonary edema.

The use of tourniquet at the local site can exacerbate pain and swelling and even give rise to gangrenous changes of the skin.

## CONCLUSION

Scorpion bites are endemic in tropical countries and can cause substantial mortality if untreated. A high grade of suspicion should exist in these parts for early recognition of the clinical features and complications. Major complications of Indian scorpion envenomation are cardiovascular compromise and autonomic chaos. Maintaining hemodynamic stability is of utmost priority in such cases in hospital or critical care setting. Prazosin has brought a revolution in the management of autonomic dysfunction. This, along with the newly introduced antivenom, has reduced mortality from venomous scorpion sting miraculously. Age-old concepts of using lytic cocktail or steroids should be avoided to mitigate potential harm.

## CLINICAL PEARLS

- Scorpion bite can lead to high mortality if not recognized and treated in time.
- The venom contains neurotoxic peptide which modulates ion channel.
- Presenting feature is severe pain in sting site along with autonomic dysfunction like elevated blood pressure bradycardia, etc.
- Systemic features may include myocarditis, encephalopathy, acute lung injury, etc.
- Autonomic storm may occur causing sweating, vomiting, hypertension, tachycardia in certain species.
- Antivenom against Indian red scorpion has resulted in significant improvement in morbidity statistics.

- Other treatment modalities include prazosin, benzodiazepine, nitroprusside, dobutamine, captopril and analgesics.
- Use of morphine, lytic cocktail, steroids, nifedipine, beta blockers are not recommended and may be potentially harmful.

## FURTHER READINGS

1. Rajarajeswari G, Sivaprakasam S, Viswanathan J. Morbidity and mortality pattern in scorpion stings. A review of 68 cases. J Indian Med Assoc. 1979;73:123-6.
2. Mahadevan S, Choudhury P, Puri RK, Srinivasan S. Scorpion envenomation and the role of lytic cocktail in its management. Indian J Pediatr. 1981;48:757-61.
3. Singhal A, Mannan R, Rampal U. Epidemiology, clinical presentation, and final outcome of patients with scorpion bite. J Clin Diagn Res. 2009;3(3):1523-8.
4. Bawaskar HS, Bawaskar PH. Scorpion sting: update. J Assoc Physicians India. 2012;60:46-55.
5. Karnad DR. Haemodynamic pattern in patients with scorpion envenoming. Heart. 1998;79:485-9.
6. Zlotkin E, Shulov AS. Studies on the mode of scorpion neurotoxins–a review. Toxicon. 1969;7:217-21.
7. Bawaskar HS, Bawaskar PH. Management of cardiovascular manifestations of poisoning by the Indian red scorpion (Mesobuthus tamulus). Br Heart J. 1992;68:478-80.
8. Mahadevan S. Scorpion sting. Indian Pediatr. 2000;37:504-14.
9. Balasubramaniam P, Murthy KRK. Liver glycogen depletion in acute myocarditis produced by scorpion venom (Buthus tamulus). Indian Heart J. 1984;36:101-6.
10. Murthy KRK, Billimora FR, Khopkar M, Dave KN. Acute hyperglycemia and hyperkalemia in acute myocarditis produced by scorpion (Buthus tamulus) venom injection in dogs. Indian Heart J. 1986;38:71-6.
11. Devi CS, Reddy NC, Lakshmidevi S, Subramaniyam YR, Reddy CRRM. Defibrination syndrome due to scorpion venom poisoning. Brit Med J. 1970;1:345-6.
12. D'Suze G, Comellas A, Pesce L, Sevcik C, Sanchez-de-Leon R. *Tityus discrepans* venom produces a respiratory distress syndrome in rabbits through an indirect mechanism. Toxicon. 1999;37:173-80.
13. Meki AR, Mohey El-Dean ZM. Serum interleukin-1 beta, interleukin-6, nitric oxide and alpha1 antitrypsin in scorpion envenomed children. Toxicon. 1998;36:1851-9.
14. Boyer LV, Theodorou AA, Berg RA, Mallie J, Arizona Envenomation Investigators, Chávez-Méndez A, et al. Antivenom for critically ill children with neurotoxicity from scorpion sting. N Engl J Med. 2009;360:2090-8.
15. Bawaskar HS, Bawaskar PH. Utility of scorpion antivenom vs prazosin in the management of severe Mesobuthus tamulus envenoming at rural setting. J Assoc Physicians India. 2007;55:14-21.

CHAPTER 105

# Snakebite

*Oendri Bhattacharyya, Ratul Seal,*
*Kaushik Hazra, Apu Adhikary*

## INTRODUCTION

Snakebites account for a substantial hospitalization and financial burden, especially in third-world countries. The World Health Organization (WHO) "estimates that approximately 5 million snakebites occur each year, out of which 2.7 million land up to be poisonous." The clinical manifestations from the poisoning can highly overlap among different classes of venomous snakes. About 81,000–1,38,000 people die from snakebites every year, and three times this number survive but may end up with permanent disabilities. Many snakebite cases go unreported owing to the limited access to healthcare as many people avail therapy from nonmedical resources. Keeping this grave scenario in mind, in 2017, the WHO included snakebite envenomation in the priority list of neglected tropical diseases and introduced a strategy in 2019 to half the number of deaths and serious disabilities by 2030 compared to the 2015 baseline data. India, which homes approximately 50% of the global snakebite cases, will play a pivotal role in achieving this target.

Snakebite occurs either while capturing the prey or in an attempt to self-defend. They are more prevalent in poor communities, predominantly in rural areas. Certain occupations are at more risk, including farmers, hunters, and herders. The incidence of snakebites also increases during the rainy season and after natural calamities. Every snakebite should be treated as a medical emergency unless one can be certain that it is from a nonvenomous variant. A delay in treatment can often lead to a fatal outcome in the case of a bite from a venomous snake. Different species carry different types of toxins, namely cytotoxin, myotoxin, neurotoxin, and hemotoxin.

## CLINICAL FEATURES

Fang marks or their pattern play no role in assessing whether the bite species was venomous or not, the quantity of venom that was injected, and the nature and severity of systemic manifestations. Hence, keeping into consideration "the big four," namely cobra, krait, Russell's viper, and saw-scaled viper, the signs and symptoms of snakebite are categorized as follows:

- *Overt bite*: 70% of snakebites are nonvenomous. Out of the 30% venomous bites, half of those are dry bites. So, in reality, we get 15% of total bites reported as venomous bites. The venomous bites may present with the following symptoms:
  - *Viper*: Progressive painful swelling, local necrosis within minutes of the bite, compartment syndrome
  - *Cobra and krait*: Neuroparalytic symptoms may be seen 30 minutes to 6 hours post bite. The sequence is as follows: "5D and 2P"—ptosis, diplopia,

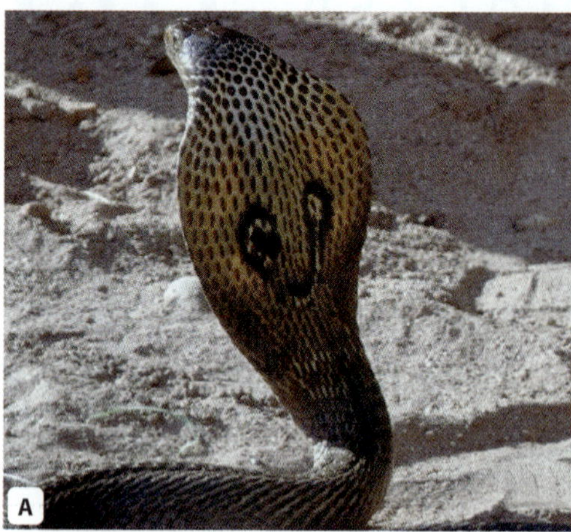
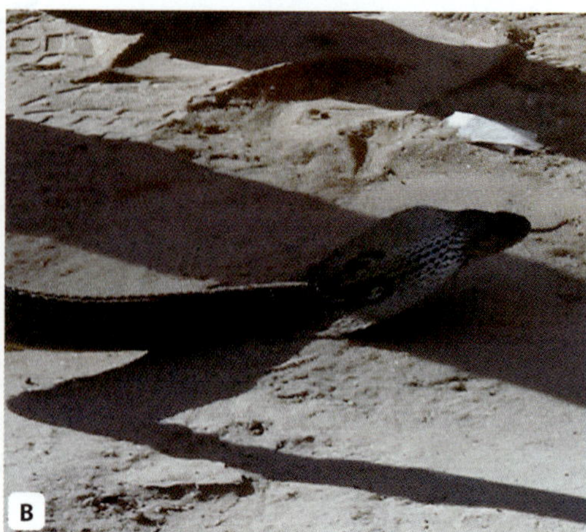

**FIGS. 1A AND B:** King Cobra.

dysarthria, dysphonia, dysphagia, and paralysis. In the case of a krait bite, symptoms may develop within minutes to as late as 36 hours post bite **(Figs. 1A and B)**.
- ○ *Russell's viper and saw-scaled viper*: Bleeding, whole blood clotting time > 20 minutes, acute renal injury, and shock
- ○ *Flat-tailed sea snakes*: Muscle pain, swelling, abnormal contraction of muscles, and compartment syndrome

- *Occult bite*: It is commonly seen in krait bites. Patients may present with indolent signs such as pain in the abdomen and vomiting with neither any neuroparalytic signs nor any local signs. Ptosis may even develop 36 hours post bite.

# STAGES OF MANAGEMENT

## First-aid Treatment

The aim of first-aid treatment is to do no harm to the patient.

## Goals

- Reassure the patient.
- Immobilize the limb by using bandages and clothes to hold the splint. This slows down the systemic absorption of the venom. The patient should be placed in the prone or left lateral position, which reduces the risk of aspiration of vomitus.
- It is absolutely contraindicated to tie tight tourniquets made of rope, belts, or strings. By doing so, the risk of ischemia and limb loss, the risk of neurotoxic blockade on opening the block, the risk of embolism in the case of viper bites, and the increased risk of hypotension are all increased. A false sense of relief also generates in the patients and kin, which delays treatment. It is advocated to immobilize from proximal to distal in the Indian scenario, as the bite-to-hospital reach time can vary from minutes to hours. In the case of a poisonous snakebite, the ligature must be removed after reaching the hospital, hospital staff and medical resuscitation provisions are available, and an intravenous (IV) access has been established, and the proximal-most ligature should be removed only after antivenom serum (ASV) has been started and overviewed by a doctor at the patient bedside.
- Cutting, washing, massaging, and suctioning of the wound area are highly dangerous, as they may assist the venom to spread in the bloodstream.

- Electrical therapy and cryotherapy have no role in snakebite first aid.
- Nothing per mouth till the patient reaches the hospital.
- Traditional measures provide no added benefit other than delaying the necessary treatment.
- One should not waste time in trying to kill or capture the snake. A picture can be taken of the snake safely for identification by an expert. However, if the snake has already been killed, it should be taken to the health care center for identification by the doctor.
- There is no role of black stones and scarification in snakebites.

## Transport to the Nearest Medical Facility

- The victim and the victim's family have to be informed about the immediate need for referral.
- The receiving center has to be informed, and the availability of ASV has to be checked.
- Transfer the patient to a higher center where mechanical ventilation and dialysis are available, only after the completion of ASV infusion.
- During transport, airway support and continuous life-supporting measures may be required.
- Do not insert nasogastric tubes routinely. It is only indicated if the patient's Glasgow Coma Scale (GCS) is poor or the gag reflex is impaired.
- Send a referral note with the details of the clinical assessment at presentation and the treatment that has been provided to the patient.

## Rapid Clinical Assessment and Resuscitation

The clinical presentation of a snakebite victim can be highly variable, depending on the age and size of the patient, the species of the snake, the quantity and toxicity of the venom, and the number and location of the bites. Effects range from systemic envenomation signs, local envenoming signs, effects of anxiety, effects of prehospital, and first-aid mismanagement. These signs are not themselves the sole criteria for administering ASV.

- CABDE approach
    - Circulation (arterial pulse, blood pressure), airway, breathing, disability of the nervous system, and exposure and environmental protection
- Clinical conditions where the patient might require urgent resuscitation
    - Any shock resulting from hypovolemia, the release of inflammatory vasoactive mediators, or anaphylactic reaction induced by the poison itself
    - Impending respiratory failure owing to progressive neuroparalytic effects of venom
    - Sudden deterioration following the removal of the proximal tourniquet
    - Sudden cardiac arrest
    - Acute renal failure
    - Septicemia complicated by local necrosis
- Clinical assessment and species diagnosis
    - In noncritical and critical patients after stabilization
        - What was the patient doing at the time of bite?
        - Determine the exact time of bite
        - Early symptoms post bite: Vomiting, bleeding from the wound site, sleepiness, drooping of eyelid, dark-colored urine, generalized weakness, tenderness, and stiffness of muscles
        - If the snake responsible can be identified
        - Determine if any possible traditional medicine was used
        - Obtain a brief medical history
- Physical examination
    - Vitals such as pulse rate, blood pressure, respiratory rate, and

20-minute whole blood clotting time test (20WBCT) have to be monitored hourly for the first 3 hours and then every 4 hours for the remaining 24 hours.
  - Close assessment is necessary of the site of the bite and signs of local envenomation.
  - Pain on passive movement, pallor, distal pulses, and hypoesthesia through the region of the sensory nerve of the affected part to rule out compartment syndrome

## INVESTIGATIONS

The 20-minute whole blood clotting test is the most reliable test of coagulation, can be done bedside, is executed in most basic healthcare facilities. A few milliliters of fresh venous blood are placed in a new, clean, and dry glass.

*Results*: If the blood has clotted within 20 minutes, there is no need for ASV at this stage. The 20WBCT needs to be repeated every hour for the next 3 hours and then every 6 hours for the next 24 hours. However, antivenom treatment should not be delayed if any evidence of spontaneous bleeding is present 20 minutes post bite, irrespective of 20WBCT results.

- *At primary health center (PHC) level*:
  - Assessment of respiratory function: Peak flow meter for adolescents and adults. If not available as per the latest guidelines for snakebite management, the "single breath count test, breath-holding time, and ability to complete one sentence in one breath" can be done.
  - Urine examination for albumin and blood by dipstick method
- *At district hospital*: All the above-mentioned tests and
  - Prothrombin time
  - Liver function test
  - Renal function test
  - Serum amylase
  - Platelet count
  - Blood sugar
  - Ultrasound of the whole abdomen
  - 12-lead electrocardiogram (ECG)
  - Two-dimensional echocardiography
- *At the tertiary care center*: All the above-mentioned tests and
  - Arterial blood gas analysis
  - Urine routine examination, red blood cell (RBC) casts, myoglobin, hemoglobin, urinary protein-creatinine ratio
  - *Cardiac enzymes*: Creatine phosphokinase (CPK), CPK-MB
  - Serum procalcitonin, blood urine, and wound culture and sensitivity

## ANTISNAKE VENOM

### Dose in Vasculotoxic and Hemotoxic Snakebites

The dosage of ASV is the same for both adults and children. There are no absolute contraindications for ASV administration. Both low-dose infusion therapy and high-dose intermittent bolus therapy have been recommended. Multiple studies from all over the world have compared intermittent bolus dosing versus a continuous low-dose infusion of antivenom. However, apart from the obvious economic advantage, there was no statistically significant difference between the efficacy of the two doses.

*Low-dose infusion therapy*: In this regimen, we divide the patients according to the species of the snake. In the case of Russel's viper, we administer 10 vials of antitoxin as bolus over 30 minutes, followed by 6-hourly infusion of 2 vials in 100 of normal saline. In the case of saw-scaled viper, the initial bolus dose comprises 6 vials. We continue this treatment for 3 days till it normalizes or till the normalization of clotting time.

*Or*

*High-dose intermittent bolus therapy*: In this regimen, irrespective of the species, we administer 10 vials of polyvalent ASV stat over 30 minutes as infusion, followed by a maintenance dose of 6 vials 6 hourly as bolus therapy till either clotting time normalizes or local edema subsides.

Sea snakebite, which is myotoxic, does not have any specific ASV nor does pit viper bite. Poisoning by the latter manifests with coagulopathy which may persist for up to 3 weeks as it does not show any response to normal Indian polyvalent ASV. Even after 30 vials of ASV infusion, if the 20WBCT is still abnormal, it needs to be assessed if further infusion of ASV will be of any more value, especially if no systemic bleeding manifestations are there.

## Dose: Neuroparalytic or Neurotoxic Envenomation

In the case of patients presenting with neurological symptoms, we infuse 10 vials of ASV over 30 minutes. However, a second dose of 10 vials is often required if the patient does not show any improvement within 1 hour. Subsequently, deterioration of neurological and cardiovascular signs would require repetition of ASV after 1–2 hours. 20 vials of ASV with the maximal dose for patients presenting with neurotoxic symptoms are recommended.

### *Monitoring of Patients on Antivenom Serum Therapy*

All patients should be watched carefully every 5 minutes for half an hour and then at 15-minute intervals for the next 2 hours for any side effects. The infusion has to be suspended temporarily at the slightest sign of any adverse reaction.

A strict intake-output chart has to be maintained and the color of urine to detect acute kidney injury early should be noted.

## Adverse Antivenom Serum Reactions

- *Early anaphylactic reaction*: It is seen 10–180 minutes of initiating infusion and is characterized by itching, urticaria, nausea and vomiting, diarrhea, abdominal colic, dry cough, and tachycardia. Severe life-threatening anaphylactic reactions may also develop, characterized by angioedema, bronchospasm, and hypotension.
- *Pyrogenic reaction*: The patient can develop fever with chills, rigor, and hypotension 1–2 hours after starting the transfusion. These reactions are due to contamination of the ASV during the manufacturing process.
- *Late serum sickness-type reaction*: It occurs 7 days after treatment, presenting with nausea, vomiting, diarrhea, fever, itching, recurrent urticarial, myalgia, arthralgia, lymphadenopathy, and, rarely, encephalopathy.

### *Prevention of Adverse Reactions Owing to Antivenom Serum*

There is a high incidence of allergic reactions owing to ASV, and adequate medical support is not always available to manage acute allergic reactions. Only few small studies show beneficial effects of prophylactic subcutaneous epinephrine prior to the administration of ASV. 0.1% of adrenaline solution at a dose of 0.25 mg is administered subcutaneously in adults.

### *Neurotoxin Envenomation*

The "atropine neostigmine challenge test" is recommended in all neurotoxic snakebites, although many institutes avoid this drug in krait bite. In this test, we push 0.6 mg of atropine intravenously, followed by 1.5 mg of neostigmine, and 0.5 mg of neostigmine can be repeated with atropine every 30 minutes up to five times. Alternatively, a fixed-dose combination of neostigmine and glycopyrrolate IV is available, which can also be used in the same scenario. The above drugs need to be tapered sequentially, hourly for 2 hours, and then 6 hourly for the next 12 hours.

Atropine neostigmine (AN) dosage schedule can be stopped if the patient has shown complete recovery from neurotoxicity, the appearance of bradycardia or fasciculation, or there is no improvement despite three doses.

Symptom resolution with atropine-neostigmine indicates a cobra bite. Failure of neurological symptoms to improve after three doses of the same within 1 hour points toward a probable krait bite. This is because the toxin from the krait acts on presynaptic calcium channel, hindering its action as a neurotransmitter. In this case, injection calcium gluconate 10% at a dose of 10 mL IV can be slowly given over 10 minutes and may be repeated every 6 hourly until the resolution of neurological symptoms, which may persist for as long as 1 week.

### *Wound Management*

Patients with a local reaction to snakebite are at a high risk of developing tetanus, and prophylaxis with antitetanus toxoid is recommended. However, a relative contraindication exists if the patient develops coagulopathy till ASV has been infused.

## FUTURE PROSPECTS

In the rapidly evolving world of medical science and technology, death due to snakebite still poses a significant cause of mortality across the globe, especially in developing nations. Small molecules such as varespladib, marimastat, and dimercaprol have shown promising results in clinical trials; however, they are yet to be implemented at a mass level. A comprehensive care model for snakebite treatment is the need of the hour, starting from society, different social organizations, electronic media, strengthening of the healthcare system, and active involvement of the policymakers and the administration.

## CLINICAL PEARLS

- India accounts for 50% of the snakebite burden across the globe.
- First-aid management is an integral part of snakebite management.
- Nonmedical resources for snakebite management should be highly discouraged.
- Antisnake venom should be made available at every level of health care.
- The introduction of small molecules such as varespladib, marimastat, and dimercaprol can revolutionize the treatment for poisonous snakebites.

## FURTHER READINGS

1. Chippaux JP. Snake-bites: appraisal of the global situation. Bull World Health Organ. 1998;76(5):515-24.
2. Suraweera W, Warrell D, Whitaker R, Menon G, Rodrigues R, Fu SH, et al. Trends in snakebite deaths in India from 2000 to 2019 in a nationally representative mortality study. Elife. 2020;9:e54076.
3. Das RR, Sankar J, Dev N. High-dose versus low-dose antivenom in the treatment of poisonous snake bites: a systematic review. Indian J Crit Care Med. 2015;19(6):340-9.
4. Premawardhena AP, de Silva CE, Fonseka MM, Gunatilake SB, de Silva HJ. Low dose subcutaneous adrenaline to prevent acute adverse reactions to antivenom serum in

people bitten by snakes: randomised, placebo controlled trial. BMJ. 1999;318(7190):1041-3.
5. Albulescu LO, Xie C, Ainsworth S, Alsolaiss J, Crittenden E, Dawson CA, et al. A therapeutic combination of two small molecule toxin inhibitors provides broad preclinical efficacy against viper snakebite. Nat Commun. 2020;15;11(1):6094. Erratum in: Nat Commun.
6. Xie C, Slagboom J, Albulescu LO, Somsen GW, Vonk FJ, Casewell NR, et al. Neutralising effects of small molecule toxin inhibitors on nanofractionated coagulopathic Crotalinae snake venoms. Acta Pharm Sin B. 2020;10(10):1835-45.
7. Snakebite in India [Internet]. World Health Organization; 2020 [cited 2023 Dec 6]. Available from: https://www.who.int/india/health-topics/snakebite South-East Asia.
8. Fairly NH. Criteria for determining the efficacy of ligatures in snakebite. Med J Aust. 1929;1: 377-94.
9. Pugh RN, Theakston RD. Fatality following use of a tourniquet after viper bite envenoming. Ann Trop Med Parasitol. 1987;81(1):77-8.
10. Bush SP. Snakebite suction devices don't remove venom: they just suck. Ann Emerg Med. 2004;43(2):181-6.
11. Davidson TM. Sam splint for wrap and immobilisation of snakebite. J Wilderness Med. 2001;12:206-7.
12. Agarwal R, Aggarwal AN, Gupta D, Behera D, Jindal SK. Low dose of snake antivenom is as effective as high dose in patients with severe neurotoxic snake envenoming. Emerg Med J. 2005;22(6):397-9.

CHAPTER 106

# Dog Bite

*Pasang Lahmu Sherpa*

## INTRODUCTION

Humans have bonded with canines for centuries and are considered as a human's best companion. Dogs lessen their worries and make them feel safer. Though this is mutually beneficial, at the same time there is also a risk of being in the vicinity for aggressive encounters leading to a potential risk of transmission of infectious disease.

The sequelae of dog bite are always focused on rabies, but other recognized sequelae are often neglected. These range from local wound infection, disfigurement, anxiety, lifetime fear and anxiety from interaction with dogs, and post-traumatic stress disorder (PTSD).

## AT-RISK POPULATION FOR DOG BITE

- *Children*: Due to their smaller size and less capacity to respond to the circumstances, majority of the dog bite occurs in children. They sustain deep wounds rather than superficial scratches or lacerations and are more often on the head and neck, with death perhaps as a result of damage to vital vessels and the child's fragile skull structure.
- *Adults*: They are more commonly bitten on the extremities, either the hands or lower limbs.

## TYPES OF BITE WOUNDS

- *Single-bite wounds*: Most recorded dog-related incidents result in a single wound.
- *Multiple wounds*: Several lacerated wounds **(Fig. 1)**

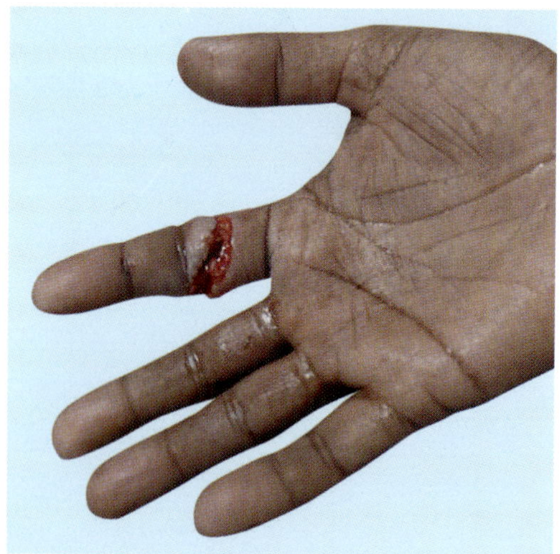

**FIG. 1:** Lacerated wound.

Bite locations are key considerations for disease transmission and clinical progression.

## COMPLICATIONS OF DOG BITE

The most dreaded complication of dog bite is rabies. Dogs are the main source of human rabies, contributing 99% of all rabies transmission to humans. Apart from this fatal disease, dogs can transmit other infections and lead to various postbite sequelae, which are often neglected.

### Rabies

Rabies is a vaccine-preventable, zoonotic viral disease which occurs in more than 150 countries and territories. In up to 99% of cases, domestic dogs are responsible for rabies virus (RABV) transmission to humans. 40% of people bitten by suspected rabid animals are children under 15 years of age. It is 100% fatal once clinical symptoms develop.

- *Modes of transmission*: Rabies is almost always transmitted through the bite or scratches of a rabid dog. Transmission can also occur if the saliva of infected animals comes into direct contact with human mucosa or fresh skin wounds. Contraction of rabies through inhalation of virus-containing aerosols or through transplantation of infected organs is described, but extremely rare. Human-to-human transmission through bites or saliva is theoretically possible but has never been confirmed. Transmission to humans via consumption of raw meat or milk of infected animals has not been confirmed till now.
- *Incubation period*: Depending on the location of bite and viral load, the incubation period for rabies is typically 2–3 months but may vary from 1 week to 1 year.
- *Symptoms*: Rabies presents with a wide variety of clinical manifestations that vary depending on multiple factors, many of which remain unknown. Initial symptoms include the following:
  - Fever
  - Pain and unusual tingling sensation at the site of bite
  - Pricking and burning sensation at the wound site
  - Other symptoms include malaise, headache, chills, pharyngitis, anorexia, diarrhea, and vomiting.
  - As the virus spreads to the central nervous system, progressive and fatal inflammation of the brain and spinal cord develops. It frequently presents with classical hydrophobia and aerophobia.
  - Two forms of rabies can manifest, namely encephalitic (furious or classical) and paralytic rabies.
    - *Furious form:* Two-thirds of human rabies cases manifest as a furious form, characterized by hyperactivity, excitable behavior, hydrophobia (fear of water), and sometimes aerophobia (fear of drafts or fresh air). Death occurs after a few days due to cardiorespiratory arrest.
    - *Paralytic form*: One-third of rabies cases present as a paralytic form. The patient develops muscle weakness and becomes paralyzed. He/she is relatively quiet and has headache and fever with muscle weakness from the onset of the disease. Coma develops slowly and eventually the patient succumbs to death.

#### *World Health Organization Exposure Categories*

The World Health Organization (WHO) categorizes RABV exposures based on relative risks, matched to a prophylaxis paradigm.

- *Category I*: It includes contact but non-RABV exposure, such as licks on intact skin or touching an animal determined to be rabid (without any break in the skin).
- *Category II*: It includes nibbling of uncovered skin, minor scratches, or

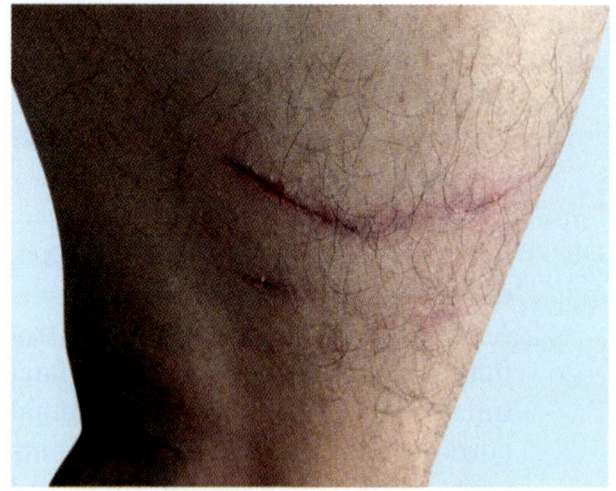

**FIG. 2:** Scratch marks from a rabid animal.

abrasions without bleeding (exposure) from rabid animals.

- *Category III*: Single or multiple transdermal bites or scratches with bleeding, contamination of mucous membrane or broken skin with saliva from animal licks, plus all types of bites from a rabid animal **(Figs. 1 and 2)**.

The proposal for a fourth category (*Category IV*) has been initiated for those exposures and bites occurring in areas of high neural density such as the face and severe exposure over the head and neck. These areas are very close to the brain and pose the greatest risk of progression of disease (shortest incubation period < 1 week) even before receiving proper intervention and treatment.

### *Treatment of Rabies*

It is important to clarify that there is no effective curative treatment against rabies once clinical signs have appeared.

The administration of rabies immunoglobulin is no longer recommended in a clinically established case as these immunoglobulins do not cross the blood–brain barrier. Treatment should have a palliative approach to administer deep sedation and avoid intubation or life-support measures. A combination of sedation and analgesia by opioids and benzodiazepines is useful to treat agitation and muscle spasms, while haloperidol is recommended to treat restlessness, agitation, hallucinations, and aggressiveness. In the case of excessive salivation, anticholinergics such as scopolamine are useful.

### *Postexposure Prophylaxis for Dog Bite*

Once clinical symptoms appear, rabies is virtually 100% fatal.

So, postexposure prophylaxis (PEP) plays a pivotal role in preventing the entry of virus into the central nervous system and death.

This first-aid measure includes immediate and thorough flushing and washing of the wound for a minimum of 15 minutes with soap and water, detergent, povidone, and iodine.

- *Category I*: Washing of exposed skin surfaces, no PEP
- *Category II*: Wound washing and immediate vaccination
- *Category III*: Wound washing, immediate vaccination, and administration of rabies immunoglobulin

### *Treatment of Wound*

Apart from thorough washing of wound, prophylaxis for tetanus and rabies is indicated for all Category II and III bites, although tetanus following a dog bite is extremely rare. The basic treatment includes wound irrigation, debridement, and presumptive antibiotics in high-risk cases.

Infiltration of human rabies immunoglobulin (HRIG) around the wound for Category III exposure is of utmost importance and should be done if anatomically feasible and at the earliest at the dose of 20 IU/kg. The remaining RIG should be injected at an intramuscular (IM) site distant from that of vaccine inoculation. It takes some time for active immunity to be triggered by vaccines; thus passive immunization with RIG can neutralize the RABV, while the active immune response develops. The rabies vaccine and

RIG combination can almost wholly prevent disease development as soon as possible. The available RIG used in treatment is mainly related to equine rabies immunoglobulin (ERIG) and HRIG derived from the serum of immunized humans.

Rabies monoclonal antibodies (mAbs) can be the best choice in rabies PEP as the supply of RIG is limited due to its cost, supply, and safety. It has broad application prospects with the advantages of high neutralizing activity, strong specificity to the corresponding target, easy to standardize production, and so on.

### *Vaccination*

Two types of vaccines are available: Nerve tissue and cell culture vaccines. The WHO recommends the replacement of nerve tissue vaccines with more efficacious, safer vaccines developed through cell culture as soon as possible.

The standard route of administration is IM. However, the intradermal route is an acceptable alternative as it is equally safe and immunogenic as the IM route and is cost-effective for developing countries as it requires less amount for both pre-exposure prophylaxis and PEP. This alternative should thus be considered in settings constrained by cost and/or supply issues.

*Pre-exposure prophylaxis* is recommended for anyone at continual, frequent, or increased risk of exposure to RABV, either by nature of their residence or occupation like veterinarians, veterinary students, and laboratory members working with samples and specimens considered high risk for rabies. The Centers for Disease Control and Prevention (CDC) and WHO recommend two doses of cell-cultured vaccines intramuscularly or intradermally on day 0 and day 3.

Periodic booster injections are recommended as an extra precaution only for people whose occupation puts them at continual or frequent risk of exposure. If available, antibody monitoring of personnel at risk is preferred to the administration of routine boosters.

The current WHO recommended guidelines for rabies PEP in an unimmunized individual in order of preference include the following:

- Two-site intradermal vaccine on days 0, 3, and 7
- One-site IM vaccine on days 0, 3, and 7 and the fourth dose between days 14 and 28
- Two-site IM vaccine on day 0 and one site on days 7 and 21

In a previously immunized individual: 1 mL × 2 doses on days 0 and 3

## Bacterial Infections

Dog bite-related disease bacterial transmission is underreported. Most of the oral flora of dogs have the potential to be pathogenic; >100 species of bacteria have been isolated from bacterial infection of dog bites.

*Incubation period* for bacterial infection of wounds: 7–10 days

### *Microbial Agents Accounted*

- Polymicrobial with a combination of aerobic and anaerobic bacteria
- The three most common microbial organisms detected were *Pasteurella*, *Staphylococcus*, and *Streptococcus*.
- Only 2% of dog bite wounds contained *Capnocytophaga canimorsus*.

### *Clinical Features*

- Pain and burning sensation at the site of bite
- Wound can be purulent without abscess formation
- Cellulitis
- Lymphangitis
- Septicemia in neglected cases
- Severe disfigurement and death due to lack of initial treatment

### *Treatment*

Most of the pathogens are susceptible to penicillin with clavulanate or doxycycline.

### Post-traumatic Stress Disorder

More than 50% of children showed evidence of complete or partial PTSD 1 month after sustaining injuries from an aggressive dog–human encounter. Younger children are at higher risk of developing PTSD symptomatology.

### Other Manifestations

- Emotional distress and anxiety
- Increased fear of dogs or unknown situation
- Nightmares

## CLINICAL PEARLS

Dog bite is one of the important problems in our community. It is critical that community members be encouraged to report and seek medical attention for any injury sustained that breaks the skin. Timely PEP saves a life.

The long-term impact of dog bites such as permanent scarring and disfigurement, infection, and pain is important; other sequelae such as post-traumatic stress or anxiety should not be overlooked.

## FURTHER READINGS

1. Gilchrist J, Sacks JJ, White D, Kresnow MJ. Dog bites: still a problem? Inj Prev. 2008;14(5): 296-301.
2. Rothe K, Tsokos M, Handrick W. Animal and human bite wounds. Dtsch Arztebl Int. 2015;112(25):433-42.
3. Griego RD, Rosen T, Orengo IF, Wolf JE. Dog, cat, and human bites: a review. J Am Acad Dermatol. 1995;33(6):1019-29.
4. McDermitt BA, Romanchak NL, Ponte CD. The management of dog bites. J Pharm Technol. 2002:18(2):63-9.
5. Both L, Banyard AC, van Dolleweerd C, Horton DL, Ma JK, Fooks AR. Passive immunity in the prevention of rabies. Lancet Infect Dis. 2012;12(5):397-407.
6. Carrieri ML, Peixoto ZM, Paciencia ML, Kotait I, Germano PM. Laboratory diagnosis of equine rabies and its implications for human postexposure prophylaxis. J Virol Methods. 2006;138(1-2):1-9.
7. de Kruif J, Bakker AB, Marissen WE, Kramer RA, Throsby M, Rupprecht CE, et al. A human monoclonal antibody cocktail as a novel component of rabies postexposure prophylaxis. Annu Rev Med. 2007;58:359-68.
8. De Benedictis P, Minola A, Rota Nodari E, Aiello R, Zecchin B, Salomoni A, et al. Development of broad-spectrum human monoclonal antibodies for rabies post-exposure prophylaxis. EMBO Mol Med. 2016;8(4):407-21.
9. World Health Organization. (2018). Rabies vaccines and immunoglobulins: WHO position. [online] Available from https://www.who.int/publications-detail-redirect/WHO-CDS-NTD-NZD-2018.04. [Last accessed September, 2023].
10. Talan DA, Citron DM, Abrahamian FM, Moran GJ, Goldstein EJC. Bacteriologic analysis of infected dog and cat bites. Emergency Medicine Animal Bite Infection Study Group. N Engl J Med. 1999;340(2):85-92.
11. Abrahamian FM, Goldstein EJC. Microbiology of animal bite wound infections. Clin Microbiol Rev. 2011;24(2):231-46.
12. Goldstein EJC. Management of human and animal bite wounds. J Am Acad Dermatol. 1989;21(6):1275-9.
13. Peters V, Sottiaux M, Appelboom J, Kahn A. Posttraumatic stress disorder after dog bites in children. J Pediatr. 2004;144(1):121-2.

CHAPTER 107

# Drowning

*Pasang Lahmu Sherpa*

## INTRODUCTION

Drowning is a serious and neglected public health threat and a major global health problem. It is a leading cause of death worldwide, particularly in low- and middle-income countries. Evidence shows that a range of interventions are effective at preventing drowning.

Drowning is one of the most important causes of death of children and young people in every region of the world, with children aged under 5 years disproportionately at risk and males twice as likely to drown as females.

## DEFINITION

Drowning is defined as the process of experiencing respiratory impairment from submersion or immersion in liquid.

## RISK FACTORS ASSOCIATED WITH DROWNING

Most instances of fatal drowning occur alone or in situations where the people surrounding the victim are either unaware of the victim's situation or unable to offer assistance.

The place of drowning (e.g., swimming pool, river, ocean) is an important consideration which informs prevention efforts as the populations and circumstances of different water sites vary. In most countries, unintentional drowning occurs more frequently at natural water sites, compared to pools or bathtubs.

### Age

Age is an important risk factor for drowning as per the global report on drowning and the risk is highest among children between 1 and 4 years of age. In South India, nearly 90% of drowning deaths among children aged 1–12 years involved water in a pot, well, or pond.

### Gender

Males are especially at risk of drowning, with twice the overall mortality rate of females. They are more likely to be hospitalized than females for nonfatal drowning. Studies suggest that the higher drowning rates among males are due to increased exposure to water and riskier behavior such as swimming alone, drinking alcohol before swimming alone, and boating.

### Access to Water

Drowning is common when access to water is easy without any standard safety measures and equipment. In Bangladesh, a national survey found that 80% of drowning among children aged under 5 years happened within

20 m of the family home—mainly in ponds, followed by ditches and water containers. Older children and adults drown further away from home, typically in natural water bodies, often while working, traveling, or collecting water.

### Other Risk Factors Associated with Drowning

- Occupation oriented near water like commercial fishing or fishing for subsistence using small boats in low-income countries are more prone to drowning. Small-scale fishing is estimated to employ around 37 million people worldwide—around 90% are in Asia.
- *Residing near water*: In low- and middle-income countries, many people settle near lakes or river banks and some are built over the water—and this, along with poor flood disaster protection, puts local people at greater risk.
- Lack of barriers or signs around water hazards such as unsafe crossings, open wells, uncovered manholes and ditches in low- and middle-income countries poses a risk.
- *Traveling on water*: Daily commuting and journeys on overcrowded and unsafe vessels that lack safety equipment or those operated by personnel not trained to deal with transport incidents.
- *Flood disasters*: The number of people exposed to hazards is rising with the increased frequency and severity of flood disasters and unplanned urbanization. Drowning risks increase with floods, particularly in low- and middle-income countries where people live in flood-prone areas and the ability to warn, evacuate, or protect communities from floods is weak or only just developing.
- Other risk factors are as follows:
  - A person under the influence of alcohol or drugs is at an increased risk of drowning.
  - Infants if left unattended or alone in water
  - Medical conditions, such as epilepsy
  - Tourists unfamiliar with local water risks and features

## PATHOPHYSIOLOGY

Following aspiration, intense laryngospasm is triggered by the presence of fluid in the oropharynx or larynx causing hypoxia and carbon dioxide retention. As the oxygen tension in the blood drops further, laryngospasm releases and the victim gasps and hyperventilates, further aspirating more liquid. This further leads to hypoxia.

In freshwater drowning, water being hypotonic compared to plasma, the water moves across the alveolar-capillary membrane into the microcirculation causing disruption of alveolar surfactant. Saltwater being hyperosmolar increases the osmotic gradient and draws fluid into alveoli, diluting surfactant. Protein-rich fluid exudates and collects into the alveoli reducing lung compliance due to damage of the alveolar-capillary membrane and shunting occurs, resulting in acute lung injury and acute respiratory distress syndrome (ARDS)-like syndrome. A high proportion of drowning patients are hypoxic and have an arterial partial pressure of oxygen ($PaO_2$)/fraction of inspired oxygen ($FiO_2$) ratio < 300 mm Hg. Hypoxia and subsequent acidosis are the most important contributing factors to increased mortality and morbidity from drowning.

Depending on the degree of hypoxemia and the resultant acidotic changes in acid-base balance, the person may develop myocardial dysfunction and electrical instability, cardiac arrest, and central nervous system (CNS) ischemia.

Large volumes of fluid aspiration are required to cause alteration in blood volume (11 mL/kg) and significant electrolyte imbalance (22 mL/kg). CNS damage can occur due to hypoxemia resulting in arrhythmia, ongoing pulmonary injury, and multiorgan dysfunction.

# CLINICAL FEATURES

## History

It is very important to evaluate the circumstances around the submersion. The classical history of drowning may not be obvious in many cases. Many patients are found submerged in water for a prolonged period. Drowning in most of the circumstances is accidental, especially in young children, when they are left unobserved near a pool, bathtub, or other natural water sources. The relevant factors that need to be considered are the age of the victim, submersion time, water temperature, water tonicity (freshwater or saltwater), degree of water contamination, interval time between rescue and resuscitation, underlying medical condition, and the possibility of alcohol or drug use by the victim.

## Clinical Examination

Symptoms could be persistent cough, wheezing, shortness of breath, disorientation, and variable level of consciousness due to hypoxia and vomiting.

Any signs of injuries such as trauma to the head and spine should be carefully examined for.

A drowning victim may be classified into four groups:

1. *Asymptomatic*: If the submersion is for a very short duration of few seconds with immediate resuscitation, the victim is likely to be asymptomatic.
2. *Symptomatic*: Cough, wheezing, hypothermia, tachycardia or bradycardia (vagal stimulation), tachypnea, dyspnea or hypoxia, vomiting, diarrhea, metabolic acidosis, altered level of consciousness, neurological deficit
3. *Cardiopulmonary arrest*: Apnea, asystole, ventricular tachycardia or fibrillation, bradycardia, immersion syndrome
4. Death

# COMPLICATIONS

Lung is the target organ in drowning. Aspiration of as little as 1–3 mL/kg of fluid can lead to significant impairment in gas exchange. The manifestations are as follows:

- *Pulmonary*:
  - Acute lung injury and ARDS
  - Chemical pneumonitis
  - Pneumonia involving organisms such as *Aeromonas*, *Burkholderia*, and *Pseudallescheria*
- *Cardiovascular*:
  - Ventricular tachycardia/fibrillation
  - Bradycardia
  - Asystole
- *CNS*:
  - Altered sensorium
  - Unconsciousness, coma
- *Others*:
  - Head trauma
  - Cervical spine injury
  - Baric injury including air embolism
- Death

# MANAGEMENT OF DROWNING

## Prehospital Care

- Call for emergency service.
- Rapid rescue and resuscitation should be done by any person witnessing the event. The victim should be removed from the water at the earliest opportunity.
- Make the victim lie on the nearest flat surface and start rescue breathing as well as chest compression at the same time.
- If any injury is suspected, then move the victim the least as possible and start cardiopulmonary resuscitation (CPR).

- Clear airways and check for any foreign bodies. Ensure airway, breathing, and circulation (ABC).
- Transport the victim to the nearest hospital for further management.

## Hospital Care

- Provide supplemental oxygen with $FiO_2$ 100%.
- If the patient is still dyspneic or oxygen saturation is still low 100% oxygen, use continuous positive airway pressure (CPAP) if available.
- If CPAP is required and not available, then intubate the patient with adequate positive end-expiratory pressure (PEEP).
- Careful physical examination for any kind of injuries like head trauma and spinal injuries
- The victim may be unconscious due to the direct effect of drowning like hypoxemia or due to the indirect effect as a result of injuries.
- Immediate blood test like complete blood count (CBC), blood sugar, electrolyte levels, lactate levels, arterial blood gas (ABG) analysis, liver function test, and renal function test. Consider a blood alcohol level and urine toxicology screen for use of drugs.
- Chest radiography to detect evidence of aspiration, pulmonary edema, segmental atelectasis due to the presence of any foreign bodies (silt or sand).
- Electrocardiography (ECG) to see if there is significant tachycardia, significant bradycardia, ventricular arrhythmias.
- Computed tomography/magnetic resonance imaging (CT/MRI) in individuals with head or spinal injuries

Management of hypoxemia is key to the management of drowning.

## Noninvasive Ventilation

The earliest report of successful use of noninvasive ventilation (NIV) dates from 1982, where 11 patients were successfully treated with CPAP.

In alert, awake, and cooperative patients, a trial of bilevel positive airway pressure (BiPAP)/CPAP is to be used to provide oxygenation before intubation is warranted.

## Mechanical Ventilation

Early intubation and mechanical ventilation may be indicated in patients who are unable to maintain adequate oxygenation via mask or CPAP or in whom airway protection is warranted.

Mechanical intubation is also indicated in patients with a decreased conscious state or cardiac arrest. The idea is to decrease ventilator-associated lung injury, and this has led to the use of a terminology known as lung protective ventilation (LPV). This practice is currently advocated for the treatment of drowning patients.

*Extracorporeal membrane oxygenation (ECMO)*: It has been beneficial in selected patients. It may be considered in patients with a lack of response to conventional mechanical ventilation or patients with persistent hypothermia with cold water drowning.

## Others

### *Treatment of Volume Depletion and Acidosis*

Due to ingestion of large volumes of fresh or saltwater, hyponatremia and hypernatremia can occur. Rapid volume expansion may be indicated using isotonic crystalloids (20 mL/kg) or colloids. Inotropic support may be required using dopamine or dobutamine.

Mild acidosis is usually corrected after correction of hypoxemia and volume restoration.

### *Therapeutic Hypothermia*

Current recommendations propose maintaining a core temperature of 32–34°C for

12–72 hours. Newer literature suggests that therapeutic hypothermia improves oxygen supply to ischemic brain areas, decreases cerebral metabolic demand, and reduces increased intracranial pressure.

### *Treatment of Cold Water Drowning*

As per the recommendation made by the panel of experts at the 2002 World Congress on Drowning, the highest priority is restoration of spontaneous circulation followed by subsequent and continuous monitoring of core or brain (tympanic) temperature. Core temperature should not be above 34°C; if so, then hypothermia should be achieved as soon as possible for 12–24 hours.

### *Prophylactic Antibiotics*

Some studies have compared the outcome of prophylactic use of antibiotics versus no antibiotic and found that the mortality rate was 7.4% versus 5.6% successively among the consecutive group. Two more studies reported no improvement from the use of prophylactic antibiotics without including outcome data.

### *Prophylactic Steroids*

The outcomes reported from seven papers for prophylactic steroids showed no benefit. Studies have shown that the mortality rates were much lower in patients not treated with prophylactic antibiotics.

### *Prophylactic Diuretics*

No clinical benefit was observed with the prophylactic use of diuretics.

## PREVENTIVE MEASURES

Drowning can be prevented with simple safety measures. Adult supervision is essential in the prevention of drowning. Preventable strategies such as teaching basic swimming and water safety skills, adopting pool fencing, close supervision, and providing water safety gears and equipment can be adopted. Public awareness regarding the risks associated with natural water and educating them to avoid alcohol while swimming are recommended.

## CLINICAL PEARLS

Drowning is a major cause of preventable death and morbidity worldwide. The mechanism of injury involves inhalation of water, lung injury, and hypoxia. The duration of immersion is important in ascertaining the clinical outcome.

Treating this lung injury and reversing the hypoxia are the cornerstone of the management of drowning.

Since there are no definitive guidelines pertaining to treatment and management of drowning, this calls for an urgent need for high-quality research on the treatment of drowning. Until and unless specific guidelines are published in treating drowning victims, prevention becomes the most effective strategy in reducing drowning mortality. It is equally necessary to train common people to give CPR as learning this skill could save someone's life.

## FURTHER READINGS

1. Idris AH, Bierens J, Perkins GD, Wenzel V, Nadkarni V, Morley P, et al. 2015 revised Utstein-style recommended guidelines for uniform reporting of data from drowning-related resuscitation: an ILCOR advisory statement. Circ Cardiovasc Qual Outcomes. 2017;10(7): e000024.
2. World Health Organization. Global report on drowning: preventing a leading killer. Geneva: World Health Organization; 2014. [online] Available from https://www.who.int/publications/i/item/global-report-on-drowning-preventing-a-leading-killer. [Last accessed September, 2023].

3. Branche C, van Beeck E. The epidemiology of drowning: summary and recommendations. In: Bierens J (Ed). Drowning: Prevention, Rescue Treatment, 2nd edition. Berlin; New York: Springer; 2014. pp. 81-3.
4. Lin CY, Wang YF, Lu TH, Kawach I. Unintentional drowning mortality, by age and body of water: an analysis of 60 countries. Inj Prev. 2015;21(e1):e43-50.
5. Bose A, George K, Joseph A. Drowning in childhood: a population based study. Indian Pediatr. 2000;37:80-3.
6. Bierens JJLM, Lunetta P, Tipton M, Warner DS. Physiology of drowning: a review. Physiology (Bethesda). 2016;31:147-66.
7. Gregorakos L, Markou N, Psalida V, Kanakaki M, Alexopoulou A, Sotiriou E, et al. Near-drowning: clinical course of lung injury in adults. Lung. 2009;187:93-7.
8. Lee KH. A retrospective study of near-drowning victims admitted to the intensive care unit. Ann Acad Med Singap. 1998;27:344-6.
9. Szpilman D, Bierens JJ, Handley AJ, Orlowski JP. Drowning. N Engl J Med. 2012;366:2102-10.
10. Dick AE, Potgieter PD. Secondary drowning in the Cape Peninsula. S Afr Med J. 1982;62:803-6.
11. Michelet P, Bouzana F, Charmensat O, Tiger F, Durand-Gasselin J, Hraiech S, et al. Acute respiratory failure after drowning: a retrospective multicenter survey. Eur J Emerg Med. 2017;24:295-300.
12. Saidel-Odes LR, Almog Y. Near-drowning in the Dead Sea: a retrospective observational analysis of 69 patients. Isr Med Assoc J. 2003;5: 856-8.
13. Kotsiou O, Pasparaki E, Bibaki E, Damianaki A, Kotsios V, Ntaoukakis E, et al. Drowning and near drowning victims in Chania area. Pneumon. 2014;27:231-5.
14. Schmidt AC, Sempsrott JR, Hawkins SC, Arastu AS, Cushing TA, Auerbach PS. Wilderness medical society practice guidelines for the prevention and treatment of drowning. Wilderness Environ Med. 2016;27:236-51.
15. Kim KI, Lee WY, Kim HS, Jeong JH, Ko HH. Extracorporeal membrane oxygenation in near-drowning patients with cardiac or pulmonary failure. Scand J Trauma Resusc Emerg Med. 2014;22:77.
16. Topjian AA, Berg RA, Bierens JJ, Branche CM, Clark RS, Friberg H, et al. Brain resuscitation in the drowning victim. Neurocit Care. 2012;17:441-67.
17. Warner DS, Bierens JJ, Beerman SB, Katz LM. Drowning: a cry for help. Anesthesiology. 2009;110(6):1211-3.
18. Hypothermia after Cardiac Arrest Study Group. Mild therapeutic hypothermia to improve the neurologic outcome after cardiac arrest. N Engl J Med. 2002;346(8):549-56.
19. Van Beeck EF, Branche CM, Szoilman D, Modell JH, Bierens JJ. A new definition of drowning: towards documentation and prevention of a global public health problem. Bull World Health Organ. 2005;83(11):853-6.
20. Modell JH, Graves SA, Ketover A. Clinical course of 91 consecutive near-drowning victims. Chest. 1976;70:231-8.
21. Orlowski JP. Prognostic factors in pediatric cases of drowning and near-drowning. JACEP. 1979;8:176-9.
22. van Berkel M, Bierens JJLM, Lie RLK, de Rooy TP, Kool LJ, van de Velde EA, et al. Pulmonary oedema, pneumonia and mortality in submersion victims; a retrospective study in 125 patients. Intensive Care Med. 1996;22:101-7.
23. Corbin DO, Fraser HS. A review of 98 cases of near-drowning at the Queen Elizabeth Hospital, Barbados. West Indian Med J. 1981;30:22-9.

CHAPTER 108

# Organophosphate Poisoning

*Subhra Sankar Sen, Smarajit Banik*

## INTRODUCTION

*Organophosphate* (OP) is a double-edged sword. On one hand, it is used as medicine and insecticide in many industries, and on the other hand, it is one of the most widely used poisons among mankind, especially in countries such as *India*, where *agriculture* still remains the main profession. *OPs* were invented in the 19th century by French chemists. They are being used since *World War II*. Around 3 million people are exposed to OP every year, among which there are about 30 lakh deaths each year.

## WHAT IS ORGANOPHOSPHATE?

*Organophosphates* are *indirect cholinergics* (*parasympathomimetics*) that act by irreversibly blocking *acetylcholinesterase* (AChE). AChE has two binding sites, one being the *esteratic site* and the other being the *anionic site*. AChE causes hydrolysis of ACh, which is bound to the anionic site. *OPs* act by forming a phosphate bond with the esteratic site while leaving behind the anionic site. But after some time, the phosphate bond is replaced by a very strong bond that is resistant to be hydrolyzed (*aging of AChE*). Thus, *OP irreversibly* blocks AChE until fresh enzymes are synthesized **(Fig. 1)**.

## WHY IS ORGANOPHOSPHATE DANGEROUS?

Organophosphate is parasympathomimetic and activates muscarinic and nicotinic receptors in our body. As they are extensively used as agricultural and household insecticide, accidental as well as suicidal and homicidal poisoning is quite common. It can enter the human body by any means, contact via intact skin, ingestion, or inhalation, and gets quickly absorbed. Local muscarinic effects occur immediately followed by systemic muscarinic and nicotinic actions.

## WHAT ARE THE CLINICAL FEATURES?

There are a number of symptoms, of which the important ones are described below:

- *Increased secretions*: Lacrimation, salivation, increased tracheobronchial secretions, sweating due to exaggerated parasympathetic effect on M3 receptors of respective glands

  However, increased gastrointestinal (GI) secretions are due to M1 receptors.
- *Miosis*: Unopposed ACh acts on the circular muscle (sphincter pupillae) of the iris and makes them contract and the pupil gets constricted. This leads to blurring of vision.

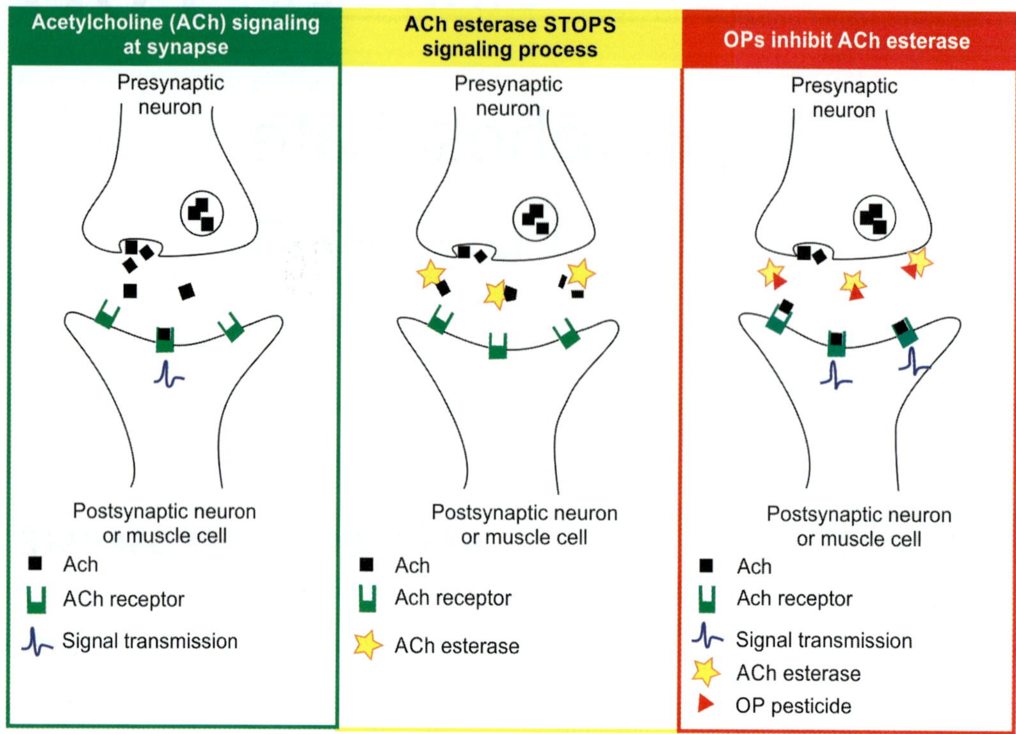


**FIG. 1:** Pathogenesis of organophosphate (OP).

- *Increased smooth muscle contraction*: This is all due to action over the M3 receptor. There is bronchoconstriction, gastrointestinal tract (GIT) contraction, detrusor contraction, and blood vessel smooth muscle contraction. These lead to a list of symptoms such as breathlessness, colic, and involuntary defecation and urination.
- *Cardiovascular*: Although there is blood vessel smooth muscle contraction, the overall effect is vasodilation due to endothelial nitric oxide synthase (eNOS) action on endothelium, which also gets stimulated via M3 receptors but in a different way by increasing calcium in endothelium. So, there is a fall in blood pressure (BP). Also, there is bradycardia, mediated by the M2 receptor.
- *Others*: Muscular fasciculations (nicotinic receptor), weakness, respiratory paralysis, irritability, disorientation, tremor, ataxia, convulsion. Death is due to respiratory failure.

## INTERMEDIATE SYNDROME

*Intermediate syndrome* (IMS) is characterized by weakness of the respiratory, neck, and proximal limb muscles. It neither appears immediately after OP exposure like the cholinergic symptoms nor is delayed as OP-induced postponed neuropathy (OPIPN). It normally appears 2–4 days after presentation when cholinergic symptoms tend to disappear.

Intermediate syndrome involves the diaphragm, intercostal muscles, neck muscles, and proximal limb muscles. Symptoms range from weakness of neck and proximal limb muscles to severe breathing difficulties, sometimes even requiring ventilator support.

Pathogenesis of IMS still remains to be unknown. But the theory of delayed release of OP from tissues and blocking of AChE has been proposed. Some suggested that it is due to the damaged pre- and postsynaptic neuron. Others found it to be muscular damage and downregulation of ACh receptors. While some experts suggested it is due to interrupted energy metabolism and calcium homeostasis, the exact pathogenesis is yet to be established.

## TREATMENT

The treatment must be started as soon as possible. It should begin with decontamination; in case of exposure to skin or mucosa, it should be washed off under running tap water and soap and the clothes should be discarded, while in case of ingestion, gastric lavage must be done if presented within 30 minutes. Charcoal can also be tried **(Fig. 2)**.

Airway should be maintained and positive pressure ventilation (PPV) should be given if needed.

Supportive measures include maintaining the BP, properly hydrating the patient, and using *diazepam* cautiously.

*Antidote of OP poisoning is atropine.* Being an anticholinergic, it counteracts the muscarinic effect of ACh. But it does not reverse muscle paralysis, which is a nicotinic action. Atropine is given at a dose of 1–3 mg intravenously (IV), doubling the dose at a regular 5-minute interval until dryness of mouth and other signs of atropinization appear. The most reliable signs are the *dilatation of pupil* and *drying of respiratory secretions.*

Up to 200 mg/day can be administered safely.

After using such a large dose of atropine, there can be psychosis in a patient. In that case, *haloperidol* can be used as treatment.

*Cholinesterase reactivator* can also be used in the treatment of OP poisoning. *Oximes* are used to ameliorate the nicotinic symptoms. *Oximes* being a positively charged molecule (having quaternary nitrogen), if administered before the *aging* of *AChE*, bind to an unoccupied anionic site of the enzyme, break the $PO_4$ bonds of OP with AChE, and render the enzyme free to act with ACh so that the excess ACh can be destroyed. Thus, the nicotinic symptoms improve.

In *India*, *pralidoxime* (2-PAM) is the most commonly used *oxime*. PAM is injected intravenously slowly at a dose of 1–2 g. Alternatively, it can be used as a loading dose of 30 mg/kg IV followed by 8–10 mg/kg/h. *Pralidoxime* has no effect on the central nervous system (CNS) symptoms as it does not penetrate the blood–brain barrier. Lower doses according to the symptoms are continued till 1–2 weeks.

Other oximes are *diacetyl-monoxime* (DAM) and *obidoxime.*

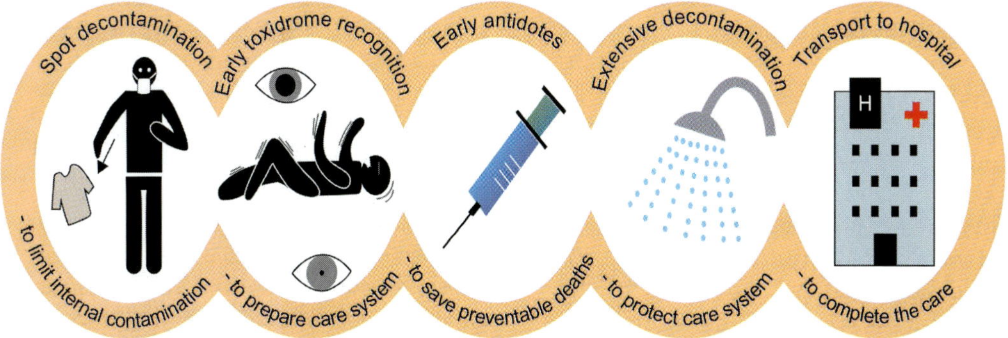


**FIG. 2:** Treatment of organophosphate (OP) poisoning in a nutshell.

## CLINICAL PEARLS

- Organophosphorus compounds are extensively used as insectisides at comprise the most common poisons used.
- They are parasympathomimetic compounds and should strongly be suspected iff patient presents with pinpointpupils , bradycardia , increased expectoration and chest crepitation.

## FURTHER READINGS

1. Sikary AK. Homicidal poisoning in India: a short review. J Forensic Leg Med. 2019;61:13-6.
2. Chen KX, Zhou XH, Sun CA, Yan PX. Manifestations of and risk factors for acute myocardial injury after acute organophosphorus pesticide poisoning. Medicine (Baltimore). 2019;98(6): e14371.
3. Peter JV, Sudarsan TI, Moran JL. Clinical features of organophosphate poisoning: a review of different classification systems and approaches. Indian J Crit Care Med. 2014;18(11):735-45.
4. Roberts D, Buckley NA. Alkalinisation for organophosphorus pesticide poisoning. Cochrane Database Syst Rev. 2005;2010(1): CD004897.
5. Peter JV, Moran JL, Graham P. Oxime therapy and outcomes in human organophosphate poisoning: an evaluation using meta-analytic techniques. Crit Care Med. 2006;34(2):502-10.

CHAPTER 109

# Paraquat Poisoning

*Uttam Kumar Nath*

## DEFINITION/INTRODUCTION

Paraquat (PQ) is a fast-acting, nonselective herbicide that kills green plant tissue on contact and through translocation inside the plant. Despite being employed on big and small farms, plantations, estates, and in non-agricultural weed control, it is extremely harmful to humans.

## PATHOGENESIS

Paraquat is metabolized by several enzyme systems. It prevents the conversion of NADP to NADPH, resulting in increased generation of ROS and nitrites. PQ also releases free-form iron from ferritin, which increases ROS generation. The highly reactive oxygen and nitrite species induce toxicity in numerous organs, but it is especially severe in the lungs because PQ is absorbed against a concentration gradient. In vitro, animal, and human research have shown that PQ can cause lipid peroxidation. Lipid peroxidation disrupts cell membrane function and may cause apoptosis. PQ is taken up against a concentration gradient into the lung, causing inflammation, leukocyte recruitment, and late pulmonary fibrosis, ultimately leading to hypoxemia.

## CLINICAL COURSE

Symptoms and signs depend upon the quantity ingested. Acute PQ intoxication is usually asymptomatic in the early stage. Irritation and numbness of the tongue and oral mucosa are generally the only symptoms in most cases within the first few days. Shortness of breath, tachypnea, lethargy, and confusion appear within 3–4 days as the lung injury progresses **(Table 1)**.

Hiccups generally occur when the ingestion amount is >100 mL. Confusion is usually accompanied by death within a few days. An acute alveolitis develops over 1–3 days followed by a secondary fibrosis. A patient typically develops increasing signs of respiratory involvement over 3–7 days and ultimately dies of severe anoxia due to rapidly progressive fibrosis up to 5 weeks later.

The incidence of acute kidney injury (AKI) secondary to PQ intoxication is approximately 50% and is usually normalized within 3 weeks.

## HOW TO MANAGE?

### Investigations

*Bicarbonate and sodium dithionite urine test*: It is a semi-quantitative bedside test to confirm systemic PQ toxicity.

**Table 1: Main symptoms and signs of acute PQ intoxication, according to the severity of intoxication.**

| *Severity of intoxication* | *Ingested amount (mL)* | *Symptoms* | *Signs* |
|---|---|---|---|
| Mild | <10 | No specific symptom | No specific sign |
| Moderate | 10–40 | • Sore tongue<br>• Shortness of breath<br>• Agitation<br>• Abdominal discomfort<br>• Head-lightness | • Tachypnea<br>• Tachycardia<br>• Increased serum creatinine<br>• Oral mucosa necrosis ("paraquat tongue") |
| Severe | >40 | • Sore tongue<br>• Shortness of breath<br>• Hiccup<br>• Agitation<br>• Confusion | • Tachypnea, tachycardia<br>• Increased serum creatinine<br>• Oral mucosa necrosis<br>• Jaundice |

*Plasma PQ concentration*: It is useful to both confirm poisoning and predict prognosis.

Serum electrolyte, renal and liver function tests, and full blood count should be done at least daily. Serum amylase and lipase should be done if patients develop abdominal pain and a raised blood sugar.

A chest radiograph should be performed if pneumomediastinum, pneumothorax, or lung fibrosis is suspected. But a simple chest radiograph has poor sensitivity and specificity for evaluating PQ-induced lung injury and a high-resolution computed tomography (HRCT) of the lungs on day 7 post-PQ ingestion may be useful in detecting early lung fibrosis or assessing long-term damage in survivors.

## Therapy

### *Medical Management*

There is no specific treatment. Resuscitation starts with the assessment and management of airway, breathing, and circulation. Mild-to-moderate hypoxia should not be routinely treated with oxygen as it will worsen oxidative stress. Hypotension is generally treated with boluses of fluids (15–20 mL/kg over 15–30 minutes) repeated as necessary. Close monitoring of fluid balance is required as renal failure commonly occurs over the first 24 hours.

#### Gastric Lavage

Gastric lavage followed by a dose of activated charcoal has been recommended for consenting patients who present within 1 hour of ingestion of PQ with a protected airway. Patients should be monitored for the development of acute renal failure, liver toxicity, respiratory failure, and mucosal injury. Early insertion of a nasogastric feeding tube is required to ensure adequate nutrition.

To relieve pain, opiates are often required. Supplementary oxygen should not be given except as a palliative measure.

#### Hemodialysis/Hemoperfusion

The reduction rate of plasma PQ levels by hemoperfusion (HP) is higher than hemodialysis (HD), but the most important consideration is starting the treatment within a few hours and the choice of method is secondary. HD could be considered in patients who have developed symptomatic acute renal failure. However, this is unlikely to change the outcome.

### *Other Treatment Options*

#### Immunosuppression

Though the clinical evidence is also very limited, the most widely studied regimen uses are cyclophosphamide, methylprednisolone, and dexamethasone.

#### Antioxidants

Several antioxidants have been investigated as possible antidotes for PQ poisoning. Human trials have been either nonexistent or insufficient, and the appropriate dose to induce this effect in humans is unclear.

*Vitamin E*: Possible processes include membrane stability of polyunsaturated fatty acids and ROS scavenging. In a human investigation, just two of nine patients receiving vitamin E (200-4,000 mg/day) survived.

Vitamin C is an antioxidant that donates an electron to free radicals, neutralizing them.

N-acetylcysteine (NAC) supplies cysteine, which is a rate-limiting factor in the synthesis of glutathione, an important antioxidant defense. NAC inhibited PQ-induced apoptosis and inflammatory responses in human lung cultures.

*Deferoxamine (DFO)*: Iron contributes significantly to the formation of ROS. However, there has been no randomized controlled study to demonstrate the efficacy of iron chelating therapy in acute PQ poisoning.

*Salicylic Acid (SA)*: In addition to its proven anti-inflammatory mechanism of inhibiting cyclooxygenase, SA exhibits a number of antioxidant properties. There have been no published human investigations thus far.

## RED FLAG SIGNS: POOR PROGNOSTIC INDICATORS

The survival rate varies according to the ingestion amount: <10 mL, almost 100%; 10–20 mL, 80–90%; 20–40 mL, 50–60%; 40–50 mL, <10%; >60 mL, <1%.

Patients who present with overt systemic toxicity on the first day [e.g., hypotension, severe hypoxia, acidosis, and low Glasgow Coma Scale (GCS)] are deadly. Renal failure, alterations on chest radiographs [ground-glass opacity (GGO) region > 50% of total lung volume is typically deadly], and gastrointestinal diseases are also poor prognostic indicators. Patients who report a "burning sensation" in their skin also have a dismal prognosis. A patient is characterized as a "survivor" if he or she survives more than three months following PQ intake with stable vital signs and lung function.

## CLINICAL PEARLS

There is no specific antidote for PQ poisoning. Relieving symptoms and treating complications are the only goals. Patients generally maintain normal levels of consciousness. Any impairment typically implies either coingestion with different chemicals (e.g., ethanol) or severe toxicity. Intensive treatment can arrest the progression of PQ lung injury in certain subgroups, despite the high death rate (80-90%).

The recommended therapeutic options include extracorporeal elimination (HP), intravenous antioxidants, fluid diuresis, and short-term cytotoxic medication treatment (e.g., steroid pulse therapy or cyclophosphamide). Early therapy is crucial, with renal protection as the primary focus.

## FURTHER READINGS

1. Moustakas M, Malea P, Zafeirakoglou A, Sperdouli I. Photochemical changes and oxidative damage in the aquatic macrophyte Cymodocea nodosa exposed to paraquat-induced oxidative stress. Pestic Biochem Physiol. 2016;126:28-34.

2. Oracz K, El-Maarouf-Bouteau H, Kranner I, Bogatek R, Corbineau F, Bailly C. The mechanisms involved in seed dormancy alleviation by hydrogen cyanide unravel the role of reactive oxygen species as key factors of cellular signaling during germination. Plant Physiol. 2009;150:494-505.
3. Gawarammana IB, Buckley NA. Medical management of paraquat ingestion. Br J Clin Pharmacol. 2021;72(5):745-57.
4. Gil H-W, Hong JR, Jang SH, Hong SY. Diagnostic and therapeutic approach for acute paraquat intoxication. J Korean Med Sci. 2014;29:1441-9.
5. Rannels DE, Kameji R, Pegg AE, Rannels SR. Spermidine uptake by type II pneumocytes: interactions of amine uptake pathways. Am J Physiol. 1989;257(Pt 1):L346-53.
6. Bus JS, Aust SD, Gibson JE. Lipid peroxidation: a possible mechanism for paraquat toxicity. Res Commun Chem Pathol Pharmacol. 1975;11:31-8.
7. Bus JS, Aust SD, Gibson JE. Paraquat toxicity: proposed mechanism of action involving lipid peroxidation. Environ Health Perspect. 1976;16:139-46.
8. Yasaka T, Ohya I, Matsumoto J, Shiramizu T, Sasaguri Y. Acceleration of lipid peroxidation in human paraquat poisoning. Arch Intern Med. 1981;141:1169-71.
9. Lee SH, Lee KS, Ahn JM, Kim SH, Hong SY. Paraquat poisoning of the lung: thin-section CT findings. Radiology. 1995;195:271-4.
10. Liu ZN, Zhao M, Zheng Q, Zhao HY, Hou WJ, Bai SL. Inhibitory effects of rosiglitazone on paraquat-induced acute lung injury in rats. Acta Pharmacol Sin. 2013;34:1317-24.
11. Cappelletti G, Maggioni MG, Maci R. Apoptosis in human lung epithelial cells: triggering by paraquat and modulation by antioxidants. Cell Biol Int. 1998;22:671-8.
12. Yeh ST, Guo HR, Su YS, Lin HJ, Hou CC, Chen HM, et al. Protective effects of N-acetylcysteine treatment post acute paraquat intoxication in rats and in human lung epithelial cells. Toxicology. 2006;223:181-90.
13. Yasaka T, Okudaira K, Fujito H, Matsumoto J, Ohya I, Miyamoto Y. Further studies of lipid peroxidation in human paraquat poisoning. Arch Intern Med. 1986;146:681-5.

CHAPTER 110

# Corrosive Poisoning

*Uttam Kumar Nath*

## DEFINITION

Corrosives are a class of compounds that destroy tissue upon contact. A wide range of chemical and physical factors can induce corrosive injuries. They include mineral and organic acids, alkalis, oxidizing agents, denaturants, certain hydrocarbons, and exothermic agents. Ingestions can be intentional, such as suicide attempts in teens and adults, or unintentional, as in most youngsters.

## WHEN TO SUSPECT?

### Clinical Clues in History and Examination

A physical examination and history should be performed to determine the caustic substance, volume, timing of admission, prehospital treatment, and cause of ingestion. Symptoms vary depending on the agent kind, quantity, and length of interaction with the tissues.

Patients may have indications of burns in the oral cavity during physical examination, however, approximately 20–45% of patients may have normal physical tests. Patients typically approach to the emergency room with a terrible burning sensation in their lips, mouth, and throat, oropharyngeal pain, hypersalivation, trouble swallowing with edema ulceration, or whitish plaques in the oral cavity, palatal mucosa, and pharynx. There may be epigastric pain and hematemesis in severe cases. Persistent chest or back pain suggests esophageal perforation and mediastinitis. One needs to suspect gastric perforation and peritonitis if there is severe abdominal pain with high temperature. These can occur after 48 hours of caustic consumption or take up to 14 days. Corrosive substance ingestion during the acute phase can produce laryngeal injury and laryngospasm, which can be accompanied by dyspnea, tachypnea, dysphonia, and aphonia. Aspiration of the caustic substance frequently results in death due to endotracheal or bronchial necrosis with mediastinitis.

## HOW TO MANAGE?

### Investigations and Treatment

#### Investigations

##### Laboratory Investigations

Laboratory testing include a full hemogram, serum electrolytes, renal function tests, liver function tests, blood grouping and crossmatching, coagulation profile, and arterial blood gas analysis.

### Radiology Investigations

Radiology tests are performed to determine the extent of the damage caused by the caustic intake.

- Chest X-rays cannot diagnose or grade injury severity, but can identify pneumothorax and pneumomediastinum abdominal.
- *X-ray*: Used to detect pneumoperitoneum. Gas under the diaphragm is indicative of an intestinal perforation.
- A computed tomography (CT) scan of the neck, chest, and abdomen is recommended when a high index of suspicion for perforation persists despite negative plain X-rays.
- Upper gastrointestinal (UGI) endoscopy, particularly flexible esophagoscopy, is the most efficient tool for visualizing the degree of esophageal injury and should be done in the first 24–48 hours following caustic ingestion in patients without perforation.

## Treatment

### Emergency Treatment

The initial objective is to keep the patient's hemodynamic condition stable. Critically sick patients with hypotension and respiratory distress should be brought to the intensive care unit, treated with inotropic support and intravenous fluid resuscitation, and closely monitored for signs of perforation. When there is respiratory distress and airway edema, endotracheal intubation should be performed immediately. Patients with an edematous and necrotic laryngopharynx will require a tracheostomy to maintain their airway.

Routine use of systemic glucocorticoids is not recommended; nonetheless, dexamethasone and prednisolone have been utilized. The patient should receive nil per os (NPO) and appropriate resuscitation. Nasogastric tube intubation, gastric lavage, administration of emetic medicines, and neutralizing agents are contraindicated because they may reflux into the esophageal injuries with perforation.

Intravenous broad-spectrum antibiotics may benefit a patient with high-grade esophageal injuries with perforation.

### Specific Treatment

Specific treatment is determined by the clinical condition and level of harm seen after a UGI endoscopy performed during the first 24–48 hours following consumption. Asymptomatic individuals with normal endoscopic examinations or grade I or IIA injuries require simply observation in the emergency room and can begin oral feedings within the first 24–48 hours.

Perforation necessitates immediate surgery, which may include an esophagectomy or gastrectomy.

*Preventing strictures*: Stricture formation is the most significant late-postcorrosive consequence, affecting up to one-third of patients after initial healing. Esophageal stricture typically appears around 2 months following the injury, especially in severe cases.

Stricture formation can be prevented or minimized by using steroids, stenting, nasogastric tube, balanced diet, and retrograde intraluminal dilatation.

*Corticosteroids*: The utility of corticosteroids in cases of acute corrosive poisoning is disputed. Endoscopic injection of triamcinolone into the stricture has been shown to be effective. However, multicentric studies have shown that corticosteroids have no meaningful effect on the prevention of postcorrosive stenosis in acute corrosive poisoning.

*Nutrition*: Because of substantial damage to the gastrointestinal tract, these patients' nutrition quickly deteriorates, and they may enter a severe hypercatabolic state. In patients with grades I and IIA damage, total parenteral nourishment is suggested for the first 24–48 hours, followed by a liquid diet until the 10th day. Patients with IIB and III damage must not consume food per os (NPO). During this time, the patient is fed via a nasogastric or nasoenteral tube, gastrostoma, or jejunostoma, as well as parenterally through a peripheral or central vein. NPO, or "esophageal rest," may remain until the 10th day following caustic intake. Intensive hyperalimentation and esophageal rest may lower the incidence of late-stage corrosive stenosis and strictures.

*Esophageal dilatation*: Retrograde intraluminal esophageal dilation is used to prevent or dilate existing esophageal narrowings. It is best to start esophageal dilatation 6 weeks after consumption. The procedure is then repeated every 2–3 months in a row.

*Sucralfate suspension*: According to subjective reports, sucralfate may reduce the percentage of postcorrosive stenosis in the UGI tract.

*Surgical Intervention*: It is indicated when there is:

- Complete stenosis that cannot be cured using traditional conservative procedures.
- X-ray testing detects esophageal or stomach defects.

### *Fistula Formation*

In cases of attempted suicide, the patient should be assessed by a psychiatrist to prevent further attempts.

## CLINICAL PEARLS

Corrosive poisoning is a severe health issue and medical emergency around the world. Urgent esophagogastroduodenoscopy is still the most widely used standard method for diagnosing and treating acute corrosive poisonings. Appropriate diet is of the utmost significance throughout treatment. Postcorrosive stenosis is the most common hidden complication. The use of corticosteroids as a treatment for acid poisoning remains contentious. Perforations during the acute or chronic phase of poisoning necessitate immediate surgical intervention.

## FURTHER READINGS

1. Gautam SK, Gupta RK, Alam A. Corrosive poisoning–an update. Indian J Med Specialities. 2018;9:160-2.
2. Hall AH, Jacquemin D, Henny D, Mathieu L, Josset P, Meyer B. Corrosive substances ingestion: a review. Crit Rev Toxicol. 2019;49(8): 637-69.
3. Cello JP, Fogel RP, Boland R. Liquid caustic ingestion spectrum of injury. Arch intern Med. 1980;140:501-4.
4. Lovejoy FH, Woolf AD. Corrosive ingestions. Pediatr Rev. 1995;16:473-4.
5. Satar S, Topal M, Kozaci N. Ingestion of caustic substances by adults. Am J Ther. 2004;11:258-61.
6. Mamede RC, De Mello Filho FV. Treatment of caustic ingestion: an analysis of 239 cases. Dis Esophagus. 2002;15:210-3.
7. Chibishev A, Pereska Z, Chibisheva V, Simonovska N. Corrosive poisonings in adults. Mater Sociomed. 2012;24(2):125-30.
8. Browne J, Thompson J. Caustic ingestion. In: Cummings CW, Flint PW, Haughey BH, Robbins KT, Thomas JR (Eds). Cummings Otolaryngology: Head & Neck Surgery, 4th edition. St Louis, MO: Elsevier Mosby; 2005. pp. 4330-41.
9. Poley JW, Steyerberg EW, Kuipers EJ, Dees J, Hartmans R, Tilanus HW, et al. Ingestion of acid and alkaline agents: outcome and prognostic value of early upper endoscopy. Gastrointest Endosc. 2004;60:372-7.
10. Leape LL, Ashcraft KW, Scarpelli DG, Holder TM. Hazard to health: liquid lye. N Engl J Med. 1971;284:578-81.
11. Korolev MP, Fedorov LE, Makarova OL. Treatment of patients with combined burn strictures of the esophagus and stomach. Vestn Khir IM I I Grek. 2005;164:70-2.
12. Mahawongkajit P. Acute management in corrosive ingestion. Dysphagia—New Advances. London: IntechOpen; 2022.

13. Kikendall JW. Caustic ingestion injuries. Gastroenterol Clin North Am. 1991;20:847-57.
14. Temir ZG, Karkiner A, Karaca J, Ortaç R, Ozdamar A. The effectiveness of sucralfate against stricture formation in experimental corrosive esophageal burns. Surg Today. 2005;35:617-22.
15. Bicakci U, Tender B, Deveci G, Rizalar R, Ariturk E, Bernay F. Minimally invasive management of children with caustic ingestion: less pain for patients. Pediatr Surg Int. 2010;26:251-5.
16. Peclova D, Navratil T. Do corticosteroids prevent oesophageal stricture after corrosive ingestion? Toxicol Rev. 2005;24:125-9.
17. Kochhar R, Kochhar S. Endoscopic balloon dilation for benign gastric outlet obstruction in adults. World J Gastrointest Endosc. 2010;2:29-35.

CHAPTER 111

# Sedative Poisoning

*Uttam Kumar Nath*

## DEFINITION

The term "sedative and hypnotic drugs" refers to many pharmacological compounds including anxiolytics, hypnotics, muscle relaxants, and anticonvulsants. Sedative hypnotic drugs are commonly used to treat anxiety and insomnia in both home and hospital settings. The most frequently abused anxiolytic is benzodiazepine (BZD).

## PATHOGENESIS

Each agent has its own specific mode of action and pharmacokinetics. BZDs and barbiturates are GABA-A receptor agonists, which are the primary neurotransmitter inhibitors in the central nervous system (CNS). Opiates operate on many receptors, including mu receptors, both centrally and peripherally, to release dopamine via increasing GABA disinhibition of dopamine release, which causes respiratory depression, coma, and death with overdoses. Antidepressants and antipsychotics cause sedation by blocking the antihistamine H1 receptor. Anticonvulsants typically increase GABA neurotransmission and induce drowsiness through this method. The primary toxic consequence that causes severe poisoning or death is global cerebral function depression, which results in coma, respiratory arrest, and pulmonary aspiration of gastric contents. The toxicity is determined by the amount of medicine consumed, its pharmacokinetics, the patient's tolerance, and the presence of other drugs.

Unexpectedly extended coma may be caused by the continued absorption of significant amounts of medication in the stomach or the emergence of long-lasting active metabolites. Typically, three to five times the average hypnotic dose induces a coma. Except for cerebellar symptoms, focal neurological indications are unusual and should alert the clinician to a different or concomitant condition. Pupillary alterations are nonspecific, but pinpoint pupils are indicative of opioid intoxication until proven otherwise.

## WHAT ARE THE POSSIBILITIES?

In BZD overdose, most of the patients are arousable and can provide relevant information themselves. Profound coma or cardiopulmonary instability should prompt the search for a coingestant. Presence of atypical or focal findings suggests other nontoxicologic causes of CNS depression.

Alcohol intoxication may be distinguished from sedative, hypnotic, or anxiolytic intoxication by the smell of alcohol on the breath and a history of recent ingestion of sedative, hypnotic, or anxiolytic medications.

In situations like cognitive impairment, traumatic brain injury, and/or delirium, an additional diagnosis of sedative, hypnotic, or anxiolytic intoxication may be appropriate even if the substance has been ingested at a low dosage.

## PATH TO DIAGNOSIS

### History and Physical Examination

Diagnosis usually is based on a history of ingestion because clinical manifestations are nonspecific. Physical examination should consist of an assessment of the patient's mental status and vital signs. Signs such as odor, pupillary changes, neuromuscular abnormalities, mental status, skin changes, temperature, blood pressure, heart rate changes, and respiratory pattern can help to establish a potential diagnosis.

An overdose of oral BZDs rarely results in toxicity unless combined with another drug. The most common manifestation of BZD toxicity is CNS depression, which can range from mild drowsiness to coma with hemodynamically stable vital signs. Respiratory depression is a rare condition. Clinically, the patient may exhibit slurred speech, ataxia, and depressed mentation, particularly if combined with another sedative. Although drowsy, these individuals are frequently arousable. Ataxia is the most common symptom of poisoning, affecting 90% of patients. Patients with renal or hepatic impairment are more likely to develop lactic acidosis. Non-BZD hypnotic overdoses with controlled-release formulations include drowsiness, hallucinations, and ataxia. Drowsiness is by far the most prevalent symptom. Coma and respiratory failure are uncommon, even overdoses of up to 40 times the recommended amount. They are more commonly linked to sleepwalking, sleep driving, eating, and other actions. When compared to other sleep drugs, zolpidem, zaleplon, and eszopiclone were associated with greater of these effects. Isolated zolpidem overdose is rarely fatal.

Overdoses of selective serotonin reuptake inhibitors/norepinephrine uptake inhibitors (SSRIs/SNRIs) rarely result in death or severe harm. All fatal overdoses include the consumption of another substance. Patients suffering from serotonin syndrome may experience anxiety, agitation, delirium, diaphoresis, tachycardia, hypertension, hyperthermia, gastrointestinal distress, tremor, muscle rigidity, myoclonus, and hyperreflexia. When used at hazardous doses, bupropion and venlafaxine can cause seizures. Even when combined with ethanol, buspirone induces minor CNS depression. The patient may experience lethargy and, on rare occasions, tonic-clonic seizures, but he or she recovers completely.

Patients with tricyclic antidepressant (TCA) overdose have a change in mental status such as drowsiness, disorientation, delirium, or delusion. Cardiac conduction delays, arrhythmias, hypotension, heat, flushing, and pupillary dilatation are prevalent. Due to the varying absorption kinetics involved in TCAs, patients may initially show normally before abruptly deteriorating. Opiate poisoning can cause depressed mental status, decreased respiration rate, hypothermia, decreased bowel sounds/movements, and/or miotic pupils. Histamine release can cause bradycardia to tachycardia, as well as hypotension.

Some antiseizure medications might cause drowsiness and possible toxicity, including Stevens–Johnson syndrome (SJS), toxic epidermal necrolysis (TEN), and drug-induced eosinophilia. Though rare, it is critical to be aware of the potential repercussions. Overdose with antihistamine phenothiazine results in cardiovascular and neurological symptoms such as sympathetic overactivity and metabolic acidosis. Diphenhydramine overdose is most commonly associated with impaired consciousness. Doxylamine poisoning is characterized by widespread complicated tachycardia, somnolence, psychotic behavior, convulsions, and agitation.

Before making a diagnosis, physicians must ensure that the signs or symptoms are not caused by another medical condition and cannot be explained by another problem, such as intoxication with another substance.

## Investigations

### *Diagnostic Strategies*

Any patient with changed mental status should have their blood glucose levels checked as away. Other lab tests include electrolytes, blood urea nitrogen (BUN), creatinine, and arterial blood gases. Qualitative immunoassays for BZDs in urine are available, but are rarely useful in emergency management. Serum medication concentrations are not readily obtainable and do not correspond with clinical severity.

*Electrocardiography (ECG), chest radiography, and plain abdomen radiographs*: Electrocardiology can offer diagnostic and prognostic data. TCA poisoning results in toxin-induced lengthening of the QRS interval. Some drugs (e.g., chloral hydrate) are radiopaque and may appear on plain abdomen radiographs.

# TREATMENT

The treatment's purpose is to keep the patient's hemodynamic stability by maintaining the airway, breathing, and circulation. Patients at high risk of respiratory failure and cardiopulmonary arrest frequently require endotracheal intubation and mechanical ventilation.

In the absence of substantial cardiorespiratory compromise, the majority of intoxications can be treated conservatively with symptomatic therapy.

*Benzodiazepine toxicity*: Decontamination with activated charcoal is not indicated in cases of isolated BZD overdose. Flumazenil, a nonspecific competitive antagonist of the BZD receptor, can be utilized in cases of acute overdose or severe toxicity. Flumazenil should be administered with caution and extra consideration to patients who are on a long-term BZD regimen since it can cause seizures.

SSRI/SNRI poisoning is treated by monitoring for signs and symptoms, with a focus on seizures, cardiac conduction abnormalities, and QT interval prolongation. BZDs can be administered to those exhibiting symptoms of serotonin syndrome or convulsions, whereas sodium bicarbonate can be administered to those exhibiting cardiac toxicity. Individuals at risk of developing torsades de pointes can receive magnesium sulfate intravenously. In addition, immediate nonsynchronized electric defibrillation is recommended for individuals with hemodynamic instability.

*Tricyclic antidepressant toxicity*: Sodium bicarbonate is the first line of treatment for patients with cardiac toxicity, and it is advised in patients with a QRS interval widening of more than 100 ms or ventricular arrhythmias. If the patient begins to experience seizures, BZDs should be provided. Activated charcoal should be used to decontaminate the gastrointestinal tract within 2 hours of consumption, unless bowel blockage, ileus, or perforation is detected.

*Opiate toxicity*: If opiate toxicity is suspected, naloxone, which is a short-acting opiate antagonist, can be administered intravenously. Any metabolic acidosis should be corrected in case of an overdose of antihistamine phenothiazines.

*Poor prognostic indicators*: Prognosis will depend on several factors, including duration, dosage, and intervention. If identified and treated, early toxicity will have a good prognosis and is manageable. A delay in care or a substantial dosage of the intoxicant can lead to a prognosis that may be extremely poor.

## CLINICAL PEARLS

Rapid identification of life-threatening toxicity could save a patient's life. Proper monitoring, correct usage, and medication adherence can help to decrease the risk of toxicity with sedative-hypnotics. Pupillary changes occur nonspecifically and vary with time. Pinpoint pupils are a sign of opioid toxicity until proven otherwise. Most intoxication can be managed conservatively with symptomatic treatment. Flumazenil is not needed in most BZD overdoses.

## FURTHER READINGS

1. Byatt C, Volans G. ABC of poisoning. Sedative and hypnotic drugs. Br Med J (Clin Res Ed). 1984;289(6453):1214-7.
2. Tsutaoka BT. Sedative hypnotic agents. In: Olson KR (Ed). Poisoning & Drug Overdose, 6th edition. New York: McGraw Hill; 2022.
3. Twyman RE, Rogers CJ, Macdonald RL. Differential regulation of gamma-aminobutyric acid receptor channels by diazepam and phenobarbital. Ann Neurol. 1989;25(3):213-20.
4. Simone CG, Bobrin BD. Anxiolytics and sedative-hypnotics toxicity. StatPearls [Internet]. Treasure Island, FL: StatPearls Publishing; 2022.
5. Gussow L, Carlson A. Sedative hypnotics. Rosen's Emergency Medicine: Concepts and Clinical Practice E-Book. Part IV. Environment and Toxicology. Section Two. Toxicology. Philadelphia, PA: Saunders; 2013.
6. Höjer J, Baehrendtz S, Gustafsson L. Benzodiazepine poisoning: experience of 702 admissions to an intensive care unit during a 14-year period. J Intern Med. 1989;226(2):117-22.
7. Zosel A, Egelhoff E, Heard K. Severe lactic acidosis after an iatrogenic propylene glycol overdose. Pharmacotherapy. 2010;30:219.
8. Barbey JT, Roose SP. SSRI safety in overdose. J Clin Psychiatry. 1998;59(Suppl. 15):42-8.
9. Graudins A, Dowsett RP, Liddle C. The toxicity of antidepressant poisoning: is it changing? A comparative study of cyclic and newer serotonin-specific antidepressants. Emerg Med (Fremantle). 2002;14(4):440-6.
10. Mason J, Freemantle N, Eccles M. Fatal toxicity associated with antidepressant use in primary care. Br J Gen Pract. 2000;50(454):366-70.
11. Catalano G, Catalano MC, Hanley PF. Seizures associated with buspirone overdose: case report and literature review. Clin Neuropharmacol. 1998;21:347-50.
12. Jang DH, Manini AF, Trueger NS, Duque D, Nestor NB, Nelson LS, et al. Status epilepticus and wide-complex tachycardia secondary to diphenhydramine overdose. Clin Toxicol (Phila). 2010;48:945-8.
13. PsychDB (Psychiatry DataBase), Sedative, hypnotic, or anxiolytic (benzodiazepine) intoxication. [online] Available from https://www.psychdb.com/addictions/sedative-hypnotics/2-intoxication. [Last accessed September, 2023].
14. Perry HE, Shannon MW. Diagnosis and management of opioid- and benzodiazepine-induced comatose overdose in children. Curr Opin Pediatr. 1996;8:243-7.

CHAPTER 112

# Datura Poisoning

*Uttam Kumar Nath*

## INTRODUCTION

Datura, often known as "thorn apple," is a hallucinogenic plant that grows naturally in temperate and tropical regions of the world and is extensively distributed in both urban and rural areas across the country. It is regarded as one of the most deadly plant species due to its highly toxic components. Datura's leaves, fruits, flowers, stem, and even roots have long been employed in folklore medicine and alternative therapies, including the treatment of epilepsy, hysteria, insanity, and heart disease, as well as fever with catarrh, diarrhea, and skin problems. However, the alkaloids responsible for both therapeutic and hallucinogenic qualities are deadly in high doses, and reckless usage frequently results in hospitalization and death.

## PATHOGENESIS

The exact medicinal dosage of Datura varies from person to person based on the patient's age, bodily strength, appetite effects, severity, and condition. The entire plant, particularly the foliage and seeds, is hazardous due to the presence of tropane alkaloids. Atropine, L-hyoscyamine, and L-scopolamine create an anticholinergic syndrome by inhibiting central and peripheral muscarinic neurotransmission. Datura's toxicity varies greatly and is unpredictable. It can occur when consumed, smoked, or absorbed topically, especially through mucosal membranes. Toxicity can vary amongst leaves and plants, as well as seasonally. The lethal dose is approximately 100–125 seeds. The fatal dose of alkaloids is around 60 mg for humans and 4 mg for 24 hours.

Classic anticholinergic poisoning occurs when a tropane alkaloid-containing plant is consumed, which contains hyoscyamine in the leaves, roots, and seeds, as well as hyoscine, atropine (DL-hyoscyamine), and scopolamine (L-hyoscine) in the roots. They compete with muscarinic acetylcholine receptors in the peripheral and central nervous systems, resulting in parasympathetic organ paralysis. Acute psychosis or delirium can result from its inhibitory impact on central nervous system receptors.

## PATH TO DIAGNOSIS

### History

Physicians in the emergency department face a hurdle when diagnosing and treating Datura intoxication. Diagnosing such cases is difficult because to the lack of routine laboratory screening tests for alkaloids, as well as the complicated and confounding symptoms of Datura intoxication. Physicians' clinical suspicion, proper knowledge, and history of Datura use are critical in the accurate and prompt diagnosis and therapy of Datura toxicity cases.

## Clinical Examination

The symptoms are characterized as "dry as a bone, red as a beet, blind as a bat, hot as a hare, and mad as a wet hen." They occur within half an hour of taking seeds, or quicker if taking a seed decoction. However, the first sign is a bitter taste in the mouth. Due to delayed stomach emptying, clinical symptoms might last up to 24–48 hours.

### *Nine D's of Datura Poisoning*

- **D**ryness of the mouth and throat, difficulty speaking, and dysphagia are all symptoms of salivation inhibition.
- **D**ilatation of cutaneous blood vessels causes the face to flush with tinged conjunctivae.
- ***Dilatation of the pupils***: The pupils are dilated and insensitive to light, and the ability to accommodate for close vision is impaired by diplopia and near blindness.
- ***Dry hot skin***: Because sweat secretion is inhibited and the heat-regulating center is stimulated, hyperpyrexia occurs, with temperatures reaching 40–42°C.
- ***Drunken gait***: A person who is staggering as if drunk, with giddiness and an unsteady gait, may have hyperreflexia and convulsions.
- ***Delirium***: The patient is initially restless, with with giddiness and unsteady gait may have hyperreflexia and convulsions.
- ***Delirium***: Patient is at first restless with a tendency to run away, agitative, violent, and confused, and later becomes delirious and is subject to visual and auditory hallucinations with a tendency to grasp imaginary objects or pick up bed clothes or pull imaginary threads from fingertips, and spontaneous laughing or crying.
- ***Drowsiness and Death***: The delirium passes off after an hour and the patient becomes drowsy. This may last for few days followed by complete recovery. Rarely, in fatal cases, the drowsiness may progress to stupor or coma and death from respiratory paralysis.

The patient may have vomiting, decreased bowel activity, and urinary retention. Respiratory failure and cardiovascular collapse were reported in severe cases. In rare cases, rhabdomyolysis and fulminant hepatitis have also been described.

## Investigations

Diagnosis is mostly based on history and clinical features. There is absence of routine laboratory screening tests for alkaloids. Investigations are done to detect the complications or other causes of the neurological symptoms which include:

- Routine blood examination—shows neutrophil leukocytosis
- Serum electrolytes, kidney and liver function tests
- *Urine screening test*: Not routinely done
- *Electrocardiography (ECG)*: To detect conduction defect and arrhythmia
- *Computed tomography (CT) scan brain*: To exclude any cerebral lesions
- *Plasma atropine concentration*: Even minute traces of atropine in blood (as low as 10 ng/mL) can be detected by gas chromatography-mass spectrometry. However, there is little or no correlation between plasma concentration and observed clinical effects.

# WHAT ARE THE POSSIBILITIES? DIFFERENTIAL DIAGNOSIS

The symptoms of Datura poisoning may be mistaken for drunkenness or heat stroke. History of alcohol intake or prolonged exposure to hot humid condition is very important.

## THERAPY

The patient needs to be treated in a quiet and dark environment. Management is primarily supportive. It comprises of stomach decontamination with activated charcoal (50 g) and magnesium sulphate (30 g) as a cathartic every 4–6 hours till the stool turns black. Gastric emptying and disinfection are crucial management measures if started early. Decreased gastrointestinal motility may have increased the efficacy of activated charcoal. Sedation with intravenous (IV) benzodiazepines to control agitation and seizure is to be given as supportive care. Hyperpyrexia is to be controlled by fluid administration and internal and external cooling methods. Tachycardia is usually responsive to crystalloids.

Physostigmine is the antidote of choice and should be administered if the patient has severe toxic symptoms such as coma, arrhythmias, hallucinations, severe hypertension, and convulsions. The adult dose is 2 mg IV, slowly, repeated if required, in 20 minutes. Continuous cardiac monitoring is required.

Respiratory failure is treated with endotracheal intubation and assisted ventilation. Catheterization of the urinary bladder and a close watch on intake and output are required.

## RED FLAG SIGNS: POOR PROGNOSTIC INDICATORS

Patients passing into deep coma with hypotension and shock and having convulsion and respiratory paralysis are poor prognostic signs. In fatal cases, death usually occurs within 24 hours.

## CLINICAL PEARLS

Diagnosis is essentially clinical. Treatment is symptomatic and supportive. Prognosis is usually favorable. In patients with acute anticholinergic and psychiatric symptoms, Datura poisoning should always be considered unless proved otherwise, and early management with decontamination should be initiated. Moistening of the tongue and a decrease in pupil size toward normal are useful therapeutic guidelines. In nonfatal situations, recovery takes a day or two, with the pupils being the last to go.

## FURTHER READINGS

1. Netmeds.com. (2021). Datura: benefits, uses, formulations, ingredients, method, dosage and side effects. [online] Available from https://www.netmeds.com/health-library/post/datura-benefits-uses-formulations-ingredients-method-dosage-and-side-effects [Last accessed September, 2023].
2. Bouziri A, Hamdi A, Borgi A, Hadj SB, Fitouri Z, Menif K, et al. Datura stramonium L. poisoning in a geophagous child: a case report. Int J Emerg Med. 2011;4:31.
3. Kurzbaum A, Simsolo C, Kvasha L, Blum A. Toxic delirium due to Datura stramonium. Isr Med Assoc J. 2001;3:538-9.
4. Arouko H, Matray M-D, Bragança C, Mpaka JP, Chinello L, Castaing F, et al. Voluntary poisoning by ingestion of Datura stramonium. Another cause of hospitalization in youth seeking strong sensations. Ann Med Interne (Paris). 2003;154:S46-50.
5. Spina SP, Taddei A. Teenagers with Jimson weed (Datura stramonium) poisoning. CJEM. 2007;9:467-9.
6. Gaire BP, Subedi L. A review on the pharmacological and toxicological aspects of Datura stramonium L. J Integr Med. 2013;11:73-9.
7. Vijay Kumar B. Review article on dhatura (Dhatura metal, Linn). Int J Recent Adv Multidiscip Res. 2015;2(2):0240-3.
8. Kadam SD, Chavhan SA, Shinde SA, Sapkal PN. Pharmacognostic review on datura. Int J Pharmacogn Chin Med. 2018;2(4):000145.

# CHAPTER 113

# Kerosene Poisoning

*Uttam Kumar Nath*

## DEFINITION

Kerosene intake is the leading cause of unintentional poisoning. This preventable health issue affects children in underdeveloped nations, resulting in significant morbidity and mortality. Kerosene is a hydrocarbon that can irritate the respiratory and neurological systems, as well as the gastrointestinal tract. Kerosene's high volatility, low viscosity, and low surface tension make it more likely to cause aspiration and severe lung injury.

## WHEN TO SUSPECT?

### Clinical Clues in History and Examination

Initially, the patient may be asymptomatic and have a history of kerosene oil exposure or ingestion. The majority of the patients smell like kerosene. Ingestion of kerosene causes a burning feeling in the mouth, followed by nausea and vomiting. Spontaneous or induced vomiting after ingestion increases the chances of aspiration with subsequent chemical pneumonitis. While most respiratory effects appear within 30 minutes of consumption, they can be delayed for up to 12–24 hours. Chemical peritonitis causes coughing, tachypnea, breathing difficulties, bronchospasm, and atelectasis. Symptomatic patients with respiratory distress and hypoxemia shortly after consumption usually develop quickly to respiratory failure. Recovery normally lasts approximately a week, although it may take longer if secondary bacterial pneumonia develops and worsens the clinical course.

Fever may appear as early as 30 minutes after consumption and last for many days. If it develops after 48 hours of intake, it indicates that a bacterial infection has grown. Central nervous system involvement affects around 25–70% of patients. Mild, transitory sleepiness is common. The patient may experience restlessness, stupor, convulsions, dizziness, euphoria, headache, visual abnormalities, and impaired memory.

### Physical Examination

Patients are feverish at the time of presentation, with tachycardia and tachypnea. Signs of respiratory discomfort may include nasal flaring, head bobbing, and the usage of auxiliary muscles. Blood pressure may be aberrant as a result of the systemic inflammatory response, and pulse oximetry may indicate hypoxia. Depending on the etiology and presentation, auscultation may reveal decreased breath sounds, diminished percussion resonance, bronchial breath sounds, crepitations, or wheezing.

## PATHOPHYSIOLOGY

Kerosene produces minimal mucosal irritation as it has poor gastrointestinal absorption. Due to irritation of the larynx and trachea, it produces choking or gagging. The choking, gagging, or vomiting induced after ingestion leads to aspiration. Kerosene oil aspiration predominantly affects the pulmonary tree, particularly the distal airways. The primary mechanism of injury is its direct toxicity and physical properties such as low viscosity, low surface tension, and high volatility, which help its easy spread over a large surface area into distal airways and tracheobronchial tree. Therefore, even small quantities of around 1 mL are potentially life-threatening. Necrotizing pneumonia is the most common pathological finding. Other changes include atelectasis, interstitial inflammation, hemorrhagic pulmonary edema, vascular thrombosis, and hyaline membrane formation. Effect on type II pneumocytes results in alveolar collapse, ventilation–perfusion mismatch, and hypoxemia. The incidence of hemorrhagic exudative alveolitis peaks 3 days after ingestion. Being volatile, kerosene also displaces oxygen from the alveoli, producing hypoxia. Inflammatory response is triggered due to chemical irritation resulting in elevation of temperature, usually within hours of exposure, not unlike sepsis. Central nervous system manifestation is due to severe hypoxemia and also due to the high lipid content of neurons that makes them vulnerable to kerosene.

## WHAT ARE THE POSSIBILITIES?

Bronchopneumonia, atelectasis, salicylate poisoning, and other toxin ingestions should be considered if exposure history is uncertain or findings are suggestive of other poisonings.

## HOW TO MANAGE?

### Investigations and Treatment

*Chest radiograph*: A chest radiograph should be performed within 4–6 hours of exposure, or sooner if there are evidence of pulmonary aspiration. Approximately 60–70% of patients exhibit radiological abnormalities. Radiological abnormalities appear in about 88% of cases within 2 hours and 98% within 12 hours of pulmonary aspiration. Radiological findings include perihilar and lung infiltration, lobar pneumonia, pulmonary cystic alterations, pneumatoceles, pleural effusion, empyema, pneumothorax, pneumomediastinum, and surgical emphysema.

Other *ancillary investigations* for symptomatic patients are as follows:

*Complete blood count*: Neutrophilic leukocytosis is commonly observed early in the clinical course. It is unrelated to the pulmonary pathology and lasts for roughly a week. Massive consumption may cause disseminated intravascular coagulopathy, and a peripheral blood smear may reveal hemolysis.

*Arterial blood gas analysis*: It first exhibits mild respiratory alkalosis and hypoxemia. If not treated, it will progress to metabolic acidosis.

Liver and kidney function testing using serum electrolytes.

*Urinalysis*: In cases of massive ingestion, there may be a presence of hemoglobinuria.

## TREATMENT

Contaminated clothing should be removed, and the skin should be properly cleansed with soap and water. There is no specific remedy. The majority of measures focus on stabilization, supportive management, and complication prevention and treatment. An asymptomatic patient with a normal radiograph should be monitored for at least 6–8 hours, with the patient remaining nil per orally (NPO). Gastric lavage should be avoided in symptomatic individuals to minimize the risk of aspiration. Activated charcoal is not particularly useful because it does not bond to kerosene. In the event of hypoxemia, supplemental oxygen should be supplied, and appropriate hydration with intravenous fluids should be maintained while on NPO throughout the initial observation period.

Corticosteroids have no beneficial effect on the course of the illness and may be harmful; hence, they are not recommended. Prophylactic antibiotics play no function unless in cases of fever recurrence after 48 hours after ingestion, leukocytosis after the first 48 hours, worsening chest radiology/symptoms, or bacterial growth discovered on sputum or tracheal aspirates. Bronchodilators (β2 agonists) can treat bronchospasm. In the event of severe respiratory distress, unresponsiveness to oxygen or bronchodilators, or changed mental status, endotracheal intubation and mechanical ventilation may be necessary. Extracorporeal membrane oxygenation may also be life-saving.

## RED FLAG SIGNS

### Poor Prognostic Indicators

Most patients with kerosene poisoning survive without sequelae. Mortality ranges from 0.7 to 7%. The prognosis depends on the volume of ingestion or aspiration and the adequacy of medical care. Lack of transport to the hospital, financial restraints, and administration of harmful first aid (forceful ingestion of coconut milk/milk/water/eggs, inducing emesis, etc.) by caregivers are poor prognostic factors. Severe malnourishment, prior lavage, hypoxemia at admission, need for ventilation, secondary sepsis, and ventilator-related complications are other factors associated with poor outcome.

## CLINICAL PEARLS

The most common presentation is respiratory symptoms. Early hospitalization with supportive management can lead to the majority of the patients being cured without any sequelae. Due to the possibility of delayed development of pneumonitis, no patient should be discharged before 6 hours after ingestion of kerosene. There is no convincing evidence for administering early steroid or antibiotic prophylaxis to prevent chemical pneumonitis and improve outcome.

## FURTHER READINGS

1. Anwar S, Rahman A, Houqe SA, Moshed A. Clinical profile of kerosene poisoning in a tertiary level hospital in Bangladesh. Bangladesh J Child Health. 2014;38(1):11-4.
2. Chowdhury MJBA, Akhter A, Maruf-Ul-Quader M, Choudhury Z, Kamrun Nahar K, Chowdhury D, et al. Clinical profile and immediate outcome of kerosene poisoning in children. IOSR J Dent Med Sci (IOSR-JDMS). 2019;18(4):59-63.
3. Litovitz T. Hydrocarbon ingestions. Entechnology. 1983;62(3):142-7.
4. Divecha CA, Tullu MS. Kerosene poisoning in children: a review. Indian J Trauma Emerg Pediatr. 2020;12(1):29-36.
5. Maheshwari A, Gulati S. Kerosene poisoning. Indian J Med Spec. 2018;9(3):163-6.
6. Gupta P. API Medicine Update, Volume 28. Mumbai: The Association of Physicians of India; 2018. p. 740.
7. Ellenhorn MJ. The hydrocarbon products. In: Ellenhorn MJ, Schonwald S, Ordog G, Wasserberger J (Eds). Ellenhorn's Medical Toxicology: Diagnosis and Treatment of Human Poisoning, 2nd edition. Baltimore: Williams & Wilkins; 1997. p. 1420.
8. Shotar AM. Kerosene poisoning in childhood: a 6-year prospective study at the Princess Rahmat Teaching Hospital. Neuro Endocrinol Lett. 2005;26(6):835-8.
9. Nagi NA, Abdulallah ZA. Kerosene poisoning in children in Iraq. Postgrad Med J. 1995;71(837):419-22.
10. Kostic MA. Poisoning. In: Kliegman R, Stanton B, Behrman RE, St Gem JW, Schor NF, Nelson WE, (Eds). Nelson Textbook of Pediatrics, 20th edition. Philadelphia: Elsevier; 2016. pp. 464-5.
11. Feng S, Goto CS. Toxic ingestions and exposures.

In: Kline MW, Blaney SM, Giardino AP, Orange JS, Penny DJ, Schutze GE, Shekerdemian LS, Rudolph AM, Rudolph CD (Eds). Rudolph's Pediatrics, 23rd edition (vol. 1). New York: McGraw-Hill Education; 2018. pp. 631-2.
12. Klein BL, Simon JE. Hydrocarbon poisonings. Pediatr Clin North Am. 1986;33(2):411-9.
13. Anas N, Namasonthi V, Ginsburg CM. Criteria for hospitalizing children who have ingested products containing hydrocarbons. JAMA. 1981;246(8):840-3.
14. Lewander WJ, Aleguas A. Hydrocarbon poisoning. In: Post TW (Ed). Up to Date. Waltham, MA: Up to Date Inc.; 2019.
15. Lee A, Bye M. Lung injury from hydrocarbon aspiration and smoke inhalation. In: Wilmott RW, Deterding R, Li A, Ratjen F, Sly P, Zar HJ, Bush A (Eds). Kendig's Disorders of the Respiratory Tract in Children, 9th edition. Philadelphia, PA: Elsevier; 2019. pp. 2313-20.
16. Mansour AZZ, Hammody A, Makki K. Kerosene poisoning in children. Int J Curr Res. 2020;12(2):10313-8.
17. Orenstein DM. Hydrocarbon pneumonia. In: Behrinan RE (Ed). Nelson Textbook of Paediatrics, 16th edition. Philadelphia: WB Saunders; 2000. pp. 1289-90.
18. Jayashree M, Singhi S, Gupta A. Predictors of outcome in children with hydrocarbon poisoning receiving intensive care. Indian Pediatr. 2006;43(8):715-9.

CHAPTER 114

# Myxedema Coma

*Rana Bhattacharjee*

## DEFINITION

Myxedema coma is a severe, life-threatening form of decompensated hypothyroidism. Myxedema crisis is a better term as some patients may present with severe drowsiness or semicoma. If not detected on time, it is associated with high mortality.

## WHEN TO SUSPECT?

This condition is typically seen in patients with prolonged uncontrolled hypothyroidism. One or more precipitating factors are usually associated. Common precipitating factors include sepsis, stroke, acute myocardial infarction, heart failure, gastrointestinal bleeding, and the use of drugs such as sedatives, amiodarone, lithium, or diuretics. Common clinical features include altered sensorium, cognitive impairment, hoarse voice, enlarged tongue, dry skin, nonpitting edema, or delayed relaxation of tendon jerk. Hypothermia may not manifest in the warm tropical climate.

## HOW TO MANAGE?

If clinical suspicion is strong, the treatment can be started awaiting biochemical confirmation.

Serum thyroxine (T4) or free T4 is low. Serum thyroid-stimulating hormone (TSH) is usually very high. Sometimes, TSH may be low, normal, or slightly elevated due to the presence of central hypothyroidism or coexistent severe nonthyroidal illness. Creatine kinase is usually very high. Hyponatremia is common. A blood count and culture and urine culture should be sent to rule out infection. Serum electrolytes and renal and liver function tests should also be obtained.

*Supportive measures*: The airway should be secured. Ventilatory support may be required in those with hypoventilation. Blankets are sometimes needed to prevent heat loss. Hypertonic saline, normal saline, dextrose normal saline, vasopressors, and/or furosemide may be used to tackle hypotension and hyponatremia.

*Thyroid hormones*: Levothyroxine should be administered orally or via a nasogastric (NG) tube. A loading dose of 500 mg is followed by a 100 mg daily dose. Intravenous forms of T4 and triiodothyronine (T3) are not available in India.

*Glucocorticoids*: Intravenous hydrocortisone is administered at a dose of 50 mg every 6 hours.

Treatment of precipitating factor(s) should be undertaken.

## CLINICAL PEARLS

- Myxedema coma is a life-threatening complication of hypothyroidism requiring prompt recognition and management.
- Appropriate supportive measures, glucocorticoid administration, and thyroid hormone replacement are the mainstay of therapy.

## FURTHER READINGS

1. Mathew V, Misgar RA, Ghosh S, Mukhopadhyay P, Roychowdhury P, Pandit K, et al. Myxedema coma: a new look into an old crisis. J Thyroid Res. 2011;2011:493462.
2. Ono Y, Ono S, Yasunaga H, Matsui H, Fushimi K, Tanaka Y. Clinical characteristics and outcomes of myxedema coma: analysis of a national inpatient database in Japan. J Epidemiol.2017;27:117-22.

CHAPTER 115

# Thyrotoxic Crisis

*Rana Bhattacharjee*

## DEFINITION

Thyrotoxic crisis is a life-threatening condition, characterized by exaggerated thyrotoxic manifestations along with one or more organ decompensation. It is associated with significant mortality.

## WHEN TO SUSPECT?

This condition is suspected when there are manifestations of severe thyrotoxicosis (tremor, palpitation, heat intolerance, excessive sweating) with features of one or more organ dysfunction such as fever, diarrhea, vomiting, atrial fibrillation, heart failure, delirium, seizure, and coma. There may be a history of precipitating factors such as poor compliance with antithyroid drugs, sepsis, or major trauma.

The Burch-Wartofsky scoring system **(Table 1)**, which is a point-based scoring system of various clinical parameters, is used for diagnosis.

## HOW TO MANAGE?

Total and free thyroid hormone levels are usually high with suppressed thyroid-stimulating hormone (TSH). Hyperbilirubinemia and transaminitis are common. Leukocytosis, hyperglycemia, and hypercalcemia can also occur. Electrocardiography (ECG) and echocardiography are often required to diagnose arrhythmias and heart failure.

*Intensive supportive care*: Management of airway, breathing, and circulation is of paramount importance. Proper use of moist oxygen and intravenous (IV) fluid is required. External cooling is needed in febrile patients (e.g., cold sponging with tepid water). Paracetamol can also be used for fever.

*Antithyroid drugs*: High dose of propylthiouracil (PTU), 500–1,000 mg bolus followed by 250 mg every 4 hours, is given orally, via a nasogastric tube, or rectally. If PTU is not tolerated, carbimazole 20 mg every 6–8 hours can be used as an alternative.

*Iodine*: Saturated solution of potassium iodide (SSKI) five drops every 6 hours may be administered 1 hour after the first dose of antithyroid drugs. Alternatively, Lugol's iodine can be administered as 10 drops every 8 hours.

*Lithium*: It can be used in patients with a history of severe adverse reactions to antithyroid drugs or iodine. The usual starting dose is 300 mg every 6 hours with subsequent adjustments to maintain serum lithium level around 1 mEq/L.

*Cholestyramine*: It can be used in the dose of 4 g every 6 hours to interrupt enterohepatic circulation of thyroxine (T4) and triiodothyronine (T3).

**Table 1: Burch–Wartofsky scoring system.**

| ***Thermoregulatory dysfunction*** | | **Points** |
|---|---|---|
| Temperature (°F) | 99–99.9 | 5 |
| | 100–100.9 | 10 |
| | 101–101.9 | 15 |
| | 102–102.9 | 20 |
| | 103–103.9 | 25 |
| | ≥104 | 30 |
| Central nervous system | Absent | 0 |
| | Mild agitation | 10 |
| | Delirium, psychosis, lethargy | 20 |
| | Seizures or coma | 30 |
| Gastrointestinal dysfunction | Absent | 0 |
| | Diarrhea, nausea, vomiting, abdominal pain | 10 |
| | Unexplained jaundice | 20 |
| ***Cardiovascular dysfunctions*** | | |
| Tachycardia (beats/min) | 90–109 | 5 |
| | 110–119 | 10 |
| | 120–129 | 15 |
| | 130–139 | 20 |
| | ≥140 | 25 |
| Heart failure | Absent | 0 |
| | Mild (edema) | 5 |
| | Moderate (bibasal rales) | 10 |
| | Severe (pulmonary edema) | 15 |
| Atrial fibrillation | Absent | 0 |
| | Present | 10 |
| History of precipitating events (sepsis, stroke, trauma, etc.) | Absent | 0 |
| | Present | 10 |
| Likelihood of thyroid storm is: Unlikely, <25; impending, 25–44; likely, 45–60; highly likely, >60 | | |

*Beta-blockers*: Orally administered propranolol 60–80 mg every 4 hours is used. Alternatively, esmolol infusion of 50–100 μg/kg/min intravenously can be used.

*Steroids*: Hydrocortisone 300 mg bolus followed by 100 mg 8 hourly for several days should be given. Subsequently, it is rapidly tapered off.

*Treatment of precipitating factors*: Identification and treatment of precipitating factors such as infection are required.

## CLINICAL PEARLS

- Thyroid storm is a life-threatening condition that warrants prompt diagnosis and management.
- The Burch–Wartofsky scoring system, which is based on various clinical parameters, is a validated way to diagnose this condition.
- Supportive measures, administration of high-dose antithyroid drugs, glucocorticoids, beta-blockers, and iodine are the mainstay of therapy.

## FURTHER READINGS

1. Burch HB, Wartofsky L. Life-threatening thyrotoxicosis: Thyroid storm. Endocrinol Metab Clin North Am. 1993;22:263-77.
2. Ross DS, Burch HB, Cooper DS, Greenlee MC, Laurberg P, Maia AL, et al. 2016 American Thyroid Association guidelines for diagnosis and management of hyperthyroidism and other causes of thyrotoxicosis. Thyroid. 2016;26(10):1343-1421.

# CHAPTER 116

# Adrenal Crisis

*Rana Bhattacharjee*

## DEFINITION

Adrenal crisis is a life-threatening condition where acute glucocorticoid with/without mineralocorticoid insufficiency leads to a variable constellation of symptoms and signs such as hypotension, lethargy, abdominal abdomen, vomiting, or psychiatric illness.

## WHEN TO SUSPECT?

A high index of suspicion is needed to diagnose this condition. It can present in many different clinical contexts.

A known patient with primary or secondary adrenal insufficiency can land up in crisis if they become noncompliant with their medications. Precipitating factors such as infection, major trauma, surgery, or any severe illness can also lead to crisis, particularly if the replacement dose is not up-titrated timely.

The above-mentioned precipitating factors can also tip the balance in a patient with undiagnosed long-standing adrenal insufficiency and induce crisis.

Bilateral adrenal hemorrhage or pituitary apoplexy can lead to acute-onset primary and secondary adrenal insufficiency, respectively.

Adrenal crisis may be precipitated when a supraphysiological dose of glucocorticoid (which is commonly used as an anti-inflammatory or immunomodulating agent) is abruptly withdrawn after long-term use (>3 weeks).

Common clinical features of the crisis include shock, anorexia, nausea, vomiting, abdominal pain, fever, lethargy, psychiatric symptoms, or coma. Some of the clinical features may point toward the etiology. Acute-onset headache and cranial nerve palsies point toward pituitary apoplexy. Diffuse hyperpigmentation indicates long-standing primary adrenal insufficiency.

## HOW TO MANAGE?

In a suspected case, blood should immediately be drawn for cortisol, electrolytes, blood count, urea, creatinine, and liver function tests. Treatment should be started immediately after sending the samples.

*Glucocorticoid*: 100 mg of hydrocortisone (HC) should be administered intravenously as a bolus, followed by 200 mg over 24 hours (either as a continuous infusion or as four divided doses). After 24 hours, the dose is reduced to 100 mg/day, either as a continuous infusion or as four divided doses till the crisis is resolved. The dose of intravenous HC in children is 50 mg/m$^2$ bolus, followed by 50–100 mg/m$^2$/day. After stabilization of the clinical condition, the HC dose is rapidly tapered to the physiological replacement dose administered orally.

*Intravenous fluids*: 1 L of normal saline or dextrose normal saline is infused rapidly. For children in shock, normal saline or dextrose normal saline is infused at the rate of 20 mL/kg, repeated up to a total of 60 mL/kg. Subsequent infusion is individualized as per the patient's need. For hypoglycemia, 2–4 mL/kg of 25% dextrose (maximum single dose 25 g) is infused slowly at a rate of 2–3 mL/min. Alternatively, 5–10 mL/kg of 10% dextrose can be infused in children aged <12 years.

Precipitating factor(s) such as sepsis must be treated.

## CLINICAL PEARLS

- Timely identification and prompt management improve the survival of a patient with adrenal crisis.
- The presenting symptoms can be nonspecific. A high index of suspicion is needed to diagnose this condition.
- Intravenous HC and fluids are the mainstay of therapy.

## FURTHER READINGS

1. Rushworth RL, Torpy DJ, Stratakis CA, Falhammar H. Adrenal crises in children: perspectives and research directions. Horm Res Paediatr. 2018;89:341-51.
2. Bornstein SR, Allolio B, Arlt W, Barthel A, Don-Wauchope A, Hammer GD, et al. Diagnosis and treatment of primary adrenal insufficiency: an Endocrine Society clinical practice guideline. J Clin Endocrinol Metab. 2016;101:364-89.

# SECTION 3

# Practitioner's Guide

CHAPTER 117

# How to Write a Prescription?

*Anirban Dalui, Satabdi Datta*

## INTRODUCTION

A prescription is a written or electronic order from a practitioner or designated agent to a pharmacist for a particular medication for a specific patient. Prescription is a medicolegal document; hence, utmost care is needed while writing a prescription. All components of a prescription should be complete. There is no global standard for prescriptions, and every country has its own regulations.

Once a patient with a clinical problem has been evaluated and a diagnosis has been reached, the practitioner can often select from a variety of therapeutic approaches. Medication, surgery, psychiatric treatment, radiation, physical therapy, health education, counseling, further consultation (second opinions), and no therapy are some of the options available. Of these options, drug therapy is by far the most frequently chosen. In most cases, this requires the writing of a prescription. A written prescription is the prescriber's order to prepare or dispense a specific treatment—usually medication—for a specific patient.

## RATIONAL PRESCRIBING

Like any other process in healthcare, writing a prescription should be based on a series of rational steps **(Fig. 1)**.

- *Make a specific diagnosis*: A specific diagnosis, even if it is tentative, is required to move to the next step. For example, in a patient with a probable diagnosis of rheumatoid arthritis, the diagnosis and the reasoning underlying it should be clear and should be shared with the patient.
- *Consider the pathophysiologic implications of the diagnosis*: If the disorder is well understood, the prescriber is in a much better position to offer effective therapy. For example, increasing knowledge about the mediators of inflammation makes possible more effective use of nonsteroidal anti-inflammatory drugs (NSAIDs) and other agents used in rheumatoid arthritis. The patient should be provided with the appropriate level and amount of information about the pathophysiology. Many pharmacies, websites, and disease-oriented public and private agencies provide information sheets suitable for patients.
- *Select a specific therapeutic objective*: A therapeutic objective should be chosen for each of the pathophysiologic processes defined in the preceding step. In a patient with rheumatoid arthritis, relief of pain by reduction of the inflammatory process is one of the major therapeutic goals that identifies the drug groups that should be

**Doctor's Name**

**Qualification (e.g., MBBS, MD)**

**Regd. No. ........................................................................................ (ALLOPATHY)**

**Full address, Contacts: (Telephone number, e-mail, etc.)**

Date..................................

Name of the patient.......................................................................................................

Address* .........................................................................................................................

Age and Sex ........................................................................Weight**.............................

Rx.

1. Name of the Medicine***

   Strength, dosage instruction, duration and total quantity***

2. – do –
3. –do –

Doctor's signature

Stamp

DISPENSED

Date: ................................Pharmacist: ..................................

Name of the pharmacy: .....................................................................

City

*Postal address/e-mail/mobile number

**For pediatric patients

***In capital letters only

Minimum size of the prescription blank should be (a) 14 × 21 cm (A5 size) and (b) XI × XI cm size

**FIG. 1:** Model prescription format proposed by the Medical Council of India for the purpose of making prescriptions by registered medical practitioners.

considered. Arresting the course of the disease process in rheumatoid arthritis is a different therapeutic goal, which might lead to the consideration of other drug groups and prescriptions.

- *Select a drug of choice*: One or more drug groups will be suggested by each of the therapeutic goals specified in the preceding step. Selection of a drug of choice among these groups follows from a consideration of the specific characteristics of the patient and the clinical presentation. For certain drugs, characteristics such as age, other diseases, and other drugs being taken (because of the risk of duplicative therapy or drug-drug interactions) are extremely important in determining the most suitable drug for the management of the present complaint. In the example of the patient with probable rheumatoid arthritis, it would be important to know whether the patient has a history of aspirin intolerance or ulcer disease, whether the cost of medication is an especially important factor and the nature of the patient's insurance coverage, and whether there is a need for once-daily dosing. Based on this information, a drug would probably be selected from the NSAID group. If the patient does not have ulcer disease but does have a need for low-cost treatment, ibuprofen or naproxen would be a rational choice.

- *Determine the appropriate dosing regimen*: The dosing regimen is determined primarily by the pharmacokinetics of the drug in that patient. For a drug such as ibuprofen, which is eliminated mainly by the kidneys, renal function should be assessed. If renal function is normal, the half-life of ibuprofen (about 2 hours) requires administration three or four times daily. The dose suggested in this book, drug handbooks, and the manufacturer's literature is 400–800 mg four times daily.
- *Devise a plan for monitoring the drug's action and determine an endpoint for therapy*: The prescriber should be able to describe to the patient the kinds of drug effects that will be monitored and in what way, including laboratory tests (if necessary) and signs and symptoms that the patient should report. For conditions that call for a limited course of therapy (e.g., most infections), the duration of therapy should be made clear so that the patient does not stop taking the drug prematurely and understands why the prescription probably need not be renewed. For the patient with rheumatoid arthritis, the need for prolonged—perhaps indefinite—therapy should be explained, including how to obtain refills.

## Elements of a Prescription (Fig. 2)

- *Date*:
    - Every prescription must bear the date on which the particular medicines are prescribed.
    - This helps the pharmacist.
        - To keep day-to-day patient records in a chronologic order, which helps the pharmacist or a physician to refer the old case in future
        - To avoid misuse of the narcotic or other habitat-forming drugs containing prescriptions by the patient a number of times for dispensing.
- *Name, age, sex, and address of the patient*:
    - Name helps the pharmacist to identify the correct patients avoiding any chance of giving the medicine to a person other than the one it is dispensed for.
    - Note: The patient's full name must be written instead of nicknames or surnames.

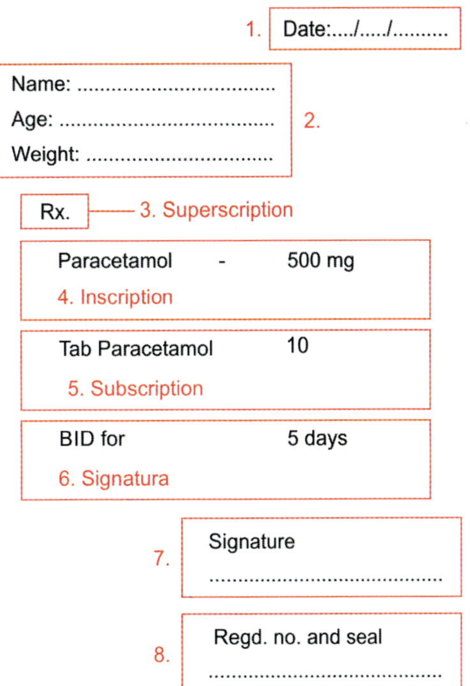


**FIG. 2:** Elements of a prescription.

  - Age of the patient becomes important in the case of pediatric (children) and geriatric (old people) cases. Because the dose of drugs in such cases varies (due to their differences in ability to metabolize drugs). Hence, dose of the drugs is calculated based on the age factor in such cases.
  - Note: In some cases, weight and height of the patients are also required.
  - Sex/gender of the patient also plays a major role in prescription because the dose of drugs may also vary based on the sex/gender of the patient (as their abilities to metabolize/respond toward drugs may vary in many cases).
  - Address of the patient is generally recorded to contact the person at a later stage or to deliver the medication personally.
- *Superscription (prescriber's details)*:
  - This part of the prescription is represented by the symbol Rx.
  - In ancient times, it was considered as a prayer to Jupiter, the God of healing, for the fast recovery of the patient.
  - Nowadays, it is used as an abbreviation for the Latin term "Take Thou" which means "you take."
  - Rx may be derived from the Egyptian "Eye of Horus" symbol denoting health or may be a symbolic appeal by the physician to the god Jupiter (God of knowledge, learning, and healing) for the prescription's success.
- *Inscription (name of drug, amount, duration, and frequency)*:
  - This is considered as the main part of the prescription order.
  - It contains the names and quantities of the prescribed ingredients.
  - In a complex prescription containing several ingredients, the inscription can be divided into the following parts:
    - Base (active medicament of therapeutic action)
    - Adjuvants (substances added to increase action of medicament/its palatability)
    - Vehicle (substance used to dissolve medicament/increase volume of preparation)
- *Subscription (direction to the pharmacist)*:
  - This part of the prescription contains directions of the prescriber to the pharmacist regarding the type and compounding of dosage form along with the number of doses to be dispensed.
  - This is important because the dose of the drug also depends on the type of the dosage form.
- *Signa (instruction to the patient)*:
  - This part of the prescription contains directions to the patient regarding the administration of the drugs.
  - It is generally represented as "Sig" on the prescription.
  - The instructions may include:
    - The quantity to be taken
    - The frequency of administration
    - The mode of administration
    - The special instructions such as dilation direction
- *Renewal instructions*:
  - In this part, the prescriber should mention whether the prescription can be renewed or not.
  - It should also include the specifications like how many times it can be renewed.
  - It is of utmost importance in the case of narcotic/other habitat-forming drugs.
- *Signature of prescriber*:
  - The signature and Regd. No of the prescriber turn the prescription into a legal and authentic order to the pharmacist.
  - This helps in preventing the use of spurious drugs.
  - Registered No is of utmost importance in prescription containing narcotic drugs.

## Prescription Writing Standards

### General

- *The patient*:
  - All drug charts and to take away (TTA) *must* include the patient's surname and given name, their date of birth, date of admission, and consultant.
  - Where dosing is weight dependent, e.g., pediatrics, low-molecular-weight heparins, or the patient is significantly under- or overweight, the weight should be documented.
- *Allergy box*:
  - Both positive and negative allergy histories and drug sensitivities *must* be documented.
  - Where allergy history is positive, symptoms of the allergy should be described.
- *Drug name*:
  - Write approved names, legibly and correctly spelt.
  - Do *not* use abbreviations.
  - Print if necessary.
- *Dose*:
  - *No* trailing zeroes (5 mg *not* 5.0 mg)
  - Quantities of 1 g or more should be written (1 g, 1.5 g, etc.).
  - Quantities < 1 g should be written in milligrams (500 mg *not* 0.5 g).
  - Quantities < 1 mg should be written in micrograms (100 µg *not* 0.1 mg).
  - When decimals are unavoidable, the decimal point *must* be preceded by another figure (0.5 mL *not* 0.5 mL).
- *Dose units*:
  - The words micrograms, nanograms, and units *must not* be abbreviated.
  - The term milliliter is abbreviated to mL, *not* cc or cm$^3$.
- *Frequency*:
  - The dose and frequency must be specified.
  - For as required prescriptions, the minimum dose interval *must* be specified (6 hours *not* qds).
- *Start date*:
  - Specify the date the drug was first prescribed/due this admission (not the date the chart is rewritten).
- *Indication*:
  - For as required prescriptions, the indication should be included.
- *Signature*:
  - Prescriptions must be signed in ink.
  - Contact numbers should be included so that prescribers can be contacted if necessary.

### Intravenous Prescriptions

- Drugs for continuous infusion should be written on an intravenous (IV) fluid prescription.
- The drug and quantity must be specified.
- The name of the infusion solution (diluent) must be specified.
- The rate of administration must be specified in mL/min or mL/h.

### Unusual Regimens

- For doses taken intermittently or at irregular intervals, boxes corresponding to doses that are not due *must* be crossed out, e.g., weekly alendronate, 3× week erythropoietin.

### Discontinuing Medications and Changing Doses

- Cross off the prescribing section of the drug chart *and* the administration section. Sign and date the chart.
- If the dose is changed, it must be rewritten with the *new* start date.

### Additional Drug Charts

- Insulin and warfarin must be prescribed on drug charts with the instruction—see insulin prescription or see anticoagulation prescription. Doses must *not* appear on two separate charts concurrently.
- Only *one* drug chart should be in use at once.

- Two drug charts are *only* permitted if the number of drugs currently prescribed exceeds the number of spaces on the chart. Where more than one chart is used, they must be labeled "1 of 2," "2 of 2," etc.
- Where two charts are necessary, they must be fastened together.

## Common Errors while Writing a Prescription

- Wrong/inappropriate drug (e.g., drugs that sound similar)
- Wrong/inappropriate dose
- Inappropriate units
- Poor/illegible prescriptions
- Failure to take account of drug interactions
- Two drugs from the same class
- Omissions
- Wrong/multiple routes [IV/subcutaneous (SC)/PO]
- Calculation errors (important in pediatrics)
- Infusions with not enough details of diluent, rate, etc.

## Significance of Date in the Prescription

- Important part of the medical record
- It can assist the pharmacist in recognizing potential problems.
- Compliance behavior can be estimated using the date of filling and refilling.
- Duration of therapy
- All the orders for controlled substances should be dated and signed on the day issued.

## What can be done to Inculcate the Practice of Writing a Sound Prescription?

- Revisit prescription writing class at the start of the internship.

***Steps or Instructions for a Good Prescription***

- Write legibly (use block letters).
- Sign and date the prescription (it is a legal document!).
- Never abbreviate drug names.
- Never use proprietary names; always use generic names.
- Use plain English for dosing directions.
- Be careful with look-alike/soundalike names, e.g., clotrimazole/ co-trimoxazole, carbamazepine/ carbimazole.
- Do not guess (check the name or the dose of the drug).
- Avoid 10-fold dosing errors; write 1 mg instead of 1.0 mg.
- Do not allow patients to prescribe for you.

- Prescription audit is to be taken up at regular intervals.
- Make it a part of medical education workshops.
- Awareness and sensitization workshops are to be conducted by the department of pharmacology.
- Clinical discussions are to be followed by a prescription writing exercise.
- Education and training of prescribers and the use of online aids are recommended.
- Introduction of automated systems or uniform prescribing charts, in order to avoid transcription and omission errors that might result in prescribing faults, is recommended.

In the government setup, due to patient overload, lack of manpower, and financial issues, the use of prescription writing software is a farfetched idea. However, it is the will to change one's attitude that is required at this point of time. Simply writing in block letters (the name of the drugs), the use of symbols (for dose frequency), the use of generic names as far as possible (brand names for combinations only), and the appropriate instructions to the patients in the prescription will suffice for a beginning.

## CLINICAL PEARLS

Prescription is an important part of the medical record.

Try to write the name of the drugs in block letters.

Mention dose frequency clearly.

Use generic names as far as possible.

Write appropriate instructions to the patients.

## FURTHER READINGS

1. Guide to good prescribing—a practical manual. [online] Available from https://ephor.nl/wp-content/uploads/2018/12/who-guide-to-good-prescribing-1.pdf.
2. Model prescription format for the purpose of making prescription by the registered medical practitioners. [online] Available from http://www.delhimedicalcouncil.org/pdf/modalprescription.pdf. [Last accessed September, 2023].
3. Kalra BS. Prescription writing: time to revisit! Neurol India. 2016;64:1106-8.
4. Velo GP, Minuz P. Medication errors: prescribing faults and prescription errors. Br J Clin Pharmacol. 2009;67:624-8.
5. Code of Medical Ethics Regulations, 2002. [online] Available from https://www.nmc.org.in/rules-regulations/code-of-medical-ethics-regulations-2002.

CHAPTER 118

# Certificates in Day-to-day Practice

*Anirban Dalui*

## INTRODUCTION

Medical certificate or doctor's certificate is a written statement from a physician or another medically qualified healthcare provider that attests to the result of a medical examination of a patient.

## PURPOSE OF MEDICAL CERTIFICATES

- Medical leave
- Medical fitness
- Certification of pregnancy/childbirth
- For insurance purposes
- Disability certification
- Determination of age
- Renewal of licenses
- Death certificate
- *Other examples*: Mental health certification and vaccine certificates

## CHARACTERISTICS OF IDEAL MEDICAL CERTIFICATE

- It should be written legibly.
- It should be written on forms designed specifically for this purpose.
- It should minimize the use of medical terms.
- It should contain the date of consultation.
- It should contain the date of certification.
- It should contain the name, age, gender, and address of the person being certified.
- It should be completed by a registered health practitioner who is authorized to do so.
- It should contain the name, designation, and registration number of the registered medical practitioner who is doing the certification.

## LEGAL IMPORTANCE

- Court of law
- Indian Penal Code (IPC): Section 197 and Section 463
- Indian Medical Council
- Civil suit for compensation

## TYPES OF CERTIFICATES

- Birth certificate
- Sickness certificate
- Fitness certificate
- Vaccination certificate
- Mental fitness certificate
- Certificate on will
- Domiciliary treatment certificate
- Life certificate

- Certifying left thumb impression
- Certificate for injury
- Certificate for Life Insurance Corporation (LIC) policy
- Certificate for withdrawing money from provident fund
- Certificate for opinion in case patient is referred for medical opinion
- Death certificate

Important points to remember when you are issuing a certificate:

- A registered medical practitioner shall maintain a Register of Medical Certificates, giving full details of certificates issued. When issuing a medical certificate, he/she shall always enter the identification marks of the patient and keep a copy of the certificate. He/she shall not omit to record the signature and/or thumbmark, address, and at least one identification mark of the patient on the medical certificates or report.
- Every physician shall display the registration number accorded to him by the State Medical Council/National Medical Council in his clinic and in all his prescriptions, certificates, and money receipts given to his patients. If he/she does not display the registration number accorded to him/her by the State Medical Council or the Medical Council of India in his clinic, prescriptions, certificates, etc., issued by him or violates the provisions of regulation.
- Physicians shall display as suffix to their names only recognized medical degrees or such certificates/diplomas and memberships/honors that confer professional knowledge or recognize any exemplary qualification/achievements.
- *Signing professional certificates, reports, and other documents*: Registered medical practitioners are, in certain cases, bound by law to give, or may from time to time be called upon or requested to give certificates, notifications, reports, and other documents of similar character signed by them in their professional capacity for subsequent use in the courts or for administrative purposes, etc. Any registered practitioner who is shown to have signed or given under his name and authority any such certificate, notification, report, or document of a similar character that is untrue, misleading, or improper is liable to have his name deleted from the Register.

## Death Certificate

The death certificate is an important and vital document because:

- It is an important legal document that certifies the death of a person.
- It explains the cause, manner, mode, and time of death.
- It is required before obtaining permission for cremation or burial from municipal authorities.
- A properly registered certificate is essential for claims of various dues such as insurance, gratuity, provident fund, family pension, and accident benefit claims.
- For execution of the will of the deceased
- For claims of movable and immovable properties
- Deletion of the name of the deceased person's name from ration card, shares, movable and immovable properties, bank account, etc.

It is a vital document for the government also because:

- It is the basis of mortality data, thus required to assess the effectiveness of health policies.
- It is helpful to provide feedback from such health policies.
- It is important for proper health planning and implementation.
- It is needed to decide the priorities for health and medical research programs.

Prerequisites for issuing a death certificate:

- It is issued free of charge. [Registration of Birth and Death Act, 1969, Section 10(3)]
- Only a single copy of death certificate is issued. The doctor/hospital should retain a carbon copy of the certificate.
- It is the duty of a registered medical practitioner or a medical officer in charge of the hospital to give information to the registrar of birth and death occurring in hospital as per the Registration of Birth and Death Act, Section 8(b).
- Any medical practitioner who refuses to give or issue a certificate under subsection 3 of section (10) of Registration of Birth and Death Act, 1969 shall be punished with a fine that may extend to 50 rupees [Section 23(3)].
- It is issued by the registered medical practitioner:
  - Who has been the medical attendant during the deceased's life
  - Has attended the patient at least once during the 7 days preceding death (as recommended by the Brodrick committee)
  - Is satisfied with the cause of death
- Death certificate is necessary even in cases of death that are stillborn/premature.
- The doctor should not sign the certificate blank, leaving the details to be filled in by someone else.
- No certificate is to be issued in case of sudden death of a person who has not been attended by the doctor before his/her death.
- In partnership practice, one doctor should not certify the case of his colleague's patient unless attended the deceased in the past.
- No certificate is issued in death, which is unexpected, unexplained, and death under suspicious circumstances.
- The death of a person under the custody of police or those residing in public institutions such as remand home, asylum, hostel, and under medical procedure, are reported to police/coroner and are subjected to postmortem.

### How to Fill Up the Death Certificate

- *Name of the deceased*: To be given in full. Do not use initials. If the deceased is an infant, not yet named at the time of death, write son of (S/O) or daughter of (D/O), followed by the names of the mother and father.
- *Age*: If the deceased is over 1 year of age, give age in complete years. If the deceased was below 1 year of age, give age in months and if below 1 month of age, in completed number of days, and if below 1 day, in hours.
- *Cause of death*: This part of the form should always be completed by the attending physician personally. The actual certificate is divided in two parts: Part-I and part-II.
  - *Part-I*: It deals with the immediate cause and the underlying cause of death. The immediate cause or the terminal event is entered here.
  - *Part-II*: It deals with other significant conditions or diseases contributed to the process of death but did not lead to it.

*Part-I*:

- Only one cause is to be entered in each line.
- *Line-a*: Immediate cause of death is entered here, such as disease/abnormality/injury/poisoning. The immediate cause is defined as the immediate or terminal event leading to death. The mode of death, such as respiratory failure and cardiac failure, is not an appropriate entry.
- *Line-b*: Next, consider whether the immediate cause is a complication of delayed result of some other cause. If so, enter the antecedent cause in part-I, line-b. The antecedent causes refer to the pathological process or injury responsible for death. Thus, it is a disease or injury that has initiated the train of morbid

events leading directly to death or it is the circumstances of the accident or violence that produced the fatal injury.

- *Line-c*: Sometimes, there will be three stages in the course of events leading to death. If so, line-c will be completed.

*Part-II*:

- Other significant conditions contributing to death but not related to disease condition causing it.

*Onset*: Complete the column for the interval between onset and death whenever possible, even if very approximate, e.g., from birth, or several years.

## Medical Fitness Certificate

### *Contents*

Following are the contents of a medical fitness certificate:

- Mention the title of the document clearly in bold letters.
- Address the certificate to the correct party (either the client's employer, insurer, etc.).
- State the date of examination.
- Provide the name and address of the medical practitioner's client/patient.
- Also, the name, designation, and address of the qualified medical practitioner should be mentioned (clinic or hospital).
- Mention the observations and any additional notes, which might be of importance to the client or their employer (such as limitations or restrictions on certain movements/activities. However, this is more relevant when the client is returning to work after an injury or illness).
- Conclude the certificate with a closing signature and the registration number of the medical practitioner.
- An additional point to note is that a copy of the medical certificate shall be retained by the doctor/medical practitioner for a period of 3 years from the date of issue.

### *Who can Issue a Medical Fitness Certificate?*

Medical fitness certificates are only issued by any MBBS graduate, provided they are registered with the state's medical council. Moreover, certain government agencies may specifically ask that you obtain a medical fitness certificate in word format from a civil surgeon.

### *Validity of a Medical Fitness Certificate*

Typically, most medical fitness certificates have a validity of 15 days. An individual must renew their certificate at the end of their term if they want to extend it beyond 15 days.

## CLINICAL PEARLS

- There are different categories of medical certificates.
- Learning to write proper medical certificates is of prime importance in daily practice.
- As it has medicolegal significance.

## FURTHER READING

1. Medical certificates: what you should know [Internet]. www.mcnsw.org.au. 2017. Available from: https://www.mcnsw.org.au/medical-certificates-what-you-should-know

CHAPTER 119

# Referral Letter: An Art

*Anirban Dalui*

## INTRODUCTION

Referral letter is an essential means of communication between primary and secondary care, giving the receiving clinician/department a detailed summary of the patient's presenting complaint and medical history to ensure a smooth transition of care. Done well, referrals provide important and timely specialist recommendations for patient care without undue burden for clinicians or patients.

The ideal behind issuing a referral is that two physicians having different experiences and expertise exchange ideas and treatment modalities targeting effective patient care at the right time and place.

As a primary care physician, an important part of working day is writing referrals. And when the physician is busy, it is easy to be tempted into writing a quick referral like this:

*Dear Gastroenterologist,*

*Thank you for seeing Mrs AB, a 45-year-old female with gastroesophageal reflux disease (GERD).*

*Regards,*

*Dr XYZ*

A referral with such brevity of information is neither helpful to your patient nor the specialist you are referring to! But do not be fooled: The length of a referral letter is not directly proportional to an increase in quality!

**Don't overdo it**

Check this one:

*Dear Gastroenterologist,*

*Thank you for seeing Mrs AB, a 45-year-old female with epigastric pain. She has had 6 months of epigastric pain, which she describes as a gnawing sensation. She rates this pain 6/10, and it occurs after most meals, lasting for 1 hour. It is worse after eating tomato-based foods and when she is stressed. The pain is relieved after drinking milk.*

| ***Past medical history*** | ***Date*** |
|---|---|
| Tonsillitis | 2005 |
| Bee sting | 2009 |
| Itch | 2009 |
| Medical certificate | 2011 |
| Stress | 2014 |
| Influenza vaccination | 2015 |
| Gallstones | 2016 |
| Cholecystectomy | 2016 |
| Obesity | 2017 |

The epigastric pain initially started when she separated from her husband 6 months ago and moved house. She does not have any associated reflux, retrosternal burning, throat pain, nausea, vomiting, diarrhea, constipation, fevers, night sweats, anorexia, loss of weight, dyspnea, orthopnea, cough, chest pain, or jaw pain. Please see details of her past medical history below.

*On examination today, her general appearance was unremarkable. Her observations: HR 65, RR 20, Temp. 36.4, BP 122/84, $O_2$ 98% RA, GCS 15, BSL 5.3. She did not have any palmar erythema, clubbing or nicotine stains on examination of her hands. Examination of her face was normal.*

*She had dual heart sounds, no heaves, thrills, or murmurs. She had good air entry in her right and left lobes posteriorly. Her abdomen was soft with epigastric tenderness. There was no guarding or rebound tenderness. Her bowel sounds were present. Her digital rectal examination was normal. I have arranged for an abdominal ultrasound and a H. pylori breath test today. My provisional diagnosis is GERD.*

*Thank you for seeing this patient.*

*Kind regards,*

*Dr XYZ*

*Issues with this referral letter*:

This referral letter is way too lengthy and is filled with superfluous information! It also does not really outline the reason for the referral. An effective referral letter is vital so your patient can be triaged and reviewed appropriately.

## COMPONENTS OF A REFERRAL LETTER

Referral letter reflects the diagnostic skills, communication skills, and professionalism of the doctor. Several studies have revealed frequent absence of an explanation for referral, medical history, clinical findings, test results, and details of prior treatment in referral letters. At the same time, clarity, legibility, and overall format are also important features of a good referral letter.

- Name of the doctor/specialty department to which referral is being sent
- Patient particulars including the vitals and other relevant statistics
- History of present illness (symptoms, onset, duration, severity, etc.)
- Differential diagnosis
- Any relevant past medical/surgical histories
- Allergy history
- Travel history
- Any invasive procedures done during the period of hospital stay
- Summary of laboratory diagnosis and other relevant tests done
- Management done till date
- Present condition of patient
- Reason for referral
- Name of referring doctor along with designation
- Legal information, including consent for treatment, mental capacity assessment, advanced decisions about treatment as discussed with the patient, lasting power of attorney, etc.
- Any information provided to the patient or his family by the referring physician.

## ISBAR FOR YOUR REFERRAL LETTERS

- *Information*:
    - Up-to-date and correct patient information
    - Your details as the referring doctor
- *Situation*
    - Relevant summary of the patient presentation
- *Background*
    - Relevant medical history
    - Current medications and any allergies
- *Assessment*
    - Relevant examination and investigation findings
- *Request*
    - Purpose of the referral
    - Using this framework, let us see if we can improve Ms AB's referral.

*A good example of a referral is as below:*

**Dr MNO**

Consultant Gastroenterologist,

Dear Sir,

[Information] RE: New Referral Mrs AB, DOB 01/01/1975, Dakhinpara, Barasat, North 24 PGs, WB

[Situation] Thank you for seeing Ms AB, a 47-year-old female with difficult-to-control GERD for your consideration of a gastroscopy.

[Background] She has had 6 months of worsening epigastric pain, worse after meals. She has not displayed any constitutional symptoms during this time. Her medical history includes obesity and a cholecystectomy in 2016. She is currently on 40 mg esomeprazole daily and does not have any allergies.

[Assessment] The only finding on physical examination is epigastric tenderness on palpation of her abdomen. Her most recent liver function tests (dated 11/5/2022) and upper abdominal ultrasound (dated 17/5/2022) were normal. A *H. pylori* breath test (dated 19/5/2022) was negative. For the past 6 months, she has been managed with 40 mg esomeprazole daily. She has also modified her diet and been trying to lose weight.

[Request] Despite this, her symptoms persist, and I would greatly appreciate your clinical review and consideration of an endoscopy to confirm this diagnosis and ensure no other pathology contributing to her symptoms.

Kind regards,

Dr XYZ, MBBS, General Physician

## BASICS OF REFERRAL

- There should be merit in the process (need-objective).
- It should be practical.
- It should be individualized to the patient.

## STEPS OF REFERRAL PROCESS

1. Establish a good relationship with the patient.
2. Explain the need for referral.
3. Set objectives for referral.
4. Explore resource availability.
5. Patients' acceptance for need of referral
6. Make prereferral treatment.
7. Facilitate and coordinate referral.
8. Evaluate and follow-up.

## TYPES OF REFERRALS

- *Routine*: Seeking expert opinion for diagnosis and prognosis, hospital admission for management of the case, seeking further investigations
- *Emergency*: Seeking on time advise from a specialist before deterioration in patient condition
- *Opportunistic*: For expert opinion, admission, investigation, and management

## MODERN CLASSIFICATION OF REFERRALS

- Interval
- Collateral
- Split referral
- Cross referral

## FACTORS AFFECTING REFERRALS

- Availability of qualified consultants
- Physician specialty
- Length of training
- Unexplained findings
- Uncertainty of diagnosis
- Patient characteristics
- Reimbursement plans

## ADVANTAGES OF REFERRAL

- *For the patient*:
  - Prompt diagnosis and treatment
  - Saves time, money, and effort
  - Better outcome
- *For the referring physician*:
  - Learning and training
  - Gaining self-confidence
  - Increased communication between healthcare staff
- *For the referred doctor (consultant)*:
  - Improved quality of management
  - Better communication

## ANOTHER SAMPLE OF A PHYSICIAN REFERRAL LETTER

*[Date]*

*Re: [Patient's Name]*

Dear Dr [Bariatric Surgeon's Name],

I am referring [patient's name] for evaluation and consideration for a weight management surgical procedure. (S)He currently weighs [# of kgs] kilograms and is [# of cm] cm tall. Her/His BMI is [BMI #]. I have been [patient's name]'s primary care physician for the past [#of yrs] years. I have supervised several of her/his weight control diets and programs. None of these have resulted in any sustained weight loss. As a result of this persistent morbid obesity, her/his comorbid conditions are becoming more difficult to manage. These comorbid conditions are as follows:

| ***Comorbidity*** | ***Duration*** | ***Medication*** |
|---|---|---|
| Hypertension | 3 years | Telmisartan, Amlodipine |
| Diabetes mellitus | 5 years | Metformin, Vildagliptin |

Losing weight will certainly make these conditions easier to manage. Since nonsurgical programs have failed to provide any long-term benefits for the patient, I feel surgery is her/his only option.

I hope you will find [patient's name] a suitable candidate for the surgical weight reduction program. It will provide a tool to assist her/him in losing weight, as well as maintain that weight loss. I anticipate that this will provide her/him with a significantly improved quality of life.

Sincerely,

[Physician signature]

Dr [Physician's Name]

## CLINICAL PEARLS

- Referral letter should be need-objective based, individualized, and practical one.
- An ideal referral letter should contain information, situation, background, assessment, and request.
- The steps of referral process, including explanation and consent, should be followed, and follow-up is always necessary.

## FURTHER READINGS

1. Tobin-Schnittger P, O'Doherty J, O'Connor R, O'Regan A. Improving quality of referral letters from primary to secondary care: a literature review and discussion paper. Prim Health Care Res Dev. 2018;19(3):211-22.
2. Eskeland SL, Brunborg C, Rueegg CS, Aabakken L, de Lange T. Assessment of the effect of an Interactive Dynamic Referral Interface (IDRI) on the quality of referral letters from general practitioners to gastroenterologists: a randomised cross-over vignette trial. BMJ Open. 2017;7:e014636.
3. Jiwa M, Dadich A. Referral letter content: can it affect patient outcomes? Br J Healthc Manag. 2013;19:140-46.
4. Zuchowski JL, Rose DE, Hamilton AB, Stockdale SE, Meredith LS, Yano EM, et al. Challenges in referral communication between VHA primary care and specialty care. J Gen Intern Med. 2015;30:305-11.

# Index

Page numbers followed by *b* refer to box, *f* refer to figure, *fc* refer to flowchart, and *t* refer to table.

## A

## B

## C

## D

## F

## G

## H

## I

## J



## K

## M

## O

## P

## S

## T

## W

## X



## Y



## Z